THE TREATMENT OF
OPIOID DEPENDENCE

THE TREATMENT OF OPIOID DEPENDENCE

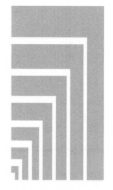

Edited by

Eric C. Strain, M.D.

Professor, Department of Psychiatry and Behavioral Sciences
Johns Hopkins University School of Medicine
Baltimore, Maryland

and

Maxine L. Stitzer, Ph.D.

Professor, Department of Psychiatry and Behavioral Sciences
Associate Director, Behavioral Pharmacology Research Unit
Director, Mid-Atlantic Node, National Drug Abuse
    Treatment Clinical Trials Network
Johns Hopkins University School of Medicine
Baltimore, Maryland

THE JOHNS HOPKINS UNIVERSITY PRESS
Baltimore

Drug dosage: The authors and publisher have exerted every effort to ensure that the selection and dosage of drugs discussed in this text accord with recommendations and practice at the time of publication. However, in view of ongoing research, changes in governmental regulations, and the constant flow of information relating to drug therapy and drug reactions, the reader is urged to check the package insert of each drug for any change in indications and dosage and for warnings and precautions. This is particularly important when the recommended agent is a new and/or infrequently used drug.

©2006 The Johns Hopkins University Press
All rights reserved. Published 2006
Printed in the United States of America on acid-free paper
9 8 7 6 5 4 3 2 1

The Johns Hopkins University Press
2715 North Charles Street
Baltimore, Maryland 21218-4363
www.press.jhu.edu

Library of Congress Cataloging-in-Publication Data

The treatment of opioid dependence / edited by Eric C. Strain and
   Maxine L. Stitzer.
     p. ; cm.
   Includes bibliographical references and index.
   ISBN 0-8018-8219-2 (alk. paper) — ISBN 0-8018-8303-2 (pbk.: alk. paper)
     1. Methadone maintenance.   2. Narcotic habit—Treatment.
   3. Buprenorphine.   I. Strain, Eric C.   II. Stitzer, Maxine L.
   [DNLM: 1. Opioid-Related Disorders—therapy.   2. Analgesics,
   Opioid—therapeutic use.   3. Methadone—therapeutic use. WM 284 T784 2005]
   RC568.M4T74 2005
   616.86'32061—dc22   2005001871

A catalog record for this book is available from the British Library.

Contents

VI SPECIAL TREATMENT ISSUES

CONTRIBUTORS

Mary M. Bailes, M.A., LCPC, *Senior Clinical Research Program Manager, Behavioral Pharmacology Research Unit, Department of Psychiatry and Behavioral Sciences, Johns Hopkins University School of Medicine, Baltimore, Maryland*

George E. Bigelow, Ph.D., *Professor, Department of Psychiatry and Behavioral Sciences, and Director, Behavioral Pharmacology Research Unit, Johns Hopkins University School of Medicine, Baltimore, Maryland*

Robert K. Brooner, Ph.D., *Professor, Department of Psychiatry and Behavioral Sciences, Johns Hopkins University School of Medicine, Baltimore, Maryland*

Mitchell J. M. Cohen, M.D., *Director, Undergraduate Medical Education, and Director, Pain Medicine Program, Department of Psychiatry and Human Behavior, Jefferson Medical College, Philadelphia, Pennsylvania*

Sandra D. Comer, Ph.D., *Associate Professor, Department of Psychiatry, Columbia University/New York State Psychiatric Institute, New York, New York*

Rosa M. Crum, M.D., M.H.S., *Associate Professor, Department of Epidemiology, Johns Hopkins Medical Institutions, Welch Center for Prevention, Epidemiology and Clinical Research, Baltimore, Maryland*

George De Leon, Ph.D., *Center for Therapeutic Community Research at National Development and Research Institute; Clinical Professor of Psychiatry, New York University School of Medicine, New York, New York*

David A. Fiellin, M.D., *Associate Professor of Medicine, Yale University School of Medicine, New Haven, Connecticut*

Michael I. Fingerhood, M.D., FACP, *Associate Professor of Medicine, Johns Hopkins University School of Medicine, Baltimore, Maryland*

Michael Gossop, Ph.D., *Professor, Head of Research, Addictions Directorate, National Addiction Centre, Maudsley Hospital, Institute of Psychiatry, London, England*

Samar A. Jasser, *Senior Medical Student, Department of Psychiatry and Human Behavior, Jefferson Medical College, Philadelphia, Pennsylvania*

Hendrée E. Jones, Ph.D., *Associate Professor, Department of Psychiatry and Behavioral Sciences, Johns Hopkins University School of Medicine, Baltimore, Maryland*

Lori Keyser-Marcus, Ph.D., *Department of Psychiatry, Virginia Commonwealth University Medical Center, Richmond, Virginia*

Michael Kidorf, Ph.D., *Associate Professor, Department of Psychiatry and Behavioral Sciences, Johns University School of Medicine, Baltimore, Maryland*

Van L. King, Jr., M.D., *Medical Director, Addiction Treatment Services, Associate Professor, Department of Psychiatry and Behavioral Sciences, Johns Hopkins University School of Medicine, Baltimore, Maryland*

Carl G. Leukefeld, D.S.W., *Professor and Director, Center on Drug and Alcohol Research, University of Kentucky, Lexington, Kentucky*

Connie A. Lowery, R.N., CARN, *Advanced Clinical Nurse Research, Department of Psychiatry and Behavioral Sciences, Johns Hopkins Bayview Medical Center, Baltimore, Maryland*

Lisa A. Marsch, Ph.D., *Senior Principal Investigator, National Development and Research Institutes, and Research Scientist, Department of Psychiatry, St. Luke's-Roosevelt Hospital Center, New York, New York*

Hope M. Smiley-McDonald, M.A., *NIMH Predoctoral Research Fellow, Department of Behavioral Science, University of Kentucky, Lexington, Kentucky*

Edward V. Nunes, M.D., *Associate Professor of Clinical Psychiatry, Research Psychiatrist, Columbia University, College of Physicians and Surgeons, New York State Psychiatric Institute, New York, New York*

Jessica M. Peirce, Ph.D., *Assistant Professor, Johns Hopkins University School of Medicine, Baltimore, Maryland*

Nancy Petry, Ph.D., *Professor of Psychiatry, University of Connecticut Health Center, Farmington, Connecticut*

Stacey C. Sigmon, Ph.D., *Research Assistant Professor, Department of Psychiatry, University of Vermont, Burlington, Vermont*

Kenneth Silverman, Ph.D., *Professor, Department of Psychiatry and Behavioral Sciences, Johns Hopkins University School of Medicine, Baltimore, Maryland*

Michele Staton, Ph.D., *Project Director, Center on Drug and Alcohol Research, University of Kentucky, Lexington, Kentucky*

Kenneth B. Stoller, M.D., *Assistant Professor, Department of Psychiatry and Behavioral Sciences, Johns Hopkins University School of Medicine, Baltimore, Maryland*

Maria A. Sullivan, M.D., Ph.D., *Assistant Professor of Clinical Psychiatry, Columbia University/New York State Psychiatric Institute, New York, New York*

Dace S. Svikis, Ph.D., *Professor, Virginia Commonwealth University, Richmond, Virginia*

Michelle Tuten, M.S.W., LCSW-C, *Clinical Research Program Supervisor, Johns Hopkins University School of Medicine, Baltimore, Maryland*

Sharon L. Walsh, Ph.D., *Professor, Department of Psychiatry and Behavioral Sciences, Johns Hopkins University School of Medicine, Baltimore, Maryland*

J. Matthew Webster, Ph.D., *Assistant Professor, Center on Drug and Alcohol Research, University of Kentucky, Lexington, Kentucky*

James P. Zacny, Ph.D., *Professor, Psychopharmacologist, Department of Anesthesia and Critical Care, University of Chicago Medical Center, Chicago, Illinois*

Preface

Since *Methadone Treatment for Opioid Dependence* was published in 1999, there has been considerable change in the treatment of opioid dependence. For example, in the United States there have been revisions in the federal regulation of methadone treatment programs, approval of buprenorphine for the treatment of opioid dependence, and the institution of office-based opioid treatment. Similarly, there has been approval and expansion of buprenorphine treatment in other parts of the world, expansion of methadone treatment into new countries, and the removal of L-alpha-acetylmethodol (LAAM) as a therapeutic option throughout the world. The past six years have seen a marked growth of our knowledge about opioid dependence and its treatment, and a new book about opioid dependence is clearly needed.

The Treatment of Opioid Dependence contains updated contents and alters the title of the first book in a manner that reflects the growth of options for treatment of opioid dependence. *Methadone Treatment for Opioid Dependence* emphasized the clinical use of methadone, given that most pharmacologic treatment for opioid dependence occurred in methadone clinics and was patterned after a model that was developed in the United States in the 1960s and early 1970s. One mark of the extent of the change in opioid addiction treatment is that the term *methadone clinic* appears to have fallen out of favor and been replaced with the more nonspecific term *opioid treatment program*. This new book retains significant portions from the first, especially with respect to methadone treatment, but it also highlights the significant expansion of treatment options. This change should not be viewed as a decrement in our support for methadone treatment—we remain firmly committed to this very effective modality of care for persons with opioid dependence.

In addition to this evolution in the pharmacologic treatments, innovation and change also continue in other aspects of treatment for opioid dependence, and this is reflected in the expansion of the content of this book. The first book had 13 chapters, whereas *The Treatment of Opioid Dependence* has 24 chapters, nearly double the original number. In part, this increase reflects the greater attention devoted to buprenorphine and other pharmacotherapies such as naltrexone and lofexidine. Several nonpharmacologic topics related to the treatment of opioid dependence have been added (e.g., office-based opioid dependence treatment, characteristics and treatment of patients with prescription opioid abuse, treatment of patients under legal restrictions, treatment of adolescents with opioid dependence). This expansion reflects the widening knowledge base and clinical experience treating opioid dependence.

In the preface for *Methadone Treatment for Opioid Dependence,* we noted that more than 100,000 people in the United States were receiving methadone treatment. This number has increased dramatically during the past six years. At this time, probably well in excess of 250,000 persons in the United States are receiving either methadone or buprenorphine for opioid dependence (with at least 200,000 of these receiving methadone), and probably at least another 250,000 persons are receiving methadone or buprenorphine in other parts of the world. (Indeed, it is estimated that at least 75,000 persons are receiving buprenorphine in France alone.) By the time this book is published, it will have been more than 40 years since methadone was first used for the treatment of opioid dependence. The treatment of opioid dependence should be viewed as a maturing medical discipline, with significant recent advances in the expansion and professionalization of these treatments. A major goal of this book continues to be an effort to provide an objective and comprehensive overview of opioid dependence treatment that uses the extensive body of research available on this modality to support clinical recommendations. Thus, we hope that colleagues in the treatment community will find this a useful resource in their clinical practice and researchers may find new clinically based questions that need empirical study.

In addition, we hope that this book will be useful to those in the public policy arena. One of our important goals is to show that there is a substantial body of research supporting the treatment of opioid dependence and that these treatments have been studied under rigorous conditions (like other commonly accepted medical treatments). We hope that this information will be used by those in governmental agencies, for example, to provide support for the continued expansion of availability and funding for treatment of opioid dependence.

Numerous friends and colleagues contributed chapters to this edition, and we are grateful that they helped on this project. Our own work has been conducted at the Johns Hopkins Behavioral Pharmacology Research Unit during the past 20 plus years. We appreciate the many patients and research volunteers who have participated in our studies of opioid dependence. These projects have been funded through a series of grants from the National Institute on Drug Abuse (NIDA), and the support of NIDA is greatly appreciated. Similarly, the Department of Psychiatry at the Johns Hopkins University School of Medicine has been an invaluable support. Finally, we would like to thank our families (Grace, Andrew, Kate, Cori, and Duncan) for their patience, support, and good cheer during the many evenings and weekends we have been working on this and other projects. We hope that this book will help to improve, expand, and mainstream in medicine the treatment of opioid dependence—the time involved was well worth the effort if this book helps to improve the care of patients with opioid dependence.

ABBREVIATIONS

AAPM	American Academy of Pain Medicine
ABA	American Bar Association
ADAM	Arrestee Drug Abuse Monitoring
ADHD	attention-deficit hyperactivity disorder
AIDS	acquired immunodeficiency syndrome
AMA	American Medical Association
APA	American Psychiatric Association
APD	antisocial personality disorder
APS	American Pain Society
ARC	Addiction Research Center
ARC	Alcohol Research Center
ASI	Addiction Severity Index
AUDIT	Alcohol Use Disorders Identification Test
AZT	Zidovudine
BDI	Beck Depression Inventory
BFC	behavioral family counseling
BMDI	Bayley Mental Development Index
BNT	behavioral naltrexone therapy
CAC	Certified Addiction Counselor
CALDATA	California Drug and Alcohol Treatment Assessment
CAP	Center for Addiction and Pregnancy
CARF	Commission on Accreditation of Rehabilitation Facilities
CDC	Centers for Disease Control and Prevention
CE	compliance enhancement
CFR	Code of Federal Regulations
CIDI-2	Composite International Diagnostic Interview–Second Edition
CINA	Clinical Institute Narcotic Assessment

CM	contingency management
CNS	central nervous system
COA	Council on Accreditation for Children and Family Services
COPD	chronic obstructive pulmonary disease
CPDD	College on Problems of Drug Dependence
CPS	Child Protective Services
CR	controlled release
CSA	Controlled Substances Act
CSAT	Center for Substance Abuse Treatment
DARP	Drug Abuse Reporting Program
DATA 2000	Drug Addiction Treatment Act of 2000
DATOS	Drug Abuse Treatment Outcome Study
DAWN	Drug Abuse Warning Network
DEA	Drug Enforcement Agency
DHHS	Department of Health and Human Services
DIS	Diagnostic Interview Schedule
DNADA	Division of Narcotic Addiction and Drug Abuse
DSM-IV	*Diagnostic and Statistical Manual of Mental Disorders,* fourth edition
DVA	Department of Veterans Affairs
ECA	Epidemiological Catchment Area
ECG	electrocardiogram
ED	Emergency Department
EDDP	2-ethylidene-1,5-dimethyl-3,3-diphenylpyrolidene
EEG	electroencephalogram
EMIT	enzyme multiplied immunoassay test
ESPAD	European School Survey Project on Alcohol and Other Drug Use
FBN	Federal Bureau of Narcotics
FPIA	fluorescence polarization immunoassay
FSMB	Federation of State Medical Boards
FTA	free treponemal antibody
GAD	generalized anxiety disorder
GAO	General Accounting Office
HAART	highly active antiretroviral therapy
HCV	hepatitis C virus
HEW	Health, Education and Welfare
HIPAA	Health Insurance Portability and Accountability Act
HIV	human immunodeficiency virus
HPV	human papilloma virus
IBT	individual-based treatment

IMM	interim methadone maintenance
INH	Isoniazid
IOM	Institute of Medicine
IOP	intensive outpatient program
IPT	interpersonal therapy
IR	immediate release
JAMA	*Journal of the American Medical Association*
JCAHO	Joint Commission on Accreditation of Healthcare Organizations
KEEP	Key Extended Entry Program
LAAM	L-alpha-acetylmethadol
LAC	Legal Action Center
LSD	lysergic acid diethylamide
MAOI	monoamine oxidase inhibitor
MAST	Michigan Alcoholism Screening Test
MDD	Medications Development Division
MRT	methadone reduction treatment
MSC	motivated stepped care
MSCA	McCarthy Scales of Children's Abilities
MTF	Monitoring the Future
NAS	neonatal abstinence syndrome
NATA	Narcotic Addict Treatment Act
NDA	New Drug Application
NDATUS	National Drug and Alcohol Treatment Unit Survey
NHSDA	National Household Survey on Drug Abuse
NIDA	National Institute on Drug Abuse
NIH	National Institutes of Health
NIMBY	not in my back yard
NIMH	National Institute for Mental Health
NMDA	N-methyl-D-aspartate
NSAID	nonsteroidal anti-inflammatory drug
NSDUH	National Survey on Drug Use and Health
NTORS	National Treatment Outcome Research Study
NTX	Naltrexone
OBOT	office-based opioid treatment
OCD	obsessive-compulsive disorder
ONDCP	Office of National Drug Control Policy
OSHA	Occupational Safety and Health Administration
OTP	opioid treatment program
PCP	phencyclidine
PHI	protected health information

PMP	prescription monitoring program
PPD	purified protein derivative
PTSD	posttraumatic stress disorder
RBT	reinforcement-based therapy
RMP	risk-management plan
SADS	Schedule for Affective Disorders and Schizophrenia
SADS-L	Schedule for Affective Disorders and Schizophrenia-Lifetime
SAMHSA	Substance Abuse and Mental Health Services Administration
SAODAP	Special Action Office for Drug Abuse Prevention
SCID	Structured Clinical Interview for DSM-IV
SES	socioeconomic status
SFP	Strengthening Families Program
SO	significant other
SSC	standard stepped care
SSRI	selective serotonin reuptake inhibitors
STD	sexually transmitted disease
$t_{1/2}$	half-life
TC	therapeutic community
TCA	Therapeutic Communities of America
TCA	tricyclic antidepressant
TEDS	Treatment Episode Data Set
TH	take home
TLC	thin-layer chromatography
TOPS	Treatment Outcome Prospective Study
TSR	Treatment Services Review
UROD	ultrarapid opioid detoxification
WOW	Weak Opioid Withdrawal scale

I

Overview of
Opioid Dependence

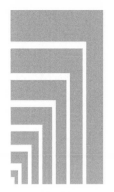

I

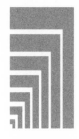

Introduction and Historical Overview

Kenneth B. Stoller, M.D., and George E. Bigelow, Ph.D.

Although it is difficult to obtain an exact number, the Office of National Drug Control Policy estimates the number of persons in the United States with "hardcore" heroin addiction to be between 750,000 and 1 million. The most commonly used medication for the treatment of opioid dependence is methadone. Methadone was not developed for the treatment of opioid dependence; it was developed in Germany during the 1940s for use as an analgesic, and it continues to be used as an effective analgesic today. Not until the 1960s did studies and reports of using methadone for the treatment of opioid dependence first begin to appear in the scientific literature.

For many years methadone was the most effective medication for the treatment of opioid dependence because it was the only medication available. Although this chapter focuses on methadone, one must realize that other medications are available and approved for the treatment of opioid dependence (such as naltrexone and buprenorphine). This chapter reviews the development of methadone for the treatment of opioid dependence and provides the more recent history of the development of these other medications.

OPIATE ABUSE BEFORE METHADONE TREATMENT
Development and Recognition of an Opioid Problem

Opioids have been abused for hundreds of years; the contemporary problems associated with opioid use are not unique to the present era. Nor has abuse of opioids been isolated to a single culture or region of the world. Since the late nineteenth century, however, the United States has often occupied a unique position in terms of total consumption and prevalence of opioid abuse, and a review of the history of opioid use in the United States provides a useful, illustrative example of the context in which methadone was developed for the treatment of opioid dependence.

During the second half of the nineteenth century, the use of opioids markedly increased in the United States (Jonnes 1996; Musto 1987)—primarily for medical use—and this increase reflected a common social and medical perception that opioids were safe and effective. In addition to being prescribed by physicians, substantial amounts of opioids were consumed, often unknowingly, in the form of patent medications marketed for a variety of maladies; manufacturers were not required to list the ingredients. At this time, most opiate addiction in the United States occurred among middle- and upper-class Caucasian women, although some opiate-containing patent medications were marketed specifically for use by children.

By the turn of the twentieth century, there were probably at least 250,000 persons with opiate addiction in the United States (1 in 300 persons), perhaps a conservative estimate. (By way of comparison, in the 1990s the prevalence of opioid dependence was estimated to be about 1 in 375 persons.) Society's perception of the safety of opioids was in flux, prompted in part by the publication of exposés, at the turn of the century, that reported the analytic results of the contents of commonly used patent medications. As the public became aware of these results, interest grew in regulating this industry, culminating in passage of the Pure Food and Drug Act of 1906.

The Pure Food and Drug Act of 1906 required manufacturers to list the contents of medications that would be shipped across state lines. The act resulted in both a withdrawal from the market of a large number of medications and a suddenly heightened awareness by consumers of the actual content of medicines previously thought to be safe. Within a few years of the act's passage, sales of these patent medications dropped by about a third, and the number of people dependent on opiates also began to drop.

As use of opiates began to decline, the perception of who was using opiates also shifted. Opiate use had previously been primarily in white middle- and upper-class women, but now illicit opiate use became associated with minorities (especially Chinese immigrants). Furthermore, although opiate use in the nineteenth century had been restricted mainly to morphine and opium, with the outlawing of opium dens, heroin became a popular form of opioid to abuse. Heroin was introduced to the public in 1898 (initially marketed as a cough suppressant and nonaddictive analgesic agent by the Friedrich Bayer Company), and in the early 1900s, this new form of opioid quickly became a popular drug of abuse for young men living in the inner cities.

Thus, by the start of the twentieth century three major changes were occurring in opiate use. First, the demographics of those addicted were changing from middle-class white women to inner-city minorities and poor, young men. Second, concurrent with this demographic shift, the overall number of people using opiates was declining. Third, opiate use largely shifted from morphine and opium to heroin.

The Harrison Narcotics Act

Despite this overall decline in drug use, political interest in limiting international opium trade was rising. This interest culminated in the Harrison Narcotics Act of 1914—federal legislation sponsored by Representative Francis Burton Harrison—which heavily taxed and regulated domestic trade in narcotics. The Harrison Act is best understood as a response to international events, in particular, to the desire to improve trade relations with China, even though it addressed domestic rather than international issues.

During the early 1900s, the United States actively participated in a series of international conferences that sought to regulate the international trade in narcotics. The United States wanted other countries to exert greater local control over the production and distribution of opiates. However, the United States was placed in an awkward position, because it could hardly argue that other nations should improve opiate-related laws when its own laws were weak and ineffective. The Harrison Act provided a federal mechanism for control of opiates (previously handled at the state level), and once the act had been passed the United States was able to confront other nations that did not have similar antiopiate laws. Although passage of the act served a useful purpose for international conferences, enforcement of the act by the Treasury Department also resulted in a further tightening of opiate use in the United States.

As the Harrison and Pure Food and Drug acts produced further control over opiate distribution and use in the United States, programs for the treatment of opiate abusers through the provision of maintenance opioids began to be established in various cities. These programs, which operated in areas such as New York, Connecticut, Ohio, Texas, and Louisiana, continued into the 1920s and can be viewed as the forerunners of methadone treatment. The provision of maintenance or detoxification opioids to persons with opiate addiction was initially deemed acceptable through rulings under the provisions of the Harrison Act (e.g., *Jin Fuey Moy v. United States*). However, subsequent interpretations of the act (e.g., *Webb et al. v. United States; United States v. Doremus*) allowed the Treasury Department to shut down programs offering such support and to arrest doctors prescribing opiates. By the mid- to late-1920s maintenance treatment for opioid dependence had effectively ended in the United States.

Prohibitive Enforcement

In 1930 the Federal Bureau of Narcotics (FBN) was established under a Commissioner of Narcotics and given the task of enforcing the Harrison Act and representing the nation in foreign conferences concerning narcotics control. Harry Anslinger led the FBN from the time of its creation until his retirement in 1962. Anslinger believed in strict enforcement of laws and the active discouragement of medical treatments for opioid dependence (such as agonist medications). Despite this strictly punitive approach to the management of opioid dependence, a review of Anslinger's tenure suggests that, under his leadership, the FBN failed to provide effective control of illicit opiate use. The FBN operated within the Treasury Department until 1968, when it was turned over to the Justice Department. This turnover was prompted, in part, by the belief that a single agency with domestic and international responsibilities would be more effective in performing enforcement duties, preventing smuggling, and, at the same time, acting as a model to other nations.

Both the use of illicit opiates and the intolerance regarding such use intensified after World War II (much as it had after World War I). There was a notable increase in heroin use in New York City—which probably had the greatest concentration of opiate addiction in the United States during this period—a trend that was apparent in other cities throughout the United States during the 1950s as well. This was in part related to the appearance of Mexican opium in major cities during this time, including New York. As the prevalence of heroin addiction rose, so did drug-related crime. Governmental action during this time culminated in the enactment of the 1956 Narcotic Control Act, which firmly established suppression of drug trafficking as the primary role of the federal government in this matter. The act imposed severe penalties for drug-related crimes, including mandatory minimum prison sentencing even for first-conviction drug charges and the threat of the death penalty for some cases.

The Transition toward Medicalization

In 1955 the American Bar Association (ABA) and the American Medical Association (AMA) joined in studying the narcotics problem, and the Joint Committee of the ABA and the AMA on Narcotic Drugs was appointed. In 1958 the committee's Interim Report recommended that an outpatient facility prescribing narcotics be established on a controlled, experimental basis. The report also criticized the intimidation of physicians by federal agents and suggested that, through maintenance therapy, crime might be prevented. The FBN aggressively criticized the Joint Committee, whose recommendations were seen as a threat that would lead to softened penalties, increased prescribing of opioids, and/or the establishment of maintenance clinics.

Increasing concern about drug use mounted in the 1960s, spawned by the increased use of heroin (as well as amphetamines and marijuana) and the emergence of new drugs such as lysergic acid diethylamide (LSD). Increased drug use during this period led to elevated morbidity and mortality associated with drug use. In New York City, by the mid-1960s, heroin-related mortality was the leading cause of death of persons between the ages of 15 and 35. Hepatitis transmitted through intravenous drug injection was increasing, as were drug-related crimes. These problems developed during a time when President John F. Kennedy was advocating increased resources for research and treatment of persons with mental illness and individuals with mental retardation. The understanding of drug addiction by those in the mental health field differed tremendously from the prevailing view at the FBN, where drug abuse was seen as a problem to be handled through more vigorous law enforcement and punishment of those breaking laws. Physicians and mental health care workers viewed addiction as a medical problem, placing the responsibility for finding solutions within the arena of health care providers and medical researchers.

Although these attitudes within the health care field had become increasingly prevalent before the 1960s, it was only with the clear failure of prohibitive enforcement that the existing approach was questioned. In 1962 the Supreme Court declared that addiction in itself was a disease not a crime (*Robinson v. California*). Subsequently, courts became more lenient, mandatory sentencing was opposed, and funding for drug abuse research increased. That year the President called for a White House conference on drug abuse, followed by the President's Advisory Commission on Narcotic and Drug Abuse (the Prettyman Commission). This commission recommended the relaxation of mandatory minimum sentences and intensified research for all aspects of narcotic abuse, including the effectiveness of outpatient dispensing of narcotics for addiction. It also recommended dismantling the FBN and making Health, Education and Welfare (HEW) responsible for distribution and research and the Justice Department responsible for the investigation of illicit trafficking. The medical profession would now determine what constituted legitimate medical treatment. This changing perception of opiate abuse as a medical disorder and not simply a problem of law enforcement prompted the study of methadone treatment in the late 1960s.

The Development of Methadone

Methadone was developed by German chemists at I.G. Farbenindustrie, as a substitute for morphine in the face of a shortage of that medication during World War II. In August 1947 the pharmaceutical company Eli Lilly and Company was granted a New Drug Application (NDA) by the Food and Drug Administration for the use of methadone as an analgesic and antitussive (anticough) medication. Its trade name for methadone was Dolophine (derived from *dolor* for pain or sorrow). Interestingly, because of the drug's link to Germany, some in the addict community came to believe that this brand name—Dolophine—was a derivative of Adolf Hitler's name.

Studies of the pharmacologic effects of methadone began appearing in the scientific literature in the late 1940s. These early studies characterized the abuse liability of methadone and indicated that it was an opioid similar to morphine in many aspects. However, methadone was also noted to differ in important ways from morphine, such as in its longer duration of action and the delay of a withdrawal syndrome produced upon sudden discontinuation of chronic dosing (see chap. 4). These early studies did not identify the therapeutic potential of methadone for the treatment of opioid dependence. But, even if this potential had been appreciated, the regulatory environment at that time most likely would have precluded its use for this indication.

Early Methadone Treatment for Opioid Dependence

Many reports on the early use of methadone for the treatment of opioid dependence begin with the work conducted in the 1960s by Vincent Dole and Marie Nyswander (fig. 1.1) at Rockefeller University in New York. Other sites also were experimenting with its use and had been doing so even before Dole and Nyswander had begun their studies. For example,

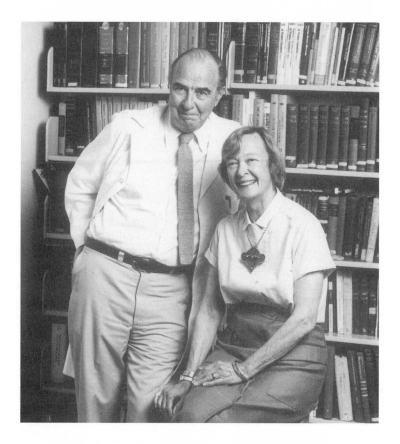

Figure 1.1. Drs. Vincent Dole and Marie Nyswander

a facility in Vancouver, British Columbia, first began experimenting with methadone as a short-term treatment for opioid dependence as early as 1959 and established a program providing extended methadone treatment in 1963 (Williams 1971). Dole and Nyswander, however, have generally been considered as the innovators of methadone treatment for opioid dependence. To understand this, it is useful to place their work in the context of time, location, and scientific success.

First, after World War II opiate use in the United States was increasing, especially in New York City. This rise occurred despite the efforts of the Treasury Department's FBN. The head of the FBN, Harry Anslinger, was a tough-talking bureaucrat who actively worked to prevent the medicalization of addiction and who tended to portray drug abuse in the United States based on his beliefs rather than on data and scientific studies.

Although Anslinger maintained that drug use was under control (through his efforts and the efforts of the FBN), by the late 1950s and early 1960s it was clear that this was not the case. Because efforts to control illicit opiate use through the prosecution of users were not successful, there was renewed interest in studying possible treatments for opioid dependence. It was not simply a fringe element of society that advocated this study of treatment; as previously described, the AMA, the ABA, the U.S. Supreme Court, and the White House itself were reevaluating how opiate abuse should best be viewed and managed.

Second, Dole and Nyswander were at a place that was receptive to their work. New York was a city with a growing population of persons with opiate addiction. Furthermore, they were in the right academic location—Rockefeller University. Despite efforts by the FBN to intimidate them, they received support in continuing their studies and treatments with the backing of the university (and its lawyers).

Finally, the ultimate importance of Dole and Nyswander's work rests on the investigations conducted and the results shown. Starting in late 1963, Dole and Nyswander began treating persons with opiate addiction on an inpatient unit at Rockefeller University. Although their early efforts had examined the potential efficacy of morphine maintenance, Dole and Nyswander observed that patients who transferred to maintenance on methadone from morphine appeared to function more effectively on methadone. This observation led to their initial studies of treating patients with methadone and to a series of published scientific reports on their success (Dole and Nyswander 1965; Dole et al. 1966a, 1966b). These results quickly gained the attention and interest of the medical community, both in the United States and in other countries, and led to the institution and rapid expansion of methadone treatment worldwide. For example, in 1969, in New York City almost 2,000 patients were in methadone treatment, whereas by 1970 the number of patients had reached 20,000. In addition, programs were begun in Sweden in 1966, Holland in 1968, Australia in 1970, Hong Kong in 1972, Italy and Switzerland in 1975, and France in 1983. In some cases, clinicians initially trained with Dole and Nyswander in New York, then returned to their home countries to begin programs that integrated methadone maintenance.

Contemporary Methadone Treatment

When methadone treatment became popular during the late 1960s and early 1970s, the medical community hoped and believed that it would provide a solution to the problems of opioid addiction. The early documented successes in methadone treatment, which occurred in small populations of selected patients treated under specific circumstances (e.g., living in a hospital, initially for extended periods), were not replicated as treatment expanded rapidly. Success rates in some clinics were quite poor, and treatment practices across clinics were highly variable. During the 1980s the previous enthusiasm for methadone treatment waned, and expansion of treatment programs virtually halted in the United States. However, not all countries had the same experience, and during this time some countries continued to develop and expand methadone treatment programs.

By the mid-1990s an estimated 250,000 patients were in methadone treatment worldwide, with the United States continuing to have the largest number of patients. In 2002, the National Survey of Substance Abuse Treatment Services estimated that there were 225,000 patients in the United States currently in methadone treatment. Although new methadone treatment programs rarely open in the United States, continued interest in methadone treatment has lead to the opening of new programs in other countries. Worldwide, the spread of human immunodeficiency virus (HIV) infection through injecting-drug use has sparked a new interest in methadone treatment, because studies in the late 1980s and in the 1990s demonstrated that methadone treatment can significantly decrease this HIV-risk behavior. As of January 1, 2004, methadone maintenance treatment is currently available in 47 countries (including pilot programs), and buprenorphine maintenance treatment is available in 28 countries (ta-

Table 1.1 **Countries with Methadone Maintenance Treatment**

Andorra	Hungary	New Zealand
Australia	Iran	Norway
Austria	Ireland	Poland
Belgium	Israel	Portugal
Bosnia and Herzegovina	Italy	Romania
Bulgaria	Kyrgyzstan	San Marino
Canada	Latvia	Serbia and Montenegro
China (Hong Kong)	Liechtenstein	Slovak Republic
Croatia	Lithuania	Slovenia
Czech Republic	Luxembourg	Spain
Denmark	Macedonia	Sweden
Estonia	Malaysia	Switzerland
Finland	Malta	Thailand
France	Mexico	United Kingdom
Germany	Nepal	United States
Greece	The Netherlands	

Table 1.2 Countries with Buprenorphine Maintenance Treatment

Australia	Greece	Portugal
Austria	Iceland	Singapore
Belgium	Indonesia	Slovak Republic
China (Hong Kong)	Israel	Slovenia
Czech Republic	Italy	South Africa
Denmark	Lithuania	Sweden
Estonia	Luxembourg	Switzerland
Finland	Malaysia	United Kingdom
France	Norway	United States
Germany		

bles 1.1 and 1.2). Many of these countries, however, do not have methadone available nationwide, and the models of treatment utilized (e.g., necessity for on-site dispensing versus pharmacy prescription) vary widely.

What Is Methadone Treatment?

The defining feature of methadone treatment is the use of the medication methadone. However, because methadone treatment is rarely limited to methadone pharmacotherapy, the label "methadone treatment" may be less than optimal because it provides undue emphasis on the pharmacologic aspects of treatment.

Thus, although methadone treatment includes a pharmacotherapy (methadone), one must recognize that methadone treatment represents both pharmacologic and nonpharmacologic therapies; it is a combination of the two, and optimal outcomes are obtained when both are delivered. Since the inception of methadone treatment, as designed by Dole and Nyswander at Rockefeller University, nonpharmacologic aspects of treatment have been included in virtually all methadone programs. The importance of these treatment components deserves special emphasis, because for most patients cessation of illicit drug use is not achieved simply by ingesting a daily dose of methadone. As stated by Vincent Dole:

> Some people became overly converted. They felt, without reading our reports carefully, that all they had to do was give methadone and then there was no more problem with the addict . . . I urged that physicians should see that the problem was one of rehabilitating people with a very complicated mixture of social problems on top of a specific medical problem and that they ought to tailor their programs to the kinds of problems they were dealing with. The

strength of the early programs as designed by Marie Nyswander was in their sensitivity to individual human problems. The stupidity of thinking that just giving methadone will solve a complicated social problem seems to me beyond comprehension (Courtwright et al. 1989, 338).

These nonpharmacologic aspects of methadone treatment are considered in other chapters of this book. They commonly include individual counseling, group therapy, and urinalysis testing. They can also include couples counseling, contingency contracting, vocational rehabilitation, education programs, parenting classes, HIV testing and counseling, primary medical care services, and assessment and treatment of comorbid psychiatric disorders. The clinic offering methadone may be best viewed as a site for the comprehensive treatment of patients with substance use disorders.

Although methadone treatment represents a combination of pharmacologic and nonpharmacologic therapies, there has been interest in the development of treatment models where methadone is provided without significant concurrent nonpharmacologic services (often referred to as "medical maintenance"). As a methadone clinic builds up a group of stable patients who are doing well, it is not uncommon for such patients to be given special privileges such as take-home doses of medication for several days each week. It is possible to transfer such patients into a modality that provides methadone and only limited nonpharmacologic treatments (such as urinalysis monitoring), if documentation for a sustained period indicates that the patients demonstrate good social functioning and absence of drug use. For most patients newly entering treatment, however, the need to address multiple problem areas related to their drug use requires treatment services beyond simply their daily dose of methadone.

History of the Development of Other Medications for the Treatment of Opioid Dependence

In addition to methadone, several other medications are available for the treatment of opioid dependence. Other medications not yet available are under development, such as those involving novel routes of administration of existing medications (e.g., depot injections, biodegradable beads, and subcutaneous implants). More details about these medications can be found in subsequent chapters, but the history of the development of these other available medications is briefly summarized here.

After methadone treatment was launched, the next medication that became available for the treatment of opioid dependence was naltrexone. During the period that methadone treatment was undergoing rapid expansion, interest in the substance abuse research and treatment communities turned to the possibility of developing an opioid antagonist for the treatment of opioid dependence. A concern was that some methadone doses meant to be taken outside the supervision of the clinic were being diverted to persons not in treatment. Therefore, an alternate medication that would have a low abuse potential was needed, and interest focused on an opioid *antagonist* (versus methadone, an opioid *agonist*). A patient maintained on an opioid antagonist medication would not experience acute effects if an abused opiate were taken (i.e., it would block the effects of heroin), and the antagonist itself should have no diversion and abuse potential (as it would not produce a subjective feeling of being high). If there was no abuse potential, then the antagonist could be prescribed and taken at home with no concern about diversion.

In 1971 President Nixon created the Special Action Office for Drug Abuse Prevention (SAODAP), a U.S. government office that predated the National Institute on Drug Abuse (NIDA). One of SAODAP's early interests (specifically included in the legislation that created SAODAP), in collaboration with the Division of Narcotic Addiction and Drug Abuse (DNADA) (located within the National Institute for Mental Health [NIMH]), was the development of an opioid antagonist. Although several possible compounds were considered, the most promising was EN-1639A (initially synthesized at Endo Laboratories), an orally active, relatively long-duration opioid antagonist subsequently named naltrexone (Julius and Renault 1976).

In the late 1970s and early 1980s, naltrexone underwent a series of studies sponsored by the U.S. government to examine both its safety and efficacy. It was eventually approved by the U.S. Food and Drug Administration (FDA) in 1984 for use in the treatment of opioid dependence in the United States. Naltrexone never gained widespread use comparable with methadone; however, studies in the early 1990s suggested it decreased alcohol use and craving in patients with alcohol dependence, and in 1995 it gained approval for this indication. Although naltrexone can be efficacious in clinical trials, effectiveness is typically limited by poor compliance. A new depot naltrexone microcapsule formulation (Depotrex, Biotek, Inc.) has been developed to overcome problems in compliance with the daily oral formulation. Results from a study by Comer and colleagues demonstrate that depot naltrexone has efficacy in blocking heroin effects for three to five weeks after injection (Comer et al. 2002). Other formulations are under development, such as Naltrel (DrugAbuse

Sciences), a naltrexone depot suspension intended for once-per-month injection.

After the approval of naltrexone in 1984, nine years passed before another medication, L-alpha-acetylmethadol (LAAM), was approved by the FDA for the treatment of opioid dependence. Initial work with LAAM actually occurred before the development of naltrexone, dating back to the late 1940s and early 1950s, and in the 1960s Merck and Company studied LAAM's possible use as an analgesic, but this indication was eventually abandoned because of the delayed onset of effects and long duration of action.

However, near the end of the 1960s Jaffe and co-workers began studying the clinical use of LAAM on a thrice-weekly basis for the treatment of opioid dependence (Jaffe et al. 1970, 1972). The results from this early work were promising and led the DNADA to sponsor, in the 1970s, further studies of LAAM for the treatment of opioid dependence. Several important clinical trials with LAAM were conducted under the sponsorship of NIDA (which grew out of the DNADA) in the mid- and late-1970s (see chap.13). But, in the 1980s LAAM languished, with little clinical research or further movement in its development or approval. In 1990 the Medications Development Division (MDD) at NIDA was created, and one of its early objectives was the approval of LAAM for the treatment of opioid dependence. In consultation with the FDA, MDD sponsored a final clinical trial with LAAM (called the Labeling Assessment Study), and in 1993 received FDA approval for LAAM.

Since the introduction of LAAM, there have been reports of cardiac-related adverse events, including QT interval prolongation, Torsades de Pointes, and cardiac arrest. In 2001, LAAM was removed from the European market and extensive packaging changes were initiated in the United States to warn and guide practitioners about these possible adverse effects. Use of LAAM was restricted to patients for whom methadone was ineffective or not tolerated, and ongoing electrocardiograph monitoring was required. Since these changes, the use of LAAM in the United States decreased dramatically, and as of 2004, the sole manufacturer of LAAM (Roxane Laboratories) ceased its sale and distribution.

While the MDD successfully completed the approval of LAAM in the 1990s, it also began sponsoring work with buprenorphine for the treatment of opioid dependence. Buprenorphine, an opioid with mixed agonist-antagonist properties, gained the attention and interest of the research and treatment communities because its unique pharmacologic profile suggested advantages over full opioid agonist medications such as methadone and LAAM (see chap. 10). Early human studies with buprenorphine were conducted in the late 1970s, with subsequent small clinical trials in the 1980s. However, it was not until the late 1980s and early 1990s that large clinical trials on the efficacy and safety of buprenorphine in the treatment of opioid dependence began to appear.

Although previous medications for the treatment of opioid dependence (methadone, naltrexone, and LAAM) had generally first been approved for use in the United States, buprenorphine was first approved for use in France in 1996. Buprenorphine has been approved for use in the treatment of opioid dependence in several other countries (including the United States) and, as of January 1, 2004, is currently available in 28 countries worldwide (table 1.2). As with naltrexone, novel, long-acting formulations of buprenorphine are under development, such as depot buprenorphine injection (Biotek, Inc.; DrugAbuse Sciences), and human pharmacology studies have shown promise with such a product (Sobel et al. 2004).

Two other pharmacotherapies used in the treatment of opioid dependence should be briefly mentioned in this overview: clonidine and lofexidine, both alpha$_2$-adrenergic agonists (see chap. 13). Clonidine is available as an antihypertensive agent in several countries, but it is generally not approved for use in the treatment of opioid dependence. However, several studies in the 1980s showed that it could be effective in attenuating opioid withdrawal, making it a popular nonopioid detoxification agent. Lofexidine is approved for opioid withdrawal in the United Kingdom (as BritLofex, Britannia Pharmaceuticals). Although the development of naltrexone, LAAM, and buprenorphine have involved substantial governmental support, it appears that lofexidine has developed primarily through the sponsorship of the private sector.

Summary

Methadone treatment represents the first pharmacotherapy targeting opioid dependence to have gained wide acceptance and availability. Although attempts were made at the turn of the twentieth century to treat opioid-dependent persons at clinics that used substitution therapies such as morphine, these clinics were relatively short lived and closed in response to political pressures. Early studies on the efficacy of methadone treatment produced markedly good outcomes, leading to the rapid expansion of methadone treatment in the United States and in other countries. Although this expansion has markedly slowed in the United States, steady expansion of methadone treatment continues throughout the world. Renewed interest in methadone treatment in the late 1980s was prompted, in part, by the rise of HIV infection among injecting-drug users and by a resurgence of interest in methadone treatment as a highly effective means for decreasing high-risk behaviors. In addition to methadone treatment, other pharmacotherapies such as naltrexone, LAAM (until recently), buprenorphine, clonidine, and lofexidine have become available for the treatment of opioid dependence in many countries. The use of these treatments continues to expand as clinicians gain familiarity with their application, and some novel formulations are under development in an attempt to improve effectiveness, decrease diversion, improve adherence, and offer more clinical options. However, despite these newer medications, methadone continues to be the most widely used pharmacotherapy for the treatment for opioid dependence.

References

Comer SD, Collins ED, Kleber HD, Nuwayser ES, Kerrigan JH, Fischman MW (2002). Depot naltrexone: long-lasting antagonism of the effects of heroin in humans. *Psychopharmacology (Berl)* 159: 351–60.

Courtwright D, Joseph H, des Jarlais D (1989). *Addicts Who Survived: An Oral History of Narcotics Use in America, 1923–1965.* Knoxville: University of Tennessee Press.

Dole VP, Nyswander M (1965). A medical treatment for diacetylmorphine (heroin) addiction. A clinical trial with methadone hydrochloride. *JAMA* 193: 646–50.

Dole VP, Nyswander ME, Kreek MJ (1966a). Narcotic blockade. *Arch Intern Med* 118: 304–9.

Dole VP, Nyswander ME, Kreek MJ (1966b). Narcotic blockade—a medical technique for stopping heroin use by addicts. *Trans Assoc Am Physicians* 79: 122–36.

Jaffe JH, Schuster CR, Smith BB, Blachley PH (1970). Comparison of acetylmethadol and methadone in the treatment of long- term heroin users. A pilot study. *JAMA* 211: 1834–6.

Jaffe JH, Senay EC, Schuster CR, Renault PR, Smith B, DiMenza S (1972). Methadyl acetate vs methadone. A double-blind study in heroin users. *JAMA* 222: 437–42.

Jonnes J (1996). *Hep-cats, Narcs, and Pipe Dreams: A History of America's Romance with Illegal Drugs.* New York: Scribner.

Julius D, Renault P (1976). Narcotic Antagonists: Naltrexone Progress Report. NIDA Research Monograph 9. Bethesda, MD: National Institutes of Health, U.S. Department of Health, Education, and Welfare.

Musto DF (1987). *The American Disease: Origins of Narcotic Control.* New York: Oxford University Press.

Sobel BF, Sigmon SC, Walsh SL, Johnson RE, Liebson IA, Nuwayser ES, Kerrigan JH, Bigelow GE (2004). Open-label trial of an injection depot formulation of buprenorphine in opioid detoxification. *Drug Alcohol Depend* 73: 11–22.

Williams HR (1971). Low and high methadone maintenance in the out-patient treatment of the hard core heroin addict. In: Einstein S, ed. *Methadone Maintenance.* New York: Marcel Dekker.

2

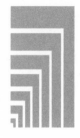

Regulatory, Cost, and Policy Issues

Kenneth B. Stoller, M.D., and George E. Bigelow, Ph.D.

With the dramatic increase in the prevalence of HIV, hepatitis B and C viruses, and tuberculosis among injecting-opiate users during the past two decades, the delivery of effective treatments for opioid dependence should be of critical importance. After four decades of experience and scientific inquiry, the efficacy and safety of methadone in the treatment of opiate dependence are indisputable. Even so, public misperception and the stigma associated with opioid dependence and treatment continue to prevail. Since the early 1970s, concern over possible diversion of methadone from treatment clinics has been a significant driving factor behind policymaking. Rather than focusing on how best to deliver treatment to those who could benefit from it, public policy has been primarily centered on controls that limit delivery. Owing to this and other issues to be discussed in this chapter, opioid-agonist treatment (especially methadone treatment) is readily available to only a small portion of individuals in need of treatment. Although this chapter focuses on methadone treatment and methadone clinics, the material covered here is generally applicable to the broader categories of opioid-agonist treatments and opioid treatment programs (OTPs).

The regulation of methadone treatment has varied over time, across countries, and among localities. Despite a recent relaxation of regulation in the United States, methadone maintenance is the medical treatment with the greatest degree of oversight. The governmental bodies and agencies involved in its regulation are numerous, as are the relevant laws and regulations. For example, in the United States mandatory oversight of methadone treatment exists at local, state, and federal levels and, since 2001, by approved accreditation bodies. Even within the federal level, multiple agencies, such as the Substance Abuse and Mental Health Services Administration (SAMHSA) and the Drug Enforcement Agency (DEA), are involved in the monitoring and oversight of methadone treatment.

This chapter, organized into three sections, addresses regulatory as well as cost and policy issues as they pertain to methadone. The first part examines regulatory issues as they pertain to the use of methadone in the United States, where the regulation of methadone treatment is uniquely complex. The largest population of methadone patients is in the United States, where the treatment originated. Methadone treatment, however, is also available in many other parts of the world, including eastern and western Asia, Australia, Canada, Europe, and the Middle East (see table 1.1). Regulatory issues in other countries where methadone is available for the treatment of opioid dependence are also briefly reviewed.

The second part of this chapter examines the cost-related issues of methadone treatment. Although regulatory and policy issues regarding methadone treatment have played a prominent role in the use and expansion of methadone treatment, cost issues also have played an important role. Numerous studies have demonstrated that methadone treatment is highly cost-effective when a broad array of beneficial outcomes is considered (e.g., decreases in crime, increases in employment). However, in countries such as the United States, it is not clear how methadone treatment will operate and be adequately reimbursed in the evolving environment of managed health care. These issues become increasingly important when government-supported services for uninsured people are decreased or withdrawn, because a large population of patients entering drug abuse treatment relies on treatment subsidized by the government.

Creative and more cost-effective mechanisms for the delivery of methadone treatment continue to be proposed and investigated. The third part of this chapter explores approaches that could lead to improved quality and access to treatment. Novel approaches to treatment are reviewed, including interim methadone maintenance, mobile treatment, methadone clinics as primary health care sites, office-based and medical maintenance models, and the use of buprenorphine. These and other approaches may be used in the future as part of a medically and economically effective delivery system. The chapter ends with discussions of the need to inform policymakers and of international experience in using systems that differ from that in the United States.

Regulatory Issues in the United States

In the United States, the extent of regulation for methadone (and more recently LAAM) is extensive and unique (Institute of Medicine [IOM] 1995). No other medications approved by the FDA in the United States have been regulated in a similar fashion. During the past decade there have been strong appeals to relax methadone regulations; substantial changes in methadone regulations have been made, but only after considerable bureaucratic process, considerable time, and with limited scope.

Federal Levels of Control

In the United States, methadone manufacturers and treatment providers currently must comply with four levels of regulatory control, the first three of which are on the level of the federal government. First, as with all prescription drugs, the manufacturing, labeling, and dispensing must meet the requirements of the FDA under the Federal Food, Drug, and Cosmetic Act. The primary intent of this first layer of control is to protect the consumer. Second, as with all schedule II controlled substances, DEA regulations govern the manufacturing, distribution, and dispensing of methadone. The objective of the DEA in this role is to prevent the diversion of drugs with abuse potential. The third level of control involves federal regulations specific to methadone (or LAAM), currently assigning oversight of methadone treatment to SAMHSA through a process of accreditation. As part of this third level of control, programs are subject to compliance with treatment standards developed by specific accreditation bodies (e.g., Commission for the Accreditation of Rehabilitation Facilities [CARF] or Joint Commission on Accreditation of Healthcare Organizations [JCAHO]) and consistent with Center for Substance Abuse Treatment (CSAT) guidelines. This third level of control deserves a detailed discussion, but first a brief review of the evolution of this tier is in order.

In 1972 methadone was approved by the FDA for use in the maintenance treatment of opioid dependence in the United States. The basic framework for methadone regulation was issued by the FDA in December 1972 and became effective in March 1973 (37 FR 26790) (IOM 1995). During this time, Congress approved a series of bills that became known as the Narcotic Addict Treatment Act (NATA) of 1974. The NATA was driven by concerns about substantial diversion of methadone to illicit channels during the rapid expansion of methadone treatment in the late 1960s and early 1970s. It established the statutory role of the Secretary of the Department of Health and Human Services (DHHS) over methadone treatment. Guidelines established by the Secretary defined a unique, third level of federal control, beyond the usual regulations (FDA and DEA) for controlled substances, and the NATA resulted in a closed system of methadone distribution that persisted through the end of the century. That is, all methadone treatment for opioid dependence was to be limited to highly regulated comprehensive treatment centers.

NATA also defined the differences between detoxification and maintenance treatments. Detoxification was defined as the use of methadone in decreasing doses to reach a drug-free state in not more than 21 days. Maintenance treatment was to be restricted to methadone treatment programs and was defined as the use of methadone "at relatively stable doses" for more than 21 days, along with social and medical services. (Notably, subsequent revisions have changed the definitions of detoxification and maintenance treatment; see chap. 9, for a discussion of current regulations regarding methadone detoxification and maintenance treatment in the United States.)

These regulations between 1972 and 1974 created a closed system of delivery, restricting treatment to *methadone treatment programs,* which provided comprehensive services for methadone detoxification or maintenance, as well as initial patient evaluation. Also defined were *methadone treatment medication units,* which were facilities within treatment programs that were restricted to dispensing methadone and collecting urine samples to test for narcotics. This system limited the dispensing of methadone to treatment programs with specific prior approval by federal and state authorities and to hospital pharmacies.

Much of the basic framework for this early and unique form of regulation for methadone treatment in the United States persisted over the next 30 years, although recent policy initiatives have been applied with the aim of improving treatment quality and access (Merrill 2002). These initiatives involve moving oversight of methadone treatment further toward the oversight in place for general medical (more specifically, psychiatric) practice. In January 2001 the federal government issued a Final Rule, repealing the existing FDA regulations (21 CFR Part 291) and enacting new SAMHSA regulations (42 CFR Part 8) entitled "Opioid Drugs in Maintenance and Detoxification Treatment of Opiate Addiction." Under this new rule, the responsibility for oversight of OTPs was transferred from the FDA to SAMHSA. The new regulatory system is based on an accreditation model, such that a treatment program is required to obtain accreditation from an approved accreditation body (table 2.1) to apply to SAMHSA for certification. This process of accreditation and certification is described in detail within these regulations. The regulations also include

Table 2.1 **Opioid Treatment Program Approved Accreditation Bodies**

Commission on Accreditation of Rehabilitation Facilities (CARF)

Council on Accreditation (COA)

Joint Commission on Accreditation of Healthcare Organizations (JCAHO)

Division of Alcohol and Substance Abuse, Washington Department of Social and Health Services

Division of Alcohol and Drug Abuse, State of Missouri Department of Mental Health

National Commission on Correctional Health Care

Table 2.2 **U.S. Federal Opioid Treatment Standards (DHHS, SAMHSA, 42 CFR Part 8, Subpart B, 8.12)**

Administrative and organizational structure (including role of Medical Director)

Continuous quality improvement (including quality assurance plan and "Diversion Control Plan")

Staff credentials

Patient admission criteria (including criteria, informed consent, treatment for persons under age 18, exceptions [pregnancy, penal release, previous treatment], detoxification episodes)

Required services (including initial medical services, special services for pregnant patients, initial and periodic assessment, counseling, drug testing)

Recordkeeping and confidentiality

Medication administration, dispensing, and use (including who may administer or dispense, permitted medications, maximum initial dose, adherence to labeling, take-home use)

Interim maintenance treatment

Note: See also chapter 9 for related information on this topic.

a section describing, in only limited detail, treatment standards by which programs must abide (table 2.2). SAMHSA delegated day-to-day responsibilities for administration of these new regulations to the CSAT, a component of SAMHSA. CSAT in turn issued more guidelines, in much more detail than provided in 42 CFR, for the accreditation of treatment programs with the aim of guiding programs to deliver the highest possible quality of treatment in a secure setting that did not put unnecessary burden on the program or patients (table 2.3).

This revised system of federal oversight, from one of strict regulation

Table 2.3 **Domains Covered in the CSAT Guidelines for the Accreditation of Opioid Treatment Programs**

Administrative organization and responsibilities
Management of facility and clinical environment
Risk management and continuous quality improvement
Professional staff credentials and development
Patient admission criteria
Patient medical and psychosocial assessment
Therapeutic dosage
Treatment planning, evaluation of progress, continuous assessment
Drug testing
Take-home medication
Withdrawal and discharge
Management of polysubstance abuse
Concurrent services
Special considerations
Care of women
Patient rights
Recordkeeping
Community relations and education
Diversion control
Research activities

to one of accreditation, is viewed as a step forward for many reasons. First, the relaxation of some previously overrestrictive rules allows for increased medical judgment in the course of treatment. For example, take-home doses for patients on a daily methadone dose of more than 100 mg are no longer prohibited. Additionally, a more generous take-home schedule allows for more appropriate, individualized care tailored for particular patient needs. Patients who have demonstrated a high degree of stability for two or more years of treatment can be given as much as a month's supply of medication to take outside of the context of the clinic. Second, the system of accreditation allows for guidelines to be updated on a regular basis, when the medical community determines that it best serves the clinical care of patients. In the past, this was only possible through the cumbersome and often interminable legislative process of changing codified regulations. Third, the system of oversight by accreditation bodies and treatment-oriented guidelines stresses the use of best clinical practice and mandates a continual process of quality improvement and outcomes measurement. In short, the bar of quality care has been raised, and the structure of this new system of federal oversight reinforces the concept of methadone as a proven and effective medical treatment.

State and Local Levels of Control

The fourth and final level of control over methadone treatment is on a more local level and involves individual states, counties, and municipalities. These local levels of government often codify their own controls, further restricting the use of methadone for the treatment of opiate addiction. At times extremely restrictive local regulations have resulted essentially in banning methadone treatment altogether in some parts of the country.

The local control of methadone treatment may itself consist of multiple layers involving state, county, and local interests in treatment programs. These entities comprise governmental agencies and local organizations and are involved in many aspects of professional practice and program operation, such as regulation, financing, licensing of practitioners, quality assurance, data collection, use of controlled substances, control of diversion, and control of illicit drugs. Beyond adhering to federal regulatory requirements, states may, and often do, impose more restrictive measures. Areas of clinical operation affected by these measures include urine collection and testing, take-home doses of methadone, issues of patient rights, recordkeeping, staffing, and admission criteria. In addition, issues involving patient registry, treatment duration, and treatment plan reviews are often addressed.

REGULATORY ISSUES IN OTHER PARTS OF THE WORLD

It is difficult to summarize the regulatory and policy issues of methadone treatment in the numerous other countries where methadone treatment is provided. At least 45 countries have methadone treatment to some extent (see table 1.1) and, as in the United States, the regulation of this treatment undergoes periodic revision in many of these countries. A brief summary of the history of methadone treatment and regulation for several countries can be found in the third edition of the Swiss Methadone Report (Uchtenhagen 1996). Additional information can be obtained online, such as from The International Center for Advancement of Addiction Treatment (The Baron Edmond de Rothschild Chemical Dependency Institute) (www.opiateaddictionrx.info/addiction/addiction03.html), or INDRO e.V., a nonprofit and nongovernmental advocacy organization based in Germany (www.indro-online.de). The INDRO Web site includes information on methadone availability for both citizens and international travelers.

Most countries that developed methadone programs in the 1970s based their model of methadone treatment on the early work done by Dole and Nyswander. For example, the first European methadone program was started in Sweden in 1966 and was essentially a replication of the model used by Dole and Nyswander in New York. However, there has been considerable variability in methadone treatment practices across countries and over time, and it is no longer unusual for some countries (such as Australia) to allow individual physicians to prescribe methadone (rather than centralized treatment programs such as those in the United States).

Although generalizations across countries about the regulation of methadone treatment should be recognized *as* generalizations, a few points do seem to appear consistently. First, most countries use oral methadone (rather than injections), and the liquid more often than tablet formulation. Second, many countries either require or recommend methadone treatment be delivered in the context of other, nonpharmacologic treatment services. Finally, it is common to find countries regulating specific aspects of methadone practice, such as dosing and urinalysis testing. Thus, the heavy regulation of methadone treatment in the United States is not unique. Many countries have made substantial efforts to find the best means for regulating methadone treatment.

COST-BENEFIT ANALYSIS OF DRUG ABUSE TREATMENT

Calculating the costs of drug abuse and its treatment and the benefits of treatment can be exceedingly complicated. Drug abuse has an impact on many areas beyond simply the individual user. Drug use disorders also have a negative impact on the family, the local and broader communities, and the society at large. Costs related to drug use include the direct cost of the drugs, lost potential earnings, decreased workforce productivity, associated medical costs, treatment costs, increased enforcement and prison costs, and drug-related theft and violence (table 2.4). In total, untreated opiate addiction in the United States costs an estimated $20 billion per year (Mark et al. 2001). However, dollar figures often fail to capture the magnitude of personal suffering, familial pain, and societal woes produced by drug use.

Fortunately, effective treatment can produce both a reduction in direct costs associated with drug use problems, as well as an array of other less financially tangible, but highly valuable, benefits at individual, familial, communal, and societal levels. That is, the justification of drug abuse treatment is not simply one of straightforward economics; patients, families, and society benefit in other highly meaningful ways.

Table 2.4   **Costs Associated with Substance Use Disorders**

Criminal justice system	Cost of police protection, prosecution, adjudication, public defense, and corrections (incarceration and parole/probation)
Victim losses	Victim expenditures on medical care, repairs of damaged property, and lost time from work that result from predatory crimes
Theft losses	Value of property or money stolen during a crime, excluding any property damage or other victim losses
Health care utilization	Economic value of avoidable inpatient, outpatient, and emergency medical and mental health care
Lost legitimate earnings	Value of legitimate productivity lost because individuals pursue income through crime or live off the resources of friends, families, and others
Income transfers	Resources moved from non-substance-abusing taxpayers to others via gifts, public assistance, or public and private disability insurance

Source: Adapted from CALDATA General Report (1994), figure 1.

The California Drug and Alcohol Treatment Assessment (CALDATA)

Before discussing the specific costs of methadone treatment, this section provides a brief review of a comprehensive cost-benefit analysis for general substance abuse treatment conducted in the early 1990s in California. The study, titled "Evaluating Recovery Services: The California Drug and Alcohol Treatment Assessment" (more commonly referred to as CALDATA), was published in 1994 (Gerstein et al. 1994). The study's objective was to evaluate the effectiveness, benefits, and costs of alcohol and drug abuse treatment. A voluntary survey was conducted of approximately 3,000 participants in 97 residential, residential "social model," general outpatient, and outpatient methadone treatment programs in 16 counties in California. Participants were in treatment or were discharged from treatment between October 1991 and September 1992 and were randomly selected to represent the nearly 150,000 statewide patients in treatment. More than 1,850 of the survey participants were successfully contacted and interviewed for follow-up after nine months.

The cost of treating these 150,000 statewide patients was $209 million, and the one-year benefits to taxpaying citizens, mostly owing to reductions in crime, were worth approximately $1.5 billion. This 1:7 average cost-benefit ratio ranged from 1:4 to greater than 1:12, depending on the treatment modality. However, it was evident that the populations served by the various modalities were very different, and assignment to type of treatment was not random. Therefore, comparisons across the modalities of the relative costs and benefits should be made with caution.

Table 2.5 gives data regarding costs and benefits of "continuing" and "discharged" methadone patients. The "methadone discharge" group comprised short-term methadone detoxification patients in addition to long-term maintenance patients who began maintenance but left treatment. All "methadone continuing" patients had been in treatment for at least four months at the time of the follow-up interview. Of all treatment modalities studied, the most favorable cost-to-benefit ratio (1:12.58) was for discharged methadone patients. However, this largely reflects the low total cost incurred per treatment episode ($405) despite a far lower (relative to the other treatment modalities) total benefit ($5,093). Total benefits reported for the methadone-continuing group were $11,112, yielding a cost-to-benefit ratio of 1:4.78. Furthermore, benefits persisted after treatment through the second year of follow-up for participants monitored longer than one year. Thus, longer-term benefits are likely to be substantially higher than outcomes found after one year.

The results from the CALDATA, in which a comparison was made of patients before and after a treatment episode, demonstrated a two-thirds decrease in criminal activity, with longer treatment duration associated with greater improvement. Alcohol and drug use fell by approximately two-fifths. Hospitalizations were reduced by about one-third, with significant improvements in other health indicators. Additionally, longer lengths of stay in treatment had a positive effect on employment.

These results from the CALDATA provide an exceedingly important message: substance abuse treatment results in remarkable savings, even

Table 2.5   **Total Benefits and Costs to Taxpayers by Treatment Modality**

	Methadone Discharge	Methadone Continuing
Average length of stay	60 days	365 days
Societal benefits per day during treatment	$20.59	$30.47
Societal benefits per day after treatment	$11.32	N/A*
Total benefits	$5,093	$11,122
Cost per day of treatment	$6.79	$6.37
Total cost per treatment episode	$405	$2,325
Net benefit (total benefits minus costs)	$4,688	$8,797
Benefit-to-cost ratio	12.58:1	4.78:1

Source: Adapted from CALDATA General Report (1994), table 35.
*N/A, not applicable (posttreatment values not applicable for continuing participants).

when patients are monitored for relatively short periods. As noted in the final report, $1 spent on treatment results in $7 in savings to taxpaying citizens who, after all, ultimately pay for publicly funded treatment. Although that benefit figure represents a variety of treatment modalities, analyses of only the methadone patients shows a benefit of $4 to $13 for every $1 spent.

Other Studies of Economic Benefits of Methadone Treatment

Other studies have shown similar substantial savings associated with methadone treatment (table 2.6). In one study of methadone treatment conducted in the late 1980s, a 16-week course of methadone maintenance therapy resulted in striking decreases in drug use, criminal activity, and economic costs to the community (Strain et al. 1993). There was a 96 percent reduction in money spent on drugs, a 96 percent reduction in days with illegal activity, and a 95 percent reduction in the amount of money obtained through illegal activities. Illegal income fell, on average, from $1,504 to $73 per month—a social benefit of $1,431 per month during treatment.

Regarding the health-related cost benefits of methadone treatment, the potential reduction in HIV transmission is of paramount importance. In November 1997, The National Institutes of Health convened a consensus development conference during which data were presented on this topic. A study was described that tracked HIV seroconversion rates over time among subjects both in and out of methadone maintenance therapy in Philadelphia, Pennsylvania, during the late 1980s and early 1990s (Merrill 1997). After four years, those who had received no treatment were 4.2 times more likely (13.5% versus 3.2%) to have seroconverted to HIV-positive than those who had received two or more years of methadone treatment. Currently, the annual incidence of seroconversion to HIV for injecting-drug users is approximately 3 percent per year, based

Table 2.6 **Methadone Treatment: Benefits**

• Reduced illicit drug consumption	• Reduced theft and property damage
• Improved general health	• Employment acquisition/maintenance
• Improved access to health care	• Decreased reliance on public assistance
• Reduced spread of infectious diseases	• Improved domestic relations
• Improved psychological well-being	• Improved childrearing
• Reduced violence	• Improved social functioning

on Centers for Disease Control and Prevention (CDC) surveillance data and other studies (for example, see Strathdee et al. 2001). Generalizing the findings from this study to the entire population of injecting-drug users, entry of all opiate-dependent persons into methadone maintenance treatment could result in a decrease of more than 50,000 individuals who would otherwise have become HIV-positive over a four-year period. The associated health care cost savings for such a decrease in HIV incidence would likely be measured in hundreds of millions of dollars per year.

Even among persons who have already contracted acquired immuno-deficiency syndrome (AIDS), methadone treatment conveys very positive and valuable benefits. A study of injecting-drug users with AIDS examined HIV-related health care utilization and costs among persons in or not in methadone treatment (Sambamoorthi et al. 2000). Consistent methadone treatment was associated with reduced total medical expenses, including those for inpatient services. Methadone-treated patients were also more likely to be taking antiretroviral agents, and among all participants receiving antiretroviral agents, those taking methadone had superior adherence. Now that highly active retroviral therapies can delay or prevent the devastating effects of HIV, interventions that enhance adherence to these highly complex medication regimens are exceedingly valuable.

Costs of Methadone Treatment

Methadone medication alone is relatively inexpensive. In the United States, a 60 mg per day dose of methadone (not including costs of medication administration, counseling, facilities, etc.) costs about $100 per year. However, annual costs for comprehensive methadone treatment can easily exceed 30 times the cost of the medication. Using 1991 data obtained from an annual survey by the Office of Applied Studies of SAMHSA (the National Drug and Alcohol Treatment Unit Survey [NDATUS]) (SAMHSA 1993), Harwood (as described in IOM [1995]) estimated that in fiscal year 1993 payments for methadone treatment from all sources totaled $480 million. Assuming that 117,000 patients were in outpatient methadone maintenance treatment during that time, the average cost per patient was $4,100 per year. Similarly, Bradley and colleagues, in a study involving three methadone treatment programs (one hospital based and two freestanding clinics), determined the average annual cost per patient to be between $3,750 and $4,400 for standard treatment (i.e., methadone pharmacotherapy plus counseling and urinalysis testing) (Bradley et al. 1994). The cost of traditional methadone treatment has not significantly changed subsequent to the publication of these studies.

Table 2.7 **Methadone Treatment: Program Costs**

• Staff wages and benefits*	• Methadone medication
• Rent and utilities	• Urinalysis testing
• Licensing and accreditation	• Security
• Medical supplies	• Documentation and recordkeeping
• Staff training	

*See chapter 9 for a discussion of the staff usually required for an opioid treatment program's operations.

This difference between the cost of medication alone and costs for full methadone treatment is a consequence of the other components of methadone treatment (table 2.7). The largest cost associated with methadone treatment is staffing of the program. (A discussion of personnel requirements for methadone treatment can be found in chap. 9.) Other costs that can represent substantial outlays include rent and utilities, security, and urinalysis testing. In the study by Bradley and colleagues (1994), expenditures for labor, professional consultants, and contracted services such as laboratory analyses amounted to 69–81 percent of the total annual cost of treatment. The extent to which supplemental services are provided can, of course, affect cost. Although the inclusion of nonpharmacologic clinical services increases the total cost, however, total benefits may also increase. In fact, provision of a moderate intensity of counseling services (versus low or high intensities) seems to be most cost-effective (Kraft et al. 1997; Puigdollers et al. 2003).

Revenue Sources for Methadone Treatment

Financing of drug abuse treatment can come from a variety of sources, including patients, insurance companies, community entities such as foundations and churches, hospitals, and most significantly, local, state, and federal governments. The primary sources of funding for methadone treatment programs in the United States are federal block grants, Medicare, Medicaid, state agencies, self-pay (out-of-pocket), and private insurance. The percent of total revenue dollars that each source contributes to methadone treatment varies among individual states and programs and is largely a function of program type (e.g., hospital based, public, for-profit, etc.), patient population, and resource availability.

There are three primary sources of public funding of substance abuse treatment (not limited to methadone) in the United States: federal Substance Abuse Prevention and Treatment block grants (administered by CSAT), Medicaid and Medicare, and state and local funding. These public funding sources account for approximately 60 percent of substance abuse treatment expenditures. According to CSAT (Mark et al. 2001; SAMHSA 2000), funds from block grants accounted for approximately 40 percent of the public funds spent on substance abuse treatment and prevention in the states. Medicaid's role in the funding of methadone treatment has been significant. Medicaid supported about 20 percent of all substance abuse treatment costs in 1997. The largest portion of spending on substance abuse treatment comes from state and local governments. When all federal sources are combined (including the federal share of Medicaid), however, it becomes evident that approximately 56 percent of publicly funded drug treatment consists of federal dollars.

Self-pay, private insurance, and, for a select group of patients, the Department of Veterans Affairs (DVA) comprise most of the remainder of payment sources. Using NDATUS data, investigators have estimated that self-pay and private insurance contribute 17 percent and 2.5 percent, respectively, of total expenditures for methadone treatment (IOM 1995). When one examines different types of treatment programs, it is evident that for-profit programs derive a significantly higher proportion of revenue from patient out-of-pocket payments than not-for-profit programs do (Batten et al. 1992; Gerstein and Harwood 1990). Regarding the Veterans Affairs system, one study found that 26 percent of all inpatients were diagnosed with a substance abuse disorder (Peterson et al. 1993), indicating a large population in need of treatment. In 1993 approximately 36 Veterans Affairs medical centers were providing methadone maintenance to 5,886 patients, or 5 percent of all U.S. methadone patients (IOM 1995). The estimated cost of this treatment was about $22 million (DVA 1993) or $3,700 per patient.

In the United States, Medicaid funding increasingly is through assignment to managed care organizations; managed care has typically taken a negative view of long-term treatments in general, and substance abuse is no exception. Psychiatric and substance abuse treatments preferred by managed care have been, and still are, oriented toward short-term crisis intervention. In part, this may be due to a lack of appreciation of drug dependence as a chronic psychiatric disorder requiring ongoing, if not lifelong, monitoring and/or treatment. Methadone maintenance, therefore, by its nature as one such long-term treatment model, is not a favored modality of treatment by managed care. When Medicaid dollars are under public control, the societal benefits of treatment such as decreases in crime enter the cost-benefit equation, making treatments with high net benefits (even if cost is high or treatment duration is long), more favorable. Decision makers in managed care, however, do not view societal benefits as being relevant to their corporate cost-benefit decisions if they do not affect their bottom line in the short run.

In time, managed care may come to appreciate more fully the value of long-term substance abuse treatment, including methadone treatment, if substance abuse treatment dollars become a part of all health care dollars (rather than "carved out" for administration by an entity outside the managed care organization). Then, managed care may recognize that failure to invest in effective, long-term treatment of addiction can result in increased total expenditures owing to medical complications from continued drug use. That is, the cost of providing effective substance abuse treatment is offset by savings in general medical utilization. For example, the projected value of avoiding the morbidity associated with a single case of HIV/AIDS is approximately $158,000 (French et al. 1996). The shorter-term (1- to 3-year span) cost offset of drug abuse treatment has also been clearly demonstrated in several prospective and retrospective cost-benefit analyses. In many of these studies, total medical care costs when drug abuse was treated (including the cost of treatment) appeared closer to costs for persons with no drug use problems than to costs for those whose drug abuse went untreated.

Treatment programs and researchers must do their part in informing managed care about the clinical and economic benefits of treatment. For example, it is useful to demonstrate decreases in risk behaviors (e.g., HIV-related) associated with treatment and to show the advantages of funding sustained treatment rather than paying for multiple, brief, costly, acute admissions. Providers also must be increasingly willing to work effectively with managed care utilization review and management staff to justify the most clinically appropriate intensity and duration of treatment (McCarty 1997). For managed care organizations, efforts to perform analyses of health care utilization and costs among one of their most costly populations, members with chronic and severe drug use disorder, is likely to confirm that provision of treatment not only reduces morbidity but also contributes toward bottom-line financial savings.

Summary of Costs, Benefits, and Financing of Methadone Treatment

Methadone treatment is the combination of pharmacologic and non-pharmacologic treatment services. Both of these aspects of methadone treatment incur costs. It is clear, however, that effective treatment using methadone maintenance results in substantial benefits that more than offset the cost of treatment. These savings from treatment not only have an impact on the individual in treatment, but they also affect taxpaying citizens and society as a whole. Zaric and colleagues assert that more than half of the benefits of methadone maintenance are actually gained by persons who do not inject drugs (Zaric et al. 2000). Expansion of outcomes research including cost-effectiveness and cost-benefit studies will help shed light on the extent to which provision of methadone maintenance results not only in the substantial improvement of the quality of life of the individual, but also in the bottom-line cost savings to society as a whole.

POSSIBLE FUTURE DIRECTIONS AND IMPLICATIONS REGARDING POLICY

Those individuals most in need of methadone treatment often do not have the resources to pay for it. Although government sources such as state and local grants often helped to underwrite the costs of methadone treatment in the past, these sources of funding are declining in many areas. Efforts in three areas may help to make this effective treatment more widely available to those who could benefit from it. First, modifications of current methadone treatment systems may lower cost while maintaining or even improving effectiveness. Second, new and innovative systems for the delivery of opioid-agonist treatment should be systematically studied and developed. And third, the benefits of methadone treatment must be effectively communicated to funding sources, policymakers, and the general public.

Modifications of Current Methadone Treatment Systems

Some changes within the current framework of treatment may result in improved efficiency of operation in existing programs. Staff optimization through organizational efficiency, introduction of computerized tracking and documentation systems, and state-of-the-art automated systems for physician ordering, dispensing, and accounting of methadone pharmacotherapy are potential means for increasing the efficiency of programs. Some larger systemwide initiatives could also result in enhanced efficiency. For example, in Baltimore, Maryland, a centralized system of "home delivery" of methadone exists for patients too infirm to come to their home clinic or for patients temporarily in subacute nursing facilities. This has replaced a previous situation where staff from each clinic was responsible for delivering their own patients' doses throughout the city themselves. Also in Baltimore, all urinalysis samples from state grant-funded programs are sent to a central reference laboratory. This has enabled substantial discounts due to the sheer number of samples submitted per year, and the laboratory bills the funding agency directly, increasing the efficiency of the enterprise. This also has allowed urinalysis results to be analyzed on a citywide basis, enabling comparisons between programs and over time. Program representatives meet monthly to discuss statistics, monitor performance in relation to benchmarks, and discuss quality improvement initiatives, in an effort dubbed *DrugStat*.

Other changes of a more novel nature could be made within existing treatment programs using proven clinical tools such as formalized behavioral contingencies (Kidorf et al. 1994; Brooner et al. 1998, 1997; Silverman et al. 1996) (see also chap. 8). The fundamental objective of a methadone maintenance clinic is to provide a context that encourages behavioral change. Use of behavioral contingency models have promise in enhancing the effectiveness of treatment by providing a structure that rewards behavioral movement toward recovery-based actions and discouraging behaviors that encourage continued drug use. Reinforcers such as take-home medication or increased hours of methadone dosing can be delivered in response to behaviors such as submitting a drug-free urinalysis sample, adhering to scheduled treatment sessions, or obtaining employment. If use of such methods is clinically effective, they could lead to an increase in the proportion of patients who are stable in their recovery and require less intensive services (e.g., decreased hours of counseling or days medicated in clinic). Clinic resources are thus freed, allowing enhanced treatment for less stable patients, increased census, or a reduction in resource expenditures.

Alternative Treatment Systems

Innovations of the type that fall outside the realm of the typical comprehensive methadone program, though controversial, are worth considering. There has been some experience with all the modalities discussed here.

Interim Methadone Maintenance

A proposal for interim methadone maintenance (IMM) in the United States was initially issued in 1989 by NIDA and the DEA, and eventually regulations for IMM were published in the revised 1993 regulations (58 FR 495) (IOM 1995). An allowance for IMM continues to exist in the current methadone regulations (42 CFR Part 8). IMM involves the dispensing of methadone on a temporary basis to individuals awaiting treatment placement in a comprehensive program. With IMM other services required by existing regulations in the United States are not required. IMM was to be provided by comprehensive treatment programs that must offer medical evaluation and service as well as counseling on HIV risk. Take-home doses are prohibited. The only program providing IMM services on a significant scale was Beth Israel in New York City; it was forced to close in 1993. Opposition to the Beth Israel program was largely based on evidence that interim treatment was not as effective as comprehensive treatment and on the fear that these less costly programs would set precedents, resulting in decreased funding for existing programs. Treatment in such limited service (or "low threshold") programs, though not as effective, has been associated with reduced heroin use and transition into comprehensive treatment (Yancovitz et al. 1991). IMM may therefore be a useful way to provide some degree of initial stabilization for individuals who cannot be placed in a comprehensive program within a reasonable period, facilitate treatment entry, and improve early clinical success after transfer to comprehensive treatment.

Mobile Methadone Treatment

Another novel method for engaging opioid-dependent individuals in treatment is through mobile treatment—a medical, van-based clinic on wheels. Mobile methadone treatment has been used in Baltimore, Maryland, and Springfield, Massachusetts (Brady 1993; Besteman and Brady 1994). All too often, neighborhoods in need of expanded treatment are intolerant of plans to introduce new facilities—a phenomenon referred to by NIMBY (not in my back yard). By bringing services into the addicted individual's neighborhood, treatment becomes more available to those not able or willing to travel, perhaps long distances, to the closest clinic with an available opening. Coordination of mobile treatment resources with needle-exchange programs may create a system whereby individuals are approached and referred to treatment, gradually initiated into the role of patient, stabilized in terms of their dependence and social situation, and eventually transferred to more traditional comprehensive clinics. There are even indications that mobile methadone treatment can have some advantages over fixed-location clinics. Greenfield and colleagues compared treatment retention for patients enrolled in a mobile methadone treatment program versus patients enrolled in fixed-site programs (Greenfield et al. 1996). On average, treatment retention for mobile program patients was much higher than for patients enrolled in fixed-site programs.

The Methadone Clinic as a Comprehensive Medical/Psychiatric Care Clinic

Substance abuse patients comprise a high-risk population with a host of prevalent comorbid medical and psychiatric problems. However, despite the high medical (including psychiatric) needs of this population, patients often slip through cracks in the health care delivery system. Referring patients from the methadone clinic to other sites for care often results in poor compliance rates in attending such off-site appointments. Methadone treatment programs that operate as sites for primary medical and/or psychiatric care address this problem by using a "one-stop shopping" model for health care delivery (Umbricht-Schneiter et al. 1994). Daily attendance for methadone administration can facilitate compliance with appointments and treatments. By using the methadone clinic as a site for primary care services, enhanced preventive and problem-oriented care can decrease the frequency of costly hospitalizations and emergency department visits. In turn, this can lead to a better quality of life for patients, as well as decreased total medical expenditures.

Office-Based and Medical Maintenance Models

Medical methadone maintenance refers to the provision of methadone maintenance services within the physical context of a general medical practice. (See chap. 12 for a more detailed description of office-based models of treatment for opioid dependence.) It was conceived as a modality that matches the intensity and types of services needed with medical care. Informed clinical judgment is used to determine the necessary intensity of treatment, as in other treatments for medical (including psychiatric) disorders.

Office-based physician prescribing with pharmacy pickup of methadone may be especially valuable for two populations: (1) socially rehabilitated patients, to further reduce contact with current abusers, and (2) residents in rural areas, where it is not feasible to require persons to travel long distances for clinic-based treatment. Although it is not commonly practiced, regulations in the United States do allow office-based treatment with methadone by individual physicians, when done in coordination with a methadone (OTP) clinic (Kreek and Vocci 2002). Although revised methadone regulations in the United States allow for up to one month's supply of methadone to be dispensed in the context of the typical comprehensive program, for some highly stable patients it may be most therapeutic, and least stigmatizing, for them to receive services altogether outside the context of a drug treatment program. Another alternative, office-based treatment using buprenorphine is discussed next.

Buprenorphine and Other Alternative Medications

Although not new as a treatment in Europe, buprenorphine is the latest pharmacotherapy for opioid addiction approved by the FDA, and as a partial agonist it appears to offer certain advantages when compared with methadone (see chaps. 10 and 11 for a review of buprenorphine's use in the treatment of opioid dependence). Buprenorphine's opioid agonist activity provides sufficient reinforcement to make it acceptable to patients, but its ceiling on the magnitude of these effects (including respiratory depression) translates to a reduced abuse liability relative to full opioid agonists, such as methadone, and greater safety. The inclusion of naloxone in the primary product currently marketed in the United States (i.e., Suboxone) may further reduce abuse liability by causing precipitated withdrawal if misused by the intravenous route by an individual with opiate dependence. This potential safety advantage and lower abuse liability led the FDA to approve buprenorphine and buprenorphine combined with naloxone as Schedule III narcotic medications. Since implementation of the Drug Addiction Treatment Act of 2000 (DATA 2000), physicians in office settings can dispense or prescribe Schedule III, IV, or V narcotic medications (including, but not limited to, buprenorphine) for the treatment of opioid dependence in the United States. DATA 2000, part of the Children's Health Act of 2000, permits physicians to provide such treatment so long as they meet specific criteria (table 2.8). The physician must obtain a federal waiver from the requirements of the NATA.

Research continues in the search for new medications and new formulations of existing medications, for example, long-acting depot forms of naltrexone and buprenorphine, for the treatment of opioid addiction. As these new medications or new formulations become available, the unique benefits of each will come to light, such as improved efficacy in subgroups, improved adherence to treatment, reduced burden of treatment, or increased acceptability.

Encouraging Changes in Resource Allocation

Probably the most important intervention the substance abuse treatment community could make toward improving the system of care delivery is to make drug abuse treatment more attractive and acceptable to the general public, as well as to policymakers and funding agencies. This can be

Table 2.8 **Physician Waiver Criteria as Specified by DATA 2000**

Hold a current state medical license
Hold a valid DEA registration number
Meet one or more of the following conditions:
- Subspecialty certification in addiction from at least one:
  - American Board of Medical Specialties
  - American Society of Addiction Medicine
  - American Osteopathic Association
- Completion of eight hours of approved training
- Investigator in a clinical trial leading to approval of a Schedule II, IV, or V narcotic drug for such treatment
- Other training or experience considered by the State medical licensing board to demonstrate ability to provide such treatment
- Other training or experience considered by the Secretary of HHS to demonstrate ability to provide such treatment

Has capacity to refer patients for appropriate nonpharmacologic therapies
Attest their practice will not exceed 30 patients in such treatment at any one time

accomplished through teaching, advocacy, and outreach to the community, as well as continued rigorous economic evaluations of the cost-effectiveness and net benefits of treatment (French 1995). Disseminating the message—to decision makers in government and managed care, and, especially, to the general public—that substance abuse treatment including methadone treatment is effective and ultimately results in net savings continues to be needed. Increasing the public's understanding of the disorder of addiction and the effectiveness of treatment will not only make it easier to expand treatment into neighborhoods in need but will also direct policymaking. It is unfortunate that politicians often find it difficult to campaign on a platform that includes increased funding to treat a segment of the population that the public views as marginal at best to immoral at worst. Publicizing the financial value of treatment is of critical importance; this information will affect those who allocate managed care dollars as well as policymakers who assign public resources and control treatment regulations. Dr. Mary Jeanne Kreek, one of the most renown and productive researchers providing critical evidence for the effectiveness of methadone, commented on this critical need, arguing that "the greatest needs with respect to methadone maintenance treatment now begin with the need to change general public attitudes and therefore the attitudes of policymakers with respect to this treatment modality" (Parrino 1993).

International Experience

Methadone treatment for opioid dependence is available in almost 50 countries worldwide, comprising 300,000 people in Europe and 20,000 in Australia. Several countries have used alternatives to the United States' *comprehensive methadone clinic* model (Farrell 1996). Some countries such as France have many patients in opioid substitution treatment using other pharmacotherapies, most commonly buprenorphine. Germany has used dihydrocodeine and codeine in opioid substitution treatment on a large scale in the recent past. Other factors differ substantially among countries, including the percent of the population in treatment, treatment entry criteria, and the manner in which the medication is dispensed or prescribed. In some countries patients are mostly enrolled in centralized methadone treatment in specialized programs with little involvement by general practitioners, whereas in other countries there is a less centralized structure. In some parts of the world, methadone dispensing is typically within the confines of the treatment program or a pharmacy, whereas elsewhere prescriptions for methadone are filled in community pharmacies with subsequent consumption outside the pharmacy. In The Netherlands, mobile methadone treatment dates from as early as 1978. The sheer number of permutations of varying factors, as well as the high rate of reform within any given country, illustrates the continued desire to improve and optimize methadone treatment, the innovations that can occur with this modality of care, and the difficulty in providing a concise and useful summary of the state of methadone practice throughout the world.

SUMMARY

Methadone maintenance is the most highly regulated of medical treatments. In the United States, a consensus panel on the treatment of heroin addiction sponsored by NIH in 1997 pointed out that federal regulations at that time prevented treatment from being tailored to the needs of the individual patient by requiring an inflexible system of delivery, unproductive paperwork, and excessive administrative costs (News & Notes 1998). The panel recommended that the regulations be eliminated and that some alternate means, such as accreditation, be instituted to ensure safe and effective practice. The revised methadone regulations, enacted in 2001, transferred oversight of treatment to SAMHSA/CSAT and moved to a system of accreditation. Future changes in the United States that would decrease unnecessary regulatory burden could include revisions that would permit more physicians and pharmacies to prescribe and dispense methadone for opiate addiction outside the confines of a comprehensive methadone program, at least to patients with sustained stability. The consensus panel on the treatment of heroin addiction also recommended that federal, state, and local agencies coordinate their efforts, target programs with poor performance for more scrutiny, reduce scrutiny for programs consistently performing well, and address the problem of slow state approval of medications.

Many studies have demonstrated that methadone treatment is cost-effective when a broad array of cost-saving measures is included (e.g., decreases in crime, increases in employment). However, it is not yet clear how methadone treatment will operate and be adequately reimbursed in the current environment of managed health care. This issue becomes increasingly important as state and federally supported insurance programs assume a greater managed care orientation.

Creative and more effective and cost-effective mechanisms for the delivery of methadone and similar treatments continue to be proposed and investigated. These alternative treatment approaches have sought to decrease costs, improve outcomes, or increase availability of treatment. They have included operations such as interim methadone maintenance, mobile methadone treatment, the designation of methadone clinics as primary care sites, and office-based practice. Cost-effective models such as contingency contracting can be integrated into existing programs, resulting in improved treatment efficacy and/or cost savings. In addition, the use of other pharmacotherapies, such as buprenorphine, or the use of alternative medication delivery systems, such as long-acting depot forms, will offer more options to patients that may at times prove more effective, less intrusive, or less costly.

Agencies that fund substance abuse treatment may see methadone treatment as an expensive intervention, especially because many benefits are indirect social costs, and not directly economical to the funding agency. To maintain and improve the availability of methadone treatment, the medical profession must demonstrate and publicize the justification for costs and explain the individual, systemic, and societal savings incurred through treatment. Effectively communicating the value of opioid substitution treatments—to the general public and to funding agencies—is critical if these treatments are to remain an available option for a significant number of patients with opioid dependence.

References
Batten H, Prottas J, Horgan CM, Simon LJ, Larson MJ, Elliott EA, Marsden ME (1992). Drug Services Research Survey, Final Report: Phase II Revised (Contract 271-90-8319/

1). Bethesda, MD: National Institute on Drug Abuse, National Institutes of Health, U.S. Department of Health and Human Services.

Besteman KJ, Brady JV (1994). Implementing mobile drug abuse treatment: problems, procedures, and perspectives. In: Fletcher BW, Inciardi JA, Horton AM, eds. *Drug Abuse Treatment: The Implementation of Innovative Approaches*. Westport, CT: Greenwood Press, 33–42.

Bradley CJ, French MT, Rachal JV (1994). Financing and cost of standard and enhanced methadone treatment. *J Subst Abuse Treat* 11: 433–42.

Brady JV (1993). Enhancing Drug Abuse Treatment by Mobile Health Services. In: Inciardi JA, Tims FM, Fletcher BW, eds. *Innovative Approaches in the Treatment of Drug Abuse: Program Models and Strategies*. Westport, CT: Greenwood Press, 35–42.

Brooner RK, Kidorf M, King VL, Stoller K (1998). Preliminary evidence of good treatment response in antisocial drug abusers. *Drug Alcohol Depend* 49: 249–60.

Brooner RK, Kidorf MS, King VL, Bigelow GE (1997). Using behaviorally contingent pharmacotherapy in opioid abusers enhances treatment outcome. In: Harris LS, ed. Problems of Drug Dependence, 1996: Proceedings of the 58th Annual Scientific Meeting of the College on Problems of Drug Dependence, Inc. Washington, DC: U.S. Government Printing Office.

Department of Veterans Affairs (1993). Annual Cost Distribution for FY 1993. Washington, DC: U.S. Government Printing Office.

Farrell M (1996). A review of the Legislation, Regulation and Delivery of Methadone in 12 Member States of the European Union: Final Report. Luxembourg: Office for Official Publications of the European Communities.

French MT (1995). Economic evaluation of drug abuse treatment programs: methodology and findings. *Am J Drug Alcohol Abuse* 21: 111–35.

French MT, Mauskopf JA, Teague JL, Roland EJ (1996). Estimating the dollar value of health outcomes from drug-abuse interventions. *Med Care* 34: 890–910.

Gerstein D, Harwood H (1990). *Treating Drug Problems*. Washington, DC: National Academy Press.

Gerstein DR, Johnson RA, Harwood HJ, Fountain D, Suter N, Mallow K (1994). Evaluating Recovery Services: The California Drug and Alcohol Treatment Assessment (CALDATA). General Report. Sacramento, CA: California Department of Alcohol and Drug Programs.

Greenfield L, Brady JV, Besteman KJ, De Smet A (1996). Patient retention in mobile and fixed-site methadone maintenance treatment. *Drug Alcohol Depend* 42: 125–31.

Institute of Medicine (1995). *Federal Regulation of Methadone Treatment*. Washington, DC: The National Academy Press.

Kidorf M, Stitzer ML, Brooner RK, Goldberg J (1994). Contingent methadone take-home doses reinforce adjunct therapy attendance of methadone maintenance patients. *Drug Alcohol Depend* 36: 221–26.

Kraft MK, Rothbard AB, Hadley TR, McLellan AT, Asch DA (1997). Are supplementary services provided during methadone maintenance really cost-effective? *Am J Psychiatry* 154: 1214–19.

Kreek MJ, Vocci FJ (2002). History and current status of opioid maintenance treatments: blending conference session. *J Subst Abuse Treat* 23: 93–105.

Mark TL, Woody GE, Juday T, Kleber HD (2001). The economic costs of heroin addiction in the United States. *Drug Alcohol Depend* 61: 195–206.

McCarty D (1997). Narcotic Agonist Treatment as a Benefit Under Managed Care. NIH

Consensus Development Conference on Effective Medical Treatment of Heroin Addiction. Bethesda, MD: National Institutes of Health.

Merrill JC (1997). Impact of Methadone Maintenance on HIV Seroconversion and Related Costs. NIH Consensus Development Conference on Effective Medical Treatment of Heroin Addiction. Bethesda, MD: National Institutes of Health.

Merrill JO (2002). Policy progress for physician treatment of opiate addiction. *J Gen Intern Med* 17: 361–68.

News & Notes (1998). Consensus panel recommends less regulation of methadone, expanded access for heroin addicts. *Psychiatr Serv* 49: 120–21.

Parrino MW (1993). State methadone treatment guidelines. Rockville, MD: Substance Abuse and Mental Health Services Administration.

Peterson K, Swindle R, Paradise M, Moos RH (1993). Substance Abuse Treatment Programming in the Department of Veterans Affairs: Staffing, Patients, Services, and Policies. Palo Alto, CA: Department of Veterans Affairs, Program Evaluation Center.

Puigdollers E, Cots F, Brugal MT, Torralba L, Domingo-Salvany A, Costas F (2003). [Methadone maintenance programs with supplementary services: a cost-effectiveness study]. *Gac Sanit* 17: 123–30.

Sambamoorthi U, Warner LA, Crystal S, Walkup J (2000). Drug abuse, methadone treatment, and health services use among injection drug users with AIDS. *Drug Alcohol Depend* 60: 77–89.

SAMHSA (1993). National Drug and Alcoholism Treatment Unit Survey (NDATUS): 1991 Main Findings Report. DHHS Pub. No. (SMA) 93-2007. Rockville, MD: Substance Abuse and Mental Health Services Administration.

SAMHSA (2000). National Expenditures for Mental Health and Substance Abuse Treatment, 1997. Rockville, MD: Substance Abuse and Mental Health Services Administration.

Silverman K, Higgins ST, Brooner RK, Montoya ID, Cone EJ, Schuster CR, Preston KL (1996). Sustained cocaine abstinence in methadone maintenance patients through voucher-based reinforcement therapy. *Arch Gen Psychiatry* 53: 409–15.

Strain EC, Stitzer ML, Liebson IA, Bigelow GE (1993). Methadone dose and treatment outcome. *Drug Alcohol Depend* 33: 105–17.

Strathdee SA, Galai N, Safaiean M, Celentano DD, Vlahov D, Johnson L, Nelson KE (2001). Sex differences in risk factors for HIV seroconversion among injection drug users: a 10-year perspective. *Arch Intern Med* 161: 1281–88.

Uchtenhagen A (1996). Swiss Methadone Report: Narcotic Substitution in the Treatment of Heroin Addicts in Switzerland. Zurich: Swiss Federal Office of Public Health.

Umbricht-Schneiter A, Ginn DH, Pabst KM, Bigelow GE (1994). Providing medical care to methadone clinic patients: referral vs on-site care. *Am J Public Health* 84: 207–10.

Yancovitz SR, Des Jarlais DC, Peyser NP, Drew E, Friedmann P, Trigg HL, Robinson JW (1991). A randomized trial of an interim methadone maintenance clinic. *Am J Public Health* 81: 1185–91.

Zaric GS, Barnett PG, Brandeau ML (2000). HIV transmission and the cost-effectiveness of methadone maintenance. *Am J Public Health* 90: 1100–1111.

3

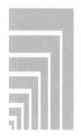

Epidemiology of Opioid Use, Abuse, and Dependence

Rosa M. Crum, M.D., M.H.S.

The class of substances described as opioids includes natural and synthetic opioid drugs such as those that are available by prescription (e.g., morphine, methadone, codeine, oxycodone, and fentanyl), as well as illicit substances such as the semisynthetic opioid, heroin [APA 2000]). This chapter reviews the epidemiology of nonmedical use, abuse, and dependence of prescription opioids first, followed by a discussion of the epidemiology of heroin use and related disorders. The focus is on the epidemiology of opioid use in the United States, because the U.S. national surveys provide several converging lines of evidence that are informative about opioid use disorders in a large, diverse population with a long history of opioid abuse. The availability of similar epidemiologic assessments from other countries is limited (e.g., national surveys from Australia) (Mills et al. 2004), and this chapter focuses on data from the United States because the United States provides the most comprehensive story of opioid use over a sustained period using relatively similar methodological approaches over time.

SOME EPIDEMIOLOGIC TERMS

Epidemiology can be described as the study of the determinants and distribution of health-related conditions in specific populations (Last 2001). Some basic terms used in epidemiology deserve attention here, because they are important to understanding some of the study data that are reported in this chapter. *Prevalence* generally is taken to represent the ratio of the total number of cases of a particular health-related condition (e.g., opioid dependence), divided by the total number of individuals in a particular population at a specific time. *Incidence* refers to the rate of occurrence of new cases of a health-related condition, divided by the total number at risk for this condition during a specified period (Mausner and Kramer 1985). Prevalence is influenced by both the incidence and duration of a disease, because it depends not only on the proportion of newly developed cases over time, but also on the length of time the disease exists in the population. In turn, the duration of the health-related condition is affected by the degree of remission and survival from the disease. Incidence represents the risk of disease, whereas prevalence is an indicator of the public health burden in the community (Mausner and Kramer 1985).

Prevalence and Incidence of Nonmedical Use, Abuse, and Dependence of Prescription Opioids

Much of the information regarding symptoms and manifestations of opioid disorders comes from studies of individuals in medical and drug treatment settings. However, many individuals who use and abuse opioid substances may not receive treatment. As a consequence, estimates of prevalence and incidence ascertained from population-based samples may reduce the potential for selection biases, which are typically present in clinic-based studies. Yet, household surveys are not able to gather information from homeless individuals or from those who may be incarcerated, populations that may have higher rates of opioid use. In addition, surveys of specialized populations, such as those conducted in schools, may also selectively miss some students including those with heroin dependence, because of their lower rates of school attendance and increased risk for school dropout. In some instances, and within specific populations or locations, other approaches to ascertaining the prevalence of hidden populations, such as those with heroin dependence, may be used effectively, such as enumeration or census methods (e.g., see Rees Davis et al. 2003). However, these methods are often restricted to local areas, such as within a specific urban neighborhood (e.g., Harlem in New York City) (Rees Davis et al. 2003). When evaluating prevalence and incidence estimates for opioid use and disorders, the limitations in data collection and sample selection should be considered. With this in mind, the following sections provide recent data available from several national surveys that indicate important trends in opioid use for the United States.

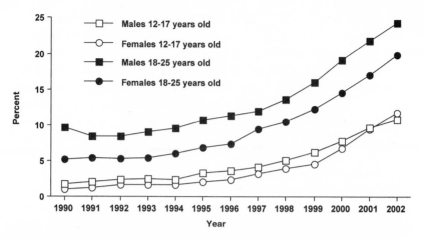

Figure 3.1. Annual prevalence of nonmedical use of prescription opioids, by age group and gender, 1990–2002. Annual prevalence estimates are the percentages of weighted sums of lifetime opioid use reported for each age group in a specific year divided by the weighted sum of all individuals within the specific age category for each year indicated. The lifetime prevalence estimates were calculated by using data gathered from the NSDUH conducted in 2002, which includes questions about prior use. The analysis of trends is based on the retrospective reports of age of first nonmedical use of prescription opioids. Data from SAMHSA 2003b.

Data from several recent surveys provide evidence that the nonmedical use of opioids available by prescription is increasing in the United States (Zacny et al. 2003). The National Survey on Drug Use and Health (NSDUH), which was formerly known as the National Household Survey on Drug Abuse (NHSDA), has been conducted by the Substance Abuse and Mental Health Services Administration (SAMHSA) since 1971. The survey is now conducted annually on more than 67,000 non-institutionalized residents of the United States, 12 years of age and older, regarding their use of alcohol, tobacco, and illicit drugs (SAMHSA 2003b). Information from the 2002 NSDUH survey indicates a trend for increasing nonmedical use of prescription opioids among youth, 12–17 years of age, and young adults, 18–25 years of age (fig. 3.1). For example, prevalence of lifetime use among individuals 12–17 years of age was 1.2 percent in 1989. Lifetime prevalence increased steadily to 9.6 percent in 2001 and most recently was estimated at 11.2 percent in 2002. Similarly, among young adults, the lifetime prevalence for the nonmedical use of prescription opioids was reported to be 6.8 percent in 1992 and most recently rose to 19.4 percent in 2001 and 22.1 percent in 2002.

As shown in figure 3.1, lifetime prevalence is generally higher among males in both age categories, although the gender difference is attenuated in the younger age group, 12–17 years of age. Because these trend analyses are based on the retrospective reports of age of first nonmedical prescription opioid use, in addition to other information provided in the 2002 survey, potential biases may be introduced by this approach, which include differential survival for those who did and did not use opioids, recall bias, and underreporting (SAMHSA 2003b). The survey data provide important information, however, that can indicate estimates for trends, which may provide information as to the public health burden of nonmedical use of prescription opioids and the health care needs that are likely to arise from the related disorders.

Some of the increase in prevalence for nonmedical use of prescription opioids may be due to the rise in the rate of new users (SAMHSA 2003b). Examination of age-specific incidence rates provided by the 2002 NSDUH indicate increases in incidence, or the onset of new use among youth, aged 12–17 years, and among young adults, aged 18–25 years (fig. 3.2). For example, the incidence or rate of the onset of new nonmedical prescription opioid users among youth aged 12–17 years was 4.5 per 1,000 person-years of exposure in 1990. In 2000, this rate had increased to 42.5 per 1,000 person-years and to 47.9 per 1,000 person-years in 2001. In 1990, the incidence of new nonmedical prescription opioid use among young adults, aged 18–25 years, was 10.9 per 1,000 person-years. The

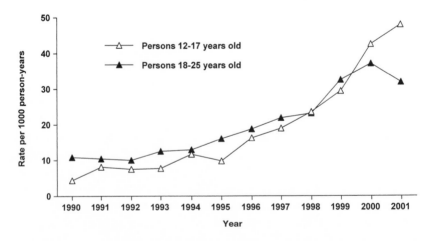

Figure 3.2.   Age-specific incidence rates per 1,000 person-years for nonmedical use of prescription opioids, 1990–2001. Rates were calculated by dividing the number of individuals with first use of nonmedical prescription opioids reported during the year indicated for each age group by the total number of person-years (in thousands) within each specific age group. Data from SAMHSA 2003a, 2003b.

rate in 2000 was 37.2 per 1,000 person-years, and 32.0 per 1,000 person-years in 2001. Again, caution should be taken in the interpretation of these results because of the potential biases discussed above, including that trends are based on the retrospective report of prior use and possible underreporting (SAMHSA 2003b). This survey, however, provides one of the principal sources of population-based data available to assess prevalence estimates and possible trends in nonmedical use of prescription opioids among adolescents and young adults in the United States.

In addition to information on the reported use of opioids, data from the NSDUH have also been used to provide estimates for the prevalence of substance use disorders, such as the nonmedical abuse of and dependence on prescription opioids. The 2002 survey provides data on the prevalence of abuse and/or dependence based on criteria from the Diagnostic and Statistical Manual of Mental Disorders, fourth edition, text revision (DSM-IV-TR) (APA 2000), for individuals using "pain relievers" (nonmedical use of prescription opioids) and other substances. Although the substance use disorder diagnoses are made based on data gathered from interviews administered by trained lay interviewers, not by clinicians treating patients, the questions utilized in the survey provide information on each of the DSM-IV-TR criteria that would normally be used by health care providers to define DSM-IV-TR substance abuse and dependence. For example, the survey items for opioid dependence included questions to assess attempts to cut down on use, tolerance, withdrawal, and other symptoms associated with opioid use (SAMHSA 2003b). The questions on abuse included those concerning problems associated with use of opioids (such as problems at work, home, and school or with family or friends) and trouble with the law due to the use of opioids. As required by DSM-IV-TR, an individual was only defined as having opioid abuse if he or she had not also met criteria for opioid dependence (SAMHSA 2003b). Results from the 2002 NSDUH indicate that the overall prior-year prevalence of dependence on prescription opioids used for nonmedical reasons was estimated to be 0.4 percent (SAMHSA 2003b). As shown in figure 3.3, however, among past-year users (individuals who reported nonmedical use of prescription opioids in the prior year), 13.7 percent met criteria for opioid abuse or dependence.

The Monitoring the Future study (MTF), initiated in 1975, is another important source of information on the assessment of prevalence and trends of substance use in the United States. It is conducted by the University of Michigan's Institute for Social Research and supported by the National Institute on Drug Abuse (Johnston et al. 2004). For example,

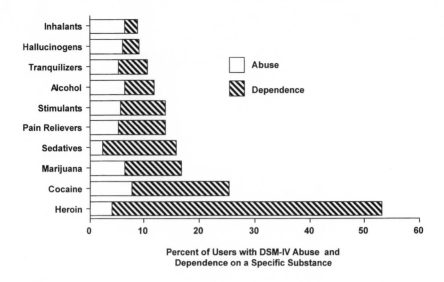

Figure 3.3. Percentage of persons fulfilling criteria for substance abuse and dependence based on DSM-IV criteria, among users of each substance in the prior year. Data from SAMHSA 2003b.

each year annual surveys of nationally representative samples of secondary students in both private and public schools are completed throughout the coterminous United States. Data on twelfth graders has been gathered since 1975, and since 1991, the surveys also have included interviews with eighth and tenth graders. In 2003, approximately 48,500 students in 392 schools were interviewed. Data gathered in the 2003 MTF also provide evidence indicating a trend toward increasing nonmedical use of prescription opioids. As illustrated in figure 3.4, lifetime prevalence of use has increased fairly steadily among twelfth graders during the past decade. Changes in the questionnaire were made in 2002, which likely explains the fluctuation in prevalence estimates observed between 2001 and 2002. In the 2002 survey, the questions on nonmedical prescription opioid use were updated in half of the questionnaires to include Vicodin, OxyContin, and Percocet as examples of opioids (talwin, laudanum, and paregoric were removed because of negligible use by 2001). In the following year, all questionnaires were updated.

Data from the MTF also indicate that specific opioids show strong increases in annual prevalence across all grades interviewed (Johnston et al. 2004). For example, in 2002, 1.3 percent of eighth graders reported using Oxycontin in the prior year. In 2003, the annual prevalence of use

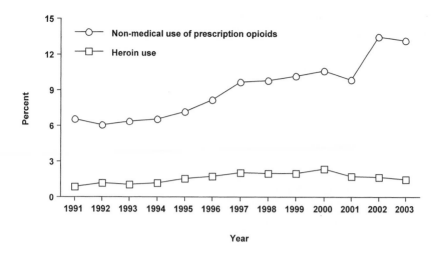

Figure 3.4. Lifetime prevalence of nonmedical use of prescription opioids and heroin use among twelfth graders, 1991–2003. Data from Johnston et al. 2004.

among eighth graders had risen to 1.7 percent. Among tenth graders, the annual prevalence of Oxycontin use was 3.0 percent in 2002 and 3.6 percent in 2003. Similar increases were noted among twelfth graders: prevalence of prior-year use was 4.0 percent in 2002 and 4.5 percent in 2003 (Johnston et al. 2004). Annual prevalence estimates have been even higher for Vicodin: among eighth graders, prior-year use was 2.5 percent in 2002 and 2.8 percent in 2003. For tenth graders, annual prevalence of Vicodin use was 6.9 percent in 2002 and 7.2 percent in 2003. Among twelfth graders, prior-year use was 9.6 percent in 2002. The annual prevalence of Vicodin use among twelfth graders had risen to 10.5 percent in 2003. Although the one-year increases in annual prevalence for each of these specific substances by school grade did not meet criteria for statistical significance, the overall absolute levels of reported use are high, and the indication of an upward trend in use is troubling. Although the MTF and the NSDUH sample different populations, and absolute values of prevalence estimates differ between the two, data from both surveys indicate consistent increases in nonmedical use of prescription opioids among young people in the United States.

Data on the nonmedical use of prescription opioids recorded in drug-related visits to hospital emergency departments in the coterminous United States is provided by the Drug Abuse Warning Network (DAWN) (SAMHSA 2003a). In a nationally representative sample, semiannual as well as annual estimates of the numbers of drug-related visits are gathered and provided under the sponsorship of the Substance Abuse and Mental Health Services Administration. A sample of the nation's nonfederal, short-stay general surgical and medical hospitals with a 24-hour emergency department are included. In the most recent report from DAWN regarding emergency department trends (SAMHSA 2003a), nonmedical use of prescription opioids was mentioned more often than any other central nervous system agent (not including anxiolytics, antidepressants, antipsychotics) in drug-related visits to emergency departments in 2002. This amounted to 10 percent of all emergency department "mentions" (all the drugs recorded during a drug-related visit to a hospital emergency department). Between 1995 and 2002, there has been a 163 percent increase in the number of hospital emergency department visits that recorded the nonmedical use of prescription opioids. From 2000 to 2002 alone, there was a 45 percent increase in emergency department visits recording nonmedical use of prescription opioids (SAMHSA 2003a). Of the specific opioids cited, oxycodone and hydroxycodone (e.g., Oxycontin, Vicodin, Percocet) were the most frequently recorded opioids, amounting to 40 percent of the narcotic analgesics recorded in drug-related visits to emergency departments in 2002 (SAMHSA 2004a).

The Treatment Episode Data Set (TEDS) provides another data set on substance use in the United States. TEDS reports on characteristics of annual admissions to treatment facilities for alcohol and drug use disorders (SAMHSA 2004b). TEDS does not include data on all substance use treatment facilities and, in general, only provides information on state-funded facilities. However, useful information is provided, in particular, on trends of admissions for individuals meeting criteria for opioid abuse and dependence. In assessing trends between 1992 and 2002, the most recent evidence from TEDS indicates a steady increase in treatment facility admissions for abuse and dependence of prescription opioids. In 1992, for 0.9 percent of admissions, the primary substance of abuse was reported as prescription opioids (including the nonmedical use of methadone). This estimate steadily rose to 2.4 percent in 2002 (SAMHSA 2004b).

PREVALENCE AND INCIDENCE OF HEROIN USE, ABUSE, AND DEPENDENCE

Some of the difficulties associated with obtaining accurate information on opiate use are mentioned above. These issues are even more of a concern with heroin use, however, because the prevalence estimates for heroin use, abuse, and dependence are lower, making some estimates unreliable, in particular, in smaller subgroups. Furthermore, the additional stigma and criminalized behavior associated with heroin use make underreporting a problem that should be kept in mind when interpreting study data.

Use of consistent sampling methodology, as is typically done in population-based annual surveys, may yet provide important information on trends of heroin use and disorders (as discussed by Hartnoll 1994). To capture samples generally missed by population-based surveys, other methods have been employed, such as studies targeting populations that are likely to have a relatively large proportion of users (e.g., prisoners, visitors to needle-exchange programs). Individuals in hidden populations are generally best recruited from settings that are natural to them, with diminished risk of being exposed (Hartnoll 1994). Snowball sampling has been used to recruit individuals from these types of social peer networks and is useful among hidden populations such as the homeless and undocumented individuals (Fry and Dwyer 2001; Humeniuk et al. 2003; Rees Davis et al. 2003). Sampling in this manner recruits individuals who are asked to name other individuals known to them, who are then included in the sample. These individuals also are asked to name acquaintances, and the sample size increases in this manner until adequate power is achieved (Last 2001). Capture-recapture methods also have been used successfully to estimate population sizes of heroin users (e.g., see Doscher and Woodward 1983 and Mastro et al. 1994). Originally employed in wildlife biology where animals were captured, tagged, and recaptured to estimate population size, capture-recapture techniques use at least two sources of population estimates and identify individuals from the population appearing in more than one of the nonrandom samples (Larson et al. 1994; Last 2001). Depending on the number of population sources available, different statistical methods can be used to avoid dependence between the sources and obtain prevalence estimates (e.g., see Brugal et al. 1999; Domingo-Salvany et al. 1995). However, these sampling methods are nonrandom and may introduce biased samples and unreliable estimates (Hook and Regal 2000; Larson and Bammer 1996). For example, some of these methods may be more likely to target individuals with heroin dependence and miss those with occasional use (Hartnoll 1994). Prior research indicates that hidden populations of heroin users are different with respect to the prevalence of heroin-related problems and in their expressed concern about their drug use behavior than those who have had contact with social service or other agencies (Robson and Bruce 1997). In this chapter, prevalence estimates are provided from U.S. population-based survey data, and the strengths and the limitations in the use of these data should be kept in mind when reviewing the findings.

Compared with estimates from reports of nonmedical use of prescription opioids, reports of heroin use are much less frequent. Prevalence estimates for lifetime use based on the 2002 NSDUH indicate that use typically increases with age, with reports of sniffing and/or snorting heroin generally being the most common route of administration (SAMHSA 2003b) (fig. 3.5). Reports of lifetime use based on the data reported in the 2002 NSDUH also have increased slightly (SAMHSA 2003b). For example, lifetime use was reported to be 0.1 percent among youth, aged 12 to 17 years, in 1990, but in 2002 it had increased to 0.4 percent. Similarly, in 1990, 0.8 percent of the young adults, aged 18 to 25 years, reported having used heroin at some time in their lifetime; whereas lifetime prevalence had doubled to 1.6 percent in 2002 (SAMHSA 2003b). As was discussed with nonmedical use of prescription opioids, this slight rise in lifetime prevalence may be related to the increase in rate of individuals who initiate heroin use. Age-specific rates of heroin use among both youth and young adults have also tended to increase since the mid-1990s, as assessed by reports from the most recent data available from the NSDUH. Rates of new heroin use in 2001 among 12 to 17 year olds was reported to be 1.6 per 1,000 person-years of exposure and 2.1 per 1,000 person-years of exposure among young adults between 18 and 25 years of age. In the population surveyed, past-year heroin dependence was reported to be 0.1 percent based on DSM-IV criteria utilized in the 2002 NSDUH (SAMHSA 2003b). Yet, among past-year heroin users (individuals who reported us-

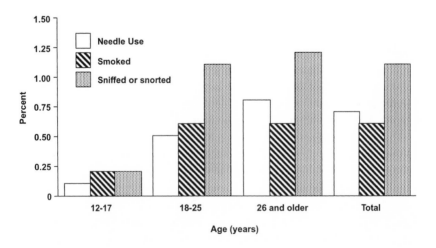

Figure 3.5. Lifetime prevalence of heroin use, by route of administration and age. Data from SAMHSA 2003b.

ing heroin in the past year), half met criteria for abuse or dependence (fig. 3.3).

Data from the MTF study also provide information on heroin use. Heroin has been one of the least-reported drugs of use, with lifetime prevalence estimates appreciably lower than those reported for nonmedical use of prescription opioids (fig. 3.4) (Johnston et al. 2004). In addition, although nonmedical use of prescription opioids is increasing, data from the MTF study sample indicate that heroin use has remained relatively stable during the past decade. This may be related to its perceived harmfulness as reported by the surveyed students. For example, in each survey conducted since 1990, when asked "How much do you think people risk harming themselves (physically or in other ways), if they use heroin once or twice?" more than 50 percent of twelfth graders indicated that they felt this was a "great risk." In 2003, 58 percent of twelfth graders felt that using heroin even once or twice was a "great risk." A total of 78.5 percent and 89.3 percent indicated that "great risk" was associated with occasional and regular heroin use, respectively. The results were similar when asked specifically about using heroin "once or twice without using a needle" and "occasionally without using a needle": 58.9 percent and 73.0 percent of twelfth graders, respectively, indicated they felt this was a "great risk." These reports of perceived harmfulness also have changed little during the past decade (Johnston et al. 2004). Rates of heroin use from the MTF differ somewhat from data provided by the NSDUH and may reflect differences in the populations sampled, as discussed previously. In addition, as mentioned above, because of the relatively low prevalence of reported heroin use in the populations surveyed, estimates will tend to be somewhat less reliable than estimates from substance use with larger reported numbers.

In the most recent report of emergency department trends based on data from DAWN, heroin "mentions" (i.e., heroin was recorded during an emergency department visit that was related to the use of an illegal substance or the nonmedical use of a legal drug) increased by 34.5 percent between 1995 and 2002 (SAMHSA 2003a). However, no statistically significant change in mentions of heroin occurred between 2001 and 2002 for the most recent DAWN surveys.

Examination of admissions to treatment facilities for substance use disorders using TEDS data from 1992 to 2002 indicate increasing trends in heroin admissions during the past decade (SAMHSA 2004b). Abuse and/or dependence of heroin accounted for 11.0 percent of treatment admissions in 1992. In 2002, 15.0 percent of admissions records indicated heroin as the primary substance of abuse.

Summary

Epidemiologic data on the patterns and trends of opioid use, abuse, and dependence can come from several sources, each providing information that can be useful to determining prevalence estimates within populations. Specific surveys have unique properties as well as potential limitations and biases. However, these types of epidemiologic data provide important information on the trends in the use of opioids and the potential public health impact of opioid disorders, as well as making available needed data for determining health policy and assessing treatment needs. Epidemiologic data can also provide valuable information on the correlates and potential predictors of opioid abuse and dependence among users. These data can help assess potential etiologic characteristics, which ultimately may enable us to better predict and prevent the occurrence of opioid use disorders.

References

APA (2000) Diagnostic and Statistical Manual of Mental Disorders, 4th ed. Text Revision. Washington, DC: American Psychiatric Association.

Brugal MT, Domingo-Salvany A, Maguire A, Cayla JA, Villalbi JR, Hartnoll R (1999). A small area analysis estimating the prevalence of addiction to opioids in Barcelona, 1993. *J Epidemiol Community Health* 53: 488–94.

Domingo-Salvany A, Hartnoll RL, Maguire A, Suelves JM, Anto JM (1995). Use of capture-recapture to estimate the prevalence of opiate addiction in Barcelona, Spain, 1989. *Am J Epidemiol* 141: 567–74.

Doscher ML, Woodward JA (1983). Estimating the size of subpopulations of heroin users: applications of log-linear models to capture/recapture sampling. *Int J Addict* 18: 167–82.

Fry C, Dwyer R (2001). For love or money? An exploratory study of why injecting drug users participate in research. *Addiction* 96: 1319–25.

Hartnoll RL (1994). Opiates: prevalence and demographic factors. *Addiction* 89: 1377–83.

Hook EB, Regal RR (2000). Accuracy of alternative approaches to capture-recapture estimates of disease frequency: internal validity analysis of data from five sources. *Am J Epidemiol* 152: 771–9.

Humeniuk R, Ali R, McGregor C, Darke S (2003). Prevalence and correlates of intravenous methadone syrup administration in Adelaide, Australia. *Addiction* 98: 413–8.

Johnston LD, O'Malley PM, Bachman JG, Schulenberg JE (2004). Monitoring the Future National Results on Adolescent Drug Use: Overview of Key Findings, 2003. Bethesda, MD: National Institute on Drug Abuse.

Larson A, Bammer G (1996). Why? Who? How? Estimating numbers of illicit drug users: lessons from a case study from the Australian Capital Territory. *Aust N Z J Public Health* 20: 493–9.

Larson A, Stevens A, Wardlaw G (1994). Indirect estimates of 'hidden' populations: capture-recapture methods to estimate the numbers of heroin users in the Australian Capital Territory. *Soc Sci Med* 39: 823–31.

Last JM (2001). *A dictionary of epidemiology.* A handbook sponsored by the International Epidemiological Association. New York: Oxford University Press.

Mastro TD, Kitayaporn D, Weniger BG, Vanichseni S, Laosunthorn V, Uneklabh T, Uneklabh C, Choopanya K, Limpakarnjanarat K (1994). Estimating the number of HIV-infected injection drug users in Bangkok: a capture—recapture method. *Am J Public Health* 84: 1094–9.

Mausner JS, Kramer S (1985). *Mausner and Bahn Epidemiology: An Introductory Text.* Philadelphia, PA: W.B. Saunders Company.

Mills KL, Teesson M, Darke S, Ross J, Lynskey M (2004). Young people with heroin dependence: findings from the Australian Treatment Outcome Study (ATOS). *J Subst Abuse Treat* 27: 67–73.

Rees Davis W, Johnson BD, Randolph D, Liberty HJ (2003). An enumeration method of determining the prevalence of users and operatives of cocaine and heroin in Central Harlem. *Drug Alcohol Depend* 72: 45–58.

Robson P, Bruce M (1997). A comparison of 'visible' and 'invisible' users of amphetamine, cocaine and heroin: two distinct populations? *Addiction* 92: 1729–36.

SAMHSA (2003a). Emergency Department Trends from the Drug Abuse Warning Network, Final Estimates 1995–2002. DHHS Pub. No. (SMA) 03-3780. Rockville, MD: Substance Abuse and Mental Health Services Administration, Office of Applied Studies.

SAMHSA (2003b). Results from the 2002 National Survey on Drug Use and Health: National Findings. DHHS Pub. No. (SMA) 03-3836. Rockville, MD: Substance Abuse and Mental Health Services Administration, Office of Applied Studies.

SAMHSA (2004a). The DAWN Report: Oxycodone, Hydrocodone, and Polydrug Use, 2002. Rockville, MD: Substance Abuse and Mental Health Services Administration, Office of Applied Studies.

SAMHSA (2004b). Treatment Episode Data Set (TEDS). Highlights—2002. DHHS Pub. No. (SMA) 04-3946. Rockville, MD: Substance Abuse and Mental Health Services Administration, Office of Applied Studies.

Zacny J, Bigelow G, Compton P, Foley K, Iguchi M, Sannerud C (2003). College on Problems of Drug Dependence taskforce on prescription opioid non-medical use and abuse: position statement. *Drug Alcohol Depend* 69: 215–32.

II

METHADONE TREATMENT
FOR OPIOID DEPENDENCE

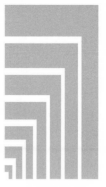

4

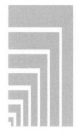

Pharmacology of Methadone

Sharon L. Walsh, Ph.D., and Eric C. Strain, M.D.

Methadone has been available for use as an analgesic for more than 60 years and as a treatment for opioid dependence for 40 years, and its pharmacologic effects have been well characterized in animals and humans. Methadone exerts its actions as an analgesic and euphoriant primarily through binding with mu opioid receptors found in the brain and the periphery. This chapter will review the pharmacologic properties of methadone and its direct effects in humans as they relate to its therapeutic actions. A brief overview of opioid receptors and basic principles of drug action are first provided as a framework for reviewing the actions of methadone.

OVERVIEW OF OPIOID RECEPTORS AND OPIOID PHARMACOLOGY

To understand the pharmacologic actions of opioid drugs, in general, and methadone, in particular, one must first become familiar with some basic principles of drug action at receptors and with the characteristics of opioid receptors. First, receptors are specially configured proteins that can produce a specific physiologic effect when activated. Opioid receptors are found on the exterior surface of cells in the brain and in the periphery. There are actually several subtypes of opioid receptors that differ in their structure, including the mu, kappa, and delta receptors. For each opioid receptor subtype, there are distinct endogenous or naturally occurring neurotransmitter substances or chemicals that interact with each receptor (e.g., beta endorphin for the mu receptor), and these subtypes exhibit differential sensitivity to exogenous opioid drugs. Central administration of these endogenous substances can produce physiologic effects similar to those produced by administration of an exogenous opioid drug, which stimulates the same receptors. Second, an opioid drug can either produce physiologic effects or block the physiologic effects mediated by a receptor, depending on whether the drug is classified as an agonist or antagonist, respectively. Each of these points will be reviewed here briefly, and the reader interested in this topic can learn more about the extensive research on opioid pharmacology and opioid receptors by reading further in one of the several excellent textbooks available on pharmacology and psychopharmacology (see Recommended Readings).

Agonists and Antagonists

Drugs that occupy a receptor and activate that receptor are called *agonists*. In general, as the dose of an agonist drug increases, the effect being measured increases until a maximal effect is achieved. Drugs that occupy a receptor and activate the receptor are said to have *intrinsic activity* at that receptor, although the degree of intrinsic activity can vary across drugs. Some agonist drugs are *partial agonists*—they occupy a receptor and activate it, but even at high doses they do not produce an effect as great as a full agonist drug, and hence the term *partial agonist,* indicating a *partial* effect (see fig. 10.1). These partial agonist drugs are said to have less intrinsic activity than a full agonist drug. Though not a focus in this chapter, the features of partial agonists are considered in chapter 10, as buprenorphine is an opioid that has partial agonist features.

A second type of drug that can occupy a receptor is an *antagonist*. These are drugs that occupy a receptor but produce no activation of that receptor—they have no intrinsic activity. Therefore, in an opioid-naive individual, an antagonist will produce no effects because it has no intrinsic activity. However, these medications can block the effects of other drugs by binding to the receptor and preventing a subsequently ingested opioid drug from binding at the same site. Moreover, administration of antagonist can result in removing a drug from the receptor in an individual who may be using opioids illicitly or therapeutically. Therefore, administration of a sufficient dose of an antagonist may reverse the effects of the agonist and/or produce withdrawal symptoms in a person who is physically dependent on an opioid agonist such as heroin.

Though not the focus of this discussion, a final feature of drug action worth mentioning is receptor affinity. Affinity is a measure of how good a fit exists between the drug and the receptor when they are bound together. Thus, even though a drug might have a low intrinsic activity (i.e., it is a partial agonist), it could have a high affinity for the receptor, making it difficult to uncouple or separate the drug from the receptor to reverse its effects. An example of this type of drug, a partial mu agonist with high affinity for the receptor, is buprenorphine, which is marketed for the treatment of opioid dependence (see chaps. 10 and 11 for further details about buprenorphine).

Multiple Opioid Receptors

The classification of a particular receptor as an opioid receptor is based on the observation that naloxone, a pure opioid antagonist, will reverse the effects of a compound acting at that receptor. Three distinct types of opioid receptors have been identified: mu, kappa, and delta receptors. It was once thought that there was another opioid receptor, called the sigma receptor, but it is now accepted that the sigma receptor is not an opioid receptor (Guitart et al. 2004). There are further subtypes for each of the three major opioid receptors, such as mu_1 and mu_2 receptors and $kappa_1$ and $kappa_3$ receptors. A review of these receptor subtypes is not necessary for understanding the pharmacologic effects of methadone, however.

The prototypic or classic mu opioid agonist is morphine (mu for morphine), although many other compounds function as agonists at the mu receptor (including methadone, heroin, opium, oxycodone, hydrocodone, and codeine, for example). Although many of these drugs primarily activate mu receptors, at sufficiently high doses they may also interact with other opioid receptors. Activation of mu receptors results in a wide variety of direct effects in humans as shown in table 4.1. The effects of primary interest that are produced by activation of mu receptors are analgesia and euphoria. In contrast, mu opioid antagonists can block or reverse the effects of morphine and other mu agonists. Naloxone (Narcan), nalmefene (Revex), and naltrexone (ReVia) are marketed and widely known for their antagonist properties; naloxone and nalmefene are commonly used to reverse narcotic overdose, whereas the much longer-acting agent naltrexone is marketed for use as an opioid-blocking treatment for heroin abuse and also for the treatment of alcoholism.

The prototypic or classic *kappa* opioid agonist is ketocyclazocine (kappa for ketocyclazocine). This drug was given to humans in past studies but was never used clinically and is no longer available for investigations. Pure kappa agonists can produce dysphoria and perceptual distortions in humans, and these problematic side effects led to a loss of interest

Table 4.1   **Effects Produced by Mu and Kappa Opioid Agonists**

Mu	
Analgesia	Miosis (pupillary constriction)
Drowsiness	Mental clouding or confusion
Constipation	Euphoria
Nausea and vomiting	Respiratory depression
Itching	

Kappa	
Analgesia (mediated primarily via the spinal cord)	Psychotomimesis
	Diuresis
Dysphoria	Sweating

Note: Effects are dose related and can vary depending on the circumstances of the person (e.g., if the person is dependent on opioids, if the person is in pain).

in developing kappa agonists for use as analgesic agents in humans. Thus, although several pure mu opioid agonists, such as morphine, are available for licensed use in humans, there are currently no pure kappa agonists that can be prescribed to humans. However, there is renewed interest in the possible use of kappa opioids in humans as possible treatments for head injury, analgesia, and cocaine dependence, and compounds with kappa agonist activity are being studied once again. Activation of kappa receptors also results in a variety of effects (table 4.1). Notably, the analgesia produced by activation of kappa receptors is not the same as that produced by activation of mu receptors. For example, animals made tolerant to the analgesic effects of a mu opioid will still experience analgesic effects from a kappa opioid. Although no pure kappa agonists are marketed, some prescribed analgesic agents, such as butorphanol (Stadol), produce their actions through activation of both mu and kappa receptors.

Delta opioid receptors are less well characterized than mu and kappa receptors, although the human receptors for all three opioid subtypes have now been cloned. Early in the discovery of delta receptors, investigators used isolated mouse vas deferens (a duct from the testicle) and found high concentrations of delta receptors in this tissue. Hence, the origin of delta is from the use of the deferens in these studies. Delta receptor activation, like mu and kappa receptor activation, can produce analgesia in animals. Although selective delta agonists and antagonists have been developed for experimental use, no pure or selective delta opioid agonists have been studied in humans to date, nor marketed for use. However, experimental delta agonists have been studied in animals and appear to be reinforcing (animals will self-administer them), suggesting that pure delta receptor agonists may have abuse potential in humans. Thus, because one of the goals of medications development with opioids is to find nonabusable analgesics, pharmaceutical companies may not find it worthwhile to pursue delta agonists either for analgesic or drug abuse treatments.

Opioid Receptor Properties of Methadone

Based on the preceding review of opioid pharmacology, the characterization of methadone as a pure mu opioid agonist can now be understood. Methadone acts on and activates mu opioid receptors, producing the characteristic profile of effects of mu opioid agonists (table 4.1). Furthermore, methadone is a full agonist and it will, therefore, produce maximal physiologic effects at sufficiently high doses. Clinically, this means that in someone who is not tolerant to the effects of opioids, severe respiratory depression and even death can occur in the case of methadone overdose.

Other Receptor-Binding Properties of Methadone

It is now recognized that, in addition to its binding properties at mu opioid receptors, methadone also acts through another neurochemical system by binding to N-methyl-D-aspartate (NMDA) receptors. NMDA receptors are part of a larger neurochemical system that is sensitive to the effects of glutamate, the major excitatory neurotransmitter in the brain. Both *d*- and *l*-methadone can bind to NMDA receptors (Gorman et al. 1997). Methadone acts as a weak antagonist at NMDA receptors. It is not yet clear whether the action of methadone at NMDA receptors contributes significantly to its clinical effects, but this is a topic of great interest because (1) NMDA receptors are now recognized as playing an important role in neuropathic pain (see Ebert et al. 1998) and (2) preclinical studies have shown that pretreatment with NMDA receptor antagonists can decrease the development of tolerance to chronically administered opioids and can suppress the expression of opioid withdrawal signs in subjects rendered physically dependent on opioids (see Herman et al. 1995 for a review of this topic).

PHARMACOKINETIC PROPERTIES OF METHADONE
Structure of Methadone

Like many other medications, methadone actually exists in two different forms or isomers, known as the *d*-form for dextrorotatory and the *l*-form

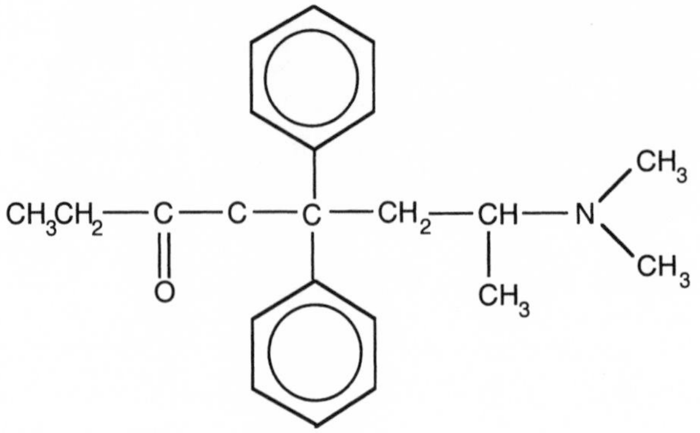

$$CH_3CH_2 - C - C - C - CH_2 - CH - N \underset{CH_3}{\overset{CH_3}{<}}$$

Methadone

Figure 4.1. The structure of methadone.

for levorotatory. When methadone is shown as a two-dimensional structure (fig. 4.1), the *d*- and *l*-forms seem identical; however, when viewed as three-dimensional structures, their conformations or configurations differ, as they are mirror images of one another. These two isomers also differ in their pharmacologic activity. *l*-Methadone is about 50 times more potent as an analgesic than *d*-methadone (Scott et al. 1948). Studies have reported that *d*-methadone can produce effects at higher doses; for example, *d*-methadone given at doses up to 1,000 mg per day can partially suppress opioid withdrawal symptoms (Fraser and Isbell 1962). The methadone formulation that is used clinically contains both the *d*- and *l*-forms ("*d,l*-methadone" or racemic methadone), although the *l*-methadone appears to account for most of the pharmacologic effects when given in typical clinical doses. Subsequent descriptions of methadone in this chapter will refer to the racemic combination or *d,l*-methadone unless otherwise specified.

Absorption, Metabolism, and Excretion

Methadone, available in tablet, liquid, and injectable forms, can be ingested orally or administered by injection (i.e., parenterally). It can also be absorbed from the buccal mucosa or mouth, although this is not the typical route for administering methadone. Methadone can be given rectally as well. The oral route of ingestion results in good bioavailability. Although estimates can vary widely between about 30 percent up to 90 percent, it is typically accepted that a dose of methadone given orally results in about 70 to 80 percent of it being circulated compared with 100 percent availability when given by an injection (see Eap et al. 2002 for review). The wide range of oral bioavailability across studies illustrates the fact that significant interindividual variability can occur, thus, highlighting the importance of individualized dosing whether for the treatment of opioid dependence or analgesia. The bioavailability of oral methadone does not markedly change as a person is stabilized on methadone or given the drug chronically.

In humans who are not physically dependent on opioids and who receive a single oral dose of methadone, methadone is typically detected in plasma within 30 minutes after ingestion, and the peak or highest concentrations of the drug occur about two to three hours after taking the dose (Inturrisi and Verebely 1972a; Meresaar et al. 1981), but peak concentrations of methadone have been observed to occur later (i.e., between four and six hours) in patients receiving methadone under chronic conditions (Inturrisi and Verebely 1972b). After a single dose, methadone blood levels decline slowly over the next 72 hours, and continued excretion of methadone and its metabolites can be found in the urine 96 hours after dosing. The half-life ($t_{1/2}$) of methadone, or the time required for one-half of the dose to disappear from plasma, is reported to be between 15 and 31 hours in humans, with most studies reporting an average $t_{1/2}$ of 24 or more hours (Verebely et al. 1975). Significant variability can occur between individuals in the $t_{1/2}$ of methadone, which can, in turn, modify the duration of its therapeutic effects. A number of factors are now recognized as important contributors to these individual differences, including genetic differences in the enzymes responsible for inactivating methadone, the pH of the urine, whether the patient is initiating treatment or has been maintained on methadone for some time, the duration of chronic exposure, and possibly gender (see Eap et al. 2002 for review). Additionally, the rate of methadone metabolism may increase for some patients stabilized on methadone for at least one month, so that the duration of its effects actually decreases (Nilsson et al. 1982). This does not occur for all patients but may occur for a significant minority of patients (perhaps about one-third) and suggests that these patients might benefit from dosing at intervals more frequent than 24 hours or should be treated with an alternate pharmacotherapy.

Methadone is extensively bound to plasma proteins (about 70–90 percent), and it also binds to proteins in tissues throughout the body. Methadone can be found in the blood and brain, and also other tissues such as the kidney, spleen, lungs, and especially the liver (Kreek et al.

1978), where concentrations of methadone are typically higher than those found in blood. This binding results in accumulation of methadone, whereby the amount of drug in the body increases in patients who received daily doses of methadone. For this reason, it is important to monitor new patients carefully who are making the transition to methadone from another opioid (either for treatment of pain or because of opioid dependence) during the early treatment period. Close monitoring during early treatment can ensure that a patient does not become overmedicated because of accumulating levels of methadone subsequent to repeated dosing. Methadone levels will also decline gradually over time when dosing is ceased because of its protein-binding capacity. Despite this gradual decline, abrupt discontinuation of methadone does lead to withdrawal signs and symptoms in those who have been maintained on methadone.

Methadone is metabolized in the liver, where it undergoes N-demethylation followed by cyclization that leads to its major metabolic product known as $M1$ (2-ethylidene-1,5-dimethyl-3,3-diphenylpyrolidene, EDDP). In addition, other metabolites of methadone have been found, including $M2$ (2-ethyl-5-methyl-3,3-diphenyl-1-pyrrolidine), produced by N-demethylation followed by cyclization and then another N-demethylation. There are several other minor metabolites of methadone, although methadone and $M1$ appear to be the primary compounds that are eliminated. Estimates suggest that approximately 10 percent of methadone is eliminated as the unchanged drug. The metabolites of methadone do not appear to exert pharmacologic activity. Methadone and its metabolites are primarily eliminated in the urine and feces, although methadone has also been found in the sweat, semen, and saliva of methadone-maintained patients. With relatively low doses of methadone, the fecal route can be a significant route of elimination for methadone and its metabolites. For higher doses, however, renal elimination predominates. Significant differences in the plasma half-life of methadone can be induced by marked changes in urinary pH. If urine is acidic, then the ratio of $M1$ to methadone decreases in urine (an increase in the clearance of the parent compound methadone); conversely, if urine is basic, there is an increase in the ratio of $M1$ to methadone (a decrease in the clearance of methadone) (Bellward et al. 1977). These observations have led some authors to suggest that purposefully reducing the pH of the urine of patients who complain that their dose is not holding them for a full 24 hours may improve therapeutic efficacy, although no known studies have systematically tested this theory.

Patients with liver disease may exhibit several changes in their metabolism of methadone. Metabolic rate may actually decrease, leading to a subsequent increase in the $t_{1/2}$ of methadone. However, patients with liver disease may have less capacity to store methadone in the liver, so that the overall pool of methadone is decreased; this decreased storage can compensate for the change in methadone $t_{1/2}$. Several other factors can influence methadone metabolism. Some evidence shows that methadone may induce or speed up its own metabolism, because the excretion of the M1 metabolite increases as a patient is stabilized on methadone. It is not clear, however, if these observations have controlled for possible variations in the pH of urine, which may account for the sometimes variable results found in such studies. Methadone metabolism is greater when methadone is taken by the oral route versus intramuscular injection. Finally, some evidence suggests that women may metabolize methadone faster then men (although this observation may again be confounded by factors such as urinary pH, and not all results from studies are consistent with this finding).

CLINICAL PHARMACOLOGY OF METHADONE

Analgesic Effects

Methadone is an effective analgesic when given either by the oral, rectal, or parenteral route of administration. The manufacturer's recommendation for initial dosing for relief of pain is between 2.5 and 10 mg given orally every three to four hours as needed; however, practical experience and published accounts of clinical experience have long suggested that these doses are excessive for initial treatment (Ettinger et al. 1979). Practice guidelines more commonly recommend an initial dose of 2.5 mg every eight hours for those patients without previous opioid experience and up to 5 mg for those patients with previous opioid exposure. Onset of analgesic effects occurs within 30–60 minutes after oral administration and around 20 minutes after parenteral administration. The peak analgesic effect produced by the parenteral route is greater than that produced by the oral route, although both oral and parenteral routes produce their peak pain relief at about one hour after administration. The duration of analgesia is somewhat greater for the oral versus parenteral route, although both oral and parenteral methadone produce analgesic effects that last about three to five hours. When given acutely by the intramuscular route, the analgesic potency of methadone is about equal to or slightly greater than the potency of morphine. The duration of analgesic effects produced by a single dose of methadone is about the same as that produced by morphine, despite the substantially longer $t_{1/2}$ for methadone. Moreover, in patients with chronic pain treated with methadone, the dosing interval can be lengthened (e.g., to 8- to 12-hour intervals) and still provide excellent pain relief.

If methadone is used in the treatment of chronic pain, then initial dosing should be based on whether the patient is already dependent on other opioids (e.g., previous treatment with morphine), the source and degree of the patient's pain, and whether oral administration is possible. Although initial doses should be relatively low and respiratory status should be monitored closely, increases of dose should be made until adequate pain relief is achieved over time. As with other actions of methadone, tolerance may develop to the analgesic efficacy of methadone after repeated exposure, necessitating dose increases in patients requiring chronic treatment.

For transferring patients to methadone for treatment of chronic pain, it is important to consider their history of prescribed opioid use to choose the correct transition dose. Although some work has suggested that oral methadone and oral morphine are equipotent, and that parenteral methadone and parenteral morphine are also equipotent, these results typically reflect results from acute rather than chronic dosing studies. In general, reports from clinical experience suggest the dose of methadone should be significantly less than the dose of morphine previously used. Reports on the conversion of patients treated with chronic hydromorphone (Dilaudid) and oxycodone to treatment with methadone suggest that methadone is also more potent than these agents. Numerous published tables are available to provide conversion information regarding the relative potency between other opioids and methadone. However, because cross-tolerance is not always complete between other opioids and methadone (i.e., the conversion is not equal in both directions), one must proceed with care to ensure that the appropriate data are used to determine the conversion dose.

The most important principles in the use of methadone for treating chronic pain are to (1) start dosing low (it is commonly recommended that the initial transition dose be about 50 percent of the equianalgesic dose of the previous opioid rather than an equivalent dose) and (2) increase the dose slowly with careful supervision and only as needed for symptomatic relief. Because of the long terminal half-life of methadone and its protein-binding characteristics, each successive dose of methadone can lead to increasing concentrations as described earlier, especially during the period when treatment is initiated and before stable levels are achieved (i.e., steady state). Moreover, the duration of the respiratory depressant effects of methadone exceed its analgesic effects, with reports indicating that a single oral dose of methadone can produce respiratory depression lasting for up to 48 hours (Olsen et al. 1977, 1981). Therefore, the risk of significant respiratory depression is heightened by too-rapid escalations of methadone dose, especially in those patients with limited opioid tolerance. With the increasing usage of methadone for the treatment of pain during the past five to eight years, there has unfortunately been a significant rise in the number of accidental fatal overdoses; these frequently occur during the early transition to methadone treatment.

Methadone offers several advantages over other medications used in the treatment of chronic pain, including its good oral bioavailability (decreasing the need for injections), its low cost, and its widely demonstrated efficacy. Because of its apparently greater analgesic potency versus other opioids when used in the treatment of chronic pain, dosing of methadone should be individualized for each patient. Although methadone is an attractive analgesic, its association with the treatment of opioid abuse may inhibit some patients from accepting it for pain relief. If a patient expresses such a concern, it should be addressed with a candid discussion about the excellent efficacy of methadone as a well-studied analgesic.

Respiratory Depressant Effects

Like other mu opioid agonists, methadone can produce respiratory depression when a dose is taken in excess of the person's level of dependence. Mu opioid agonists can produce respiratory depression by inhibiting the sensitivity of cells in the brainstem, which normally provide automatic control of respiration by monitoring circulating carbon dioxide levels. It has been reported that a single dose of methadone, in a nontolerant individual, can produce respiratory depression that may last for up to 48 hours. If an appropriately low starting dose is used, significant respiratory depression should not result from methadone dosing. Moreover, respiratory depression is not typically problematic in patients who are chronically treated with methadone at therapeutic doses. In nontolerant individuals, however, methadone administration can lead to respiratory failure and death. It is also important to avoid concomitant administration of medications that may prolong the half-life of methadone, as this can lead to increased risk of respiratory depression. The concurrent use of alcohol or sedatives such as benzodiazepines or barbiturates can also increase the risk of respiratory depression. If respiratory depression results from methadone dosing, reversal with an opioid antagonist such as intravenous naloxone should be instituted.

Other Physiologic Effects

Acute doses of methadone produce pupillary constriction (miosis); this a telltale sign of opioid use that can be assessed in clinical settings and law enforcement. In humans without physiologic dependence on opioids, pupillary constriction can persist for 24 hours after a single dose. In methadone-maintained patients, pupils are partially constricted on a chronic basis, although pupil size will fluctuate during the daily dosing cycle, decreasing after dose ingestion and increasing between doses (reflecting the rise and fall in methadone plasma concentrations). Opioids are generally considered to have a high degree of cardiovascular safety, but recent studies have focused on the potential for methadone to modify the cardiac rhythm, specifically to prolong the QTc interval, which could lead to potentially dangerous changes in conduction (see chap. 6). Data, thus far, suggest that higher doses of methadone may pose a greater risk for this than lower doses; however, future studies should further elucidate this relationship. Studies evaluating the effects of chronic methadone dosing on blood pressure have yielded equivocal results, with evidence of both slight increases and slight decreases in systolic and diastolic blood pressure. Regardless of the direction, the magnitude of these changes is modest and not likely to be of clinical importance. There is no evidence to suggest that methadone is hepatotoxic or harmful to the liver.

Methadone, like other mu opioid agonists, can cause nausea and vomiting after acute administration, especially in a nontolerant person. Tolerance tends to develop to this effect during chronic treatment in patients who are susceptible to the nausea-producing properties of methadone. Methadone can cause significant itchiness of the skin, in part, due to histamine release; other histamine-related effects can include flushing, sweating, and increased skin temperature. Another common problematic, but not dangerous, side effect associated with methadone administration is constipation. Constipation occurs because methadone inhibits peristaltic movement in the gut, slowing the transit of food through the intestines while simultaneously increasing the muscular tone of the anal sphincter. Constipation can become severe for some individuals during chronic treatment and is best treated by a change in diet, although pharmacologic aids and fiber supplements are sometimes needed.

Psychological Effects

In subjects who have a history of opioid dependence but are not currently opioid dependent, acute doses of 10–60 mg of oral methadone produce increased ratings of liking and euphoria. The euphoriant effects of methadone have been shown to be qualitatively similar to those of morphine (Jasinski and Preston 1986). These effects peak during the first five hours after the dose is ingested and dissipate within 24 hours. These doses also produce sedation in nondependent individuals and this sedation is characterized, in part, by "nodding" or head bobbing. Patients receiving chronic methadone treatment do not typically experience sedation or lethargy at low methadone doses; however, at higher doses (e.g., 100 mg orally per day) patients can report increased ratings of lethargy, weakness, and decreased motivation (Martin et al. 1973). These effects are usually of a mild magnitude, and clinical experience suggests patients are able to function well when maintained on doses of methadone in this range. Despite the development of tolerance to many of methadone's actions during chronic treatment, it has been shown that patients will choose to self-administer supplemental methadone doses when given the opportunity (Stitzer et al. 1983). This suggests that the reinforcing or euphoric properties of methadone are still detectable even in chronically maintained and tolerant patients.

Effects on Psychomotor and Cognitive Function

Acute doses of methadone given to nondependent individuals have been shown to impair psychomotor performance, and the extent of the impairment increases as a function of dose. It has long been accepted, however, that tolerance to these acute effects occurs when patients receive chronic dosing with methadone. Indeed, early studies suggested that methadone maintenance did not produce impairments in psychomotor reaction time, attention, or other measures of intellectual functioning (Gordon 1970; Lombardo et al. 1976). However, these studies have been criticized for having inadequate control conditions or making comparisons to inadequately matched subjects. More recent studies have suggested that methadone maintenance may lead to impairments in the performance of some tasks of psychomotor and cognitive speed (Mintzer and Stitzer 2002; Specka et al. 2000), whereas function on other performance and memory tasks is unimpaired. It is unclear how the impairments observed in laboratory-based studies may relate to impairment in the natural environment. No studies, to date, have reported gross impairments of psychomotor and cognitive function. One recent study compared individuals maintained on methadone, buprenorphine, or LAAM (another long-acting opioid no longer available), compared with control subjects on simulated driving. No differences were found between the groups who were in opioid-dependence treatment compared with the control group on driving performance (Lenne et al. 2003), and these results were consistent with past studies examining the effects of methadone on driving. Together, the findings from these studies suggest that there may be modest impairments in some performance tasks but largely indicate that methadone-maintained patients can function well in work and social environments.

THERAPEUTIC PROPERTIES OF METHADONE FOR TREATING OPIOID DEPENDENCE

Opioid Blockade or Cross-tolerance

One feature of methadone that makes it a useful medication in the treatment of opioid dependence is that methadone maintenance produces blockade or cross-tolerance to the effects produced by other ingested mu agonist opioids (such as heroin or morphine). One of the first scientific papers on methadone's clinical use in the treatment of opioid dependence included a report on the blockade effects of methadone (Dole et al. 1966). In that paper, methadone was reported to decrease the euphoria produced by intravenous injection of other opioids, such as morphine, and the magnitude of the blockade was increased at higher doses of methadone.

Similar results have been shown in a variety of studies that have, either directly or indirectly, assessed the blockade abilities of methadone. In one early study, inpatient subjects with histories of opioid dependence, but who were not currently opioid dependent, were allowed to "earn" intravenous doses of 4 mg of hydromorphone each day by riding an exercise bicycle (Jones and Prada 1975). The amount of hydromorphone self-administered was determined before they started on methadone (i.e., at baseline) and then determined repeatedly over time as the methadone treatment dose was increased. Methadone dosing was initiated at 5 mg per day and increased over six weeks to a final dose of 100 mg per day. Before methadone treatment started, essentially all subjects were riding the exercise bike and earning all the hydromorphone available. As methadone treatment was initiated and the dose gradually increased, the amount of riding and hydromorphone self-administration, the self-reported "liking" for hydromorphone, and the change in pupillary diameter produced by an injection of hydromorphone all decreased. After about four weeks of maintenance on 100 mg of methadone, there were days when none of the subjects in the study rode the bike (although there were still occasional days when one person rode the bike to earn an injection). Thus, this study showed how maintenance on an adequate dose of methadone could produce a blockade to the effects of an injection of an opioid, resulting in marked and sustained decreases in opioid use.

Other studies have shown that subjects maintained on 30 mg of methadone daily report drug effects from 10 mg of intramuscular hydromorphone, but that subjects maintained on 60 mg of methadone daily report essentially no drug effects from this same dose of hydromorphone. A more recent study examined the ability of methadone to blunt or block the effects of intravenous heroin and found that the degree of blockade produced by methadone increased at successively higher methadone maintenance doses from 30 to 60 to 120 mg per day (Donny et al. 2002). This study also found that, even at the highest methadone dose of 120 mg per day, the ability to block heroin was substantially lower 48 hours after dosing than 24 hours after dosing, supporting the need for daily dosing with methadone to achieve this blockade. These results demonstrate that methadone can block the effects of opioids and that higher methadone doses produce greater blockade than lower doses. The ability of methadone to produce blockade of other opioids is considered to be the critical feature that leads to its ability to suppress or reduce the use of illicit opioid abuse during maintenance therapy. Similar to the observation that the degree of opioid blockade is positively related to methadone dose in the laboratory, the reduction of illicit opioid use in clinical populations is positively related to methadone maintenance dose (Strain et al. 1993). That opioid blockade by methadone maintenance may be incomplete is suggested by some residual opioid use observed during treatment.

Withdrawal Suppression

Another pharmacologic feature of methadone important to its therapeutic efficacy in the treatment of opioid dependence is its ability to suppress the signs and symptoms of opioid withdrawal. This characteristic of methadone was first demonstrated in a study conducted in the 1940s (Isbell et al. 1948), in which inpatient subjects were maintained on daily morphine and then abruptly had their morphine discontinued. Thirty-two hours later, when they were in moderate to severe withdrawal, subjects received an injection of methadone. Injection of methadone resulted in marked and immediate decreases in withdrawal that persisted for at least 10 hours (the length of time observations were recorded) and suppressed a period of withdrawal longer than that achieved with an injection of morphine. The ability of methadone to suppress withdrawal makes patients comfortable, especially at the start of treatment when they are first attempting to initiate abstinence from heroin use. Laboratory studies suggest that methadone is effective at suppressing withdrawal signs and symptoms at fairly low doses (e.g., 30 mg), whereas higher doses of methadone may be needed to produce sufficient cross-tolerance to suppress opioid drug use.

Summary

Methadone is a full agonist whose effects are mediated through activation of the mu opioid receptor system. Methadone also acts as an antagonist in the NMDA receptor system. Like other mu opioid agonists, methadone is an effective analgesic and can also produce an array of side effects when given to nondependent humans, including pupillary constriction, respiratory depression, sedation, nausea, and vomiting. It is important to start dosing with methadone at a low dose and to increase slowly and under supervision to avoid the risk of adverse effects, especially in patients with an uncertain level of dependence. Tolerance develops to many of the direct effects of methadone when it is given under chronic dosing conditions. Several pharmacologic features of methadone make it particularly useful for the treatment of opioid dependence. These features include its good bioavailability through the oral route, thus permitting easy dosage administration (typically, through a liquid vehicle); its long $t_{1/2}$, so that dosing can occur on a once-per-day basis; its effective suppression of the opioid withdrawal syndrome, improving compliance with treatment; and its cross-tolerance to the effects of illicit opioids, decreasing the use of illicit opioids when patients are maintained on methadone.

Recommended Readings

Bigelow GE, Preston KL. Opioids. In *Psychopharmacology: The Fourth Generation of Progress,* Bloom FE and Kupfer DJ, eds., 1731–44. New York: Raven Press, 1995.

Cooper JR, Bloom FE, Roth RH. *The Biochemical Basis Of Neuropharmacology,* 8th ed. New York: Oxford University Press, 2003.

Jaffe JH. Opiates: Clinical Aspects. In *Substance Abuse: A Comprehensive Textbook,* 2nd ed. Lowinson JH, Ruiz P, Millman RB, and Langrod JG, eds., 186–94. Baltimore: Williams and Wilkins, 1992.

Preston A. *The Methadone Briefing.* London, U.K.: Island Press, 1996.

Reisine T., Pasternak G. Opioid analgesics and antagonists. In *Goodman and Gilman's The Pharmacological Basis of Therapeutics,* 9th ed. Hardman JG, Limbird LE, Molinoff PB, Ruddon RW, Goodman Gilman A, eds., 521–56. New York: McGraw Hill, 1996.

References

Bellward GD, Warren PM, Howald W, Axelson JE, Abbott FS (1977). Methadone maintenance: effect of urinary pH on renal clearance in chronic high and low doses. *Clin Pharmacol Ther* 22: 92–99.

Dole VP, Nyswander ME, Kreek MJ (1966). Narcotic blockade. *Arch Intern Med* 118: 304–9.

Donny EC, Walsh SL, Bigelow GE, Eissenberg T, Stitzer ML (2002). High-dose methadone produces superior opioid blockade and comparable withdrawal suppression to lower doses in opioid-dependent humans. *Psychopharmacology (Berl)* 161: 202–12.

Eap CB, Buclin T, Baumann P (2002). Interindividual variability of the clinical pharmacokinetics of methadone: implications for the treatment of opioid dependence. *Clin Pharmacokinet* 41: 1153–93.

Ebert B, Thorkildsen C, Andersen S, Christrup LL, Hjeds H (1998). Opioid analgesics as noncompetitive N-methyl-D-aspartate (NMDA) antagonists. *Biochem Pharmacol* 56: 553–9.

Ettinger DS, Vitale PJ, Trump DL (1979). Important clinical pharmacologic considerations in the use of methadone in cancer patients. *Cancer Treat Rep* 63: 457–9.

Fraser HF, Isbell H (1962). Human pharmacology and addictiveness of certain dextroisomers of synthetic analgesics: I. d-3-hydroxy-N-phenethylmorphinan. II. d-3-methoxy-N-phenethylmorphinan. III. d-methadone. *Bull Narc* 14: 25–35.

Gordon NB (1970). Reaction-times of methadone treated ex-heroin addicts. *Psychopharmacologia* 16: 337–44.

Gorman AL, Elliott KJ, Inturrisi CE (1997). The d- and l-isomers of methadone bind to the non-competitive site on the N-methyl-D-aspartate (NMDA) receptor in rat forebrain and spinal cord. *Neurosci Lett* 223: 5–8.

Guitart X, Codony X, Monroy X (2004). Sigma receptors: biology and therapeutic potential. *Psychopharmacology (Berl)* 174: 301–19.

Herman BH, Vocci F, Bridge P (1995). The effects of NMDA receptor antagonists and nitric oxide synthase inhibitors on opioid tolerance and withdrawal. Medication development issues for opiate addiction. *Neuropsychopharmacology* 13: 269–93.

Inturrisi CE, Verebely K (1972a). Disposition of methadone in man after a single oral dose. *Clin Pharmacol Ther* 13: 923–30.

Inturrisi CE, Verebely K (1972b). The levels of methadone in the plasma in methadone maintenance. *Clin Pharmacol Ther* 13: 633–7.

Isbell H, Wilker A, Eisenman AJ, Daingerfield M, Frank K (1948). Liability of addiction to 6-dimethylamino-4,4-diphenyl-3-heptanone (methadon, "amidone" or "10820") in man. *Arch Intern Med* 82: 362–92.

Jasinski DR, Preston KL (1986). Comparison of intravenously administered methadone, morphine and heroin. *Drug Alcohol Depend* 17: 301–10.

Jones BE, Prada JA (1975). Drug-seeking behavior during methadone maintenance. *Psychopharmacologia* 41: 7–10.

Kreek MJ, Oratz M, Rothschild MA (1978). Hepatic extraction of long- and short-acting narcotics in the isolated perfused rabbit liver. *Gastroenterology* 75: 88–94.

Lenne MG, Dietze P, Rumbold GR, Redman JR, Triggs TJ (2003). The effects of the opioid pharmacotherapies methadone, LAAM and buprenorphine, alone and in combination with alcohol, on simulated driving. *Drug Alcohol Depend* 72: 271–8.

Lombardo WK, Lombardo B, Goldstein A (1976). Cognitive functioning under moderate and low dosage methadone maintenance. *Int J Addict* 11: 389–401.

Martin WR, Jasinski DR, Haertzen CA, Kay DC, Jones BE, Mansky PA, Carpenter RW (1973). Methadone: a reevaluation. *Arch Gen Psychiatry* 28: 286–95.

Meresaar U, Nilsson MI, Holmstrand J, Anggard E (1981). Single dose pharmacokinetics and bioavailability of methadone in man studied with a stable isotope method. *Eur J Clin Pharmacol* 20: 473–8.

Mintzer MZ, Stitzer ML (2002). Cognitive impairment in methadone maintenance patients. *Drug Alcohol Depend* 67: 41–51.

Nilsson MI, Anggard E, Holmstrand J, Gunne LM (1982). Pharmacokinetics of methadone during maintenance treatment: adaptive changes during the induction phase. *Eur J Clin Pharmacol* 22: 343–9.

Olsen GD, Wendel HA, Livermore JD, Leger RM, Lynn RK, Gerber N (1977). Clinical effects and pharmacokinetics of racemic methadone and its optical isomers. *Clin Pharmacol Ther* 21: 147–57.

Olsen GD, Wilson JE, Robertson GE (1981). Respiratory and ventilatory effects of methadone in healthy women. *Clin Pharmacol Ther* 29: 373–80.

Scott CC, Robbins EB, Chen KK (1948). Pharmacologic comparison of the optical isomers of methadon. *J Pharmacol Exp Ther* 93: 282–6.

Specka M, Finkbeiner T, Lodemann E, Leifert K, Kluwig J, Gastpar M (2000). Cognitive-motor performance of methadone-maintained patients. *Eur Addict Res* 6: 8–19.

Stitzer ML, McCaul ME, Bigelow GE, Liebson IA (1983). Oral methadone self-administration: effects of dose and alternative reinforcers. *Clin Pharmacol Ther* 34: 29–35.

Strain EC, Stitzer ML, Liebson IA, Bigelow GE (1993). Dose-response effects of methadone in the treatment of opioid dependence. *Ann Intern Med* 119: 23–27.

Verebely K, Volavka J, Mule S, Resnick R (1975). Methadone in man: pharmacokinetic and excretion studies in acute and chronic treatment. *Clin Pharmacol Ther* 18: 180–90.

5

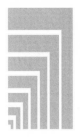

Beginning and Ending Methadone Dosing: Induction and Withdrawal

Eric C. Strain, M.D.

In general, there are three phases to methadone dosing for a patient: dose induction (the phase during which the patient starts on methadone), dose stabilization or maintenance (the phase during which the patient receives a stable dose of methadone), and dose withdrawal or detoxification (the phase during which methadone is gradually decreased and then discontinued). This chapter reviews methadone dosing during induction and withdrawal. A separate chapter (chap. 6) is devoted to issues associated with methadone stabilization, including a review of evidence that methadone is effective and that this efficacy is dose related.

METHADONE DOSE INDUCTION

Before starting a patient on methadone, it is necessary to determine whether the patient qualifies for methadone treatment. This topic is addressed in chapter 9 and will not be repeated here. Subsequent recommendations in this chapter assume that the patient has been adequately evaluated and fulfills the necessary criteria for treatment with methadone.

The goal of methadone dosing in the induction phase is to provide relief from opioid withdrawal, but unfortunately, initial doses of methadone may fail to "hold" the patient for 24 hours because insufficient levels have accumulated in tissue stores. Surprisingly, very little research has been done on the best way to start a patient on methadone. In the initial work by Dole and Nyswander, methadone was first given to inpatients using doses of 10–20 mg twice daily and gradually increased over a period of four weeks to a total daily dose of 50–150 mg (and then eventually changed to a single daily dose). Early in the development of methadone treatment, a similar process of initial twice-per-day dosing, but done on an outpatient basis, was shown to be equally effective as inpatient induction (Cheung and Pugliese 1973; Nichols et al. 1971). It is possible that the use of methadone on a twice-daily basis at the beginning of induction provides better relief from withdrawal during the first days of treatment, because it may take 5–10 days for methadone to accumulate in tissues (IOM 1995). However, it is usually not practical to administer doses twice daily during outpatient treatment, and one study found that split dosing at the start of treatment was no more effective than single daily dosing (Goldstein 1971).

Other early investigators adopted procedures using a single daily dose, and with a quicker induction. For example, Goldstein administered 30 mg of methadone on the first day of treatment and then increased the dose by 10 mg per day until a daily dose of 100 mg was achieved (Goldstein 1970). This type of schedule is generally well tolerated, although some patients become excessively drowsy and have other side effects, such as constipation and increased sweating, with such relatively rapid schedules (Freymuth 1971; Goldstein 1970). Goldstein ultimately modified his schedule so that 10-mg dose increases occurred every other day rather than every day, which decreased reports of drowsiness.

Because no double-blind controlled studies have examined the optimal dose-induction procedure for methadone, we must rely on clinical experience. In general, this experience suggests that patients dependent on short-acting opioids tolerate doses of 20–40 mg of methadone on the first day of treatment without adverse effects. If possible, the patient should be monitored for several hours after the first dose, and a second dose (5–10 mg) can be administered if there is evidence that opioid withdrawal resumes (Payte and Khuri 1993). Subsequent dosing can be increased by increments of 5–10 mg. The rate of increase can vary, and a determination of this rate should include daily clinical assessments of the patient. Slow rates of increase, such as 10-mg dose increases once per week, are usually well tolerated and safe. A disadvantage to such slow increases, however, is that patients may continue illicit opiate use because of withdrawal and may drop out of treatment. Goldstein's procedure of rapid dose increases (10-mg increases every day) probably represents the extreme in rapid dose induction on an outpatient basis and may produce drowsiness as an unwanted side effect (Goldstein 1970). Thus, an intermediate schedule (e.g.,

10 mg every other day) is recommended. However, additional research would be useful to determine whether patients might do better by rapidly increasing their dose during the first few days of treatment.

A final clinical point regarding methadone induction should be made. On the first day of methadone treatment, it is good clinical practice to monitor patients after their first doses of methadone. Patients with a clear history of current opioid dependence should tolerate the first methadone dose without problems. Occasionally, however, some patients will react with excessive sedation following this first day's dose; therefore, it is important to monitor the patient for at least one to two hours afterward. There are rare reports of higher rates of methadone-overdose deaths in the first weeks of treatment (Buster et al. 2002; Caplehorn and Drummer 1999; Caplehorn 1998; Vormfelde and Poser 2001), suggesting a need for careful supervision during the methadone induction period.

Close monitoring is also important to ensure initial doses are not too low. Patients who have objective evidence of continued or worsening opioid withdrawal two hours after their first dose of methadone could receive a second, smaller dose of methadone (5 or 10 mg) later that day.

METHADONE DOSE WITHDRAWAL

Patients who benefit from stable maintenance on methadone and who qualify for maintenance treatment may never undergo methadone withdrawal. Indefinite maintenance treatment can be clinically indicated and appropriate for such patients, especially if previous attempts at methadone withdrawal have resulted in a relapse to drug use. Methadone withdrawal may be indicated in selected cases, however.

Several studies have examined the optimal procedure for medically supervised withdrawal using methadone (also know as detoxification, although technically patients are not undergoing a process of toxin removal). Issues associated with methadone withdrawal include the length of time and rate of methadone withdrawal, the optimal size of decrease in methadone dose, whether the dose should be decreased in equal intervals or at some other rate (such as a percentage of the previous dose), and whether patients should be informed about the details of their withdrawal schedule. Each of these points is addressed in the following sections.

Length of Time and Rate of Methadone Withdrawal

Several studies have examined different periods during which methadone is withdrawn; in general, results from these studies show that better out-

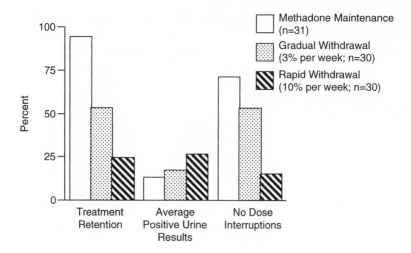

Figure 5.1. Representative results from a double-blind outpatient clinical trial comparing gradual (3% per week) and rapid (10% per week) methadone withdrawal schedules to methadone maintenance. All results are percentages. Treatment retention was based on the number of subjects who completed the 30-week study. The average percentage of positive urine test results was calculated from urine samples collected twice weekly and tested for morphine and quinine. The percentage of subjects with no dose interruption was based on requests submitted for interruptions in the dosing schedule (either an increase in methadone dose or no decrease in that week's dose of methadone); interruptions lasted for one week. Adapted from Senay et al. 1977.

comes are associated with longer lengths of time during which methadone is withdrawn. For example, patients receiving a 10-day withdrawal had higher peak withdrawal scores and higher dropout rates after withdrawal was completed when compared with patients receiving a 21-day withdrawal (Gossop et al. 1989). Similarly, for outpatients randomly assigned to either a three- or six-week methadone withdrawal, better results during treatment were found for the patients in the six-week withdrawal group (e.g., for treatment retention and percentage of opioid-positive urine samples), although these benefits were not sustained during post-treatment follow-up (Sorensen et al. 1982).

Finally, Senay and colleagues conducted an elegant double-blind study examining the relative efficacy of a 10-week withdrawal from methadone (i.e., dose reductions of 10% per week), a more gradual 30-week withdrawal (i.e., 3% per week), and continued methadone maintenance (Senay et al. 1977). In that study patients could request interruptions in their withdrawal, either as a temporary increase in methadone dose for one week or as a stabilization in the schedule for one week. Results from the study show that patients in the 10 percent per week reduction group had higher rates of treatment dropout (76% versus 47% for the 3% per week group dropped out before the end of the 30-week study), requested more detoxification schedule interruptions, and had a higher rate of opioid-positive urine samples than did patients in the maintenance and gradual dose-reduction groups (fig. 5.1). Thus, the study concludes that a gradual 3 percent methadone dose reduction per week is more efficacious than a more rapid 10 percent weekly reduction.

Size of Changes in Methadone Dose

Most studies examining methadone withdrawal have examined dose decreases that occur at some fixed rate, such as the 10 percent weekly decrease used in the study by Senay et al. (1977). That is, dose decreases are 10 percent of a patient's starting methadone dose. Thus, if a patient were on 50-mg dose of methadone, decreases would be 5 mg per week using such a schedule. Early in the withdrawal, a 5-mg dose decrease would represent a small percentage of the previous week's dose (i.e., in the first week 5 mg is 10% of 50 mg, in the second week 5 mg would be 11% of 45 mg, and in the third week 5 mg is 13% of 40 mg). However, by the end of the 10-week period, 5 mg will represent a significant proportion of the previous week's dose (i.e., in the ninth week 5 mg would be 50% of the previous week's dose of 10 mg). Would an alternate schedule, in which dose decreases become smaller as the withdrawal progresses, provide better treatment outcomes?

Strang and Gossop (1990) examined this question in a 10-day inpatient methadone withdrawal study. In that study one group of patients received daily dose reductions representing 10 percent of their *starting dose,* and another group received daily dose reductions representing 20 percent of their *previous day's dose.* For the latter dosing group, large decreases occurred during the first few days of the withdrawal, whereas much smaller absolute dose reductions occurred at the end of the withdrawal. Results showed self-reports of opioid withdrawal symptoms for the two groups were quite similar, both in terms of the time course and in the peak withdrawal produced (which occurred three days after the end of the withdrawal). Thus, variations in dose taper schedules may have less impact than duration of withdrawal.

However, similar investigations comparing alternate forms of withdrawal schedules have not been conducted on an outpatient basis or over longer periods. Because most methadone withdrawal is done with outpatients over longer periods, studies under these circumstances are needed

Table 5.1 **Examples of Methadone Withdrawal Schedules**

Day in Treatment	Week in Treatment	21-Day Schedule		91-Day Schedule		182-Day Schedule	
		Lower Dose	Higher Dose	Lower Dose	Higher Dose	Lower Dose	Higher Dose
1	1	30	40	40	40	40	40
2	1	30	38	40	40	40	40
3	1	30	36	50	50	50	50
4	1	25	34	50	60	50	60
5	1	25	32	60	70	60	70
6	1	25	30	60	70	60	70
7	1	20	28	60	80	60	80
8	2	20	26	60	80	60	80
9	2	20	24	60	80	60	80
10	2	20	22	60	80	60	90
11	2	15	20	60	80	60	90
12	2	15	18	60	80	60	90
13	2	15	16	60	80	60	90
14	2	10	14	60	80	60	100
15	3	10	12	60	80	60	100
16	3	10	10	60	80	60	100
17	3	10	8	60	80	60	100
18	3	5	6	60	80	60	100
19	3	5	4	60	80	60	100
20	3	5	2	60	80	60	100
21	3	0	0	60	80	60	100
22–28	4			54	72	60	100
29–35	5			48	64	60	100
36–42	6			42	56	60	100
43–49	7			36	48	57	95
50–56	8			30	40	54	90
57–63	9			24	32	51	85
64–70	10			18	24	48	80
71–77	11			12	16	45	75
78–84	12			6	8	42	70
85–91	13			0	0	39	65
92–98	14					36	60
99–105	15					33	55
106–112	16					30	50
113–119	17					27	45
120–126	18					24	40
127–133	19					21	35
134–140	20					18	30
141–147	21					15	25
148–154	22					12	20
155–161	23					9	15
162–168	24					6	10
169–175	25					3	5
176–182	26					0	0

to establish whether there are clinically significant differences across alternate types of withdrawal schedules. Until such work has been done, it is recommended that methadone dose decreases occur at a fixed percentage of the starting dose. Table 5.1 provides examples of 21-, 91-, and 182-day methadone withdrawal schedules for a patient who is initially dependent on illicit opioids.

Informing the Patient about the Withdrawal Schedule and Self-Regulation of Methadone Withdrawal

Several studies have examined outcome in methadone withdrawal when withdrawals are done under blind (i.e., patients are unaware of the dosing schedule) versus open conditions (i.e., patients are aware of their daily dose and changes being made) (Green and Gossop 1988; Senay et al. 1977; Stitzer et al. 1981). In general, these studies show outcomes are better when patients are aware of the details of their dosing withdrawal schedule. In studies comparing who decides the rate of withdrawal (staff versus the patient), researchers have generally found no advantage in allowing patients to determine their methadone withdrawal schedule (Senay et al. 1984; Stitzer et al. 1981).

Efficacy of Methadone Withdrawal and Predictors of Treatment Success

If successful outcome from methadone withdrawal is defined as abstinence from opioids after completion of the withdrawal, then the overall efficacy of methadone withdrawal is quite poor. In the early years of methadone treatment there was particular interest in withdrawal, and there were several reports on clinical experience in attempting to taper and discontinue methadone medication (Cushman and Dole 1973; Gearing 1970; Kremen 1973; Stimmel et al. 1973). In general, although occasional reports suggested that methadone withdrawal could be successful (Cushman and Dole 1973), most of these and similar studies (Maddux et al. 1980; Sorensen et al. 1982; Stimmel et al. 1977; Stitzer et al. 1983; Wilson et al. 1975) reported high rates of relapse to opioid use during and after the completion of methadone withdrawal. A Cochrane Review of methadone withdrawal concluded that methadone is effective at decreasing the severity of the withdrawal syndrome but that relapse is quite common after the completion of the withdrawal (Amato et al. 2004).

Despite these outcomes, renewed interest is shown periodically in the potential efficacy of methadone withdrawal. Most recently, this has been prompted in part by the idea that it might be possible to improve outcomes by enhancing the nonpharmacologic treatment delivered during the withdrawal period. A randomized, outpatient clinical trial comparing methadone maintenance treatment with methadone withdrawal, with the latter including a rich set of concurrent individual and group therapy services, found that patients receiving withdrawal did poorly on several outcome measures, including treatment retention and rates of heroin use (Sees et al. 2000). Another study utilizing vouchers to reinforce abstinence during methadone withdrawal did find promising results (Robles et al. 2002), suggesting that use of behaviorally based treatments during withdrawal may be more effective in improving methadone withdrawal outcomes.

Although many patients relapse to opioid use after withdrawal from methadone, rates of illicit opioid use are generally lower than those before methadone treatment (Strain et al. 1994). Success following methadone withdrawal is not related to prewithdrawal rates of illicit opioid use (Stitzer et al. 1983), nor the prewithdrawal dose of methadone (Gossop et al. 1987). Although the likelihood of patients' achieving complete initial abstinence is higher if the withdrawal is done on an inpatient rather than an outpatient basis (Gossop et al. 1986), posttreatment outcomes seem to be similar whether the treatment setting is inpatient or outpatient (Maddux et al. 1980; Wilson et al. 1975).

Rapid Opioid Withdrawal Using General Anesthesia

The subjective discomfort associated with opioid withdrawal and the high rate of relapse to illicit opioid use during methadone withdrawal has led to the development of procedures that withdraw methadone over relatively short periods while maintaining a patient under general anesthesia. In many cases the patient is transitioned from methadone to the opioid antagonist naltrexone while sedated. This technique generally has been called "ultrarapid opioid detoxification" (UROD) (O'Connor and Kosten 1998).

Although UROD is not a new procedure (Loimer et al. 1988), interest in it increased in the late 1990s, especially when for-profit UROD clinics began opening in the United States, Israel, and elsewhere (Brewer et al. 1998; Stephenson 1997). Reports on the efficacy of UROD began to appear in the scientific literature around this time; they suggest that outcomes from this treatment are variable, in part, because of different definitions of success. When defined with the narrow goal of achieving initial abstinence at the end of the procedure, UROD appears to be very successful; but, if the goal of treatment is maintenance of abstinence, then UROD appears to be no more effective than other procedures for withdrawing opioids such as methadone detoxification (Bochud Tornay et al. 2003; Cucchia et al. 1998; Gold et al. 1999; Krabbe et al. 2003). Some reports suggest UROD can be associated with relatively good long-term outcomes (Albanese et al. 2000; Elman et al. 2001; Laheij et al. 2000), although these reports tend to contain small numbers of patients or descriptive outcomes with no control conditions.

UROD can also be expensive, and of particular concern have been reports on complications associated with UROD (Allhoff et al. 1999; Hamilton et al. 2002; O'Connor and Kosten 1998; Stephenson 1997). For these reasons (cost, potential risks, and questionable long-term efficacy), there appears to have been a decrease in UROD use in more recent years.

SUMMARY AND CONCLUSIONS REGARDING METHADONE INDUCTION AND WITHDRAWAL

Starting a patient on methadone is relatively simple. Once it has been determined that the patient qualifies for methadone treatment, a first-day dose of 20–40 mg can be given. If a low dose is used (i.e., 20 mg), then there is the option of giving a second, smaller dose on the same day. Subsequent dose increases of 5–10 mg every other day should be given, until the patient is either stabilized on an adequate maintenance dose or there is evidence of excessive dosing. There is relatively little variability in the procedures used for methadone dose induction.

By contrast, there is considerable variability in the procedures used for methadone withdrawal. Several lessons can be drawn from the studies of methadone withdrawal reviewed in this chapter. First, for many patients methadone withdrawal does not result in sustained, complete abstinence from illicit opioid use, but it can result in a decrease in opioid use (compared with pretreatment levels of use) after completion of the withdrawal. Second, little benefit is derived from conducting the withdrawal on an inpatient versus outpatient service; although initial rates of abstinence are higher for inpatients (because they are under constant supervision), long-term rates of abstinence do not appear to be any better. Third, better outcomes are associated with more gradual withdrawal schedules accomplished over longer periods. Thus, a 90-day withdrawal is better than a 21-day withdrawal, and a 180-day withdrawal is probably even better. Finally, in general, it is better if methadone withdrawals are not done blindly; that is, it is better to inform patients about the dosing changes in their withdrawal. With these methods, patients can be comfortably and successfully inducted onto methadone, and outcomes for withdrawal can be optimized.

References

Albanese AP, Gevirtz C, Oppenheim B, Field JM, Abels I, Eustace JC (2000). Outcome and six month follow up of patients after Ultra Rapid Opiate Detoxification (UROD). *J Addict Dis* 19: 11–28.

Allhoff T, Renzing-Köhler K, Kienbaum P, Sack S, Scherbaum N (1999). Electrocardiographic abnormalities during recovery from ultra-short opiate detoxification. *Addict Biol* 4: 337–44.

Amato L, Davoli M, Ferri M, Gowing L, Perucci CA (2004). Effectiveness of interventions on opiate withdrawal treatment: an overview of systematic reviews. *Drug Alcohol Depend* 73: 219–26.

Bochud Tornay C, Favrat B, Monnat M, Daeppen JB, Schnyder C, Bertschy G, Besson J (2003). Ultra-rapid opiate detoxification using deep sedation and prior oral buprenorphine preparation: long-term results. *Drug Alcohol Depend* 69: 283–8.

Brewer C, Williams J, Carreno Rendueles E, Garcia JB (1998). Unethical promotion of rapid opiate detoxification under anaesthesia (RODA). *Lancet* 351: 218.

Buster MC, van Brussel GH, van den Brink W (2002). An increase in overdose mortality during the first 2 weeks after entering or re-entering methadone treatment in Amsterdam. *Addiction* 97: 993–1001.

Caplehorn JR, Drummer OH (1999). Mortality associated with New South Wales methadone programs in 1994: lives lost and saved. *Med J Aust* 170: 104–9.

Caplehorn JRM (1998). Deaths in the first two weeks of maintenance treatment in NSW in 1994: identifying cases of iatrongenic methadone toxicity. *Drug Alcohol Rev* 17: 9–17.

Cheung MW, Pugliese AC (1973). A hospital-based methadone program. Ambulatory induction phase. *J Med Soc N J* 70: 571–3.

Cucchia AT, Monnat M, Spagnoli J, Ferrero F, Bertschy G (1998). Ultra-rapid opiate detoxification using deep sedation with oral midazolam: short and long-term results. *Drug Alcohol Depend* 52: 243–50.

Cushman P, Dole VP (1973). Detoxification of rehabilitated methadone-maintained patients. *JAMA* 226: 747–52.

Elman I, D'Ambra MN, Krause S, Breiter H, Kane M, Morris R, Tuffy L, Gastfriend DR (2001). Ultrarapid opioid detoxification: effects on cardiopulmonary physiology, stress hormones and clinical outcomes. *Drug Alcohol Depend* 61: 163–72.

Freymuth HW (1971). Rapid induction of methadone maintenance in heroin addicts. *J Med Soc N J* 68: 729–32.

Gearing FR (1970). Successes and failures in methadone maintenance treatment of heroin addiction in New York City. Proceedings Third National Conference on Methadone Treatment, sponsored by National Association for the Prevention of Addiction to Narcotics (NAPAN) and cosponsored by National Institute of Mental Health, New York City, 2–16.

Gold CG, Cullen DJ, Gonzales S, Houtmeyers D, Dwyer MJ (1999). Rapid opioid detoxification during general anesthesia: a review of 20 patients. *Anesthesiology* 91: 1639–47.

Goldstein A (1970). Dosage, duration, side effects: blind controlled dosage comparisons with methadone in 200 patients. Proceedings of the Third National Conference on

Methadone Treatment, sponsored by National Association for the Prevention of Addiction to Narcotics (NAPAN) and cosponsored by National Institute of Mental Health, New York City, 31–37.

Goldstein A (1971). Blind dosage comparisons and other studies in a large methadone program. *J Psychedelic Drugs* 4: 177–81.

Gossop M, Bradley B, Phillips GT (1987). An investigation of withdrawal symptoms shown by opiate addicts during and subsequent to a 21-day in-patient methadone detoxification procedure. *Addict Behav* 12: 1–6

Gossop M, Griffiths P, Bradley B, Strang J (1989). Opiate withdrawal symptoms in response to 10-day and 21-day methadone withdrawal programmes. *Br J Psychiatry* 154: 360–3.

Gossop M, Johns A, Green L (1986). Opiate withdrawal: inpatient versus outpatient programmes and preferred versus random assignment to treatment. *Br Med J (Clin Res Ed)* 293: 103–4.

Green L, Gossop M (1988). Effects of information on the opiate withdrawal syndrome. *Br J Addict* 83: 305–9.

Hamilton RJ, Olmedo RE, Shah S, Hung OL, Howland MA, Perrone J, Nelson LS, Lewin NL, Hoffman RS (2002). Complications of ultrarapid opioid detoxification with subcutaneous naltrexone pellets. *Acad Emerg Med* 9: 63–68.

IOM (1995). *Federal Regulation of Methadone Treatment*. Washington, DC: National Academy Press.

Krabbe PF, Koning JP, Heinen N, Laheij RJ, van Cauter RM, De Jong CA (2003). Rapid detoxification from opioid dependence under general anaesthesia versus standard methadone tapering: abstinence rates and withdrawal distress experiences. *Addict Biol* 8: 351–8.

Kremen E (1973). New choices for methadone maintenance patients: planned, voluntary long-term detoxification. Proceedings of the Fifth National Conference on Methadone Treatment. Washington, DC: National Association for the Prevention of Addiction to Narcotics, 667–74.

Laheij RJ, Krabbe PF, de Jong CA (2000). Rapid heroin detoxification under general anesthesia. *JAMA* 283: 1143.

Loimer N, Schmid R, Presslich O, Lenz K (1988). Naloxone treatment for opiate withdrawal syndrome. *Br J Psychiatry* 153: 851–2.

Maddux JF, Desmond DP, Esquivel M (1980). Outpatient methadone withdrawal for heroin dependence. *Am J Drug Alcohol Abuse* 7: 323–33.

Nichols AW, Salwen MB, Torrens PR (1971). Outpatient induction to methadone maintenance treatment for heroin addiction. *Arch Intern Med* 127: 903–9.

O'Connor PG, Kosten TR (1998). Rapid and ultrarapid opioid detoxification techniques. *JAMA* 279: 229–34.

Payte JT, Khuri ET (1993). Principles of methadone dose determination. In: Parrino MW, ed. State Methadone Treatment Guidelines (Treatment Improvement Protocol (TIP)), 47–58. Rockville, MD: U.S. Department of Health and Human Services.

Robles E, Stitzer ML, Strain EC, Bigelow GE, Silverman K (2002). Voucher-based reinforcement of opiate abstinence during methadone detoxification. *Drug Alcohol Depend* 65: 179–89.

Sees KL, Delucchi KL, Masson C, Rosen A, Clark HW, Robillard H, Banys P, Hall SM (2000). Methadone maintenance vs 180-day psychosocially enriched detoxification for treatment of opioid dependence: a randomized controlled trial. *JAMA* 283: 1303–10.

Senay EC, Dorus W, Goldberg F, Thornton W (1977). Withdrawal from methadone maintenance. Rate of withdrawal and expectation. *Arch Gen Psychiatry* 34: 361–7.

Senay EC, Dorus W, Showalter C (1984). Methadone detoxification: self versus physician regulation. *Am J Drug Alcohol Abuse* 10: 361–74.

Sorensen JL, Hargreaves WA, Weinberg JA (1982). Withdrawal from heroin in three or six weeks. Comparison of methadyl acetate and methadone. *Arch Gen Psychiatry* 39: 167–71.

Stephenson J (1997). Experts debate merits of 1-day opiate detoxification under anesthesia. *JAMA* 277: 363–4.

Stimmel B, Goldberg J, Rotkopf E, Cohen M (1977). Ability to remain abstinent after methadone detoxification. A six-year study. *JAMA* 237: 1216–20.

Stimmel B, Rabin J, Engel C (1973). The prognosis of patients detoxified from methadone maintenance: a follow-up study. Proceedings of Fifth National Conference on Methadone Treatment, 270–4. Washington, DC: National Association for the Prevention of Addiction to Narcotics.

Stitzer ML, Bigelow GE, Liebson IA (1981). Comparison of three outpatient methadone detoxification procedures. In: Harris LS, ed. Problems of Drug Dependence, 1981. Proceedings of the 43rd Annual Scientific Meeting, Committee on Problems of Drug Dependence, 239–45. Rockville, MD: Department of Health and Human Services, National Institute on Drug Abuse.

Stitzer ML, McCaul ME, Bigelow GE, Liebson I (1983). Treatment outcome in methadone detoxification: relationship to initial levels of illicit opiate use. *Drug Alcohol Depend* 12: 259–67.

Strain EC, Stitzer ML, Liebson IA, Bigelow GE (1994). Outcome after methadone treatment: influence of prior treatment factors and current treatment status. *Drug Alcohol Depend* 35: 223–30.

Strang J, Gossop M (1990). Comparison of linear versus inverse exponential methadone reduction curves in the detoxification of opiate addicts. *Addict Behav* 15: 541–7.

Vormfelde SV, Poser W (2001). Death attributed to methadone. *Pharmacopsychiatry* 34: 217–22.

Wilson BK, Elms RR, Thomson CP (1975). Outpatient vs hospital methadone detoxification: an experimental comparison. *Int J Addict* 10: 13–21.

6

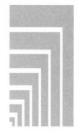

Methadone Dose during Maintenance Treatment

Eric C. Strain, M.D.

Despite more than 35 years of clinical use of methadone for the treatment of opioid dependence, appropriate dosing remains controversial. For virtually all other classes of pharmacotherapies used in medicine, such as antibiotics, antihypertensives, and antidepressants, clear guidelines exist for appropriate drug dosing. Even medications used to treat other substance use disorders, such as nicotine replacement products for smoking cessation, have well-established recommendations for dosing. However, the average dose of methadone can vary widely, with some clinics practicing low-dose philosophies and others using high doses. For example, a survey published in 1990 by the U.S. General Accounting Office (GAO) of dosing practices in 24 methadone programs in eight states of the United States found that average daily maintenance doses ranged from 21 to 68 mg (GAO 1990). A more recent survey of methadone-dosing practices in the United States found average dose levels had increased, but that 13 percent of patients received doses of less than 40 mg per day (D'Aunno and Pollack 2002). Similar evidence of dosing practices in other countries is not readily available, so it is not clear if the wide variations in methadone dosing are unique to the United States.

The many studies and reports on methadone dosing generally fall into one of two categories: surveys of the methadone dose used in treatment settings and controlled clinical trials. Surveys report results from the use of methadone in clinical settings, in which patients and staff are aware of the doses used, doses are individualized based on each patient's clinical response, and the effectiveness of dose can be influenced by nonpharmacologic treatments provided. Controlled clinical trials, on the other hand, provide a more focused assessment of medication effect conducted under conditions in which treatment is standardized (rather than individualized) across patients. Although the methods of controlled clinical trials are different from usual clinical practice, it is encouraging that studies looking at methadone dosing show similar outcomes whether data are collected from surveys of community treatment clinics or controlled clinical trials in treatment research clinics.

The primary question behind the issue of methadone dosing is whether higher doses are more effective than lower doses: if 50 mg per day is good, is 100 mg per day even better? Underlying this question, however, is the assumption that methadone is effective in treating opioid dependence. This assumption can be tested by finding out whether patients receiving active methadone have better outcomes than those receiving placebo. Although this chapter's main focus is on treatment outcome across active methadone doses, it is also important to answer this more fundamental question.

This chapter has three sections. The first section, a historical overview of methadone dosing, helps place subsequent issues into a larger context. The second section examines the efficacy of methadone treatment based on surveys. The third section reviews controlled clinical trials of methadone dosing—first as compared with placebos, then trials that have tested different doses of methadone. Finally, this last section addresses a series of topics related to methadone dosing such as the value of predictors of treatment outcome, the use of methadone blood levels in treatment, and the side effects that can be associated with methadone. The chapter concludes with recommendations regarding the optimal dosing of methadone.

HISTORICAL OVERVIEW TO METHADONE DOSING

One of the first evaluations of methadone's effects in humans was published in 1948 by a team of investigators from the U.S. Public Health Service Hospital in Lexington, Kentucky (Isbell et al. 1948). This report described a set of studies, including the assessment of direct addiction to methadone in 15 former morphine addicts. Methadone was given by injection four times daily, and daily doses reached as high as 600–800 mg per day in two subjects. However, at this high dose signs of toxicity, which were not described specifically, appeared and therefore the dose was decreased to 200–400 mg per day. Thus, results from this early study show that humans can tolerate remarkably high doses of methadone when the dose is gradually increased under careful supervision.

Although the first clinical use of methadone for the treatment of opioid dependence is generally associated with reports in the early 1960s by Vincent Dole, Marie Nyswander, and Mary Jeanne Kreek (as described subsequently), methadone treatment was, in fact, piloted in Canada in the late 1950s and early 1960s (Williams 1971). In 1959 the Narcotic Addiction Foundation of British Columbia began dispensing methadone for brief, 12-day detoxifications, and in early 1963 expanded this program to include a more prolonged period of outpatient methadone treatment. The average methadone dose used in this expanded program was 40 mg per day.

However, this early use of methadone for the outpatient treatment of opioid dependence gained little attention in the medical treatment and research communities. Not until studies by Dole, Nyswander, and Kreek were published in the American Medical Association's journal *JAMA* did methadone treatment gain widespread attention and interest. These studies were conducted at the Rockefeller Institute in New York in the 1960s. Small groups of patients were admitted to an inpatient research ward where they lived for relatively long periods (i.e., 6 weeks) (Dole and Nyswander 1965). Doses of methadone were initially given twice daily, starting at 10–20 mg per dose, and gradually increased over several weeks to stabilization doses of 50–150 mg per day (although doses as high as 180 mg were reported). Clearly, these techniques (long inpatient hospitalizations, divided doses, gradual escalation of doses over time, intensive supervision of treatment by physicians and staff) are not typical of today's methadone treatment. Outcomes were good, both with respect to elimination of illicit drug use and with regard to other, non-drug-related measures such as employment.

After these promising results, several scientific papers reported on outcomes from the use of different doses of methadone in more controlled clinical trials conducted in the 1970s. In addition, reports by clinicians about their experience with low- versus high-dose methadone were published. These papers reported on the evaluation of a variety of widely dispersed daily methadone doses. Conclusions from these studies as well as numerous other methadone-dosing studies and surveys are described next.

METHADONE'S EFFICACY: EVIDENCE FROM SURVEYS

There have been several investigations of methadone efficacy utilizing surveys of methadone clinics, as well as clinicians' reports of their experience with methadone dosing. This section provides a review of results from several of these reports.

Drug Abuse Reporting Program (DARP)

The DARP assessed patients entering a variety of treatment modalities in the United States, including methadone maintenance treatment, between 1969 and 1973. Patients were subsequently followed for various periods (e.g., 12-year follow-up reports for patients with opioid dependence were summarized in a book by Simpson and Sells [1990]). In general, results from the DARP show that three different treatment interventions—methadone maintenance, therapeutic communities, and outpatient drug-free counseling—are all effective for opioid dependence. Patients in each of these modalities did better than patients who only attended an intake assessment but failed to follow through with treatment, or patients who received a detoxification without follow-up treatment. Furthermore, results from the DARP showed favorable outcomes when patients remained in treatment for at least three months; those who remained in the three effective modalities for less than three months had outcomes similar to those who just went through intake alone or detoxification alone. Finally, outcomes from the DARP showed that the longer patients remained in treatment, the better the outcomes. Note that the DARP did not evaluate different methadone doses; therefore, conclusions about different outcomes for different methadone doses cannot be drawn from these reports. However, the DARP does provide results from an early, large survey showing methadone treatment is effective.

Treatment Outcome Prospective Study (TOPS)

The TOPS was a survey of drug abuse treatment outcome for the period 1979–1981, and it shared many features of the DARP (Hubbard et al. 1989). Like the DARP, patients entering treatment programs were assessed (i.e., patients were not randomly assigned to particular treatments), a variety of treatment modalities were evaluated (including methadone maintenance), and follow-up assessments were conducted at regular intervals. The TOPS assessed patients enrolled in 37 treatment programs in ten cities in the United States.

The TOPS did collect data about methadone dosing. After three months in methadone treatment, 40 percent of patients were receiving methadone doses below 30 mg per day, and doses were highly variable across treatment programs. Despite these relatively low doses, results from the TOPS indicate marked improvements associated with methadone treatment, especially for those patients who remained in treatment longer. Whereas the DARP results suggested 3 months as the minimum time needed to effect positive changes with methadone treatment, the TOPS found that at least 6–12 months of treatment were needed. Among patients receiving methadone who stayed in treatment for at least three months, 64 percent had regular (weekly or daily) heroin use in the year before treatment entry (with the remaining one-third primarily using other opioids or transferring from another methadone program). Three to five years after their episode of methadone treatment, this 64 percent had decreased to about 18 percent who were regular heroin users.

Drug Abuse Treatment Outcome Study (DATOS)

The DATOS is a survey study that is similar in design and methods to the DARP and the TOPS. It was conducted in the United States between 1991 and 1993 and assessed 10,010 admissions to 96 different substance abuse treatment programs. In addition to outpatient methadone treatment, which comprised 29 of the programs surveyed, the DATOS study also sampled patients entering three other treatment modalities: long-term residential, outpatient drug-free, and short-term inpatient treatment (Flynn et al. 1997). Unlike the DARP and TOPS projects, primary results from DATOS have not been published in a single book but have appeared in numerous journal articles and include both one- and five-year follow-up assessments (Hubbard et al. 1997).

With respect to methadone treatment, results from the DATOS provide further support for the effectiveness of this treatment (Flynn et al. 2003). For example, 89 percent of patients receiving methadone reported weekly or more frequent heroin use in the year before treatment entry; at the time of the one-year follow-up, this had decreased to 28 percent (Hubbard et al. 1997). Better outcomes were associated with remaining in treatment for more than one year (Simpson et al. 1997). However, information from the DATOS about methadone treatment outcome as a function of methadone dose has not yet been presented.

Effectiveness of Methadone Maintenance Treatment Study

Unlike the previous three reports, the Effectiveness of Methadone Maintenance Treatment Study (sometimes referred to as the Ball and Ross study), conducted in the mid-1980s, examined specifically and only methadone treatment. In this study, six methadone programs in three East Coast cities of the United States (Baltimore, New York, Philadelphia) were intensively investigated (Ball and Ross 1991). The programmatic aspects of each clinic as well as the patients in each program were evaluated. Patients were assessed while in their methadone program, and then followed for one year, with a second assessment at the end of that year, regardless of whether they were still in treatment at the program.

The results provide a wealth of descriptive information about the characteristics of methadone programs as well as the patients in methadone treatment. There were wide variations in dosing practices among the six programs, with mean doses as low as 26 mg in one program and as high as 66 mg in another. Aggregating the results for all programs, most patients were prescribed a daily methadone dose between 30 and 69 mg, and the average dose for all patients evaluated was 47 mg per day. Notably, methadone dose level was inversely related to self-reported heroin use in the 30 days before the follow-up interview; that is, patients receiving higher doses of methadone reported fewer days of heroin use. Methadone dose was not associated with all outcome measures assessed in this study, however (e.g., cocaine use, days of criminal activity).

Institute for Social Research Survey

The Institute for Social Research Survey, first conducted in the fall of 1988, was a survey of 172 methadone treatment programs in the United States (D'Aunno and Vaughn 1992). Follow-up surveys were conducted in 1990, 1995, and 2000 (D'Aunno and Pollack 2002), although these did not include all the original 172 programs and had some new programs added. Results from this survey show that although the majority of doses prescribed have been in the 40- to 79-mg range, since 1988 there has been a steady increase in the proportion of patients treated with higher doses of methadone ($\geq$80 mg), and a corresponding decline in the proportion of patients treated with lower doses (fig. 6.1). For example, in 1988 nearly one-half of patients (45%) received daily doses of less than 40 mg; this had declined to 13 percent by 2000. Correspondingly, whereas only 6 percent of patients were receiving daily doses of 80 mg or higher in 1988, this had increased to 32 percent by the year 2000. The results from this

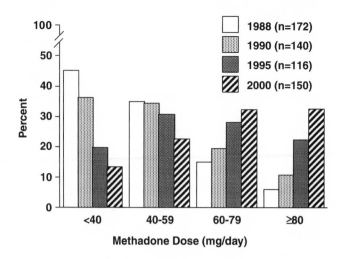

Figure 6.1. Methadone-dosing practice over time from surveys conducted in the United States. Numbers shown for each year are the number of treatment programs surveyed. Data from D'Aunno and Pollack 2002.

survey provide highly useful data on the changing dosing practices in the United States.

National Treatment Outcome Research Study (NTORS)

The surveys described above were all conducted in the United States. In contrast, the NTORS was carried out in the United Kingdom between March and July of 1995 and assessed 1,075 patients at entry to one of 54 treatment programs (Gossop et al. 1998). Of these 54 programs, 16 were methadone maintenance clinics (458 patients), and a further 15 were methadone reduction programs (209 patients). Follow-up assessments have been reported for six-month (Gossop et al. 1997, 1999), one-year (Gossop et al. 2000), two-year (Gossop et al. 2001, 2003b), and four- to five-year outcomes (Gossop et al. 2003a).

Drawing on a sample of 240 patients who were maintained on methadone , the NTORS found the mean methadone maintenance dose was 52 mg, with a small percentage of patients (6%) receiving less than 30 mg per day, the majority (71%) receiving between 30–60 mg per day, and nearly one-quarter (23%) receiving more than 60 mg per day (Gossop et al. 2001). Higher doses of methadone were associated with less heroin use (Gossop et al. 2003c), and methadone reduction treatment (detoxification) was associated with poorer outcomes when compared with maintenance treatment (Gossop et al. 2001). Although the primary impact of methadone treatment as assessed by the proportion of patients able to achieve abstinence from heroin tended to occur in the first year of treatment, further improvements in the proportion of patients maintained on methadone who achieved heroin abstinence continued at even four to five years after treatment entry (Gossop et al. 2003a). These results demonstrating the efficacy of methadone treatment in the United Kingdom nicely complement work from other countries and show the efficacy of methadone treatment need not be viewed as specific to a particular culture.

Other Survey Studies

A multitude of other reports have examined the relationship between methadone treatment and outcome based on results from naturalistic studies. In general, these studies have shown that higher doses result in better treatment retention (Caplehorn and Bell 1991; Craig 1980) and lower rates of illicit opioid use (Bell et al. 1995; Caplehorn et al. 1993; Hartel et al. 1995), but not all studies have uniformly found such results (Maddux et al. 1991; Siassi et al. 1977). Negative studies have often involved smaller numbers of patients; therefore, these exceptions may be attributed to such study limitations.

Conclusions from Survey Studies

These survey studies provide valuable information about the use of methadone treatment in community-based treatment clinics. Their strength lies in the large numbers of patients assessed and the inclusion of other treatment modalities that can function as comparison conditions. Overall, results from survey studies produce two conclusions: first, methadone treatment is effective (as measured by treatment retention and reduction in illicit opioid use), and second, higher methadone doses are more effective than lower doses. The limitations of survey studies, however, can best be addressed through controlled clinical trials. The next section reviews results from these complementary studies of methadone's efficacy.

METHADONE'S EFFICACY: EVIDENCE FROM CONTROLLED CLINICAL TRIALS

Controlled clinical trials seek to determine a medication's "true" effect, uninfluenced by expectations and biases (e.g., special encouragement or discouragement from staff), and the type or intensity of nonpharmacologic treatments. Therefore, they use special procedures, including double-blind dosing (neither patients nor staff are allowed to know what doses are being given to individual patients), random assignment to treatments, and standardized counseling interventions. In actual practice, the effectiveness of a medication may be better or worse than what is shown in clinical trials because of the operation of the factors that are controlled in clinical trials. The first half of this section is a review of controlled clinical trials in which active methadone was compared with placebo methadone. Only a limited number of such placebo-controlled studies have been conducted, however. The second half of this section reviews controlled clinical trials testing the relative efficacy of different doses of methadone, a research topic that has been studied much more extensively.

Methadone Compared with Placebo

There are only two known placebo-controlled studies examining the efficacy of methadone treatment. Although this is somewhat surprising, it is understandable, given the history of the development of methadone for opioid dependence. Most early methadone clinical trials implicitly accepted the premise that methadone worked, in part, because there were no other available effective medications for opioid dependence at the time of methadone's development. In addition, placebo-controlled studies in the treatment of opioid dependence could be difficult to implement if the design required patients to start on placebo, because the inevitable opioid withdrawal would result in high rates of dropout from the study. However, one must bear in mind that the robust outcomes found in early studies of methadone treatment may have partly reflected the enthusiasm and intensive attention given to patients by the investigators, as acknowledged by the authors of these reports. Thus, how patients respond when given placebo medication would be of great interest, because the relative efficacy of only nonpharmacologic factors, such as counseling, could then be quantified.

The first placebo-controlled study was conducted in Hong Kong between 1972 and 1975. In this study, 100 opioid abusers enrolled in a double-blind clinical trial (Newman and Whitehill 1979). All subjects were initially hospitalized for two weeks and stabilized on 60 mg of methadone daily. On discharge from the hospital, patients assigned to the placebo group received dose reductions of 1 mg per day for 60 days and then were maintained on placebo. Patients maintained on methadone could have double-blind dose adjustments, with a maximum daily dose of 130 mg. The mean dose at the end of the first year of the study was 97 mg for the maintenance group (range, 30–130 mg).

At the end of 32 weeks, only 10 percent of the placebo group remained in the study versus 76 percent of the methadone group. Most of the patients in the placebo group were removed from the study because of persistent illicit opioid use based on urine testing, although a substantial proportion of patients in the placebo group also dropped out of the study and treatment. In addition to evidence of better treatment retention and lower rates of illicit opioid use for patients receiving methadone maintenance, rates of criminal activity were markedly lower for patients in the methadone than in the placebo group.

Thus, results from this study provide strong evidence that methadone is superior to placebo in the outpatient treatment of opioid dependence. One liability to this study is that the nonpharmacologic treatment was poorly described; the report does note that staff had no prior experience with methadone treatment. Thus, placebo response rates might have been higher if patients had received nonpharmacologic treatment from staff familiar with counseling opioid-dependent patients. Also, because patients in the placebo group knew they could get active methadone if they dropped out, these results support the conclusion that active methadone treatment is not just acceptable, but desirable to opioid-dependent individuals.

The second placebo-controlled study of methadone treatment was conducted in Baltimore, Maryland, in the late 1980s. In this study, 247 opioid-dependent subjects enrolled in a treatment/research clinic (Strain et al. 1993a, 1993b). This study has no inpatient portion; patients were not in treatment at the time of study entry and were actively abusing illicit opioids. Participants were admitted directly to methadone treatment and randomly assigned to one of three dose groups: 0, 20, or 50 mg per day. All subjects were initially maintained on methadone, with dose adjustments made during the first six weeks so that final stabilization doses were achieved during week 6 of treatment. Patients assigned to the 0-mg dose group received a gradual dose taper during the first six weeks and were maintained on double-blind placebo medication thereafter. The stable dosing period lasted 14 weeks for all participants. In addition, all study participants received individual therapy from an experienced counselor, were given the opportunity to participate in group therapy, and had access to on-site primary care medical services.

Results from this study clearly showed that patients receiving 50 mg of methadone per day did better than those who received 0 mg per day (fig. 6.2). About 20 percent of patients receiving placebo methadone, however, remained in treatment through the 14 weeks of the study, suggesting that significant elements of methadone treatment reside in its non-

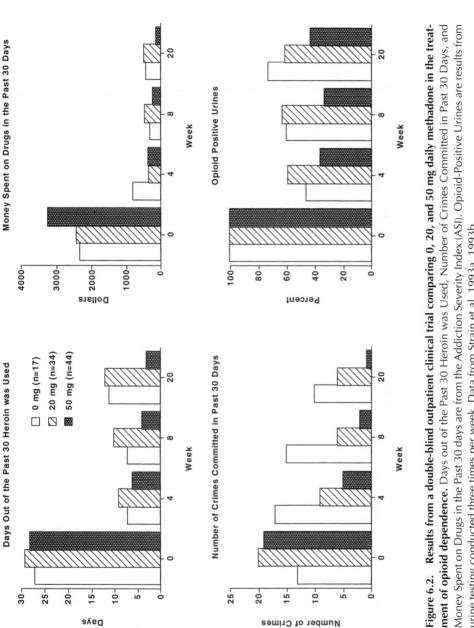

Figure 6.2. Results from a double-blind outpatient clinical trial comparing 0, 20, and 50 mg daily methadone in the treatment of opioid dependence. Days out of the Past 30 Heroin was Used, Number of Crimes Committed in Past 30 Days, and Money Spent on Drugs in the Past 30 days are from the Addiction Severity Index (ASI). Opioid-Positive Urines are results from urine testing conducted three times per week. Data from Strain et al. 1993a, 1993b.

pharmacologic aspects (e.g., nursing contact, counseling). Finally, this study found methadone treatment also produced improvements in a broad array of other areas beyond illicit opioid use (Strain et al. 1993b). These improvements were seen for patients on doses of both 50 and 0 mg of methadone, but the greatest improvements occurred for patients assigned to the 50-mg dose group. Thus, for example, the number of crimes committed decreased dramatically, as did illegal income and days of illegal activity. Such dramatic reductions in criminal activity are one of the most important benefits to society associated with methadone treatment. In addition, self-reports showed marked reductions in depressive symptoms and reductions in complaints of withdrawal symptoms (although these complaints did rise again over time for patients in the 0-mg dose group). Overall, the two controlled clinical trials described provide compelling evidence that methadone is superior to placebo in the outpatient treatment of opioid dependence.

Methadone Dose Effects

Results from survey studies show that higher doses seem to produce better outcomes than lower doses. This section reviews the relationship between specific methadone doses and treatment outcome. Although methadone would be expected to produce favorable outcomes on measures of illicit opiate use, other outcome measures associated with a lifestyle of illicit drug use also have been examined in several of these studies and are reviewed. This is not an exhaustive review of the methadone-dosing literature; rather, selected topics and illustrative studies are presented. Results from single-blind studies of methadone dosing are reviewed first, followed by outcomes from double-blind studies.

Outcomes from Single-Blind Methadone-Dosing Studies

Several reports have been based on single-blind studies of methadone treatment. Single-blind studies are not as methodologically rigorous as double-blind studies, because staff having contact with study patients may know the dose assignment. Thus, it is possible for staff biases to influence outcome in single-blind studies, and it is also possible staff may inadvertently (or intentionally!) inform patients about their dose assignment, which can introduce biases held by the patients themselves.

Two of these studies examined doses of 30, 50, and 100 mg (Garbutt and Goldstein 1972; Goldstein 1970), a third tested doses of 40, 80, and 160 mg per day (Goldstein and Judson 1973), and a more contemporary fourth study compared 50 and 80 mg (Rhoades et al. 1998). Results from these clinical trials suggest that differences among widely different doses are only slight. Thus, there was no difference between doses of 30, 50, and 100 mg with respect to treatment retention, and only a minimal difference between 50 and 80 mg (when clinic visit frequency was twice per week), although patients in higher-dose groups had somewhat lower rates of opioid-free urines. Another surprising observation was that 80- and 160-mg doses produced very similar outcomes on measures of both treatment retention and heroin use.

Conclusions from Single-Blind Studies of Methadone Dosing

These single-blind studies are of interest, especially because the early studies frequently concluded that there were few significant clinical differences between high and low doses of methadone—an observation that probably contributed to the eventual decision to use lower doses of methadone in some treatment programs. One must recognize, however, that these studies have methodological limitations and that the question of the relative efficacy of different methadone doses is best addressed in more rigorous, double-blind clinical trials.

Outcomes from Double-Blind Studies of Methadone Dosing

Several well-designed and conducted double-blind clinical trials of methadone dosing have been conducted, and seven of these studies are briefly summarized here (table 6.1). Several other early studies testing methadone dose in double-blind clinical trials were also conducted (Berry and Kuhn 1973; Jaffe 1971) and are included in table 6.1. Note, however, that some of these studies have other methodological limitations despite their use of double-blind dosing; the limitations of earlier studies are well summarized in the review by Hargreaves (1983).

Some double-blind studies that compared more than one methadone dose were conducted to answer questions other than about methadone's dose-related efficacy, but nevertheless they provide valuable information on the topic of dosing. For example, in the early 1970s an important double-blind study of methadone dose effects was conducted as part of the assessment of the efficacy of LAAM for the treatment of opioid dependence (Ling et al. 1976). This was a multisite Veterans Affairs cooperative study comparing LAAM with two doses of methadone, 50 and 100 mg per day. Four hundred thirty patients enrolled in the 40-week study (288 of these were on methadone). With respect to treatment retention,

Table 6.1 **Summary of Double-Blind Methadone-Dosing Studies**

Study	Total Number of Patients*	Methadone Doses Studied	Treatment Retention	Illicit Opioid Use
Jaffe 1971	63	Varied; averages were 36 mg and 100 mg	No difference between groups	No difference between groups
Berry and Kuhn 1973	52	50 mg and 100 mg	No difference between groups	No difference between groups
Ling et al. 1976	288	50 mg and 100 mg	100 mg had slightly better retention	100 mg had less illicit opioid use
Johnson et al. 1992	109	20 mg and 60 mg	60 mg had better retention	60 mg had less illicit opioid use
Kosten et al. 1993	69	35 mg and 65 mg	No difference between groups	No difference between groups
Strain et al. 1993a	166	20 mg and 50 mg	50 mg had better retention	50 mg had less illicit opioid use
Banys et al. 1994	38	40 mg and 80 mg	No difference between groups	Trend for 80 mg to have less illicit opioid use
Ling et al. 1996	150	30 mg and 80 mg	80 mg had better retention	80 mg had less illicit opioid use
Schottenfeld et al. 1997	58	20 mg and 65 mg	65 mg better (but unknown if significant)	65 mg had less illicit opioid use
Strain et al. 1999	192	Range of 40–50 mg and 80–100 mg	No difference between groups	80–100 mg had less illicit opioid use
Johnson et al. 2000	110	20 mg and range of 60–100 mg	60–100 mg had better retention	60–100 mg had less illicit opioid use

*Total number of patients who received methadone in the study.

the 100-mg group had slightly better retention than the 50-mg group at the end of the 40 weeks (52 and 42%, respectively). Similarly, results from urine testing for opioids showed that the 100-mg group did better than the 50-mg group. Notably, differences between the two methadone dose conditions were not great, but the results from this study did provide evidence that differential outcome between 50 and 100 mg of methadone can occur.

Five studies that tested the efficacy of buprenorphine included two methadone groups for comparison, so some conclusions regarding the efficacy of different doses of methadone can be drawn from these studies. Four studies examined outcomes for patients assigned to fixed doses within the same general range: 20 versus 60 mg of methadone per day (Johnson et al. 1992), 20 versus 65 mg per day (Schottenfeld et al. 1997), 35 versus 65 mg per day (Kosten et al. 1993), and 30 versus 80 mg per day. (Ling et al. 1996). All but Kosten et al. (1993) found both significantly better treatment retention and lower rates of opioid-positive urines for patients in the higher- versus the lower-dose groups. Significantly better results for the higher-dose group were also found in a fifth study that compared patients randomly assigned to either a fixed dose of 20 mg or a flexible dose that could range between 60 and 100 mg of methadone per day (Johnson et al. 2000).

A study by Strain and colleagues specifically examined the efficacy of different methadone doses (discussed in a previous section, as the study also included a placebo group) and included a comparison between 20 and 50 mg of methadone per day (Strain et al. 1993a, 1993b). Results from the study showed differences in treatment retention between the 20- and 50-mg dose groups, with the higher dose having better treatment retention than the lower dose. At the end of the 20-week study, 52 percent of patients in the 50-mg dose group were still in treatment, compared with 42 percent of patients in the 20-mg dose group. Subjects in this study provided urine samples for testing three times per week—an intensive schedule that is highly sensitive to detecting any illicit drug use, but relatively insensitive to detecting changes in drug use. There was a significantly lower rate of opioid-positive urine samples for the 50-mg dose group (56%) compared with the 20-mg dose group (68%) (fig. 6.2). Results for patients in the 20-mg group were not equivalent to those for patients in the placebo group. The 20-mg group had better treatment retention than the 0-mg group and lower rates of opioid use. Thus, the study shows that even a low dose of methadone can exert some beneficial effects.

A follow-up to the fixed-dose comparison described above (Strain et al. 1993a) examined the efficacy of moderate-dose methadone (40–50 mg per day) versus high-dose methadone (80–100 mg per day) using a flexible dosing procedure (Strain et al. 1999). Patients randomly assigned to the moderate-dose group were initially stabilized on 40 mg of methadone per day but could receive double-blind dose increases (to a maximum dose of 50 mg per day) if they continued to have opioid-positive urine samples. Similarly, patients assigned to the high-dose group were initially stabilized on 80 mg of methadone per day, but could receive double-blind dose increases (to a maximum dose of 100 mg per day) if they continued to have opioid-positive urine samples. Average doses were 46 and 90 mg per day for each of the groups. Results from this study showed there was no difference in treatment retention for the moderate- versus high-dose conditions, but that there was a significantly lower rate of opioid-positive urine samples for the high-dose group.

Double-Blind Studies of Methadone Dosing: Conclusions and Recommendations

The controversy regarding optimal methadone dosing becomes more understandable after reviewing results from clinical trials that have attempted to address whether higher doses of methadone are more effective than lower doses. The limited number of such studies, along with the strong recommendations from early single-blind studies that little difference exists between moderate- and high-dose methadone, provided little reason to challenge the wide variations in dosing found across treatment clinics.

However, the double-blind studies suggest there can be benefits in using higher (e.g., 80 mg and above) as compared with lower-dose methadone, with the primary benefit being a more substantial decrease in illicit opioid use. It is also very clear from the research that even moderate doses of 50–60 mg are better than low doses of 20–30 mg per day, based both on measures of treatment retention and on rates of illicit opioid use as determined by urine testing.

A few other points are worth discussing. First, no controlled clinical trials have assessed doses of methadone greater than 100 mg per day, although intriguing results from laboratory research show that doses greater than 100 mg may be necessary to provide complete blockade of heroin effects in many patients (Donny et al. 2002). It may be possible to achieve better outcomes with such higher doses of methadone, but more research is needed on this point. Second, extrapolating from well-designed and well-conducted clinical trials to actual clinical use should be done with caution. Outcomes could actually be better in clinical practice when features of a clinical trial such as double-blind dosing are not present, when more intensive nonpharmacologic treatments are used and when dosing is adjusted based on the purity and quantity of heroin being used by a particular patient. Thus, results from these double-blind studies may represent conservative estimates of treatment outcomes obtained under artificial circumstances without individualized treatment for each patient. On the other hand, some features of clinical trials, in particular, standardization of some interventions, may produce outcomes better than those likely to be seen in clinical practice.

Nevertheless, the results from these studies, along with other reviewed work (i.e., the various survey studies that have been conducted), suggest that substantial clinical gains, as defined by treatment retention and decreases in opioid-positive urine samples, can be achieved by raising doses from 20 mg per day to at least 50 mg per day. Further decreases in illicit opioid use can occur if the dose is increased up to a maximum of 100 mg per day or more. Thus, a target dose of at least 50 mg per day is clinically indicated, and doses of 100 mg per day or higher should be strongly considered, especially for patients who continue using illicit opioids during treatment.

ISSUES RELATED TO METHADONE DOSING

Predicting Outcome in Methadone Treatment and Patient-Treatment Matching

Patient-treatment matching can be defined as a proactive process in which the individual characteristics of a patient are addressed by specific aspects of the treatment service (Strain 2004). In general, studies of patient-treatment matching for patients with substance abuse disorders have failed to identify matching variables or matching procedures that have high clinical utility and are cost-effective. Most studies of patient-treatment matching have enrolled patients with a variety of substance abuse disorders (Gottheil et al. 2002; McLellan et al. 1997; Thornton et al. 1998) rather than specifically opioid dependence, and the few studies limited to opioid dependence have not yielded promising results (Belding et al. 1997, 1995).

Although our current knowledge about treatment-matching factors is limited, there are some patient characteristics that have been associated with better versus worse outcomes, and some early treatment responses have been identified that seem to be clinically useful for predicting subsequent behavior in usual-care methadone treatment (McLellan 1983).

The characteristic most consistently associated with treatment outcome is age: older patients tend to have better outcomes than younger patients. In addition, race (being nonwhite) and marital status (being married) are often associated with better treatment outcomes. Other characteristics sometimes associated with poor treatment outcome can include a history of criminal activity, psychological problems, and poor employment history (Farley et al. 1992; McLellan 1983).

In addition to these pretreatment factors, in-treatment predictors can influence treatment outcome. Thus, some features of the treatment itself, such as higher methadone dose, as reviewed above, and greater amounts of counseling services (McLellan et al. 1993; Strain et al. 1998) are associated with better outcomes. Finally, early treatment success or lack thereof, as determined through assessments such as urine testing and counseling attendance, can be highly predictive of subsequent treatment performance (Morral et al. 1999; Strain et al. 1998). For example, the amount of illicit opioid use detected in urine testing during the first two treatment weeks correlates with subsequent rates of opioid-positive urine samples, and a similar relationship between the first weeks of cocaine-positive urine samples and continued cocaine use has also been found (Strain et al. 1998). These relationships suggest that intensive urine monitoring for illicit drug use during the first weeks of methadone treatment may be useful in determining which patients should be assigned to continued intensive counseling and urine monitoring and which need not be monitored as closely. For example, patients who have no cocaine use during the first two weeks of treatment as assessed by urine testing are less likely to have subsequent cocaine use later in treatment.

Conclusions Regarding Patient-Treatment Matching and Predictors of Methadone Treatment Outcome

Although the idea of patient-treatment matching is intuitively attractive, the research on this topic is very limited with respect to opioid dependence and methadone treatment, and unfortunately, no clear clinical recommendations can be made regarding patient-treatment matching. Several patient characteristics are often associated with methadone treatment success, including age, marital status, and race, although none of these can definitively predict good treatment outcome. Similarly, some in-treatment factors, such as dose of methadone, amount of counseling contact, and early in-treatment drug use, can be associated with subsequent treatment success. However, none of these in-treatment factors are definitively associated with success.

Methadone Blood Levels

For some medications, blood levels can be used to determine the optimal dosing of the medication. Indeed, for many medications such as certain anticonvulsants and antidepressants, well-defined ranges for optimal therapeutic effects have been determined and dosing is titrated to achieve a blood level in that range. Given the wide variations in methadone dosing used in clinical practice, it is a logical step to ask whether differences in clinically assigned doses may reflect individual differences in absorption or metabolism such that patients with good clinical response end up with similar blood levels of methadone. Details regarding methadone's pharmacodynamic and pharmacokinetic effects can be found in chapter 4.

This section provides a review of the role of methadone blood levels in the management of patients.

Several studies have examined blood levels in patients receiving chronic doses of methadone and found that there are marked individual differences in these blood levels (Eap et al. 1998, 2002; Holmstrand et al. 1978; Horns et al. 1975; Kreek 1973b). For patients maintained on a stable dose of methadone, some evidence suggests that better outcomes are associated with trough (24-hour postdose) plasma concentrations greater than 150–200 ng/ml (Holmstrand et al. 1978; Loimer and Schmid 1992; Tennant et al. 1983), while levels below 50 ng/ml appear to be related to poor treatment outcome (Bell et al. 1988). However, not all studies have found that poor treatment outcome is associated with low methadone plasma levels (Torrens et al. 1998). Trough plasma levels greater than 250 ng/ml for the active enantiomer of methadone (R or l) may be a more effective measure than levels that assess both the R and S (or d) enantiomers of methadone (Eap et al. 2000). Note that methadone blood levels peak around the eighth day of dosing and then decline over subsequent days, so determinations should not be made before treatment has been ongoing for three to four weeks (Holmstrand et al. 1978).

In addition to variations during the initial time of stabilization on methadone, blood levels can also change if a patient is treated with certain other medications (see table 18.1 in chap.18). Thus, for example, enzyme-inducing medications such as phenobarbital or phenytoin can lower blood levels (Bell et al. 1988; Tong et al. 1981), as can the tuberculosis treatment medication rifampin (Kreek et al. 1976) and certain antiretrovirals (Boffito et al. 2002; McCance-Katz et al. 2003). Interactions with other medications that may be prescribed to patients receiving methadone maintenance such as antidepressants and antihypertensives have not been well characterized, although some evidence indicates that such medications may alter methadone's effects (Plummer et al. 1988).

It may be particularly useful under certain circumstances to obtain methadone blood levels. For example, sometimes patients report that their dose of methadone fails to provide adequate, 24-hour suppression of withdrawal. The clinician should check first for concurrent treatment with enzyme-inducing medications, as discussed above. However, rapid declines in blood levels have been found in some patients not treated with such medications (Tennant 1987), and some patients with higher CYP 3A4 activity may require higher doses of methadone (Shinderman et al. 2003). For patients who complain their dose does not provide 24-hour suppression of withdrawal, several methadone blood level tests done over a 24-hour period may show a rapid decline in blood levels that reveals a plausible biological basis for the self-reports (Nilsson et al. 1983; Walton et al. 1978). Such patients may benefit from a split (twice per day) dosing of methadone, so that their blood levels can be maintained at a more stable level.

Under most circumstances, however, methadone blood levels are not routinely used in clinical practice. Their use is probably best reserved for specialized conditions, such as when patients who are receiving an appropriate dose of methadone continue to report inadequate dosing and appear to be in opioid withdrawal when they return to the clinic, or when patients need treatment for other conditions with a medication that can alter methadone blood levels.

Methadone Side Effects (Table 6.2)

Overview to Methadone's Side Effects

The use of methadone in the treatment of opioid dependence is safe and entails few side effects. Formerly opioid-dependent subjects enrolled in the first human laboratory study of methadone were maintained on methadone for several weeks or months and intensively monitored for effects (Isbell et al. 1948). The most common effect initially noted was sedation, which occurred during the first days of methadone administration; tolerance quickly developed to this effect. Constipation was also noted, but tolerance did not develop to this effect. In addition, subjects showed mild decreases in heart rate (about 10 beats per minute) and respiratory rate (about 4 breaths per minute). Systolic blood pressure was slightly decreased during the first few months of methadone administration but then increased during subsequent months to levels that were still within the normal range. Thus, results from this first study show methadone produced no significant adverse side effects.

The first report by Dole and Nyswander (1965) noted only constipation and self-reported increased sweating as side effects to methadone treatment, which is especially significant given the intensive monitoring of these patients (e.g., bone marrow biopsies in four patients, blood and urine tests). Other early studies of methadone also reported constipation, excessive sweating, and sexual difficulties (Goldstein 1970; Kreek et al. 1972).

More systematic studies of the side effects of methadone have tended to replicate these early results. Thus, physiologic measures such as blood pressure, heart rate, respiratory rate, and pupil diameter tend to have mild decreases with chronic methadone dosing, whereas body temperature shows a mild increase (Gritz et al. 1975; Martin et al. 1973). All these ef-

Table 6.2 Side Effects Associated with Methadone Treatment

Changes in systolic blood pressure*
Constipation
Decrease in ejaculate volume
Decrease in heart rate[†]
Decrease in hemoglobin and hematocrit[†]
Decrease in pupil diameter[†]
Decrease in respiratory rate[†]
Decrease in seminal vesicular and prostatic secretions
Increase in sweating
Lower serum testosterone in males
Sedation[‡]
Sleep disturbances (primarily insomnia)
Slowing on EEG

*Direction varies depending on length of time taking methadone.
[†]Mild and not clinically significant.
[‡]Tolerance develops to this effect.

fects appear to be small and clinically insignificant. Mild decreases in hemoglobin and hematocrit associated with chronic methadone treatment can occur (i.e., a decrease of about 2.5–3.0 in hematocrit), but, again, these changes do not appear to be clinically significant (Martin et al. 1973).

Methadone and Cardiac Conduction

Methadone's effect on cardiac conduction deserves special mention. Two primary factors have generated interest in methadone's effect on the electrocardiogram (ECG) and especially on possible conduction abnormalities. The first is the observation that LAAM appears to produce prolongation of the QTc interval and in rare cases conduction abnormalities (Deamer et al. 2001). The second is the occasional use of very high methadone doses in clinical practice, which may increase risk of opioid-induced conduction abnormalities. Indeed, there are three reports of torsades (a type of abnormal heart rhythm associated with prolongation of the QTc interval) found in patients treated with methadone: 17 patients treated with a mean daily dose of 397 mg (Krantz et al. 2002), 3 patients treated with daily doses of 650–880 mg (Walker et al. 2003), and 3 other patients treated with doses greater than 200 mg per day (Gil et al. 2003). It appears that methadone-induced prolongation of the QTc interval may be dose related (Kornick et al. 2003; Martell et al. 2003), so the risk of arrhythmias may increase as methadone dose increases. Although the long history of safety with daily methadone use provides reassuring evidence that the risk of adverse effects by methadone on cardiac conduction is probably quite rare, these case reports suggest that caution should be exercised when higher doses of methadone are used and when methadone is provided to a patient with other risk factors for the development of conduction abnormalities (e.g., certain other medications).

Methadone and Immune Functioning

Methadone treatment is associated with lowered rates of behaviors such as injection drug use; engaging in such behaviors can otherwise place a person at risk for acquiring infectious diseases (Baker et al. 1995; Caplehorn and Ross 1995; Metzger et al. 1993). Thus, methadone treatment can serve a highly useful function in lowering the risk of contracting infectious illnesses such as HIV. At the same time, some preclinical evidence shows that methadone itself may produce detrimental changes in immune function that could raise susceptibility to these diseases once a patient is exposed (Li et al. 2002; Suzuki et al. 2002; Thomas et al. 1995). Clinical studies of methadone's effects on immune function are limited, however, and show mixed results (Quang-Cantagrel et al. 2001; Zajicova et al. 2004). Given the high rate of infectious diseases for patients in methadone treatment, clarification on whether methadone has clinically significant immune-compromising effects is needed. Until such clarification is obtained, the beneficial effects of methadone treatment on high-risk behaviors should be considered substantial and compelling.

Methadone and Sexual Side Effects

Studies of methadone and sexual side effects have predominantly been conducted in men. Surveys in patients receiving methadone generally find between 11 percent and 33 percent of men self-reporting sexual problems (Espejo et al. 1973; Hanbury et al. 1977). Serum testosterone levels are lower than normal in men maintained on methadone (Cicero et al. 1976), and although testosterone levels are also lower in subjects who use heroin regularly (Mendelson et al. 1975), levels may be lower yet in men maintained on methadone.

Ejaculate volume and seminal vesicular and prostatic secretions can also be markedly reduced in men maintained on methadone (Cicero et al. 1976), and these physiologic effects may contribute to patient complaints of decreased sexual functioning. Evidence indicates, however, that rates of sexual activity in men return to baseline (that is, to premethadone and preopioid dependence levels) as time on methadone progresses (Martin et al. 1973). Comparable data on rates of sexual activity in women are not available.

Methadone Treatment and Liver Function

Patients with opioid dependence often have liver disease before entering methadone treatment; therefore, the assessment of changes in liver function status owing to methadone use can be confounded by preexisting dysfunction. In addition, concurrent alcohol abuse while in methadone treatment can lead to new-onset liver disease that can be wrongly attributed to methadone. When these factors are taken into consideration, no evidence for hepatotoxic effects of methadone is found in studies of liver function for patients maintained on methadone (Kreek 1973a; Kreek et al. 1972; Novick et al. 1993).

Methadone Treatment and Cognitive/Performance Measures

Several early studies that examined methadone's potential to produce impairments in cognitive and/or performance measures found no significantly different scores on tests of intellectual functioning when patients maintained on methadone were compared with abstinent patients. Nor were there any differences in performance on psychomotor tasks such as reaction time (Gordon 1970; Gordon et al. 1967; Gritz et al. 1975; Rothenberg et al. 1977). An extensive and exceedingly thorough review of different opioids and their effects on cognition and performance likewise found little evidence that methadone produced clinically significant impairments, although this conclusion had to be qualified due to limitations in many of the methadone studies (Zacny 1995).

However, several contemporary studies employing more sophisticated testing batteries have shown that methadone treatment can be associated with impairments in some types of cognitive functioning and motoric performance (Curran et al. 2001; Darke et al. 2000; Mintzer and Stitzer 2002). Studies of cognition and performance for persons maintained on methadone can be extremely hard to interpret, because outcomes may be influenced by confounding factors such as other drug use and history of head injury, factors that can make it difficult to define appropriate comparison groups. Furthermore, impairments identified on sophisticated laboratory tests of cognitive ability may have minimal relevance to patients' ability to perform the normal activities of daily living.

In this regard, methadone has a long history of use on an outpatient basis with no marked abnormalities identified in cognition or performance. Nevertheless, these findings of possible subtle impairments in patients maintained on methadone could provide information that is highly useful for understanding the chronic effects of opioids and the underlying relationship between processes of cognition and the opioid system.

Conclusions Regarding Side Effects of Methadone

Methadone has been extensively used for the treatment of opioid dependence throughout the world. This extensive clinical experience provides considerable information about methadone's side effects. Based on this experience, there appear to be three clinically significant side effects to methadone: constipation, increased sweating, and sexual dysfunction. Several other effects have been noted, but tolerance typically develops to these effects, and some represent clinically insignificant changes. Higher doses of methadone may have side effects that could be significant (e.g., on cardiac function or cognitive/performance abilities), although further characterization of such is needed to understand their clinical significance. Overall, methadone's mild side-effects profile is one of its attractive features: overall, it is a very safe and well-tolerated medication.

SUMMARY AND CONCLUSIONS REGARDING METHADONE DOSING AND TREATMENT OUTCOME

Results both from surveys of methadone use in the treatment of opioid dependence and from controlled clinical trials demonstrate that methadone is an effective medication that produces excellent retention in treatment and favorable outcomes both directly related to drug use (i.e., decreases in illicit opioid use) and indirectly related to drug use (e.g., decreases in criminal activity). Even very low doses of methadone (e.g., 20 mg per day) can produce better retention than placebo methadone. Outcomes can be substantially improved by using doses greater than 20 mg per day, however, and initial stabilization doses in methadone maintenance should probably be *at least 50–60 mg per day*. For patients who do not respond in this dose range (i.e., fail to stop illicit opiate use), further increases *up to at least 100 mg per day should be considered,* because there is considerable individual difference in the response to different doses of methadone. In addition, assessment using methadone blood levels may be indicated, especially if a patient appears to be experiencing withdrawal before their next dose of methadone. Overall, methadone is a very safe and well-tolerated medication with few side effects, although additional research on the safety and clinical benefits of doses greater than 100 mg would be useful.

References

Baker A, Kochan N, Dixon J, Wodak A, Heather N (1995). HIV risk-taking behaviour among injecting drug users currently, previously and never enrolled in methadone treatment. *Addiction* 90: 545–54.

Ball JC, Ross A (1991). *The Effectiveness of Methadone Maintenance Treatment*. New York: Springer-Verlag.

Banys P, Tusel DJ, Sees KL, Reilly PM, Delucchi KL (1994). Low (40 mg) versus high (80 mg) dose methadone in a 180-day heroin detoxification program]. *J Subst Abuse Treat* 11: 225–32.

Belding MA, Iguchi MY, Lamb RJ (1997). Stages and processes of change as predictors of drug use among methadone maintenance patients. *Exp Clin Psychopharmacol* 5: 65–73.

Belding MA, Iguchi MY, Lamb RJ, Lakin M, Terry R (1995). Stages and processes of change among polydrug users in methadone maintenance treatment. *Drug Alcohol Depend* 39: 45–53.

Bell J, Chan J, Kuk A (1995). Investigating the influence of treatment philosophy on outcome of methadone maintenance. *Addiction* 90: 823–30.

Bell J, Seres V, Bowron P, Lewis J, Batey R (1988). The use of serum methadone levels in patients receiving methadone maintenance. *Clin Pharmacol Ther* 43: 623–9.

Berry GJ, Kuhn KL (1973). Dose-related response to methadone: reduction of maintenance dose. *Proc Natl Conf Methadone Treat* 2: 972–9.

Boffito M, Rossati A, Reynolds HE, Hoggard PG, Back DJ, Di Perri G (2002). Undefined duration of opiate withdrawal induced by efavirenz in drug users with HIV infection and undergoing chronic methadone treatment. *AIDS Res Hum Retroviruses* 18: 341–2.

Caplehorn JR, Bell J (1991). Methadone dosage and retention of patients in maintenance treatment. *Med J Aust* 154: 195–9.

Caplehorn JR, Bell J, Kleinbaum DG, Gebski VJ (1993). Methadone dose and heroin use during maintenance treatment. *Addiction* 88: 119–24.

Caplehorn JR, Ross MW (1995). Methadone maintenance and the likelihood of risky needle-sharing. *Int J Addict* 30: 685–98.

Cicero TJ, Meyer ER, Bell RD, Koch GA (1976). Effects of morphine and methadone on serum testosterone and luteinizing hormone levels and on the secondary sex organs of the male rat. *Endocrinology* 98: 367–72.

Craig RJ (1980). Effectiveness of low-dose methadone maintenance for the treatment of inner city heroin addicts. *Int J Addict* 15: 701–10.

Curran HV, Kleckham J, Bearn J, Strang J, Wanigaratne S (2001). Effects of methadone on cognition, mood and craving in detoxifying opiate addicts: a dose-response study. *Psychopharmacology (Berl)* 154: 153–60.

D'Aunno T, Pollack HA (2002). Changes in methadone treatment practices: results from a national panel study, 1988–2000. *JAMA* 288: 850–6.

D'Aunno T, Vaughn TE (1992). Variations in methadone treatment practices. Results from a national study. *JAMA* 267: 253–8.

Darke S, Sims J, McDonald S, Wickes W (2000). Cognitive impairment among methadone maintenance patients. *Addiction* 95: 687–95.

Deamer RL, Wilson DR, Clark DS, Prichard JG (2001). Torsades de pointes associated with high dose levomethadyl acetate (ORLAAM). *J Addict Dis* 20: 7–14.

Dole VP, Nyswander M (1965). A medical treatment for diacetylmorphine (heroin) addiction. A clinical trial with methadone hydrochloride. *JAMA* 193: 646–50.

Donny EC, Walsh SL, Bigelow GE, Eissenberg T, Stitzer ML (2002). High-dose methadone produces superior opioid blockade and comparable withdrawal suppression to lower doses in opioid-dependent humans. *Psychopharmacology (Berl)* 161: 202–12.

Eap CB, Bertschy G, Baumann P, Finkbeiner T, Gastpar M, Scherbaum N (1998). High interindividual variability of methadone enantiomer blood levels to dose ratios. *Arch Gen Psychiatry* 55: 89–90.

Eap CB, Bourquin M, Martin J, Spagnoli J, Livoti S, Powell K, Baumann P, Deglon J (2000). Plasma concentrations of the enantiomers of methadone and therapeutic response in methadone maintenance treatment. *Drug Alcohol Depend* 61: 47–54.

Eap CB, Buclin T, Baumann P (2002). Interindividual variability of the clinical pharmacokinetics of methadone: implications for the treatment of opioid dependence. *Clin Pharmacokinet* 41: 1153–93.

Espejo R, Hogben G, Stimmel B (1973). Sexual performance of men on methadone maintenance. *Proc Natl Conf Methadone Treat* 1: 490–3.

Farley TA, Cartter ML, Wassell JT, Hadler JL (1992). Predictors of outcome in methadone programs: effect of HIV counseling and testing. *AIDS* 6: 115–21

Flynn PM, Craddock SG, Hubbard RL, Anderson J, Etheridge RM (1997). Methodological overview and research design for the Drug Abuse Treatment Outcome Study (DATOS). *Psychol Addict Behav* 11: 230–43.

Flynn PM, Joe GW, Broome KM, Simpson DD, Brown BS (2003). Recovery from opioid addiction in DATOS. *J Subst Abuse Treat* 25: 177–86.

GAO (1990). Methadone Maintenance: Some Treatment Programs Are Not Effective; Greater Federal Oversight Needed. Washington, DC: U.S. General Accounting Office.

Garbutt GD, Goldstein A (1972). Blind comparison of three methadone maintenance dosages in 180 patients. Proceedings of the Fourth National Conference on Methadone Treatment, San Francisco, 411–14. New York: National Association for the Prevention of Addiction to Narcotics.

Gil M, Sala M, Anguera I, Chapinal O, Cervantes M, Guma JR, Segura F (2003). QT prolongation and Torsades de Pointes in patients infected with human immunodeficiency virus and treated with methadone. *Am J Cardiol* 92: 995–7.

Goldstein A (1970). Dosage, duration, side effects: blind controlled dosage comparisons with methadone in 200 patients. Proceedings of the Third National Conference on Methadone Treatment, sponsored by National Association for the Prevention of Addiction to Narcotics (NAPAN) and cosponsored by National Institute of Mental Health, New York City, 31–7.

Goldstein A, Judson BA (1973). Efficacy and side effects of three widely different methadone doses. Fifth National Conference on Methadone Treatment, 21–44. Washington, DC: National Association for the Prevention of Addiction to Narcotics.

Gordon NB (1970). Reaction-times of methadone treated ex-heroin addicts. *Psychopharmacologia* 16: 337–44.

Gordon NB, Warner A, Henderson A (1967). Psychomotor and intellectual performance under methadone maintenance. Committee on Problems of Drug Dependence, Minutes of the Twenty-Ninth Meeting, Lexington, KY, 5136–44. Washington, DC: National Academy of Sciences-National Research Council.

Gossop M, Marsden J, Stewart D, Edwards C, Lehmann P, Wilson A, Seger G (1997). The National Treatment Outcome Research Study in the United Kingdom: six month follow-up outcomes. *Psychol Addict Behav* 11: 324–37.

Gossop M, Marsden J, Stewart D, Kidd T (2003a). The National Treatment Outcome Research Study (NTORS): 4–5 year follow-up results. *Addiction* 98: 291–303.

Gossop M, Marsden J, Stewart D, Lehmann P, Edwards C, Wilson A, Segar G (1998). Substance use, health and social problems of service users at 54 drug treatment agencies. Intake data from the National Treatment Outcome Research Study. *Br J Psychiatry* 173: 166–71.

Gossop M, Marsden J, Stewart D, Lehmann P, Strang J (1999). Methadone treatment practices and outcome for opiate addicts treated in drug clinics and in general practice: results from the National Treatment Outcome Research Study. *Br J Gen Pract* 49: 31–4.

Gossop M, Marsden J, Stewart D, Rolfe A (2000). Patterns of improvement after methadone treatment: 1 year follow-up results from the National Treatment Outcome Research Study. *Drug Alcohol Depend* 60: 275–86.

Gossop M, Marsden J, Stewart D, Treacy S (2001). Outcomes after methadone maintenance and methadone reduction treatments: two-year follow-up results from the National Treatment Outcome Research Study. *Drug Alcohol Depend* 62: 255–64.

Gossop M, Stewart D, Browne N, Marsden J (2003b). Methadone treatment for opiate dependent patients in general practice and specialist clinic settings: outcomes at 2-year follow-up. *J Subst Abuse Treat* 24: 313–21.

Gossop M, Stewart D, Marsden J (2003c). Treatment process components and heroin use outcome among methadone patients. *Drug Alcohol Depend* 71: 93–102.

Gottheil E, Thornton C, Weinstein S (2002). Effectiveness of high versus low structure individual counseling for substance abuse. *Am J Addict* 11: 279–90.

Gritz ER, Shiffman SM, Jarvik ME, Haber J, Dymond AM, Coger R, Charuvastra V, Schlesinger J (1975). Physiological and psychological effects of methadone in man. *Arch Gen Psychiatry* 32: 237–42.

Hanbury R, Cohen M, Stimmel B (1977). Adequacy of sexual performance in men maintained on methadone. *Am J Drug Alcohol Abuse* 4: 13–20.

Hargreaves WA (1983). Methadone dosage and duration for maintenance treatment. In: Cooper JR, Altman F, Brown BS, Czechowicz D, eds. Research on the Treatment of Narcotic Addiction: State of the Art. Rockville, MD: U.S. Department of Health and Human Services.

Hartel DM, Schoenbaum EE, Selwyn PA, Kline J, Davenny K, Klein RS, Friedland GH (1995). Heroin use during methadone maintenance treatment: the importance of methadone dose and cocaine use. *Am J Public Health* 85: 83–8.

Holmstrand J, Anggard E, Gunne LM (1978). Methadone maintenance: plasma levels and therapeutic outcome. *Clin Pharmacol Ther* 23: 175–80.

Horns WH, Rado M, Goldstein A (1975). Plasma levels and symptom complaints in patients maintained on daily dosage of methadone hydrochloride. *Clin Pharmacol Ther* 17: 636–49.

Hubbard RL, Craddock SG, Flynn PM, Anderson J, Etheridge RM (1997). Overview of 1-year follow-up outcomes in the Drug Abuse Treatment Outcome Study (DATOS). *Psychol Addict Behav* 11: 261–78.

Hubbard RL, Marsden ME, Rachal JV, Harwood HJ, Cavanaugh ER, Ginzburg HM (1989).

Drug Abuse Treatment: A National Study of Effectiveness. Chapel Hill: The University of North Carolina Press.

Isbell H, Wilker A, Eisenman AJ, Daingerfield M, Frank K (1948). Liability of addiction to 6-dimethylamino-4,4-diphenyl-3-heptanone (methadon, "amidone" or "10820") in man. *Arch Intern Med* 82: 362–92.

Jaffe JH (1971). Further experience with methadone in the treatment of narcotic users. In: Einstein S, ed. *Methadone maintenance,* 29–43. New York: Marcel Dekker.

Johnson RE, Chutuape MA, Strain EC, Walsh SL, Stitzer ML, Bigelow GE (2000). A comparison of levomethadyl acetate, buprenorphine, and methadone for opioid dependence. *N Engl J Med* 343: 1290–97.

Johnson RE, Jaffe JH, Fudala PJ (1992). A controlled trial of buprenorphine treatment for opioid dependence. *JAMA* 267: 2750–5.

Kornick CA, Kilborn MJ, Santiago-Palma J, Schulman G, Thaler HT, Keefe DL, Katchman AN, Pezzullo JC, Ebert SN, Woosley RL, Payne R, Manfredi PL (2003). QTc interval prolongation associated with intravenous methadone. *Pain* 105: 499–506.

Kosten TR, Schottenfeld R, Ziedonis D, Falcioni J (1993). Buprenorphine versus methadone maintenance for opioid dependence [see comments]. *J Nerv Ment Dis* 181: 358–64.

Krantz MJ, Lewkowiez L, Hays H, Woodroffe MA, Robertson AD, Mehler PS (2002). Torsade de pointes associated with very-high-dose methadone. *Ann Intern Med* 137: 501–4.

Kreek MJ (1973a). Medical safety and side effects of methadone in tolerant individuals. *JAMA* 223: 665–8.

Kreek MJ (1973b). Plasma and urine levels of methadone. Comparison following four medication forms used in chronic maintenance treatment. *N Y State J Med* 73: 2773–7.

Kreek MJ, Dodes L, Kane S, Knobler J, Martin R (1972). Long-term methadone maintenance therapy: effects on liver function. *Ann Intern Med* 77: 598–602.

Kreek MJ, Garfield JW, Gutjahr CL, Giusti LM (1976). Rifampin-induced methadone withdrawal. *N Engl J Med* 294: 1104–6.

Li Y, Wang X, Tian S, Guo CJ, Douglas SD, Ho WZ (2002). Methadone enhances human immunodeficiency virus infection of human immune cells. *J Infect Dis* 185: 118–22.

Ling W, Charuvastra C, Kaim SC, Klett CJ (1976). Methadyl acetate and methadone as maintenance treatments for heroin addicts. A veterans administration cooperative study. *Arch Gen Psychiatry* 33: 709–20.

Ling W, Wesson DR, Charuvastra C, Klett CJ (1996). A controlled trial comparing buprenorphine and methadone maintenance in opioid dependence. *Arch Gen Psychiatry* 53: 401–7.

Loimer N, Schmid R (1992). The use of plasma levels to optimize methadone maintenance treatment. *Drug Alcohol Depend* 30: 241–6.

Maddux JF, Esquivel M, Vogtsberger KN, Desmond DP (1991). Methadone dose and urine morphine. *J Subst Abuse Treat* 8: 195–201.

Martell BA, Arnsten JH, Ray B, Gourevitch MN (2003). The impact of methadone induction on cardiac conduction in opiate users. *Ann Intern Med* 139: 154–5.

Martin WR, Jasinski DR, Haertzen CA, Kay DC, Jones BE, Mansky PA, Carpenter RW (1973). Methadone: a reevaluation. *Arch Gen Psychiatry* 28: 286–95.

McCance-Katz EF, Rainey PM, Friedland G, Jatlow P (2003). The protease inhibitor lopinavir-ritonavir may produce opiate withdrawal in methadone-maintained patients. *Clin Infect Dis* 37: 476–82.

McLellan AT (1983). Patient characteristics associated with outcome. In: Cooper JR, Altman F, Brown BS, Czechowicz D, eds. Research on the Treatment of Narcotic Addiction: State of the Art. Rockville, MD: U.S. Department of Health and Human Services.

McLellan AT, Arndt IO, Metzger DS, Woody GE, O'Brien CP (1993). The effects of psychosocial services in substance abuse treatment. *JAMA* 269: 1953–9.

McLellan AT, Grissom GR, Zanis D, Randall M, Brill P, O'Brien CP (1997). Problem-service 'matching' in addiction treatment. A prospective study in 4 programs. *Arch Gen Psychiatry* 54: 730–5.

Mendelson JH, Meyer RE, Ellingboe J, Mirin SM, McDougle M (1975). Effects of heroin and methadone on plasma cortisol and testosterone. *J Pharmacol Exp Ther* 195: 296–302.

Metzger DS, Woody GE, McLellan AT, O'Brien CP, Druley P, Navaline H, DePhilippis D, Stolley P, Abrutyn E (1993). Human immunodeficiency virus seroconversion among intravenous drug users in- and out-of-treatment: an 18-month prospective follow-up. *J Acquir Immune Defic Syndr* 6: 1049–56.

Mintzer MZ, Stitzer ML (2002). Cognitive impairment in methadone maintenance patients. *Drug Alcohol Depend* 67: 41–51.

Morral AR, Belding MA, Iguchi MY (1999). Identifying methadone maintenance clients at risk for poor treatment response: pretreatment and early progress indicators. *Drug Alcohol Depend* 55: 25–33.

Newman RG, Whitehill WB (1979). Double-blind comparison of methadone and placebo maintenance treatments of narcotic addicts in Hong Kong. *Lancet* 2: 485–8.

Nilsson MI, Gronbladh L, Widerlov E, Anggard E (1983). Pharmacokinetics of methadone in methadone maintenance treatment: characterization of therapeutic failures. *Eur J Clin Pharmacol* 25: 497–501.

Novick DM, Richman BL, Friedman JM, Friedman JE, Fried C, Wilson JP, Townley A, Kreek MJ (1993). The medical status of methadone maintenance patients in treatment for 11–18 years. *Drug Alcohol Depend* 33: 235–45.

Plummer JL, Gourlay GK, Cherry DA, Cousins MJ (1988). Estimation of methadone clearance: application in the management of cancer pain. *Pain* 33: 313–22.

Quang-Cantagrel ND, Wallace MS, Ashar N, Mathews C (2001). Long-term methadone treatment: effect on CD4+ lymphocyte counts and HIV-1 plasma RNA level in patients with HIV infection. *Eur J Pain* 5: 415–20.

Rhoades HM, Creson D, Elk R, Schmitz J, Grabowski J (1998). Retention, HIV risk, and illicit drug use during treatment: methadone dose and visit frequency. *Am J Public Health* 88: 34–9.

Rothenberg S, Schottenfeld S, Meyer RE, Krauss B, Gross K (1977). Performance differences between addicts and non-addicts. *Psychopharmacology (Berl)* 52: 299–306.

Schottenfeld RS, Pakes JR, Oliveto A, Ziedonis D, Kosten TR (1997). Buprenorphine vs methadone maintenance treatment for concurrent opioid dependence and cocaine abuse [see comments]. *Arch Gen Psychiatry* 54: 713–20.

Shinderman M, Maxwell S, Brawand-Amey M, Golay KP, Baumann P, Eap CB (2003). Cytochrome P4503A4 metabolic activity, methadone blood concentrations, and methadone doses. *Drug Alcohol Depend* 69: 205–11.

Siassi I, Angle BP, Alston DC (1977). Maintenance dosage as a critical factor in methadone maintenance treatment. *Br J Addict Alcohol Other Drugs* 72: 261–8.

Simpson DD, Joe GW, Brown BS (1997). Treatment retention and follow-up outcomes in the Drug Abuse Treatment Outcome Study (DATOS). *Psychol Addict Behav* 11: 294–307.

Simpson DD, Sells SB (1990). *Opioid addiction and treatment: a 12-year follow-up*. Malabar, FL: Robert E. Krieger Publishing Company.

Strain EC (2004). Patient-treatment matching and opioid addicted patients: past methods and future opportunities. *Heroin Addict Relat Clin Prob* 6 (3): 5–16.

Strain EC, Bigelow GE, Liebson IA, Stitzer ML (1999). Moderate- vs high-dose methadone in the treatment of opioid dependence: a randomized trial [see comments]. *JAMA* 281: 1000–5.

Strain EC, Stitzer ML, Liebson IA, Bigelow GE (1993a). Dose-response effects of methadone in the treatment of opioid dependence. *Ann Intern Med* 119: 23–27.

Strain EC, Stitzer ML, Liebson IA, Bigelow GE (1993b). Methadone dose and treatment outcome. *Drug Alcohol Depend* 33: 105–17.

Strain EC, Stitzer ML, Liebson IA, Bigelow GE (1998). Useful predictors of outcome in methadone-treated patients: results from a controlled clinical trial with three doses of methadone. *J Maintenance Addictions* 1: 15–28.

Suzuki S, Carlos MP, Chuang LF, Torres JV, Doi RH, Chuang RY (2002). Methadone induces CCR5 and promotes AIDS virus infection. *FEBS Lett* 519: 173–7.

Tennant FS, Jr. (1987). Inadequate plasma concentrations in some high-dose methadone maintenance patients. *Am J Psychiatry* 144: 1349–50.

Tennant FS, Jr., Rawson RA, Cohen A, Tarver A, Clabough D (1983). Methadone plasma levels and persistent drug abuse in high dose maintenance patients. *Subst Alcohol Actions Misuse* 4: 369–74.

Thomas PT, House RV, Bhargava HN (1995). Direct cellular immunomodulation produced by diacetylmorphine (heroin) or methadone. *Gen Pharmacol* 26: 123–30.

Thornton CC, Gottheil E, Weinstein SP, Kerachsky RS (1998). Patient-treatment matching in substance abuse. Drug addiction severity. *J Subst Abuse Treat* 15: 505–11.

Tong TG, Pond SM, Kreek MJ, Jaffery NF, Benowitz NL (1981). Phenytoin-induced methadone withdrawal. *Ann Intern Med* 94: 349–51.

Torrens M, Castillo C, San L, del Moral E, Gonzalez ML, de la Torre R (1998). Plasma methadone concentrations as an indicator of opioid withdrawal symptoms and heroin use in a methadone maintenance program. *Drug Alcohol Depend* 52: 193–200.

Walker PW, Klein D, Kasza L (2003). High dose methadone and ventricular arrhythmias: a report of three cases. *Pain* 103: 321–4.

Walton RG, Thornton TL, Wahl GF (1978). Serum methadone as an aid in managing methadone maintenance patients. *Int J Addict* 13: 689–94.

Williams HR (1971). Low and high methadone maintenance in the out-patient treatment of the hard core heroin addict. In: Einstein S, ed. *Methadone Maintenance.*, New York: Marcel Dekker.

Zacny JP (1995). A review of the effects of opioids on psychomotor and cognitive functioning in humans. *Exp Clin Psychopharmacol* 3: 432–66.

Zajicova A, Wilczek H, Holan V (2004). The alterations of immunological reactivity in heroin addicts and their normalization in patients maintained on methadone. *Folia Biol (Praha)* 50: 24–28.

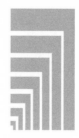

7

Counseling and Psychosocial Services

Michael Kidorf, Ph.D., Van L. King, M.D., and
Robert K. Brooner, Ph.D.

Drug abuse treatment programs offering opioid agonist treatments such as methadone are ideal settings in which to incorporate counseling and other psychosocial services that can maximize the effectiveness of medication treatments. They are also valuable sites for evaluating methods by which these nonpharmacologic services can maximize the effectiveness of medication. The typical structure of methadone treatment, which involves long-term intervention with frequent clinic attendance, supports the feasibility of implementing psychosocial treatments. Indeed, the necessity of counseling to address the complex problems of drug abusers was recognized by the founders of methadone treatment, and counseling has been a standard part of this therapeutic modality since its inception. Nevertheless, the availability of counseling does not guarantee that patients will use it regularly or effectively, and patient adherence to counseling is a highly pertinent service-delivery issue in methadone treatment.

Psychosocial treatments are useful for addressing the myriad of problems that drug abusers may bring with them to treatment. Most treatment-seeking opioid abusers engage in extensive use of nonopioid drugs, most have severe family and social problems including employment difficulties, and many have comorbid psychiatric disorders (Brooner et al. 1997; Havassy et al. 1991; Platt 1995). These are problems that can respond to supplemental, nonpharmacologic interventions, and the structure of methadone treatment provides an opportunity to expose patients to various psychosocial interventions, to intensively assess response, and to monitor this response for prolonged periods.

However, psychosocial services are surprisingly underused in methadone treatment. Although poor funding often limits the scope and intensity of a program's services, many patients fail to attend even once-per-week counseling sessions. The failure of patients to receive adequate counseling is costly to both patients and treatment programs. Partially treated patients often continue to use drugs during treatment, and in many programs, this leads to eventual discharge (Gill et al. 1992). Staff can become highly demoralized when surrounded by patients who continue using drugs, and both patients and staff may come to the mistaken conclusion that treatment is ineffective.

These and related issues associated with the nonpharmacologic aspects of methadone treatment are addressed in this chapter. The purpose of this chapter is twofold. It begins with a review of evidence that counseling and group therapies are effective treatments for patients who are dependent on opioids and receiving methadone. Although these are clearly effective treatments, they are only effective when actually delivered to patients. The issue of adherence to the nonpharmacologic aspects of methadone treatment is a prominent and common difficulty in methadone programs. Thus, the second aim of this chapter is to describe a service-delivery model designed to encourage patients to attend scheduled counseling sessions consistently. This service-delivery model, which we refer to as motivated stepped care (MSC) (Brooner and Kidorf 2002), involves the structured integration of pharmacologic treatments (i.e., methadone), verbal-expressive forms of therapy, and simple behavioral interventions to enhance attendance at counseling sessions. It conceptualizes drug use as a highly specific, goal-directed behavior motivated by the expected positive consequences of use (McHugh and Slavney 1998), such as temporary feelings of tranquility or euphoria, heightened pleasure from social activities, and cognitive dampening of self-doubts and ruminations over life problems. Drug use is then a decision on the part of the individual—positive consequences outweighing negative consequences—rather than simply a behavior driven by "uncontrollable" cravings or symptoms of physical dependence.

Methadone targets symptoms associated with physical dependence (e.g., withdrawal), whereas MSC concurrently focuses on helping the patient recognize the results from his or her decision to continue using drugs and aids the patient and staff by providing a clear set of consequences associated with continued drug use. This approach emphasizes the patient as the central agent capable of and responsible for continued drug use or abstinence and is a highly effective service-delivery model that can be implemented within the usual budgetary constraints of existing programs.

INDIVIDUAL COUNSELING

Individual counseling has long been a routine component of treatment with methadone, though many programs describe these interventions as ancillary to the dispensing of methadone. Ball and Ross provide normative data on the counseling practices of six methadone programs (Ball and Ross 1991). They found that about 50 percent of the patients received at least one 20- to 60-minute counseling session per week. In addition, patient-to-counselor caseloads ranged from 25:1, which can enhance meaningful integration of pharmacologic and psychosocial treatments, to 70:1, which shifts the primary focus of treatment onto the medication. Ten types of individual counseling services were identified in the Ball and Ross study, ranging from initial intake sessions to brief (often unscheduled) counseling contacts and more specialized psychological and vocational services.

More than a cursory outline of the responsibilities of individual counselors is beyond the scope of this chapter. The Center for Substance Abuse Treatment (CSAT) (Kauffman and Woody 1995) and the National Institute on Drug Abuse (Mercer and Woody 2000) provide a useful and comprehensive approach for counselors involved in the treatment of opioid abusers receiving methadone. In brief, counselors at the start of treatment should assess patients for patterns of polydrug use and identify problems in other life areas, such as housing, social, family, legal, and occupational functioning. The assessment should also lead to a good appreciation of the individuality of patients and the historical and cultural influences reflected in the logic and purpose of their behavior. Effective counseling also requires frequent review of the treatment plan and any associated contingencies. This work is powerfully enhanced by repeated education about the rationale and purpose for the treatment plan and any changes in it during the course of therapy. Careful education about the treatment plan can reduce the patient's conception of treatment as a mysterious force beyond their control or influence.

Counselors should work with patients to identify and prioritize problem areas in the treatment plan to establish a rational and orderly approach to their resolution. Cessation of all drug use should be the primary treatment goal; other problem areas (e.g., employment, familial) may be most successfully addressed in the context of meaningful reduction in drug use and periods of confirmed abstinence. Nevertheless, problems presenting significant barriers to recovery (e.g., excessive idle time resulting from unemployment) might be addressed concurrently with the initial goal of complete abstinence. Many patients attempt to find single solutions to multiple overlapping problems, often leading to failure and demoralization; this yields further "evidence" to the patient that counseling is useless. Counselors should limit this problem by helping patients separate complex overlapping problems into smaller units, which increases the likelihood of success. These recommendations are supported by the available literature, indicating that counselors are most effective when they engage patients in regular counseling early in the treatment process (Gossop et al. 2003; Simpson et al. 1995), when they establish good therapeutic rapport (Allison and Hubbard 1985; Joe et al. 2001), and when they remain organized and consistent in their clinical approach to problem identification and resolution (McLellan et al. 1988).

A present-oriented counseling focus using cognitive-behavioral and problem-solving strategies is a useful framework for administering individual counseling. In general, counselors should use nonconfrontational and supportive techniques with patients struggling to meet the demands of the treatment program. Several good models for this orientation are available, but the overall approach is best summarized in the book *Motivational Interviewing* by Miller and Rollnick (1991). This book outlines several motivational principles that provide an excellent context for behavior change. Equally important is the need for counselors to express empathy through reflective listening and to communicate respect for the suffering endured by patients and the conflict over continued use evident among those seeking treatment. It is not difficult to express appropriate respect to patients. Respect is easily communicated by listening closely to all concerns, by providing timely responses to questions, and by keeping all scheduled appointments or contacting patients in advance when scheduling changes are required.

How effective is individual counseling for opioid abusers receiving methadone therapy? This question was studied by McLellan and colleagues at the University of Pennsylvania (McLellan et al., 1993). Opioid abusers entering treatment ($N = 92$), all of whom received a steady methadone dose of 60–90 mg during a six-month study period, were randomly assigned to one of three counseling conditions: methadone only (low intensity), methadone plus standard counseling (medium intensity), and methadone plus standard counseling enhanced by other clinical services (high intensity). Counselors of patients receiving low-intensity services had minimal contact with patients and neither the counselor nor the patients received weekly urinalysis testing results. In the medium-intensity condition, counselors scheduled one session per week for patients during the first month, and increased or decreased the rate of counseling based on weekly urinalysis results. They could also award take-home privileges to those who were drug free and employed. Counselors of patients receiving high-intensity services scheduled individual counseling sessions in a manner similar to those providing medium intensity and also referred patients to other professional services available within the clinic, including sessions with a psychiatrist, employment counselor, and family therapist.

Data on the number of scheduled or attended counseling sessions by patients in each group were not presented. Instead, a brief interview measure called the Treatment Services Review (TSR) (McLellan et al. 1992) was used to assess the number of times various content areas (e.g., drug use, employment, psychiatric, legal) were discussed with staff. The counseling manipulation was delivered as intended; that is, patients receiving high-intensity services discussed both drug use and psychiatric issues with staff more frequently than patients receiving medium-intensity services, and patients receiving medium-intensity services discussed these issues with staff more frequently than patients receiving low-intensity services. Results showed counseling produced significant differences in treatment outcome. For example, patients receiving high-intensity services had greater rates of consecutive weeks of opioid and cocaine abstinence, as determined from urine testing (table 7.1). Some patients in the low-intensity condition (30%) performed well without counseling. However, most performed poorly and needed to be therapeutically transferred to the medium-intensity condition after three months (fig. 7.1). Patients transferred to the medium-intensity condition showed significant reductions in both cocaine and opiate use after only four weeks of more intensive counseling.

The results of this study show that counseling can dramatically im-

Table 7.1 **Dose-Effect of Psychosocial Services in Methadone Treatment**

Group*	% of patients with opiate abstinence for			% of patients with cocaine abstinence for		
	8 weeks[†]	12 weeks[†]	16 weeks[†]	8 weeks[†]	12 weeks[†]	16 weeks[†]
Low	31	22	0	31	25	22
Medium	100	59	28	89	59	34
High	94	74	55	94	74	45

Source: Adapted from McLellan et al. 1993.
*Refers to the level of intensity of nonpharmacologic treatment services provided; see text for details.
[†]Weeks of continuous abstinence as determined by urine testing.

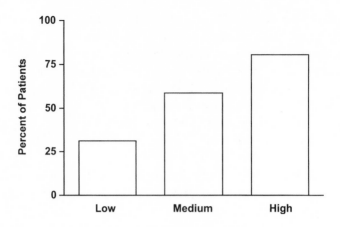

Figure 7.1. **Proportions of methadone-maintained patients with treatment success at different levels of psychosocial services.** Success was predefined as needing protective transfer out of the original, randomly assigned condition because of continued drug use or three emergency situations. Patients receiving high-intensity services had the best treatment outcome, and those receiving medium-intensity services performed better than those receiving low-intensity services. Adapted from McLellan et al. 1993.

prove the outcome of methadone treatment. Note, however, that a subset of patients in all study conditions performed well, suggesting that the amount of counseling needed to maximize therapeutic response varies from patient to patient. In addition, reductions in drug use observed in the study were attained even though the number of counseling sessions received by patients in the medium- and high-intensity groups seemed modest. Patients receiving high-intensity services had an average of only nine drug use discussions per month, and discussion of other important topic areas (e.g., vocational, social, psychiatric) was even less frequent. Because patients were not required to attend the additional counseling services, the continued drug use in both the medium- and high-intensity groups may have resulted partly from failure to access the additional services offered in the study. It is therefore possible that the favorable outcomes achieved in this study could be improved if patients were to attend extra counseling sessions each week.

GROUP COUNSELING AND SKILLS TRAINING

Many methadone programs offer group-counseling services. Groups are useful for educating patients about drug abuse and the associated risk of HIV infection and about twelve-step programming, and for providing general support and the opportunity for discussion. Furthermore, group therapy is an ideal way to deliver skills-training material efficiently and effectively. Well-written manuals are available on many group therapy topics and can be used by counselors to improve the quality and consistency of material presented in group formats (Daley and Mercer 2002). Traditionally, optimal group size is five to ten patients (Yalom 1975), but this number can be increased to about 14 when groups are structured and skills oriented and the counselor is experienced in group-based interventions. Group counseling is an extremely cost-effective intervention that allows many patients to receive treatment at one time. When possible, patients should be grouped heterogeneously to increase interest and patient involvement; for example, male and female patients who are still using drugs should be grouped with those who are recently abstinent. It is important that basic group rules (e.g., arriving on time, listening to others, giving constructive feedback) are routinely reviewed and consistently followed to maximize the effectiveness of group counseling. Despite the general popularity of this intervention, relatively few data exist about the efficacy of group counseling for patients in opioid substitution treatment. There is sufficient evidence in work with alcohol-dependent patients, however, to warrant the general view that group-based interventions are effective conduits to behavior change, especially groups that enhance skills for abstinence and coping with stressful life events (Chaney 1989). In fact, group-based coping-skills training may be particularly effective with patients exhibiting high levels of psychiatric severity and antisocial behaviors (Cooney et al. 1991).

Coping-Skills Training and Relapse Prevention

Coping-skills training is perhaps best conducted in a group setting. The group leader asks participants to identify a number of "high-risk" occasions, especially those which focus on interpersonal stressors (e.g., interpersonal conflict; pressures to drink), and helps the group generate potential responses to these situations. After an appropriate coping response is identified, the group leader teaches the new skill via role-play. Patients model the group leader's behavior and subsequently receive feedback from the leader and other group participants. The use of videotaping is particularly helpful for providing feedback and maintaining patient interest. We have found it very useful to use situations that naturally occur in the clinic setting as the content for role-playing. For instance, patients might role-play situations in which they are informed that their urine test was drug positive or that their clinic privileges were temporarily withdrawn. After patients have completed the group training, the group leader and other staff are in a position to observe directly the patient's performance of the new skills in the face of conflicts naturally occurring in the clinic.

The primary aim of coping-skills groups is to provide patients with the cognitive and social tools essential to abstain from drug use. There also has been interest in the development of groups that teach relapse prevention, thereby targeting individuals who are either abstinent on a stable or decreasing methadone dose, or who have successfully withdrawn off methadone and are drug free. Implicit to this approach is the consideration of opioid dependence as a chronic relapsing disorder that requires proactive and ongoing treatment. In fact, it could be argued that many patients make maximal use of the group content when they are drug free and have achieved some stability, though often at this time patients believe that their work is done and "reward" themselves by leaving the group. This problem is often reinforced by staff who further withdraw support once the patient is drug free. Continued staff encouragement of patients to pursue treatment even during periods of abstinence is consistent with the original intention of relapse-prevention models (Marlatt and Gordon 1985), which was to help break the cycle of relapse by identifying and changing internal and external factors contributing to the decision to use drugs.

Khantzian and colleagues, for instance, describe a type of group therapy (i.e., modified group therapy for substance abusers) that utilizes a psychodynamic approach to help patients understand how their psychological vulnerabilities and emotional reactions affect the probability of relapse (Khantzian et al. 1992). Group leaders communicate empathy and encourage the sharing of experiences to help patients manage feelings of isolation and low self-worth. The four major areas of group focus are self-care, relationship conflicts, self-esteem, and affect regulation. Using a more behavioral approach, McAuliffe (1990) developed a relapse-prevention group based on a conditioning model of addiction. Patients in this group learn alternative responses to environmental stimuli that trigger decisions to use opioids. Group members also attend self-help meetings and participate in social activities with group members and former drug abusers who are currently abstinent. McAuliffe (1990) published evidence for the effectiveness of this group in the United States and in Hong Kong, although a host of methodological confounds (including the lack of appropriate control groups) makes the results difficult to interpret. Finally, a group developed by Rawson and colleagues that combines coping-skills and relapse-control training and provides guided instruction on the neuropsychological consequences of recovery (e.g., withdrawal, craving) has shown some efficacy (Magura et al. 1994; Rawson et al. 1990).

Job-Skills Training

In addition to modifying drug use behavior directly, an important goal for any type of drug abuse treatment is to help patients initiate lifestyle changes consistent with abstinence. Although this could be accomplished indirectly through coping-skills and relapse-prevention training, a more direct route is to convey the skills necessary to pursue treatment goals that have been traditionally associated with drug abstinence and stability. One of the more important lifestyle changes for many opioid abusers is to find and maintain employment. Full-time employment provides necessary structure and responsibility and is not surprisingly associated with good drug abuse treatment outcome (Kidorf et al. 1994; McLellan et al. 1981; Platt 1995). Opioid abusers represent a particularly good population for teaching job-seeking skills. In a study of outpatients dependent on opioids, not knowing how to look for work was a primary factor differentiating patients who did and did not secure employment within a three-year period (Hermalin et al. 1990). Furthermore, the criminal and drug use history of opioid abusers tends to render them relatively unattractive to potential employers, and their occupational interests often fall notably short of their academic skills or employment experience (Silverman et al. 1995). These factors probably cause these individuals considerable frustration in their pursuit of employment and might further serve to reduce the likelihood of their continuing to search for jobs on their own.

Hall and colleagues showed that drug abusers could be taught skills that led to successful employment (Hall et al. 1981). They developed a job-seekers workshop that was tested in two groups of heroin addicts. In this study, patients receiving methadone maintenance ($N = 60$) were assigned to either a job-seekers skills training group or to a job-seeking information control group. Patients were recruited from four different drug abuse clinics and had expressed interest in attaining employment. Patients in the job-seekers skills-training group attended group workshops that taught skills for networking and using the telephone, completing applications, and responding to questions during job interviews. The primary dependent measure was employment, which was generally verified through paycheck or time clock stubs. The results showed that more experimental subjects (52%) than control subjects (30%) were employed at the three-month follow-up. This difference was not significant owing to the small sample but nevertheless demonstrates that a behavioral skills program can help many motivated patients attain employment. The data do not indicate, however, the impact of this treatment on patients who might be more ambivalent about pursuing employment. That only 60 patients were identified across four treatment programs suggests that the majority of unemployed patients were uninterested in pursuing enhanced support for attaining work.

There is also evidence that contingency management can supplement job-skills training to motivate job seeking and acquisition. Kidorf and colleagues evaluated an intervention that required unemployed patients ($N = 36$) who had participated in methadone maintenance for over a year to attend intensive counseling to help resolve ambivalence toward job seeking (Kidorf et al. 1998). Those who remained unemployed after ten weeks of additional counseling started a 21-day methadone dose taper until employment was found. The results showed that 75 percent of these patients secured paid or volunteer employment and maintained the position for at least one month; most continued working throughout the six-month follow-up. A subsequent study showed that when this intervention was implemented as clinicwide policy, over 90 percent of the program census ($N > 200$) was either working or involved in other productive activity (e.g., vocational rehabilitation, adult education) (Kidorf et al. 2004).

In sum, group counseling can be highly effective and easily applied in community treatment clinics. Many patients can be treated at the same time, which is especially helpful because most community clinics have limited resources and large patient-to-staff ratios. Group counseling with drug abusers is perhaps most effective when it is structured (i.e., manualized) and skills oriented, two features that make groups relatively easy for counselors to administer. Although an emphasis on skills training is based on the more established alcoholism literature, some studies (Hall et al. 1981; Magura et al. 1994) provide support for its effectiveness with opioid abusers. Adherence to group-counseling sessions can be a problem; however, several studies have shown that attendance can be dramatically improved by offering limited methadone take-home privileges or other clinic-based incentives specifically based on counseling attendance (see Kidorf and Stitzer 1999, for a review). Clinic-based incentives may also be used to supplement counseling to strengthen outcomes. Note that high-intensity group counseling has been tolerated as well as less intensive care. Thus, it appears that patients receiving methadone will meet the treatment expectations established by the clinic.

INDIVIDUAL PSYCHOTHERAPY

We describe psychotherapy here as a form of verbal-expressive therapy in which a trained individual develops a professional relationship with a patient and uses psychological principles to modify or remove problematic thoughts, feelings, and behaviors. In many respects, opioid abusers are good candidates for psychotherapy. Virtually all patients entering treatment are highly conflicted and demoralized by their continued use of drugs despite compelling reasons to stop. They respond to treatment staff with considerable trepidation, often avoiding the very treatments that can make sense out of their continued motivations to use drugs. These problems are not unique to drug abusers. Patients with other psychiatric problems (e.g., eating disorders) present with similar clinical features. The psychotherapeutic techniques used to help those patients can also be helpful to patients struggling with drug dependence (Andersen 1984).

Little systematic study of the effectiveness of psychotherapy with drug abusers has been done, however. The reasons for this may be attributed to both the patients and the treatment providers. First, opioid abusers are usually uninterested in pursuing psychotherapy. This is apparently a long-standing problem; more than four decades ago Nyswander commented on the small percentage of drug abusers in the New York City area who responded to the availability of professional psychotherapy (Nyswander et al. 1958). Second, opioid abusers, by definition, engage in behaviors such as drug use and drug seeking that strongly compete with therapy attendance and subsequent development of a therapeutic relationship. Many also exhibit cognitive impairment and other deficits that limit the processing of therapeutic content. Third, many opioid abusers lack the financial resources necessary to complete successfully a course of psychotherapy. Finally, psychologists, psychiatrists, and other mental health professionals typically do not receive the necessary training required to conduct psychotherapy with this population.

In the late 1970s the National Institute of Drug Abuse (NIDA) funded two large-scale studies to evaluate the effects of psychotherapy on the treatment outcome of opioid abusers receiving methadone treatment (Rounsaville et al. 1983; Woody et al. 1983). In the Woody et al. (1983) study, 110 patients were recruited and randomly assigned to one of three treatment groups: supportive-expressive therapy plus standard drug counseling (SE), cognitive-behavioral therapy plus standard drug counseling (CB), and standard drug counseling only (DC). Supportive-expressive therapy (Luborsky 1984) is an analytically oriented psychotherapy that uses patient-therapist interactions to identify relationship themes. Cognitive-behavioral therapy (Beck 1976) is a directive psychotherapeutic technique in which the therapist helps a patient identify and modify those thought processes and decisions that result in continuation of problem behaviors. Delivery of these psychotherapies was carefully integrated into the routine of methadone delivery and counseling services typically offered at the clinic. For instance, therapists worked in offices located in the clinic, remained in communication with the study patients' counselors, and promptly contacted patients who missed scheduled appointments. Across conditions, patients attended approximately 57 percent of scheduled counseling sessions.

The results showed that, on average, patients in all treatment groups improved in most outcome measures over time. The two psychotherapy conditions appeared to be particularly effective in modifying non-substance-related treatment outcome. Modest reductions in self-reported drug use were observed in each of the treatment conditions, although any between-group differences were not sustained by the time a six-month follow-up was conducted. Additional analyses from this study showed that patients diagnosed with antisocial personality disorder (APD) and no other psychiatric disorder evidenced only minimal gains from psychotherapy (Woody et al. 1985). A follow-up study that controlled for the amount of counseling services provided across study conditions provided additional support for the effectiveness of psychotherapy (Woody et al. 1995).

In the second study (Rounsaville et al. 1983), male opioid abusers with another Axis I psychiatric disorder were randomly assigned to short-term interpersonal therapy (IPT; $N = 37$) or to a comparison condition ($N = 35$). The primary goal of IPT (Klerman et al. 1984) is to help patients develop more effective strategies for dealing with interpersonal problems. Patients assigned to the comparison condition were referred to a once-per-month meeting with a psychiatrist. Patients in both conditions attended other scheduled individual- and group-counseling sessions, although overall compliance rates were not reported.

In contrast to the Woody et al. (1983) study, the specialized psychotherapy was not well integrated into the usual procedures of the clinic. The settings in which the routine methadone treatment and specialized psychotherapy was provided were physically separated. This separation may have affected both recruitment into the study and psychotherapy attendance rates for those who chose to participate. Indeed, an extremely high study-dropout rate was observed: only 38 percent of the IPT group and 54 percent of the comparison group completed the six-month study. Most of the treatment outcome data followed suit and compared unfavorably with the results of the Woody et al. (1983) clinical trial. Although patients in both study conditions demonstrated clinical improvement over time, only a few meaningful between-group differences emerged.

Several tentative conclusions can be drawn from these studies. The results offer mixed support for the efficacy of psychotherapy with opioid abusers. Both of the Woody studies (Woody et al. 1983, 1995) demonstrate that the inclusion of psychotherapy is associated with reductions in drug use and psychiatric symptom reporting and that treatment gains are often sustained after discontinuing the service. This latter result supports the findings of studies with other populations of substance abusers that have shown the long-term benefits of specialized psychotherapy (Carroll et al. 1994). Although similar results were not obtained in the Rounsaville et al. (1983) study, the specialized therapy services were offered outside of the routine methadone treatment clinic and results may have been confounded by this procedure. Finally, the effects of specialized therapy will likely be proportional to the rate of exposure to the treatment. The positive outcomes in the Woody et al. (1983, 1995) studies were obtained despite poor overall adherence to the psychotherapy intervention. The patients in the Rounsaville et al. (1983) study received even less of the planned psychotherapy. These facts suggest that improvement from specialized psychotherapies could be enhanced by ensuring that patients receive a larger "dose" of the treatment.

Family-Based Therapies

The families of opioid abusers are rarely included in the treatment process in any meaningful or structured way. This is particularly unfortunate because both the family of origin and immediate family may provide powerful environmental incentives for reduction in drug use. Many of the reasons for underutilization of family-based therapies are similar to those responsible for the limited use of professional individual psychotherapy. Drug abuse counselors are rarely trained to provide marital or family interventions, whereas professionally trained therapists are costly and most programs cannot offer the service within existing budgets. It is likewise difficult to refer patients to other settings routinely offering family services because relatively few patients have adequate insurance or money to pay for the treatment. The general reluctance of both patients and family members to become involved in family-based treatments (Stanton and Todd 1982) is an additional disincentive for implementing these interventions with opioid abusers. It is illogical to expend the limited financial resources of a program to offer family therapy if no patients will participate. This is an unfortunate situation because available research shows that including family members in drug abuse treatment has many potential benefits (Stanton and Shadish 1997).

The goal of family therapy is to improve the psychological functioning of the family system (or couple), thereby positively influencing other treatment outcome variables such as drug use and treatment retention. In this section, we first present the two most widely used family-based interventions: family therapy and conjoint (marital) therapy. We conclude by presenting a third option that involves bringing drug-free significant others (including family members) into treatment to act as "community monitors" of patient adherence to the treatment plan.

Family Therapy

Kaufman presents four models of family psychotherapy: (1) structural-strategic therapy (Minuchin 1974); (2) behavior therapy; (3) systems therapy (Bowen 1971); and (4) psychodynamic therapy (Kaufman 1989). Of these models, structural-strategic therapy has enjoyed the most empirical support with opioid abusers receiving methadone substitution (Stanton and Todd 1982). Structural-strategic therapy is a short-term, goal-oriented, nonconfrontational intervention that helps families develop new adaptive strategies for dealing with recurrent problems. The therapist is responsible for devising a treatment plan with objective outcome criteria, including reduction of drug use and enhancing participation in constructive activity. Kaufman (1989) describes several other structural strategies that might be used by the therapist to enhance the effectiveness of family treatment, including affiliating with the family system, transforming complicated problems into workable goals, encouraging patients to speak directly to each other (and not about each other), and respecting patients' feelings and family boundaries.

To test the efficacy of a structural-strategic approach, Stanton and Todd randomly assigned young male opioid abusers (<36 years old) receiving methadone treatment to one of four groups (Stanton and Todd 1982). In the paid family therapy condition ($N = 21$), each family member received $5 for attending therapy sessions and received extra money if the patient submitted drug-negative urine samples. In the unpaid family therapy condition ($N = 25$), family members were encouraged to participate, but monetary incentives were not given for attendance or abstinence. Two additional comparison conditions were used: a family movie treatment condition ($N = 19$), in which movies of family interactions across different cultures were viewed on a weekly basis, and a no treatment control condition ($N = 53$). Treatment was delivered once per week for 10 weeks, but additional sessions could be scheduled in crisis situations. All patients were scheduled for weekly counseling independent of group therapy sessions.

Study results supported the efficacy of the therapy. Patients in the paid and unpaid therapy conditions reported a higher proportion of opioid-free days (81% and 76%, respectively) than those in family movie and nonfamily control conditions (66% and 62%, respectively). This was true as well when days free of nonopioid drugs were considered (88% and 85% for paid and unpaid family therapy groups versus 79% and 75% for family movie and nonfamily groups). These promising results for drug use were seen despite striking differences in the compliance rates of patients participating in these two conditions. All family members in the paid family therapy condition, for example, attended at least four sessions of treatment, and most (81%) completed the scheduled ten sessions. In the unpaid condition, however, almost one half (48%) did not attend even four sessions, and only 40 percent completed the ten sessions. In fact, the compliance rate of patients in the unpaid family therapy condition was less than that of patients in the family movie condition, in which 94 percent of the patients attended at least six sessions and 56 percent of the patients completed ten sessions. Differences in drug use observed immediately after treatment were maintained over the one-year follow-up period, although there were no between-group differences in attainment of more constructive drug-free social activity at any point during the study.

These results demonstrate that family therapy can reduce the drug use of outpatients who are opioid dependent and receiving methadone treatment. Although the Stanton and Todd (1982) study tested the efficacy of structural-strategic therapy, it seems reasonable to hypothesize that other professionally delivered family treatments (e.g., behavioral, psychodynamic) would also have positive effects. What is not as clear, however, is how family therapy might affect the treatment outcome of older drug abusers who are likely to be more estranged from their families of origin. The investigators also do not present strategies for dealing with ongoing cocaine use, which is much more prevalent now than when the study was conducted. The comparison between paid and unpaid therapy conditions demonstrated that the intervention of paying patients and family members to attend sessions produced significant increases in rates of adherence, although surprisingly marginal differences in rates of drug use. Again, the poor attendance of patients in the unpaid family therapy condition points to the difficulties in attracting patients and family members to this type of treatment. In fact, the investigators describe a large subset of eligible patients who were never included in the study because they did not permit family contact.

Conjoint Therapy

There has been renewed interest in the evaluation of behavioral conjoint therapy (BCT) for opioid abusers. Much of this work is based on studies in the area of alcohol abuse and dependence that demonstrate the benefits of this approach for reducing total alcohol consumption (McCrady et al. 1986; O'Farrell et al. 1985), enhancing treatment retention (Zweben et al. 1983), and maintaining treatment gains over time (O'Farrell et al. 1993; see O'Farrell and Fals-Stewart 2000 for a review). The standard package for opioid abusers includes abstinence contracting, communication skills training, and shared recreational activity. The goal is to reduce drug use and facilitate positive and mutually reinforcing social interaction. An important component of BCT is the utilization of a non-drug-using partner to monitor treatment and reinforce positive behaviors. For instance, the partner might monitor naltrexone ingestion (versus disulfiram monitoring for alcoholics), attendance to self-help meetings, and performance of other behaviors conducive to maintaining abstinence from drugs. In addition, the partner might provide reinforcement (reciprocal verbal praise, intimate behavior, cooking meals, etc.) contingent on observable changes of behavior.

Fals-Stewart and colleagues (1996) evaluated the effectiveness of BCT on drug use and the relationship satisfaction of male patients receiving methadone maintenance and their non-drug-using female partners. Patients were randomly assigned to receive either BCT (plus individual counseling) or twice weekly individual counseling. The results showed that patients assigned to the BCT condition exhibited less drug use during the four-month assessment period; differences in heroin use were maintained throughout the study, although differences in cocaine use diminished over time. BCT patients also expressed significantly more relationship satisfaction over the course of study participation. Note that these positive findings were observed within the context of excellent counseling adherence; patients in both study groups attended more than 80 percent of their scheduled sessions. These results are quite promising and suggest that the benefits of BCT that are well documented in the treatment of alcoholism may generalize to opioid abusers receiving methadone maintenance.

Of course, important differences exist between opioid and alcohol abusers that may limit the widespread use of this intervention with patients receiving methadone maintenance. Perhaps most problematic is that most drug abusers entering treatment are not involved in stable romantic relationships (Kidorf et al. 1997), thus limiting this intervention to a smaller number of patients with steady partners. But even this group is often involved with partners who are actively drug dependent or significantly impaired by other psychiatric problems (Kaufman 1985). In the Fals-Stewart et al. (1996) study cited above, well over a third of the male patients involved in a conjoint relationship cohabitated with a female who had substance abuse or psychiatric problems. It is likely that such partners would have difficulty complying with the many requirements of intensive behavioral conjoint therapy. Consequently, this intervention is used infrequently in community drug abuse treatment programs (Fals-Stewart and Birchler 2001), although the use of a stable significant other to actively monitor and support treatment behavior has potential to help a wider range of opioid abusers. The manner in which such an intervention might be implemented in a methadone substitution program is described next.

Significant-Other Monitoring

The previously described family-based interventions are applicable for patients who either have an intact family or who are involved in a stable romantic relationship. These interventions focus on improving family functioning as a means to affect important areas of treatment outcome such as drug use and retention. The problem, of course, is that the skills needed to deliver family-based interventions are highly specialized and require considerable training and supervision, which is rarely available to staff in drug abuse treatment programs. Yet, family members might alternatively be utilized to monitor and support the patient's efforts to meet goals that have been established in his or her treatment plan. In this way, family involvement more closely resembles a community reinforcement approach (Azrin 1976; Azrin et al. 1994; Hunt and Azrin 1973), which emphasizes control of external reinforcers as a means of modifying drug use. Studies using this approach with substance abusers have utilized family and spousal support to enhance adherence to disulfiram and naltrexone therapy, provide social and other reinforcement contingent on abstinence, and help patients become involved in social activities that compete with substance use (Azrin et al. 1982, 1994; Hunt and Azrin 1973; Sisson and Azrin 1986; Fals-Stewart and O'Farrell 2003). This model has also been applied successfully to the treatment of substance abusers in an approach called network therapy (Galanter 1993; Galanter et al. 1997). In this therapy, selected drug-free family members or friends are enlisted into the therapy process to provide ongoing support and to promote attitude and behavior change in the patient.

A treatment model that involves support from the social network can also be adapted to opioid abusers receiving methadone substitution by utilizing drug-free family members or friends to support community-based treatment goals. One particularly important goal is for patients to become more involved in drug-free activities and to develop more extensive drug-free social support outside of the clinic. Research showing a strong association between positive social support and reduced risk for relapse to opioid use and many other substances (Havassy et al. 1991; Wasserman et al. 2001) supports the aggressive pursuit of this goal. Enhancing social support can be pursued by having drug-free significant others lead patients into drug-free activities and then monitoring their involvement in these settings. In fact, simply including a drug-free individual as part of the treatment functions as an important step to instituting more regular involvement with drug-free social support. An advantage to this approach is that it does not require the same degree of experience necessary to conduct traditional family or marital therapy and can therefore be more easily implemented in drug abuse treatment clinics.

One might think that the biggest stumbling block to this approach is that patients do not have any drug-free individuals in their lives to bring into treatment. Although this is a common belief among treatment staff, it appears to be a misconception strongly encouraged by the patients. Kidorf and colleagues showed that 85 percent of the patients targeted for this intervention both identified drug-free significant others and involved them in the treatment plan when doing so ensured continued treatment in the program (Kidorf et al. 1997). Patients and their significant others were required to attend a significant-other group for six weeks; this group focused on strategies for enhancing social support outside of the clinic, and almost 80 percent of all scheduled sessions were attended. Although other treatment outcome data were not presented in this study, the results clearly show that opioid abusers will bring significant others into treatment *if* the program is committed to the intervention.

IMPLICATIONS OF THE COUNSELING AND THERAPY LITERATURE

This review has important practical implications for staff working in opioid treatment programs. The inclusion of individual counseling was found to add significantly relative to outcomes achieved with methadone medication alone. In addition, patients exposed to more counseling achieved better outcomes than those receiving less counseling. We believe that counselors should rely primarily on a nonconfrontational interaction style that conveys support, builds rapport, and motivates patients to identify the reasons for maintaining their drug use and how they will change the process of deciding to use drugs. Group counseling appears to be most effective when it is structured and skills oriented and represents a cost-sensitive method for increasing counseling intensity. Skills developed in the group setting can be evaluated in a patient's natural interactions with staff and other patients in the treatment setting. Patients who continue to use drugs despite increased counseling intensity, and those with high levels of psychiatric distress and familial problems, will likely achieve additional therapeutic benefit from attending specialized individual- or group-based psychotherapies and family therapy. Contingency management strategies using clinic-based incentives can be used to improve counseling attendance and strengthen treatment outcomes attained through psychosocial interventions (see chap. 8). And finally, adherence to community-based treatment goals established within the program can be optimized for all patients with the help of significant-other monitoring.

This chapter has also pointed to the limited interest and poor attendance of patients to the individual- and group-based treatments reviewed. Many of the major clinical trials described previously either failed to report actual rates of counseling attendance or provided data showing modest to poor rates of compliance (table 7.2). It is likely that many patients and some program staff perceived these interventions, from individual and group counseling to the specialized therapies, as ancillary to the methadone (Kidorf et al. 1995). This detail was brought out explicitly in studies evaluating the effectiveness of specialized psychotherapies. Attendance rates were higher when the therapy was offered within the methadone treatment program (Woody et al. 1983, 1985) than when similar services were offered outside of the methadone treatment setting (Rounsaville et al. 1983). Yet in these studies by Woody and colleagues, only 50 percent of the patients attended scheduled psychotherapy sessions. The low rates of attendance reported in most studies make it almost impossible to evaluate the true impact of routine counseling and specialized psychotherapies on rehabilitation when the interventions are delivered on an intermittent schedule in an unpredictable manner.

This body of literature further suggests that verbal persuasion is insufficient to enhance initial compliance with these interventions, especially among patients with severe problem profiles characterized by multiple drug use disorders and severe psychiatric and social problems. Even though considerable attention is directed toward studies attempting to

Table 7.2   Rates of Adherence to Scheduled Counseling and Therapy Sessions across Selected Studies

Study	Type of Therapy	Length of Therapy (wks)	Scheduled Sessions	Attended Sessions	Adherence Rate (%)
Stanton and Todd 1982	Family (paid)	10	10	4–10	Unknown
	Family (unpaid)	10	0	0–10	Unknown
Woody et al. 1983	Individual counseling	24	24	17	71
	Individual counseling + supplementary psychotherapy	24	48	24	50
Rounsaville et al. 1983	Individual/group counseling	24	Unknown	Unknown	Unknown
	Individual/group counseling + supplementary psychotherapy	24	Unknown	Unknown	Unknown
McLellan et al 1993	Individual counseling	24	14–44	Unknown	Unknown
Magura et al. 1994	Individual counseling + group counseling	24	120–144	Unknown	Unknown
Woody et al. 1995	Individual counseling + supplementary counseling	24	48	23	48
	Individual counseling + supplementary psychotherapy	24	48	26	54
Iguchi et al. 1996	Group counseling (with incentives)	12	8	4.8	60
	Group counseling (without incentives)	12	8	0	0
Fals-Stewart et al. 2001	Couples counseling	12	12	9	75

match patients to specific verbal and behavioral therapies (McLellan et al. 1980, 1983, 1997; Strain 2004), the larger problem facing programs is how to get patients to regularly attend even routine counseling much less enhanced or specialized forms of treatment. The magnitude of this problem is profound and severely limits the effectiveness of available psychosocial and medication treatment for drug abuse. The remainder of this chapter reviews a treatment service-delivery approach that is capable of significantly enhancing counseling attendance in opioid substitution programs.

MOTIVATED STEPPED CARE

A new service-delivery model instituted in our treatment program several years ago links the continued delivery of methadone and other treatment services with attendance to scheduled counseling sessions (motivated stepped care, MSC) (Brooner and Kidorf 2002). This is a rational approach for fully integrating the pharmacologic and psychosocial treatment elements of a drug abuse rehabilitation program (NIDA 1995) and follows the basic principles of an adaptive treatment approach for patients with chronic health problems that require some level of clinical attention over many months or years (Murphy and McKay 2004; Murphy et al. 2001). Patients who use illicit drugs or alcohol, or miss scheduled counseling sessions, are advanced to higher steps of weekly counseling intensity. The most intensive step of care (described in more detail below) involves at least nine hours of weekly individual and group-counseling services, and includes weekly sessions with a drug-free significant other who helps monitor adherence to the treatment plan. Patients who choose to miss scheduled counseling at this highest step of care begin a 30-day methadone dose taper that is stopped only after one week of full treatment adherence and submission of a drug-negative urine sample. Patients who reach a methadone dose of 0 mg are discharged from the program, but are also offered rapid readmission to the program contingent only on agreeing to attend all their counseling sessions.

MSC borrows heavily from the psychosocial literature of effective treatments for drug abuse and other motivated disorders and aspects of the community reinforcement model that incorporate drug-abstinent family members as community monitors and reinforcers of therapeutic progress. The progression of intensity of counseling services also borrows from stepped models of care that have been strongly advocated for the treatment of many psychiatric disorders, including alcohol abuse (Newman 2000; Sobell and Sobell 2000). Stepped-care treatment is initiated at a "least restrictive" level that is intensified only after evidence of poor treatment response. Thus, each patient is matched to the minimum amount of treatment necessary to achieve a good clinical outcome. This model has the potential to be highly cost-effective because the most intensive and specialized treatments are scheduled only for those doing poorly at lower levels of care, making it particularly well suited for opioid substitution programs that need to optimize the use of often limited resources.

MSC addresses a potential weakness in stepped models of care that assume more intensive schedules of service will be consistently attended by individuals who are already missing routine counseling sessions. Our review of the literature demonstrates that opioid abusers are generally poorly adherent to psychosocial interventions offered at minimal, let alone enhanced levels of care, but that behavioral reinforcement can significantly improve rates of adherence. MSC was developed based on empirical data and clinical impression suggesting patients might be motivated to reduce drug use and engage more fully in psychosocial treatments if doing so is linked to continued availability of medication (Dolan et al. 1985; Kidorf and Stitzer 1993; McCarthy and Borders 1985). This procedure is consistent with the well-known behavioral principle that a less desirable (and therefore low frequency) behavior such as counseling attendance can be reinforced and increased when it results in access to another more desirable behavior such as ingestion of a methadone dose.

The Structured Steps of Care

MSC offers a progression of counseling services in which both the quantity or "dose" of individual and group counseling and the clinical specialization of the treatment provider is enhanced for patients who are consistently drug positive or who consistently miss scheduled counseling sessions and reduced for patients who are drug negative and regularly attend counseling sessions. All patients are educated about the structured steps of care when initially applying for treatment and again on the day of admission; the treatment model is then regularly reviewed with patients by the treatment staff. The careful attention paid to educating and reeducating the patient about the treatment methods used in the program ensures that they remain aware of the consequences of continued drug use and failure to attend scheduled counseling sessions. The structural and dynamic aspects of this approach produce a predictable response to the changing clinical status of patients and therefore enhances individualized care. The escalating intensities of weekly counseling also have the added value of improving the daily structure of drug-using patients whose day-to-day lives are often disorganized and chaotic.

The program uses four distinct levels of weekly counseling based on the patient's most recent clinical status. These steps of care and the movement from one to another of these steps are described below (fig. 7.2). All changes in counseling steps are based on highly objective behaviors (i.e., rates of positive urine specimens and rates of counseling attendance) and are monitored weekly by senior clinical staff.

All new admissions to the program begin treatment in step 2, where they are required to attend one individual counseling session per week (30 minutes) and an eight-session drug education group. Patients at this step are therefore required to attend approximately 1.5 hours of counseling per week during the first eight weeks of care and about 30 minutes of individual counseling thereafter. Patients who remain stable at this step for several months (i.e., no drug use, compliant with counseling, and engaged in productive occupational, educational, or community activities) may be referred to step 1, which represents a limited version of medical maintenance in that patients are required to come to the program as infrequently as one to two times per month for medication and counseling (King et al. 2002).

Patients in step 2 who are drug positive and/or miss a scheduled counseling session during two consecutive weeks are advanced to step 3, where they are scheduled to attend one individual counseling session and two to four group sessions per week for a maximum of four weeks (i.e., 3.5–4.5 hours of counseling per week). The counseling groups are primarily skills oriented and manual guided, including relapse-control, job-skills training, stress management, role recovery, coping skills, and time management. These interventions are provided by senior clinical staff who thereby directly support the efforts of primary counselors to improve the patient's functioning. The primary counselor, in consultation with their supervisor and with input from the patient, selects from the list of available groups those that have the greatest apparent relevance to the patient's continued drug use. Patients who are attending all scheduled counseling and are drug negative during any two consecutive weeks in step 3 are referred back to step 2 for continuing care.

Patients in step 3 who continue to use drugs and miss counseling sessions are advanced to step 4 for eight weeks. At this point, patients are scheduled for two individual counseling sessions (30 minutes each) per week and between seven and nine group-counseling sessions, including twice per week cognitive-behavioral therapy and a mandatory significant-other group. In total, patients in step 4 are required to attend approxi-

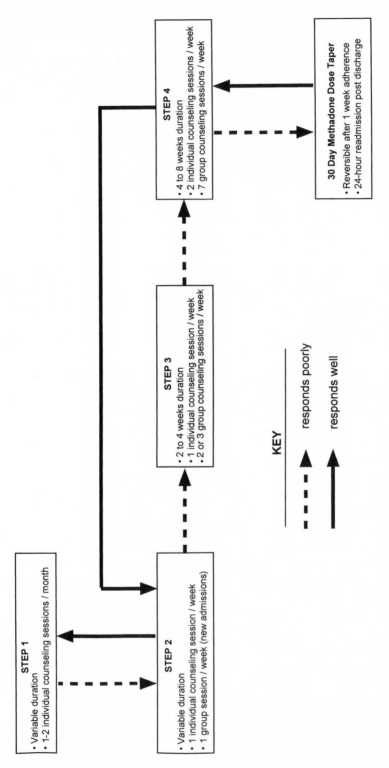

Figure 7.2. **The motivated stepped care (MSC) delivery system.** Patients begin treatment in step 2 and are advanced to higher or lower steps of care based on urinalysis results and counseling attendance. Patients who continue to test drug positive and/or miss counseling sessions in step 4 start a 30-day methadone dose taper that is reversed after one week of full program adherence. Those who reach a methadone dose of 0 mg are rapidly readmitted to step 4 care. Adapted from Brooner and Kidorf 2002.

mately 9–11 hours of counseling per week. As mentioned earlier, a significant other is incorporated to monitor the patient's involvement in specific aspects of the treatment plan outside the clinic to improve the extent of drug-free social supports. And to further enhance adherence to step 4 counseling requirements, those who miss scheduled sessions are placed on a series of escalating time restrictions for receiving methadone until one full week of adherence is attained. Patients who are drug-free and attending all counseling sessions during any four consecutive weeks in step 4 graduate to step 2.

Patients in step 4 who choose to continue missing scheduled counseling and use drugs are placed on a 30-day methadone dose taper in preparation for discharge. This discharge follows considerable direct evidence of the patient's unwillingness to follow the clearly articulated and predictable plan of care. Although it is always tempting to maintain these patients in treatment despite their obvious unwillingness to follow the treatment plan, doing so can seriously dilute the potency of treatment by letting patients continually avoid those services most likely to have a positive impact on their ongoing decisions to use drugs. Patients who choose to taper from methadone in preparation for discharge from the program are nonetheless encouraged to begin attending counseling sessions in the hopes that the methadone taper and impending discharge from the program will motivate them to follow the treatment plan. Many patients begin attending their counseling sessions during this period and therefore discontinue the medication taper. The medication dose in these patients is returned to the pretaper maintenance level after achieving one week of full counseling attendance. Those who elect to complete withdrawal from the medication are guaranteed rapid (i.e., 24 hour) readmission to the program if they attended at least 50 percent of their scheduled counseling sessions during the dose taper and agree to reenter treatment at step 4; those who miss more than 50 percent of their scheduled sessions can return to step 4 after seven days. Discharge from the program is therefore used as a discrete, reversible therapeutic intervention whose goal is to encourage patients to fully participate in aspects of their treatment plan previously ignored. This discharge procedure should reduce the likelihood of patients cycling through one after another methadone treatment program with little apparent benefit.

Overall, this service-delivery system has several important advantages: (1) it systematically lays out treatment expectations for patients and staff, which are uniform for all patients; (2) it focuses on improving individual- and group-counseling attendance, elements of treatment that have the best chance of identifying and altering the patient's decisions that result in high rates of drug use and other life problems; (3) it ensures that poorly performing patients receive additional and more specialized services; and (4) it provides all patients with the opportunity for rapid readmission simply by agreeing to follow the well-articulated plan of care.

Results from a recently completed clinical trial evaluating the efficacy of MSC support these claims (Brooner et al. 2004). One hundred twenty-seven patients were randomly assigned to either the MSC or standard stepped-care (SSC) condition. Patients in both conditions were referred to higher levels of counseling based on drug use and counseling adherence, as detailed earlier. However, the contingencies associated with step 4 participation were introduced only for patients in the MSC condition; SSC patients could remain in treatment independent of their rates of counseling attendance and drug use. Patients assigned to SSC, but who missed more than 50 percent of their scheduled groups or submitted over 50 percent drug-positive urine samples during the first 90 days of care, were therapeutically transferred to the MSC condition. The large proportion of SSC patients therapeutically transferred required main analyses to be limited to the first 90 days of study participation. The results showed that MSC patients were less likely to meet criteria for therapeutic transfer (43% versus 79%, $p < .001$) and had considerably higher rates of adherence to individual, group, and significant-other community support sessions (fig. 7.3). Although the two groups of new admissions did not sig-

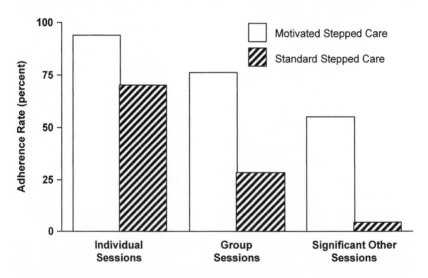

Figure 7.3. Patients assigned to the motivated stepped care (MSC) condition attended a higher proportion of individual, group, and significant other sessions than those assigned to the standard stepped-care (SSC) condition. Brooner et al. 2004.

nificantly differ in rates of drug-positive urine samples submitted during the first 90 days of treatment, SSC patients who were therapeutically transferred to the MSC condition after 90 days of high rates of ongoing drug use evidenced significant reductions in the proportion of both opiate-positive (0.40 versus 0.26, $p < .001$) and cocaine-positive (0.52 versus 0.40) urine samples. The retention rate among patients in both study conditions was excellent (95%) and showed no between-group differences. These results provide support for maximizing the efficacy of methadone pharmacotherapy for drug abuse by integrating it with appropriate levels of psychosocial treatments and meaningful behavioral incentives to enhance delivery of those services.

Summary

Drug abusers entering treatment programs that provide methadone typically present with several current drug use diagnoses, often have other comorbid psychiatric diagnoses, and have other medical and psychosocial problems that methadone has little efficacy for and was never intended to treat. Many psychosocial interventions have shown promise in treating these problems and thereby adding substantially to the benefits of methadone. Individual drug abuse counseling, in particular, has been shown to actively promote less drug use and overall better outcomes. Group therapy represents an efficient and potentially effective method for delivering education and skills-training interventions. Specialized psychotherapies may be beneficial for some patients if offered under conditions that maximize utilization. Family therapy, behavioral conjoint therapy, and significant-other monitoring also appear to be promising interventions for drug abusers, and these deserve more attention. It is problematic that patients often lack interest in these services and frequently miss counseling sessions when offered them. Patient adherence can be improved by implementing a new service-delivery model (i.e., MSC) that escalates counseling requirements for partial and poor responders and imposes a taper from methadone and discharge from the clinic as an ultimate motivator to change patient behavior.

Together, the approaches described represent a mixture of techniques designed to improve motivation for behavior change, to teach coping and decision-making skills needed to initiate and sustain abstinence, and to enhance non-drug-using sources of support and reinforcement. Although a minimal amount of counseling service is required for certification in the United States by the federal Center for Substance Abuse Treatment (CSAT), clinics should anticipate the need for additional therapeutic services to effectively respond to the daunting range and severity of problems expressed by patients dependent on drugs, keeping in mind that procedures to motivate patient attendance are often necessary to maximize treatment outcome and improve the cost-benefits and -effectiveness of these services.

References

Allison M, Hubbard RL (1985). Drug abuse treatment process: a review of the literature. *Int J Addict* 20: 1321–45.

Andersen AE (1984). Anorexia nervosa and bulimia: biological, psychological, and sociocultural aspects. In: Galler JR, ed. *Nutrition and Behavior*. New York: Plenum Publishing Corporation.

Azrin NH (1976). Improvements in the community-reinforcement approach to alcoholism. *Behav Res Ther* 14: 339–48.

Azrin NH, McMahon PT, Donohue B, Besalel VA, Lapinski KJ, Kogan ES, Acierno RE, Galloway E (1994). Behavior therapy for drug abuse: a controlled treatment outcome study. *Behav Res Ther* 32: 857–66.

Azrin NH, Sisson RW, Meyers R, Godley M (1982). Alcoholism treatment by disulfiram and community reinforcement therapy. *J Behav Ther Exp Psychiatry* 13: 105–12.

Ball JC, Ross A (1991). *The Effectiveness of Methadone Maintenance Treatment*. New York: Springer-Verlag.

Beck AT (1976). *Cognitive Therapy and the Emotional Disorders*. Guilford, CT: International University Press.

Bowen M (1971). Family therapy and family group therapy. In: Kaplan H, Sadock B, eds. *Comprehensive Group Therapy*. Baltimore, MD; Williams and Wilkins.

Brooner RK, Kidorf M (2002). Using behavioral reinforcement to improve methadone treatment participation. *Sci Pract Perspect* 1: 38–48.

Brooner RK, Kidorf MS, King VL, Stoller KB, Peirce JM, Bigelow GE, Kolodner K (2004). Behavioral contingencies improve counseling attendance in an adaptive treatment model. *J Subst Abuse Treat.* 27: 223–232.

Brooner RK, King VL, Kidorf M, Schmidt CW, Jr., Bigelow GE (1997). Psychiatric and substance use comorbidity among treatment-seeking opioid abusers. *Arch Gen Psychiatry* 54: 71–80.

Carroll KM, Rounsaville BJ, Nich C, Gordon LT, Wirtz PW, Gawin F (1994). One-year follow-up of psychotherapy and pharmacotherapy for cocaine dependence. Delayed emergence of psychotherapy effects. *Arch Gen Psychiatry* 51: 989–97.

Chaney EF (1989). Social skills training. In: Hester RK, Miller WR, eds. *Handbook of Alcoholism Treatment Approaches: Effective Alternatives*, 206–21. New York: Pergamon.

Cooney NL, Kadden RM, Litt MD, Getter H (1991). Matching alcoholics to coping skills or interactional therapies: two-year follow-up results. *J Consult Clin Psychol* 59: 598–601.

Daley DC, Mercer D (2002). Drug Counseling for Addiction: The Collaborative Cocaine Treatment Model. NIH Pub. No. 02-4381. Bethesda, MD: National Institute on Drug Abuse.

Dolan MP, Black JL, Penk WE, Robinowitz R, DeFord HA (1985). Contracting for treatment termination to reduce illicit drug use among methadone maintenance treatment failures. *J Consult Clin Psychol* 53: 549–51.

Fals-Stewart W, Birchler GR (2001). A national survey of the use of couples therapy in substance abuse treatment. *J Subst Abuse Treat* 20: 277–83; discussion 285–6.

Fals-Stewart W, Birchler GR, O'Farrell TJ (1996). Behavioral couples therapy for male substance-abusing patients: effects on relationship adjustment and drug-using behavior. *J Consult Clin Psychol* 64: 959–72.

Fals-Stewart W, O'Farrell TJ (2003). Behavioral family counseling and naltrexone for male opioid-dependent patients. *J Consult Clin Psychol* 71: 432–42.

Fals-Stewart W, O'Farrell TJ, Birchler GR (2001). Behavioral couples therapy for male methadone maintenance patients: effects on drug using behavior and relationship adjustment. *Behav Ther* 32: 391–411.

Galanter M (1993). *Network Therapy for Drug and Alcohol Abuse.* New York: Guilford Press.

Galanter M, Keller DS, Dermatis H (1997). Network therapy for addiction: assessment of the clinical outcome of training. *Am J Drug Alcohol Abuse* 23: 355–67.

Gill K, Nolimal D, Crowley TJ (1992). Antisocial personality disorder, HIV risk behavior and retention in methadone maintenance therapy. *Drug Alcohol Depend* 30: 247–52.

Gossop M, Stewart D, Marsden J (2003). Treatment process components and heroin use outcome among methadone patients. *Drug Alcohol Depend* 71: 93–102.

Hall SM, Loeb P, LeVois M, Cooper J (1981). Increasing employment in ex-heroin addicts II: methadone maintenance sample. *Behav Ther* 12: 453–60.

Havassy BE, Hall SM, Wasserman DA (1991). Social support and relapse: commonalities among alcoholics, opiate users, and cigarette smokers. *Addict Behav* 16: 235–46.

Hermalin JA, Steer RA, Platt JJ, Metzger DS (1990). Risk characteristics associated with chronic unemployment in methadone clients. *Drug Alcohol Depend* 26: 117–25.

Hunt GM, Azrin NH (1973). A community-reinforcement approach to alcoholism. *Behav Res Ther* 11: 91–104.

Iguchi MY, Lamb RJ, Belding MA, Platt JJ, Husband SD, Morral AR (1996). Contingent reinforcement of group participation versus abstinence in a methadone maintenance program. *Exp Clin Psychopharmacol* 4: 315–321.

Joe GW, Simpson DD, Dansereau DF, Rowan-Szal GA (2001). Relationships between counseling rapport and drug abuse treatment outcomes. *Psychiatr Serv* 52: 1223–9.

Kauffman JF, Woody GE (1995). Matching treatment to patient needs in opioid substitution therapy. DHHS Pub. No. (SMA) 95-3049. Washington, DC: U.S. Government Printing Office.

Kaufman E (1985). Family systems and family therapy of substance abuse: an overview of two decades of research and clinical experience. *Int J Addict* 20: 897–916.

Kaufman EF (1989). *Family therapy in substance abuse treatment. Treatment of Psychiatric Disorders.* Washington, DC: American Psychiatric Association.

Khantzian EJ, Halliday KS, Golden S, McAuliffe WE (1992). Modified group therapy for substance abusers: a psychodynamic approach to relapse-prevention. *Am J Addict* 1: 67–76.

Kidorf M, Brooner RK, King VL (1997). Motivating methadone patients to include drug-free significant others in treatment: a behavioral intervention. *J Subst Abuse Treat* 14: 23–8.

Kidorf M, Hollander JR, King VL, Brooner RK (1998). Increasing employment of opioid dependent outpatients: an intensive behavioral intervention. *Drug Alcohol Depend* 50: 73–80.

Kidorf M, Neufeld K, Brooner RK (2004) Combining stepped care approaches with behavioral reinforcement to motivate employment in opioid-dependent outpatients. *Subst Use Misuse*. 39: 2215–38.

Kidorf M, Stitzer ML (1993). Contingent access to methadone maintenance treatment: effects on cocaine use of mixed opiate-cocaine users. *Exp Clin Psychopharmacol* 1: 200–6.

Kidorf M, Stitzer ML, Brooner RK (1994). Characteristics of methadone patients responding to take-home incentives. *Behav Ther* 25: 109–21.

Kidorf M, Stitzer ML, Griffiths RR (1995). Evaluating the reinforcement value of clinic-based privileges through a multiple choice procedure. *Drug Alcohol Depend* 39: 167–72.

Kidorf MS, Stitzer ML (1999). Contingent access to clinic privileges reduced drug abuse in methadone maintenance patients. In: Higgins S, Silverman K, eds. *Motivating Behavior Change among Illicit-Drug Abusers: Contemporary Research on Contingency Management Interventions*. Washington, DC: American Psychological Association Books.

King VL, Stoller KB, Hayes M, Umbricht A, Currens M, Kidorf MS, Carter JA, Schwartz R, Brooner RK (2002). A multicenter randomized evaluation of methadone medical maintenance. *Drug Alcohol Depend* 65: 137–48.

Klerman GL, Weissman MM, Rounsaville BJ, Chevron ES (1984). *Interpersonal Psychotherapy of Depression*. New York: Basic Books.

Luborsky L (1984). *Principles of Psychoanalytic Psychotherapy: A Manual for Supportive-Expressive (SE) Treatment*. New York: Basic Books.

Magura S, Rosenblum A, Lovejoy M, Handelsman L, Foote J, Stimmel B (1994). Neurobehavioral treatment for cocaine-using methadone patients: a preliminary report. *J Addict Dis* 13: 143–60.

Marlatt GA, Gordon JR (1985). *Relapse Prevention*. New York: The Guilford Press.

McAuliffe WE (1990). A randomized controlled trial of recovery training and self-help for opioid addicts in New England and Hong Kong. *J Psychoactive Drugs* 22: 197–209.

McCarthy JJ, Borders OT (1985). Limit setting on drug abuse in methadone maintenance patients. *Am J Psychiatry* 142: 1419–23.

McCrady BS, Noel NE, Abrams DB, Stout RL, Nelson HF, Hay WM (1986). Comparative effectiveness of three types of spouse involvement in outpatient behavioral alcoholism treatment. *J Stud Alcohol* 47: 459–67.

McHugh PR, Slavney PR (1998). *The Perspectives of Psychiatry, 2nd ed*. Baltimore, MD: Johns Hopkins University Press.

McLellan AT, Alterman AI, Cacciola J, Metzger D, O'Brien CP (1992). A new measure of substance abuse treatment. Initial studies of the treatment services review. *J Nerv Ment Dis* 180: 101–10.

McLellan AT, Arndt IO, Metzger DS, Woody GE, O'Brien CP (1993). The effect of psychosocial services in substance abuse treatment. *JAMA* 269: 1953–9.

McLellan AT, Ball JC, Rosen L, O'Brien CP (1981). Pretreatment source of income and response to methadone maintenance: a follow-up study. *Am J Psychiatry* 138: 785–9.

McLellan AT, Grissom GR, Zanis D, Randall M, Brill P, O'Brien CP (1997). Problem-service 'matching' in addiction treatment. A prospective study in 4 programs. *Arch Gen Psychiatry* 54: 730–5.

McLellan AT, Luborsky L, Woody GE, O'Brien CP, Druley KA (1983). Predicting response to alcohol and drug abuse treatments. Role of psychiatric severity. *Arch Gen Psychiatry* 40: 620–5.

McLellan AT, O'Brien CP, Kron R, Alterman AI, Druley KA (1980). Matching substance abuse patients to appropriate treatments: a conceptual and methodological approach. *Drug Alcohol Depend* 5: 189–95.

McLellan AT, Woody GE, Luborsky L, Goehl L (1988). Is the counselor an "active ingredient" in substance abuse rehabilitation? An examination of treatment success among four counselors. *J Nerv Ment Dis* 176: 423–30.

Mercer DE, Woody GE (2000). An Individual Drug Counseling Approach to Treat Cocaine Addiction: The Collaborative Cocaine Treatment Study Model. NIDA Therapy Manuals for Addiction. USDHS Pub. No. 00-4380. Rockville, MD: National Institute on Drug Abuse.

Miller WR, Rollnick S (1991). *Motivational Interviewing.* New York: The Guilford Press.

Minuchin S (1974). *Families and Family Therapy.* Cambridge, MA: Harvard University Press.

Murphy SA, McKay JR (2004) Adaptive treatment strategies: an emerging approach for improving treatment effectiveness. *Clin Sci.* winter-spring: 4–13.

Murphy SA, van der Laan MJ, Robins J, CPPRG (2001). Marginal mean models for dynamic regimes. *J Am Stat Assoc* 96: 1410–23.

Newman MG (2000). Recommendations for a cost-offset model of psychotherapy allocation using generalized anxiety disorder as an example. *J Consult Clin Psychol* 68: 549–55.

NIDA (1995). Integrating Behavioral Therapies with Medications in the Treatment of Drug Dependence. NIH Pub. No. 95-3899. Rockville, MD: National Institute on Drug Abuse.

Nyswander M, Winick C, Bernstein A, Brill L, Kaufer G (1958). Treatment of the narcotic addict: workshop, 1957. 1. The treatment of drug addicts as voluntary outpatients; a progress report. *Am J Orthopsychiatry* 28: 714–27; discussion 727–9.

O'Farrell TJ, Choquette KA, Cutter HS, Brown ED, McCourt WF (1993). Behavioral marital therapy with and without additional couples relapse prevention sessions for alcoholics and their wives. *J Stud Alcohol* 54: 652–66.

O'Farrell TJ, Cutter HS, Floyd FJ (1985). Evaluating behavioral marital therapy for male alcoholics: effects on marital adjustment and communication from before to after treatment. *Behav Ther* 16: 147–67.

O'Farrell TJ, Fals-Stewart W (2000). Behavioral couples therapy for alcoholism and drug abuse. *J Subst Abuse Treat* 18: 51–54.

Platt JJ (1995). Vocational rehabilitation of drug abusers. *Psychol Bull* 117: 416–33.

Rawson RA, Obert JL, McCann MJ, Smith DP, Ling W (1990). Neurobehavioral treatment for cocaine dependency. *J Psychoactive Drugs* 22: 159–71.

Rounsaville BJ, Glazer W, Wilber CH, Weissman MM, Kleber HD (1983). Short-term interpersonal psychotherapy in methadone-maintained opiate addicts. *Arch Gen Psychiatry* 40: 629–36.

Silverman K, Chutuape MA, Svikis DS, Bigelow GE, Stitzer ML (1995). Incongruity between occupational interests and academic skills in drug abusing women. *Drug Alcohol Depend* 40: 115–23.

Simpson DD, Joe GW, Rowan-Szal G, Greener J (1995). Client engagement and change during drug abuse treatment. *J Subst Abuse* 7: 117–34.

Sisson RW, Azrin NH (1986). Family-member involvement to initiate and promote treatment of problem drinkers. *J Behav Ther Exp Psychiatry* 17: 15–21.

Sobell MB, Sobell LC (2000). Stepped care as a heuristic approach to the treatment of alcohol problems. *J Consult Clin Psychol* 68: 573–9.

Stanton MD, Shadish WR (1997). Outcome, attrition, and family-couples treatment for drug abuse: a meta-analysis and review of the controlled, comparative studies. *Psychol Bull* 122: 170–91.

Stanton MD, Todd TC (1982). *The Family Therapy of Drug Abuse and Addiction.* New York: The Guilford Press

Strain EC (2004). Patient-treatment matching and opioid addicted patients: past methods and future opportunities. *Heroin Addict Relat Clin Prob* 6 (3): 5–16.

Wasserman DA, Stewart AL, Delucchi KL (2001). Social support and abstinence from opiates and cocaine during opioid maintenance treatment. *Drug Alcohol Depend* 65: 65–75.

Woody GE, Luborsky L, McLellan AT, O'Brien CP, Beck AT, Blaine J, Herman I, Hole A (1983). Psychotherapy for opiate addicts. Does it help? *Arch Gen Psychiatry* 40: 639–45.

Woody GE, McLellan AT, Luborsky L, O'Brien CP (1985). Sociopathy and psychotherapy outcome. *Arch Gen Psychiatry* 42: 1081–6.

Woody GE, McLellan AT, Luborsky L, O'Brien CP (1995). Psychotherapy in community methadone programs: a validation study. *Am J Psychiatry* 152: 1302–8.

Yalom ID (1975). *The Theory and Practice of Group Psychotherapy.* New York: Basic Books.

Zweben A, Pearlman S, Li S (1983). Reducing attrition from conjoint therapy with alcoholic couples. *Drug Alcohol Depend* 11: 321–31.

8

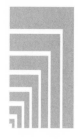

Contingency Management Therapies

Maxine L. Stitzer, Ph.D., Nancy Petry, Ph.D., and
Kenneth Silverman, Ph.D.

Methadone is an effective but incomplete treatment for opioid dependence. Even if illicit opioid use is brought under control, numerous problems remain to be addressed in the methadone maintenance population,
not the least of which is use of other drugs of abuse, such as cocaine. To
address these psychosocial and drug use problems, counseling has always
been included as a part of methadone treatment. Chapter 7 reviews the
various types of counseling and psychosocial treatments that have been
used and evaluated.

Within the panoply of therapy interventions, contingency management is one of the most effective and generally useful. Contingency management procedures may be loosely considered motivational interventions
designed to promote a clinically desirable behavior change. Under these
procedures, patients are offered some attractive options (e.g., a clinic privilege or prize) contingent on performing a clinically desired target behavior (e.g., drug abstinence as verified by drug-free urinalysis results). This
type of contingency often increases the frequency of the therapeutically
desired behavior, thereby accomplishing an important goal of treatment.
In addition to their proven effectiveness, contingency management procedures have considerable versatility because they can be used to increase
a wide range of desirable behaviors, from counseling attendance to compliance with medication regimens (e.g., daily ingestion of antiretroviral
medications).

Contingency management procedures are firmly rooted in an extensive body of basic and applied research in learning and conditioning. This body of research has not only guided the development of these procedures but, if the underlying principles are understood, can also be useful to practitioners in applying contingency management procedures to novel clinical situations and problems. This chapter briefly discusses the underlying rationale for contingency management procedures and then presents a review of controlled studies that have assessed the effectiveness of contingency management techniques in the treatment of patients receiving methadone. The final section of the chapter contains clinical recommendations for designing and implementing contingency management programs in the treatment of patients receiving methadone.

Rationale for Contingency Management Interventions

The approach taken in treatment of any disorder reflects, at least in part, the way the therapist views the underlying causes of the disorder. For example, the twelve-step approach to treatment is based on the concept that drug abuse is a disease over which the individual has little or no control. This concept implies that the drug abuser must seek outside help (i.e., from a higher power) to overcome the ravages of the disease. Contingency management approaches stem from a different view of the origins of drug abuse. Specifically, in this approach, drug abuse is viewed as a learned behavior, supported by the biological reinforcing effects of drugs. This behavior can then be counteracted by applying principles of behavior management, including reward and punishment.

The term *operant* refers to behavior that changes the environment by operating or acting on it. In a behavioral approach to drug abuse, the behaviors involved in drug seeking are viewed as operant behaviors that result in ingestion of a drug. The consequences of an operant behavior determine whether the behavior will occur under similar circumstances in the future. In the terminology of operant conditioning, consequences are classified as *reinforcing* if they increase the likelihood that a behavior will occur in the future, and *punishing* if they decrease the likelihood that the behavior will occur again. In the research laboratory, where these principles were first recognized, the dispensing of food pellets after a rat's lever press usually results in more lever pressing. The fact that many humans escalate their drug use over time after initial drug exposure indicates that drugs can act as reinforcers for humans. However, the fact that not all humans who try drugs become abusers means that modifying predispositions and circumstances exist that determine who will and who will not become a drug abuser after exposure to the reinforcing effects of drugs. In addition, humans may differ on just how reinforcing they find drug effects both initially and with repeated use over time.

The reinforcing power of drugs is not restricted to humans but can be clearly demonstrated in other animal species, including monkeys, dogs, rodents, birds, and marine mammals. Much research has shown that animals, given the opportunity in a laboratory setting, will self-administer the same drugs that are abused by humans (Griffiths et al. 1980). This evidence supports a biological basis for drug reinforcement. In support of this concept of biological reinforcement, we also know that drugs act on certain regions of the brain, which are the same regions that control pleasurable sensations derived from biological reinforcers, including food, water, and sex (Koob and Bloom 1988; Koob and Le Moal 1997). The biological basis of drug reinforcement is what makes drug use such a compelling option for some people, and it also underlies much of the difficulty people have when trying to stop using drugs. Research has also shown that behaviors maintained by drug reinforcement are similar to behaviors maintained by other reinforcers such as food, water, and social contact. Specifically, the frequency of the behavior will change (i.e., increase or decrease) if its consequences change. For example, drug self-administration can be decreased by presenting a punishing event that is also contingent on drug-seeking or drug-taking responses, or if drug use results in immediate loss of other valued reinforcers.

The identification of drug use as an operant behavior and drugs as biological reinforcers has affected our understanding and the clinical treatment of drug abuse. Most important, with respect to this chapter, these views have led to systematic efforts to decrease drug use by manipulating the consequences of drug use versus abstinence. During the past 25 years, treatment researchers and treatment providers have been arranging consequences to drug use and related behaviors in efforts to decrease drug use and increase more productive activity. Such programs are called *contingency management* programs.

Contingency Management Interventions in Methadone Treatment

The methadone clinic is a place well suited for the implementation of therapeutic contingency management programs, in part, because methadone tends to retain patients in treatment for extended periods, allowing sufficient time to implement and fully evaluate contingency management interventions. Equally important, methadone itself or features of its delivery (dose size, dosing frequency, take-home doses) can be used as re-inforcers in contingency management programs to promote desirable changes in behavior. In addition, other reinforcers such as cash payments, voucher payments (point systems), or drawings for on-site prizes can be administered in the methadone clinic. As a result of these circumstances, much of what we know about contingency management interventions in drug treatment has been learned from treating patients receiving metha-done.

Contingency management interventions can be specified by defining four major dimensions: (1) the *target behavior,* which is the behavior the therapist wants to change (e.g., attend counseling sessions); (2) the *conditions* (antecedents) under which the target behaviors are to occur (e.g., every Monday at 2:00 p.m. with no reminders from program staff); (3) the *reinforcer* (e.g., one bus token); and (4) the *contingency,* which specifies the rules according to which reinforcers can be earned for produc-ing the target behavior (e.g., one bus token for each counseling session at-tended). Contingency management interventions conducted in metha-done programs have varied in all these main dimensions. For the purpose of this chapter, we have grouped contingency management procedures by the reinforcers used to emphasize the therapeutic resources available to clinicians for changing the behavior of patients receiving methadone.

Contingent Methadone

The continued opportunity to receive methadone can function as a rein-forcer, and this opportunity can be incorporated into contingency man-agement procedures. For example, in an early study of this type (described in chap. 17), Liebson and colleagues required patients with chronic alco-holism to take disulfiram as a condition of continuing methadone main-tenance treatment and showed that in a controlled design study, this could be an effective intervention for managing patients with alcoholism (Lieb-son et al. 1978).

McCarthy and Borders studied a "structured" methadone delivery system versus a usual care control treatment in 69 patients (McCarthy and Borders 1985). The goal was to prevent excessive drug use during treat-ment. Thus, if patients in the structured group delivered drug-positive urine samples during four or more consecutive months, they were placed on irreversible methadone withdrawal and forced to leave the program. Patients in the unstructured treatment condition continued to receive methadone treatment regardless of their drug use. At the end of the 12-month evaluation period, the structured group achieved significantly more drug-free months (63%) than the unstructured treatment group (49%). A comparison between the first- and last-month urine samples showed greater treatment improvement by patients in the structured treatment (14 vs. 3 patients improved). The structured program also retained more patients (53%) during the full 12 months than the unstructured treatment (30%). Thus, the study showed that placing even modest expectations on patients and backing these up with contingencies had a beneficial effect on treatment outcome.

Kidorf and Stitzer used continued treatment access to motivate new methadone-treated patients to stop their drug use at the beginning of treatment (Kidorf and Stitzer 1993). Study patients ($N = 44$) were enrolled in a 90-day premaintenance probationary program. Those randomly assigned to contingent treatment were required to submit two consecutive weeks of cocaine-free urine samples during their first seven weeks of treatment to gain entry into a two-year maintenance program. Noncontingent patients gained access to the program independent of urinalysis results. Fifty percent of patients in the contingent group versus 14 percent of patients in the noncontingent group submitted two consecutive weeks of drug-free urine samples during the seven-week probationary period.

These and other studies (Dolan et al. 1985) have shown that the threat of treatment termination can effectively motivate a therapeutic behavior change in patients receiving methadone. (A more refined version of this approach—motivated stepped care—is described in chap. 7.) One shortcoming of these studies, however, is that they did not evaluate the status of terminated patients. Although the procedures involving threat of treatment termination clearly provide a structure and motivation that is helpful to some patients, those who leave the program may be worse off than if they had continued in methadone treatment, even if they continued in treatment with poor performance on typical treatment outcome measures. Potential adverse effects in terminated patients need more study, in particular, because these procedures are widely used and because adverse consequences of treatment termination can be serious, including HIV infection and premature death.

Methadone Dose Changes

Methadone's reinforcing effects can also be harnessed by providing short-term methadone dose increases or decreases contingent on the occurrence or nonoccurrence, respectively, of target responses. Two studies that used this approach have shown that methadone dose changes can be effective for motivating behavior change.

In a methadone detoxification study by Higgins and colleagues, 39 participants were randomly assigned to contingent, noncontingent, or control treatment groups (Higgins et al. 1986). After having been stabilized on 30 mg per day of methadone in the first three weeks, all participants received identical gradual methadone dose reductions (i.e., withdrawal) during the eight-week study intervention phase. As their methadone dose decreased, members of the contingent and noncontingent groups could obtain daily methadone dose supplements of up to 20 mg, but patients in the contingent group qualified for the dose supplements only if they provided an opioid-free urine sample. Figure 8.1 shows that during the second half of the evaluation phase, the percentage of opioid-positive urine samples was significantly lower for the contingent group (14%) than for either the noncontingent (38%) or control (50%) groups. Thus, the study showed that the opportunity to receive extra methadone during a detoxification could prevent relapse to opioid use, but this was

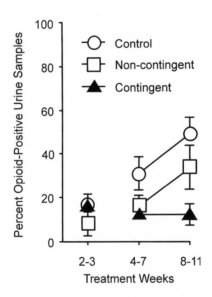

Figure 8.1. Opioid-dependent patients (N = 39) were stabilized on 30 mg per day methadone; then they were given an eight-week withdrawal during which they were randomly assigned to experimental conditions. Some could request and receive methadone dose increases up to 20 mg per day independent of their drug use (noncontingent); some could request and receive the same dose increases only if their most recent urine tested negative for opiates (contingent); the remainder (controls) could not receive any dose increases. Mean (± SEM) percentage opioid-negative urine samples are shown for each group during study weeks 2–3 (stabilization), 4–7 (early withdrawal), and 8–11 (late withdrawal). Higgins et al. 1986.

true only if the extra dose was given contingent on submitting opioid-free urine samples. This study provides a powerful demonstration that the contingency (not the dose increase per se) is the critical element for an effective intervention.

Another study (Stitzer et al. 1986) used dose change as either a reward (patients could receive dose increases for providing drug-free urine samples) or a punishment (patients received dose decreases for submitting drug-positive urine samples) to determine whether one system might work better than the other. After a 10-week baseline, study patients ($N = 20$) were randomly assigned to the increase or decrease procedure. Doses were adjusted weekly (by 5–15 mg) based on urine test results and could fluctuate up and down for both groups. The dose-increase group could go as high as 160 percent of their starting dose but never went below their baseline dose, whereas the dose-decrease group could go as low as 40 percent of their starting dose but never went above that original dose. Both dose-change procedures resulted in significantly more negative urine samples during the contingent phase (42%) than during the baseline phase (13%). This study showed that contingencies involving small methadone dose changes (5–15 mg per week) could be effective for some patients in motivating abstinence from supplemental drug use when incorporated into a structured contingency plan. The specific nature of the dose-change procedure did not seem to matter. Note, however, that more study dropouts occurred when the dose-decrease procedure was used. Therefore, the precaution about potential adverse effects of treatment termination procedures that were discussed previously also applies to interventions that involve methadone dose reductions.

Methadone Split Dosing

A final variation on the theme of dose alteration contingencies is split dosing. This is a procedure in which participants receive half of their daily dose during the clinic's morning hours and the other half-dose during the clinic's evening hours. Split dosing is inconvenient and mildly aversive for patients; thus, they may be willing to change behavior to avoid the procedure. Kidorf and Stitzer investigated the procedure in 16 polydrug-abusing patients who had not responded previously to contingent take-home interventions (Kidorf and Stitzer 1996). Study patients participated in both experimental and control procedures at different times. For the control condition, treatment was as usual. In the experimental condition, urine samples were collected on Mondays and Thursdays. Patients testing positive on a Monday were placed on split dosing for Monday, Tuesday, and Wednesday. Patients testing positive on a Thursday were placed on split dosing for Thursday and Friday. Split dosing was not in effect during the weekends. Study patients could also earn a take-home dose for each drug-negative urine sample submitted during the study. While in the experimental condition, patients submitted significantly more drug-free urine samples (29%) than during the baseline (12%) or control (9%) conditions. However, patients were often not fully compliant with the split-dosing procedure and ended up taking only half their dose.

Dose-Change Summary

This section has shown that contingent dose changes, both increases and decreases, can be an effective method to motivate behavior change in patients receiving methadone. This information must be counterbalanced, however, against the known importance of maintaining patients on an adequate stable methadone dose to achieve successful outcomes (see chap. 6) and the potential adverse effects of treatment termination. Clinicians should be aware of the potential disadvantages of any contingencies that involve methadone dose reduction, because these can lead to increased drug use or treatment dropout. This caution would also apply to the split-dose procedure because patients frequently did not take both halves of their dose, even though both were available. On the other hand, contingent dose increases could be a useful clinical strategy to motivate targeted changes in behavior.

Take-Home Methadone Doses

The requirement for daily ingestion of methadone imposes a burden on patients who must travel to the clinic seven days per week to obtain their dose. To ease this burden, patients may be given one or more "take-home" doses of methadone so that they can ingest some of their doses in the convenience of their home. Survey research with patients receiving methadone (e.g., Chutuape et al. 1998; Stitzer et al. 1977) has indicated that take-home dosing is the most highly desired privilege available at the methadone clinic. Furthermore, take-home doses are an ideal reinforcer for use in contingency management procedures, because they are a discrete commodity that can be delivered to the patient after each instance of the desired target behavior. In addition, there is no evidence that take-home doses lose potency as a reinforcer with repeated use in contingency programs; on the contrary, patients may find them more desirable after experiencing their benefits. Overall, take-home doses are a potent positive reinforcer available within the routine operation of the opioid treatment program.

A New Way to Use Take-Home Privileges

In the operation of a typical opioid treatment program, take-home privileges are often reserved for patients who have been drug free for a prolonged period (e.g., 90 days or more; see table 9.4), and employment may also be required. Take-home doses have been used differently in the research described below, in which they are used as reinforcers to promote behavior change in patients who would not typically be awarded take-home privileges because of their ongoing drug use. To enhance the ability of the take-home dose to function as a reinforcer, these studies have typically required a relatively small amount of behavior change (e.g., attendance at a single counseling session; two-week periods of abstinence) before awarding a take-home dose. The studies outlined below, then, describe a different way of utilizing take-home privileges to promote behavior change and evaluate their ability to promote the desired behavior change.

Clinic Behavior Targets

Contingent take-home privileges can be used to enhance participation in drug treatment activities. For example, one study showed that patients were more likely to keep their clinic fees up-to-date by paying their fees weekly on Wednesday to receive a Thursday take-home dose (Stitzer and Bigelow 1984a). Several other studies have shown that contingent take-home doses can increase attendance at regularly scheduled drug abuse counseling (Stitzer et al. 1977) or supplemental counseling sessions (Iguchi et al. 1996; Kidorf et al. 1994). The study by Kidorf and colleagues is especially noteworthy because patients did not have to attend the extra therapy sessions, and when no reinforcers were offered, only 7 percent of sessions were attended. However, when a single take-home dose could be earned for each attendance, there was a 10-fold increase in compliance, with 75 percent of scheduled sessions attended. Similarly, Iguchi and colleagues demonstrated that a take-home incentive program had a dramatic impact on the attendance rate of patients receiving methadone at a special group therapy program (Iguchi et al. 1996). Subjects in the contingent take-home group attended 60 percent of the scheduled group therapy sessions on average, whereas only a single session was attended by any member of the control group that did not receive take-home doses for attendance.

Drug Use Targets

Take-home doses can also be used to promote abstinence from cocaine, benzodiazepines, and other supplemental drugs that patients use during treatment. Two similar studies investigated the effectiveness of contingent take-home privileges in methadone maintenance patients (Iguchi et al. 1996; Stitzer et al. 1992). After a stabilization and baseline evaluation period, study patients were randomly assigned to a group receiving take-home doses contingent on drug-free urine samples or to a control/comparison condition. In the Stitzer study, control patients received take-home doses delivered independently of their behavior; in the Iguchi study, comparison patients received take-homes for attending special group therapy sessions. In both studies, under the contingent protocol, the first take-home dose was earned after two weeks of urine samples free of all common drugs of abuse that could be detected (except alcohol and marijuana), and an additional take-home dose was authorized after each successive two-week drug-free period up to a maximum of three (Stitzer study) or four (Iguchi study) take-home doses per week. One take-home dose was forfeited for each drug-positive urine sample, and two more drug-free weeks were required to regain lost take-home privileges.

Both studies showed that take-home doses effectively promoted abstinence among a portion of methadone maintenance patients. Specifically, about one-third of patients (30–40%) showed clinical improvement on measures of drug use when exposed to the contingent take-home procedures. Patients who received take-home doses under noncontingent procedures tended to worsen on measures of drug use during the study. This suggests that a contingent take-home procedure, in addition to promoting clinic improvement in some patients, can prevent deterioration of treatment performance in other patients who do not have an obvious positive response to the intervention.

Another study, conducted by Silverman and colleagues, has further demonstrated the ability of abstinence-contingent take-home doses to improve treatment outcomes (Silverman et al. 2004). Patients were selected for this study based on evidence of stimulant abuse at treatment intake (i.e., cocaine-positive urine samples). During the yearlong study, some patients ($N = 26$) could receive three take-home methadone doses per week if their urine samples tested negative for both opiates and cocaine. The comparison group ($N = 26$) received usual care without the opportunity to earn take-home doses. Figure 8.2 shows that the contingent take-home group submitted significantly more cocaine-free urine samples than the comparison group (about 35% vs. 15% negative, respectively, through-

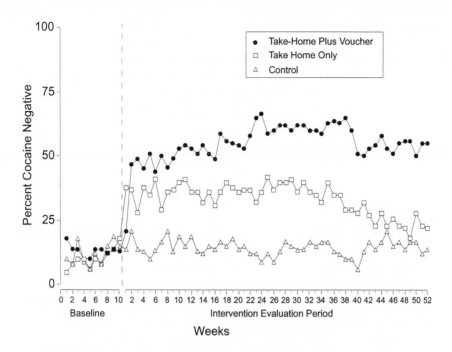

Figure 8.2. Percentage of urine samples testing negative for cocaine during a 52-week contingency management study. Methadone maintenance patients with evidence of ongoing cocaine abuse were randomly assigned to conditions in which they could earn up to three take-home doses per week for evidence of sustained abstinence from both opioids and cocaine (take-home only; $N = 26$), where they could earn take-home doses plus up to $120 per week in vouchers (take-home plus vouchers; $N = 26$), or where no abstinence-contingent benefits were available (usual care control; $N = 26$). Data from Silverman et al. 2004.

out the study), and similar urinalysis results were seen for opiate use. This study is important because it confirms earlier reports about the benefits of abstinence-contingent take-home doses of methadone, it extends the time frame of the evaluation over a full year, and it shows that the benefits apply to the group of patients who are of most concern to clinicians—those who abuse cocaine at treatment entry.

The findings reviewed above make an important point. Clearly, not all patients will respond to contingent take-home interventions with clinically meaningful improvement; overall, these studies suggest that only about one-third of patients will make behavior changes large enough to be clinically meaningful. However, the use of contingency management programs may be an important step in the prevention of treatment performance deterioration among those patients who do not dramatically improve their drug use behavior. This suggests that there are important benefits to having such programs in place to sustain overall performance of a clinic population. This conclusion is derived from research studies using intensive urine surveillance schedules (thrice weekly testing) and offering rapid initiation of take-home privileges for evidence of recent abstinence. Whether the same conclusion applies to the more usual clinical situations in which urine surveillance is less frequent and in which more prolonged periods of drug-free time may be required to earn take-home doses is a question that needs to be answered through additional research.

Monetary Reinforcers

In many ways, monetary reinforcers are ideal for use in contingency management procedures: money is a reinforcer that can be exchanged for an infinite variety of goods and services and it has universal appeal. Unlike take-home privileges, the magnitude of a monetary reinforcer (i.e., amount of money offered) can be varied continuously over an almost limitless range of values without risking satiation. The one disadvantage of money is its limited availability to treatment programs for use in contingency management procedures. The studies reviewed in the next sections have evaluated the efficacy of money as a reinforcer. If money were shown to work much better than other reinforcers, then it would be worthwhile for treatment systems to attempt the removal of barriers to its use.

Cash Payments

Several early studies showed the benefits of offering cash payments to patients who submit drug-free urine samples (between $4 and $15 per urine sample) during methadone withdrawal (Hall et al. 1979; McCaul et al. 1984) or maintenance (Stitzer et al. 1982) treatment. All these studies showed better outcomes on measures of drug use for patients who could receive cash benefits for providing drug-free urine samples. For example, the study by Stitzer and colleagues targeted benzodiazepine use in patients who exhibited chronic illicit use of these drugs, which were very popular among patients receiving methadone in the 1970s and 1980s. During the intervention, patients were given a choice of reinforcers for providing benzodiazepine-free urine samples. Choices were (a) $15 in cash, (b) two methadone take-home doses, or (c) two opportunities to self-regulate their methadone dose by up to ±20 percent. Reinforcers were available twice weekly and were delivered immediately after the urinalysis test was completed. The group as a whole had a significantly higher rate of benzodiazepine-negative urine samples during the intervention (43%) than during the pre- (4%) or postbaseline (8%) periods. Five of the ten participants were abstinent throughout most of the three-month intervention. Patients chose money on 63 percent of the occasions when reinforcers were earned and take-home doses on the remaining occasions.

Overall, these studies point to the utility of money as an effective reinforcer to promote and sustain abstinence in drug abusers during both detoxification and maintenance treatment. Because the studies were conducted some time ago, however, they provide little guidance about the amount of cash that might be necessary to sustain clinically meaningful improvement in the current economy. Furthermore, there is a concern that providing cash for abstinence could have an unwanted adverse effect on drug use if patients decide to use the cash to purchase drugs. It is widely assumed among clinicians that having money in hand frequently leads to drug use for some drug abusers. Both reports from drug abusers themselves (Kirby et al. 1995) and correlations observed between access to money and use of drugs (Shaner et al. 1995) provide support for this assumption. To circumvent this potential unwanted side effect of cash payments, more recent studies using monetary reinforcement have turned to a system of voucher incentives that are described next.

Voucher Incentive Programs

In voucher incentive programs, patients are offered the chance to earn money for providing drug-free urine samples. However, money is not paid as cash; rather, patients can use the money to purchase goods or services, with the only restriction being that the items selected must be consistent with basic necessities of living or with the treatment plan. These purchases can include payment of rent or utility bills, payment of clinic fees, and the purchase of a wide variety of retail items. Clinic staff make the actual purchases and arrange delivery. Thus, the procedure, designed with patient safety in mind, is somewhat labor intensive for staff.

Higgins and colleagues (Higgins et al. 1991, 1994, 2003) developed and tested the voucher-based reinforcement procedure that has been used most widely to date. The program was initially developed for the treatment of cocaine abusers applying to an outpatient treatment research clinic in Burlington, Vermont. This procedure has two notable features. First, the payment schedule (based on thrice weekly urine testing) was specifically designed to promote sustained abstinence. The initial cocaine-free urine sample was worth a relatively small sum of money ($2.50), but each successive drug-free urine sample was worth progressively more money. Thus, the longer the patient remained continuously abstinent, the more valuable their abstinence became. Furthermore, should a patient relapse, the money schedule reset to its original low value and the patient had to begin the procedure again to accumulate drug-free time and increase the associated cash value of abstinence. Second, it was possible to earn a substantial total amount—$1,155 for continuous abstinence during the three-month program. This total amount was arrived at somewhat arbitrarily but embodies the concept that the amount offered should be sufficiently large that drug-abusing patients perceive it as a worthwhile alternative to the drug they are foregoing.

Silverman and colleagues have shown that this voucher reinforcement program is highly effective for eliminating the use of cocaine (Silverman et al. 1996b, 2004) and opioids (Silverman et al. 1996c) in patients receiving methadone who use these drugs during treatment, and they have also shown that the same voucher-based reinforcement concept could support attendance of unemployed patients receiving methadone at an on-site job-skills training program (Silverman et al. 1996a). In the first study, patients (N = 37) who showed ongoing cocaine use during treatment were randomly assigned to either the abstinence reinforcement procedures described previously or to a control group that received vouchers on a noncontingent basis independent of their drug use. Overall rates of cocaine-free urine samples during the 12-week intervention averaged 50 percent for the contingent reinforcement group during most study weeks, compared with rates of about 10 percent cocaine-free urine samples delivered by the control group. Patients receiving vouchers for cocaine-free urine samples maintained impressive durations of cocaine abstinence; these patients were continuously abstinent for five weeks, on average, compared with one week for control subjects and 47 percent of patients exposed to the voucher condition achieved six or more weeks of sustained cocaine abstinence.

A more recent study, whose results are shown in figure 8.2, allowed patients identified as cocaine abusers to begin earning vouchers for cocaine-free urine samples at any point during a one-year intervention, with a maximum of three take-home doses per week also available for evidence of sustained opiate and cocaine abstinence (Silverman et al. 2004). The take-home plus voucher group had excellent outcomes throughout the intervention, with about 60 percent cocaine-negative urine samples submitted by the group as a whole. Furthermore, 52 percent of the patients treated with take-home plus vouchers achieved six months or more of continuous cocaine abstinence, which was true for only 8 percent of the take-home-only patients and none of the usual care control patients. Although costly (patients could earn up to $120 per week once they entered the fixed pay portion of the program after demonstrating about eight weeks of continuous abstinence), this study shows that addition of an abstinence reinforcement treatment can produce impressive outcomes in patients receiving methadone who have concurrent stimulant abuse.

These studies show that vouchers can exert a powerful influence on use of a single drug—cocaine or heroin—and can promote sustained abstinence in about half of patients who chronically abuse these drugs during treatment. Furthermore, high magnitude voucher reinforcers can be considerably more effective in their ability to suppress ongoing drug use compared with abstinence-contingent take-home doses of methadone. However, the cost of vouchers and staff time in their administration and management, as used in research to demonstrate the efficacy of these abstinence reinforcement procedures, is a significant barrier to practical use of these techniques in the routine practice of community-based opioid treatment programs.

Drawing for Prizes: Fishbowl Procedure

More recently, a technique has been developed that awards the chance to win prizes as the reinforcer rather than vouchers (Petry et al. 2000). This procedure is based on the same principles as voucher techniques, in that the reinforcers are monetary based and the chances of winning prizes increases with periods of sustained abstinence. However, rather than earning a voucher for each negative urine sample submitted, the patient earns the chance to draw a slip of paper from a fishbowl, and the slips of paper are associated with varying magnitudes of prizes. The probability of winning a prize is usually about 50 percent, such that half of the time patients draw a slip that is not associated with a prize. Most winning slips indicate a small prize has been won, and patients receive their choice of a variety of items worth about $1 in value (e.g., coupons for fast food restaurants, choice of a candy bar, a bus token, minor clothing items such as socks, etc.). For about 8 percent of draw occasions, a patient can win a larger prize worth up to $20 in value (e.g., the choice of a walkman, a watch, a pot-and-pan set, a sweatshirt, etc.). One slip of paper in the bowl is a jumbo prize, worth up to $100 in value (e.g., a television, DVD player, large radio, etc.).

Two studies utilizing this technique have been conducted in methadone programs thus far. In the first study, Petry and Martin randomly assigned 42 patients receiving methadone who were abusing cocaine to receive usual care with or without the chance to win prizes (Petry and

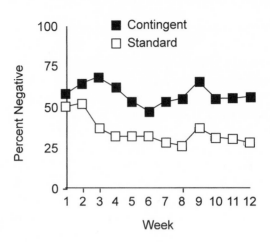

Figure 8.3. Percentage of urine samples testing negative for both opioids and co-caine during each study week. Data are shown for patients assigned to a contingent abstinence incentive procedure that targeted both drugs ($N = 19$) or to standard care ($N = 23$). Results are derived from two or three urine samples per week provided by each subject. Petry and Martin 2002. Copyright 2002 by the American Psychological Association. Reprinted with permission.

Martin 2002). The investigators wanted the patients to stop using both opiates and cocaine and devised a reinforcement schedule to help them meet this goal. Thus, in the incentive condition patients earned a draw if their urine sample tested negative for cocaine or for opiates. If the urine sample tested negative for both cocaine and opiates, the patient earned two draws that day. In addition, bonus draws could be earned under an escalating schedule for successive samples that tested negative for both target drugs. Over a 12-week period, patients could earn up to a total of 234 draws if they provided twice-weekly samples negative for both drugs. As shown in figure 8.3, the percentage of samples that were negative for both cocaine and opioids was significantly higher in the incentive condition relative to the standard treatment group; 48 percent of patients in the contingent group were able to achieve at least a week of consecutive abstinence from both substances versus 16 percent of patients in the standard treatment group. Furthermore, the beneficial effects of the contingent intervention persisted throughout a 12-week follow-up period.

In a second study using the fishbowl technique, 77 patients receiving methadone who were dependent on cocaine received standard treatment that included frequent urine testing and were randomly assigned to abstinence-contingent reinforcement or a control condition (Petry et al. Forthcoming). In the reinforcement condition, patients earned draws from the fishbowl during their group therapy session if they had submitted a cocaine-free urine sample that day and attended their assigned group therapy sessions. Patients in the contingent condition submitted more cocaine-negative samples and attended more groups than patients in standard control treatment. As in the prior study, patients in the contingency management condition showed reduced cocaine use throughout a three-month posttreatment follow-up period, and the best predictor of a cocaine-negative sample at the follow-up was the duration of continuous abstinence achieved during treatment.

In both of these studies, the average value of prizes earned per patient was less than $150 during a 12-week intervention period. Data from these studies suggest that this prize reinforcement procedure is efficacious in modifying the behaviors, including drug use behaviors, of patients receiving methadone who were dependent on cocaine. Given the relative low cost of the procedure, it may be affordable for use in community-based settings.

CLINICAL RECOMMENDATIONS

We have reviewed a range of contingency management interventions developed and tested in clinical research settings, most of which have been effective in addressing clinical problems in methadone programs. A variety of reinforcers, including contingent availability of methadone treatment, short-term methadone dose alterations, methadone take-home privileges, cash payments, monetary-based voucher incentives, and on-site prizes have been shown to promote behavior change effectively. The reviewed studies led to the following clinical recommendations.

Take-Home Privileges

A contingent methadone take-home program based on urinalysis results can be a useful addition in the operation of an opioid treatment program. Take-home doses can also be offered to patients for achieving specific therapeutic target behaviors, such as counseling attendance, when appropriate. A contingency agreement written for a patient who could earn take-home doses of methadone is shown in figure 8.4.

Dose Alterations

Methadone dose alterations should be approached with caution, in particular, dose decreases, because of the demonstrated need for adequate

Figure 8.4.   A sample contingency agreement for a patient earning take-home doses of methadone.

doses to maintain good treatment response and because of the danger of enhanced treatment dropout for patients receiving low doses. However, more refined methods for making continued treatment contingent on improved performance have been developed recently (see chap. 7 for an example of such a treatment program), and these methods may ultimately prove to be useful. In addition, contingent dose increases may be used effectively to promote behavior change.

Money-Based Incentives

Reinforcers that involve monetary payments or prizes are clearly effective and should be used according to the resources of the clinic. It would behoove practitioners to become innovative in identifying desirable reinforcers, such as food vouchers, bus tokens, and movie passes, that can be obtained, sometimes through donations from community sources, and that could be awarded to patients who achieve targeted therapeutic goals.

OTHER ISSUES IN THE CLINICAL USE OF CONTINGENCIES
Individual Contingency Contracting

One of the issues that clinic directors and staff must decide is whether to offer contingent incentive programs to all patients or to specific targeted patients in the form of individual contingency contracts. Standardized clinicwide procedures have the advantage of being easier to implement while treating all patients equally. However, considering that patients vary widely in their baseline performance on a number of outcome dimensions, and thus have different treatment needs and goals, some individualized contracting is recommended as a useful strategy. Note, however, that even in the research previously discussed in this chapter, the patients selected for study were often those who exhibited poor performance on the target behavior of interest in the study and, therefore, were in need of the therapy interventions being tested.

Factors to Consider in Devising Contingent Interventions

The examples derived from the research studies presented in this chapter should be useful guides in designing contingency management programs for clinical practice. The effectiveness of interventions can significantly depend on the detailed methods used in implementation. Practitioners who are interested in trying the procedures described here should discuss such details with other clinicians who have successfully used contingency interventions, consult with researchers who develop such interventions, and read further about using contingency procedures (DeRisi and Butz 1975; Sulzer-Azfoff and Meyer 1991) to understand fully the nuances of the procedures. Further, manuals are now available that describe voucher (Bud-

Table 8.1 Elements of a Contingency Management Intervention

Element	Definition	Examples
Target behavior	Specific behavior that can be observed and measured	• Attend counseling sessions • Pay clinic fee • Abstain from drugs
Antecedents	Specifies when, where, and how target behavior is to be performed	• Attend group Mondays at 4:00 P.M. • Pay $30 each Wednesday • Submit drug-free urine sample on randomly selected weekday
Consequences	Reward delivered if target behavior is observed	• Earn one take-home dose • Earn $10 fee rebate • Earn 10-mg dose increase • Earn $10 food coupon
Contingency	Rules for earning rewards	• One reinforcer for each instance of target behavior • One reinforcer for each fourth instance of target behavior • One reinforcer for randomly selected instance of target behavior (1 of 6)

ney and Higgins 1998) and prize-drawing (Petry and Stitzer 2002) procedures. Even with these precautions, experience shows that programs modeled after previously effective interventions will not always be effective when applied in new situations. In general, when a contingency management intervention fails to achieve the desired change in behavior, manipulations can be made in any or all of the procedure's four key elements: (1) the *target behavior*; (2) the *antecedent stimuli* that are intended to set the occasion for the target behavior; (3) the *reinforcer*; and (4) the *contingency* or rules according to which reinforcers can be earned for emitting the target behavior (table 8.1). In the following sections, we discuss some of the common pitfalls encountered in designing contingency management interventions and suggest strategies that can be used to improve the chances of success.

Target Behaviors

One advantage of contingency management interventions is that they set clear expectations for behavior change. Thus, it is important that target behaviors be clearly specified, objectively defined, easily observed, and readily quantified to avoid any confusion about what is expected. One potential pitfall in implementing these procedures, however, is that the specified target behavior may be one that the patient has never performed or is not even capable of performing. In this case, the therapist may be setting the patient up for failure. For example, a counselor may arrange a contingency in which the patient earns a take-home methadone dose for every ten job applications they complete. However, this intervention may fail if the patient lacks the necessary reading skills to identify potential jobs in the newspaper or the reading, spelling, and writing skills needed to complete an application. Alternatively, a patient may fail to demonstrate the target behavior (e.g., complete ten job applications) if another incompatible behavior occurs at very high frequencies and precludes the occurrence of the target behavior. For example, if a patient is using drugs at very high rates and consequently spends a substantial proportion of each day seeking drugs, there may be little time left for job hunting. Thus, the target behavior (i.e., treatment goal) must be realistic and obtainable for the patient.

If a patient fails to earn rewards because the patient never performs the target behavior, remedial strategies should be used to address the underlying problem. If a patient lacks the prerequisite skills needed to complete job applications (i.e., reading, writing, and spelling), the target behavior may be changed to something within the patient's abilities. For example, the patient could be directed to jobs that do not use these skills, either in the application process or on the job. Alternatively, the target behavior could be changed completely, for example, to focus on concrete steps leading toward enrolling in a literacy program (see Petry et al. 2001 for a listing of possible target behaviors).

Antecedent Stimuli

To be reinforced, a response may have to be emitted in a particular place, at a particular time, and under a specified set of circumstances. For example, patients may need to provide a drug-free urine sample under supervision of a laboratory technician every Monday, Wednesday, and Friday at the clinic site, between 8:00 a.m. and 12 p.m. to receive a methadone take-home dose. In other words, only under some specific circumstances would a drug-free laboratory report be reinforced. For this contingency to have reliable effects, it is essential that the conditions under which a particular behavior does (or does not) lead to reinforcement be clearly understood by the patients. These so-called antecedent conditions are sometimes specified as instructions to the patients that are presented orally or in written format, such as in the clinic procedures outline or treatment consent form. Because at times the conditions may be complex, a strategy sometimes used to guarantee that they are clearly understood is to give the patient brief tests on the rules they must follow to earn reinforcers and to provide additional explanation and examples as needed.

Reinforcers

What serves as a reinforcer may vary from one person to another or even across time and circumstances in the same person. A take-home methadone dose, for example, may not have the same reinforcing value for someone who owns a car as for someone who does not, for someone who holds a job as for someone who does not, and so on. Although contingency management interventions may utilize consequences that appear desirable, such as take-home methadone doses or monetary vouchers, the ability of those consequences to serve as reinforcers cannot be assumed. Contingency management interventions may fail if the consequences provided for emitting the target behavior do not serve as reinforcers for the treated individuals or if they do not maintain their reinforcing effectiveness over time.

Identifying Reinforcers

It can be useful to identify events that will serve as reinforcers for many patients by surveying the opioid treatment program population. During these surveys, patients are asked to rate their interest in different potential reinforcers that the clinic might provide, to rank their interest in a list of potential reinforcers, or to make specific choices between pairs of reinforcers (Kidorf et al. 1995; Stitzer and Bigelow 1978). Take-home methadone doses have been consistently rated as the top priority in previous surveys of this type. In cases in which counselors want to develop individual contracts, it may also be useful to ask an individual patient what rewards he or she would like to work for and to negotiate from a starting point suggested by the patient.

Reinforcer Magnitude

It is clear from previous research in animals and in humans that magnitude is an important determinant of reinforcer efficacy (Stitzer and Bigelow 1983, 1984b). Once a potentially effective reinforcer is identified, it is important to deliver it in an amount sufficient to motivate behavior change. For example, a 2-mg methadone dose increase may be ineffective, whereas a 10- or 20-mg increase would prompt a behavioral response. Negotiating the magnitude as well as the type of reinforcer with the patient is probably the best way to proceed. Alternatively, the therapist may offer the maximum size reward that is considered clinically feasible. Although the fishbowl procedure may engender beneficial results with relatively low costs, even this procedure loses its efficacy when the value or frequency of tangible rewards becomes too low (Petry et al. 2004).

Rules of the Contingency

The *contingency* in a contingency management intervention is the rule specifying that the reinforcer will be delivered only if the target behavior occurs and will not be available if the behavior does not occur. Contingency rules can vary along several dimensions, but two dimensions seem particularly critical: the immediacy and the schedule of reinforcement.

Immediacy of Reinforcement

It is very important that reinforcers closely follow behavior in time. Research in animals and in humans has shown that reinforcing effectiveness decreases as the delay between the occurrence of the behavior and presentation of the reinforcer increases (Gonzalez and Newlin 1976). Therefore, in contingency management programs, it is important to ensure that patients receive reinforcers as soon as possible after the target behavior. If a contingency management program fails, a clinician may consider whether there are substantial delays in reinforcement that could be reduced.

Schedule of Reinforcement

Most studies described in this chapter delivered a reward every time the target behavior occurred (e.g., every drug-free urine sample delivered, every counseling session attended). Another way to deliver rewards is with a schedule of intermittent reinforcement (i.e., when only some instances of the behavior are reinforced). The prize-drawing procedure devised by Petry is an excellent example, but there are other ways this principle can be achieved. For example, rather than reinforcing each drug-free urine sample, a contingency management program could randomly select and test one urine sample from those provided over two to three consecutive weeks and use this test as a basis for awarding take-home methadone doses. Although such a schedule has not actually been tested in drug abuse interventions, it should be effective based on the principles of learning and conditioning, which show that large amounts of behavior can be maintained with intermittent reinforcement (Kazdin 1973). Intermittent schedules of reinforcement also make more efficient use of resources. Remember, though, that they could fail if the patient achieves the target response too infrequently to receive reinforcement. To address this, patients could be started on a frequent reinforcement schedule with each drug-free urine sample earning the reinforcer, then shifted to an intermittent schedule after the behavior (abstinence) is established. Ideally, the requirement for reinforcement could be gradually increased over time, thereby reinforcing longer and longer periods of abstinence.

Summary

Evidence from laboratory and clinical research supports the idea that drug use is an operant behavior, maintained in large part by the biologically reinforcing effects produced by drugs of abuse. Drug seeking and drug taking, however, can also be influenced by other consequences that are imposed in a therapeutic context. Contingency management treatment programs are designed to alter the consequences of drug-related behaviors. In most cases, reinforcing consequences are programmed for objectively defined and clinically desirable target behaviors. The studies reported in this chapter demonstrate the clinical efficacy and utility of contingency management procedures in the treatment of drug abuse problems. Taken together, the results clearly show that drug use can be reduced when positive consequences (take-homes privileges, dose increases, money) are offered for abstinence or when aversive consequences (dose decreases, treatment termination) are made contingent on continued drug use; however, aversive procedures may cause treatment dropout and associated adverse outcomes. These examples should be useful guides in designing contingency management programs for clinical practice—either clinicwide contingency programs or contracts with individual patients designed to promote attainment of tailored treatment goals. Furthermore, if clinicians understand the principles underlying these contingency management examples, they can use their creativity and clinical insight to make alterations in the target behavior, antecedent conditions, nature or magnitude of the reinforcer, or contingency relationship to tailor interventions to their own patients and maximize the efficacy of their own clinical interventions.

References

Budney AJ, Higgins ST (1998). A Community Reinforcement Plus Vouchers Approach: Treating Cocaine Addiction. DHHS Pub. No. 98-4309. Rockville, MD: U.S. Department of Health and Human Services.

Chutuape MA, Silverman K, Stitzer ML (1998). Survey assessment of methadone treatment services as reinforcers. *Am J Drug Alcohol Abuse* 24: 1–16.

DeRisi WJ, Butz G (1975). *Writing Behavioral Contracts: A Case Simulation Practice Manual.* Champaign, IL: Research Press.

Dolan MP, Black JL, Penk WE, Robinowitz R, DeFord HA (1985). Contracting for treatment termination to reduce illicit drug use among methadone maintenance treatment failures. *J Consult Clin Psychol* 53: 549–51.

Gonzalez F, Newlin R (1976). Effects of delayed reinforcement on performance under IRT > t schedules. *J Exp Anal Behav* 26: 221–35.

Griffiths RR, Bigelow GE, Henningfield JE (1980). Similarities in animal and human drug-taking behavior. In: Mello NK, ed. *Advance in Substance Abuse,* 1–90. Greenwich, CT: JAI Press.

Hall SM, Bass A, Hargreaves WA, Loeb P (1979). Contingency management and information feedback in outpatient heroin detoxification. *Behav Ther* 10: 443–51.

Higgins ST, Budney AJ, Bickel WK, Foerg FE, Donham R, Badger GJ (1994). Incentives improve outcome in outpatient behavioral treatment of cocaine dependence. *Arch Gen Psychiatry* 51: 568–76.

Higgins ST, Delaney DD, Budney AJ, Bickel WK, Hughes JR, Foerg F, Fenwick JW (1991). A behavioral approach to achieving initial cocaine abstinence. *Am J Psychiatry* 148: 1218–24.

Higgins ST, Sigmon SC, Wong CJ, Heil SH, Badger GJ, Donham R, Dantona RL, Anthony S (2003). Community reinforcement therapy for cocaine-dependent outpatients. *Arch Gen Psychiatry* 60: 1043–52.

Higgins ST, Stitzer ML, Bigelow GE, Liebson IA (1986). Contingent methadone delivery: effects on illicit-opiate use. *Drug Alcohol Depend* 17: 311–22.

Iguchi MY, Lamb RJ, Belding MA, Platt JJ, Husband SD, Morral AR (1996). Contingent reinforcement of group participation versus abstinence in a methadone maintenance program. *Exp Clin Psychopharmacol* 4: 315–21.

Kazdin AE (1973). Intermittent token reinforcement and response maintenance in extinction. *Behav Ther* 4: 386–91.

Kidorf M, Stitzer ML (1993). Contingent access to methadone maintenance treatment: effects on cocaine use of mixed opiate-cocaine users. *Exp Clin Psychopharmacol* 1: 200–6.

Kidorf M, Stitzer ML (1996). Contingent use of take-homes and split-dosing to reduce illicit drug use of methadone patients. *Behav Ther* 27: 41–51.

Kidorf M, Stitzer ML, Brooner RK, Goldberg J (1994). Contingent methadone take-home doses reinforce adjunct therapy attendance of methadone maintenance patients. *Drug Alcohol Depend* 36: 221–6.

Kidorf M, Stitzer ML, Griffiths RR (1995). Evaluating the reinforcement value of clinic-based privileges through a multiple choice procedure. *Drug Alcohol Depend* 39: 167–72.

Kirby KC, Lamb RJ, Iguchi MY, Husband SD, Platt JJ (1995). Situations occasioning cocaine use and cocaine abstinence strategies. *Addiction* 90: 1241–52.

Koob GF, Bloom FE (1988). Cellular and molecular mechanisms of drug dependence. *Science* 242: 715–23.

Koob GF, Le Moal M (1997). Drug abuse: hedonic homeostatic dysregulation. *Science* 278: 52–58.

Liebson IA, Tommasello A, Bigelow GE (1978). A behavioral treatment of alcoholic methadone patients. *Ann Intern Med* 89: 342–4.

McCarthy JJ, Borders OT (1985). Limit setting on drug abuse in methadone maintenance patients. *Am J Psychiatry* 142: 1419–23.

McCaul ME, Stitzer ML, Bigelow GE, Liebson IA (1984). Contingency management interventions: effects on treatment outcome during methadone detoxification. *J Appl Behav Anal* 17: 35–43.

Petry NM, Martin B (2002). Low-cost contingency management for treating cocaine- and opioid-abusing methadone patients. *J Consult Clin Psychol* 70: 398–405.

Petry NM, Martin B, Cooney JL, Kranzler HR (2000). Give them prizes, and they will come: contingency management for treatment of alcohol dependence. *J Consult Clin Psychol* 68: 250–7.

Petry NM, Martin B, Simcic F (Forthcoming). Prize reinforcement contingency management for cocaine dependence: integration with group therapy in a methadone clinic. *J Consult Clin Psychol*.

Petry NM, Stitzer ML (2002). Contingency Management: Using Motivational Incentives to Improve Drug Abuse Treatment. Training Series 6. New Haven, CT: Yale University Psychotherapy Development Center.

Petry NM, Tedford J, Austin M, Nich C, Carroll KM, Rounsaville BJ (2004). Prize reinforcement contingency management for treating cocaine users: how low can we go, and with whom? *Addiction* 99: 349–60.

Petry NM, Tedford J, Martin B (2001). Reinforcing compliance with non-drug-related activities. *J Subst Abuse Treat* 20: 33–44.

Shaner A, Eckman TA, Roberts LJ, Wilkins JN, Tucker DE, Tsuang JW, Mintz J (1995). Disability income, cocaine use, and repeated hospitalization among schizophrenic cocaine abusers—a government-sponsored revolving door? *N Engl J Med* 333: 777–83.

Silverman K, Chutuape MA, Bigelow GE, Stitzer ML (1996a). Voucher-based reinforcement of attendance by unemployed methadone patients in a job skills training program. *Drug Alcohol Depend* 41: 197–207.

Silverman K, Higgins ST, Brooner RK, Montoya ID, Cone EJ, Schuster CR, Preston KL (1996b). Sustained cocaine abstinence in methadone maintenance patients through voucher-based reinforcement therapy. *Arch Gen Psychiatry* 53: 409–15.

Silverman K, Tobles E, Mudric T, Bigelow GE, Stitzer ML (2004). A randomized trial of long-term reinforcement of cocaine abstinence in methadone-maintained patients who inject drugs. *J Consult Clin Psychol* 72: 839–54.

Silverman K, Wong CJ, Higgins ST, Brooner RK, Montoya ID, Contoreggi C, Umbricht-Schneiter A, Schuster CR, Preston KL (1996c). Increasing opiate abstinence through voucher-based reinforcement therapy. *Drug Alcohol Depend* 41: 157–65.

Stitzer M, Bigelow G (1978). Contingency management in a methadone maintenance program: availability of reinforcers. *Int J Addict* 13: 737–46.

Stitzer M, Bigelow G, Lawrence C, Cohen J, D'Lugoff B, Hawthorne J (1977). Medication take-home as a reinforcer in a methadone maintenance program. *Addict Behav* 2: 9–14.

Stitzer ML, Bickel WK, Bigelow GE, Liebson IA (1986). Effect of methadone dose contingencies on urinalysis test results of polydrug-abusing methadone-maintenance patients. *Drug Alcohol Depend* 18: 341–8.

Stitzer ML, Bigelow GE (1983). Contingent payment for carbon monoxide reduction: effects of pay amounts. *Behav Ther* 14: 647–56.

Stitzer ML, Bigelow GE (1984a). Contingent methadone take-home privileges: effects on compliance with fee payment schedules. *Drug Alcohol Depend* 13: 395–9.

Stitzer ML, Bigelow GE (1984b). Contingent reinforcement for carbon monoxide reduction: within-subject effects of pay amount. *J Appl Behav Anal* 17: 477–83.

Stitzer ML, Bigelow GE, Liebson IA, Hawthorne JW (1982). Contingent reinforcement for benzodiazepine-free urines: evaluation of a drug abuse treatment intervention. *J Appl Behav Anal* 15: 493–503.

Stitzer ML, Iguchi MY, Felch LJ (1992). Contingent take-home incentive: effects on drug use of methadone maintenance patients. *J Consult Clin Psychol* 60: 927–34.

Sulzer-Azfoff B, Meyer GR (1991). *Behavior Analysis for Lasting Change.* Austin, TX: Holt, Rinehart and Winston.

9

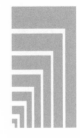

Practical Issues of Program Organization and Operation

Mary Bailes, L.C.P.C., and Connie Lowery, R.N., C.A.R.N.

This chapter addresses a number of practical issues encountered in the organization and management of a methadone treatment clinic. These issues include the physical organization of the clinic, staffing patterns, assessment of patient eligibility for treatment, management of problematic patient behaviors, accreditation of the treatment clinic, and interactions between the clinic and surrounding community. These topics are brought together within a single chapter, as they are interrelated and all are important for the operation of a successful treatment program. Further, in the United States, many of the issues addressed in this chapter are consistent with new federal and state regulations that require programs to meet accreditation standards.

CERTIFICATION AND ACCREDITATION

In January 2001, the U.S. Substance Abuse and Mental Health Services Administration (SAMHSA) finalized the new code of federal regulations addressing opioid treatment standards (Code of Federal Regulations, 42 Part 8, 2001). These new regulations continue to require opioid treatment programs (OTPs) to seek certification from the Secretary of Health and Human Services, but approval for certification is now contingent on the program obtaining accreditation from an approved body. In 2004, SAMHSA recognized six accrediting bodies to which an OTP can apply for accreditation (table 9.1).

Table 9.1 **Opioid Treatment Program Accreditation Bodies for the United States, 2004**

Commission on Accreditation of Rehabilitation Facilities (CARF)
  4891 East Grant
  Tucson, Arizona 60181
  Web site: www.carf.org
  Telephone: 520-325-1044   Fax: 520-318-1129

Council on Accreditation (COA)
  120 Wall Street, 11th Floor
  New York, New York 10005
  Web site: www.coanet.org
  Telephone: 212-797-3000   Fax: 212-797-1428

Joint Commission on Accreditation of Healthcare Organizations (JCAHO)
  One Renaissance Boulevard
  Oakbrook Terrace, Illinois 60181
  Web site: www.jcaho.org
  Telephone: 630-792-5800   Fax: 630-792-5005

Division of Alcohol and Substance Abuse
  Washington Department of Social and Health Services
  P.O. Box 45330 (Mail Stop 45330)
  Olympia, Washington 98504-5330
  Web site: www1.dshs.wa.gov/dasa
  Telephone: 360-438-8065   Fax: 360-407-5318

Division of Alcohol and Drug Abuse
  Missouri Department of Mental Health
  1706 East Elm Street
  P.O. Box 687
  Jefferson City, Missouri 65102
  Web site: www.dmh.missouri.gov/ada
  Telephone: 573-522-2372   Fax: 573-751-7814

National Commission on Correctional Health Care
  1300 W. Belmont Avenue
  Chicago, Illinois 60657
  Web site: www.ncchc.org
  Telephone: 773-880-1460 ext. 284   Fax: 773-880-2424

Source: U.S. Department of Health and Human Services, Substance Abuse and Mental Health Services Administration. Center for Substance Abuse Treatment, Division of Pharmacologic Therapies, January 24, 2004.

Accreditation ensures that programs are consistently evaluated based on standards designated in federal guidelines for the operation of opioid agonist treatment. The features of program operation covered here and the regulations addressed in chapter 2 cover most issues that a program in the United States needs to consider to become successfully accredited and certified for operation as an opioid treatment program. Although these standards reflect the requirements for the operation of OTPs in the United States, the issues reviewed in this chapter (e.g., the organization and staffing of a clinic, the management of patients) are relevant to all clinic operations and are not unique to the United States.

PRACTICAL ISSUES REGARDING THE ORGANIZATION OF AN OPIOID TREATMENT PROGRAM

Issues Surrounding Clinic Location

Opioid treatment programs should ideally be located in places that are easily accessible to the target population of opiate abusers and served by public transportation so that patients can easily comply with treatment requirements that may include daily attendance. However, programs do not always have the luxury of a wide range of location choices. The treatment of drug abuse is often plagued by social stigma and misconceptions that have a negative impact on a community's willingness to allow the establishment of a treatment program in their neighborhood. This attitude, sometimes referred to as "not in my back yard," or the NIMBY syndrome, is not unique to substance abuse treatment programs but also affects other health and social services agencies, and many community-based programs face an uphill battle in trying to find an appropriate location for service delivery. Indeed, even patients in an OTP who report methadone has had a positive impact on their lives also report strong negative perceptions of methadone treatment (Stancliff et al. 2002).

Even though considerable research has demonstrated reductions in drug use and other problems (e.g., the number of days of criminal activity) following enrollment in an OTP, a community's perception of substance abusers and substance abuse treatment at times fails to appreciate the overall good accomplished by treatment clinics (Ball et al. 1975; Ball and Ross 1991; Nurco et al. 1984). Accreditation standards outline the need to design treatment services in collaboration with communities served by the opioid treatment program. In particular in situations where community concern or resistance exists, the program director needs to actively work with the community to address concerns and resolve problems to the mutual satisfaction of everyone concerned (Genevie et al. 1988). Specifically, the program director should work with community members, informing and teaching them about the effectiveness of treatment and pointing out that the clinic provides services that ultimately benefit members of the local community, both those being directly served by the treatment program and those who are indirectly affected by reductions in drug use within the community. Further, in being responsive to community concerns, it is important for the OTP to actively work on preventing patients from loitering, dealing drugs, prostituting, or engaging in other criminal activity.

In addition to working with community members to promote acceptance of treatment programs operating within the community, there also may be novel ways to deliver treatment that address some community concerns while enhancing the feasibility of treatment delivery. For example, a mobile program that administers opioid agonist medications while also providing access to medical and counseling staff may better serve opiate-dependent patients residing in rural areas. To date, the feasibility of mobile treatment has been established primarily in pilot programs operated in urban areas where they can provide a solution to zoning problems and community objections (Brady 1993; Besteman and Brady, 1994; Wiebe and Huebert 1996).

Issues Surrounding Program Environment

The needs and safety of both patients and staff are vital in the design of the treatment facility. Entry from the street to the clinic should provide easy accessibility for physically disabled or elderly patients or staff members. If the program is not at street level, provisions should be made for elevator access. Ramps and wide hallways are necessary for patients who require a wheelchair. The importance of facilitating a smooth flow of patient traffic throughout the building should be given thoughtful consideration when designing a clinic (Lowinson and Millman 1979).

Clinic staff should be provided with a well lit, secured parking area located near the facility. If this is not possible, staff should have the option to request security transport to their vehicles, in particular, if the facility is located in an isolated area or program hours extend into the night.

It is equally important to provide convenient parking accommodations to patients, but patient and staff parking should be in separate locations. Accessible parking should be offered for the elderly or patients with disabilities. Security staff should monitor parking areas, and some facilities may be equipped with 24-hour video monitoring. If this is not feasible, security personnel, to ensure that patients are not loitering, stealing, or engaging in other illegal activities, should patrol parking areas frequently.

Within the clinic, restricted areas such as a medical records storage room, supply storage area, and administrative offices should be positioned away from the entrance to the clinic and the mainstream of traffic. More frequently used rooms such as counselors' offices, laboratories, rest rooms, and the finance office should be located so that patients may easily access them. Caution should be taken to position computers in a way that protected health information (PHI) can only be read by appropriate personnel (Legal Action Center 2003).

The space of the clinic itself should be well appointed and sufficiently large to serve the needs of the patients while providing an environment conducive to a therapeutic, counseling relationship. Fire extinguishers, smoke or fire detectors, and a sprinkler system should be placed throughout the clinic according to fire codes. Patient areas such as the restroom should be in compliance with the regulatory code for persons with disabilities and should provide tilted mirrors and insulated padding on exposed pipes under sinks. Adequate space should be provided to conduct medical evaluations, dispense medications, and provide private counseling. Regulations regarding the storage of opioid agonist medications vary between countries; in the United States the Drug Enforcement Administration (DEA) has final authority and will provide consultation regarding a program's security policies, procedures, and equipment to ensure compliance with regulations.

Consideration should be given during the design phase of the opioid treatment program to enable adequate observation of patient traffic and security (Lowinson and Millman 1979). Some programs employ the services of security personnel to monitor patient behavior in and around the program. The use of security mirrors to prevent blind spots within the building can be helpful in providing staff with an easy view of patients waiting for an appointment or to complete other clinic activity, such as submitting a urine specimen or paying clinic fees (Ball and Ross 1991). Video monitoring may augment security.

Signs and memos are important in providing direction for patients both outside and within the clinic. A clinic may be reluctant to have large outdoor signs because of potential community reactions. It is essential, however, that the clinic take responsibility for clearly notifying patients of changes in parking, hours, traffic patterns, and additional issues that may affect attendance. Notifications such as signs and posted memos should be designed with the particular needs of the clinic's treatment population in mind (e.g., adolescents, the elderly, non-English speakers). Designated smoking areas should be clearly defined, if applicable.

Finally, it is extremely important that the physical facility be well maintained and present a professional atmosphere. Thus, areas both inside and outside the clinic should be kept clean, damage from vandalism, such as graffiti, should be promptly repaired, and the facility should undergo regular maintenance and painting. The image presented by the clinic delivers an important message to patients, staff, and the community that the clinic is operated in a professional manner, that the people who work there and receive treatment there take pride in the operation, and that the attitude of professionalism, as exemplified by the care of the physical facilities, extends to the delivery of care provided to the patients.

Organization of Space within the Outpatient Clinic

The Entrance and/or Waiting Area

The entrance or waiting area should provide patients with educational materials. Pamphlets and booklets may be obtained inexpensively or sometimes may be obtained free from governmental health departments or other associations, such as the American Cancer Society or local domestic violence centers. Patients should be provided with such information to familiarize themselves with community resources. If the clinic is affiliated with a hospital, patients also should be made aware of hospital services available to them. Clinic staff may prepare their own educational or inspirational reading material for patients and present materials on bulletin boards near areas of congregation, such as the dosing windows. In addition, patients may be given the opportunity to participate in the creation of bulletin board displays.

Counseling Space

The optimal design for an outpatient treatment clinic allocates a private office for each counselor. Offices should be sufficiently insulated so that conversations cannot be overheard in a neighboring office or in the hallway. The counselor's office should be comfortable and well lit; it should provide adequate space for a desk, a chair for the counselor, and at least one other chair. Ideally, the second chair should allow face-to-face conversation between the counselor and patient without a desk or other furniture in the way. The office should be arranged with safety in mind; staff should have easy access to the exit in case a patient becomes agitated (as discussed later in this chapter). Ideally, each counselor should have a computer for recordkeeping, patient notes, and access to Internet referral resources. Storage space such as a filing cabinet and shelving are necessary for organization and storage of hard-copy records. In the United States, protected health information (PHI) must be stored in keeping with HIPAA and federal confidentiality regulations (CFR 42 Part 2).

When space is a concern, a group-counseling room may also serve as the clinic conference room. This room should be large enough to accommodate staff meetings, training events, and group therapy sessions. Resources such as a television and a videotape recorder can be kept in this room, because videos can be used effectively for both staff training and didactic presentations to patients. In addition, videotaping and reviewing counseling sessions can be highly useful for supervision and training with counseling staff (Powell 1993). It is important to remember that videotaping a patient requires written consent by the patient.

Dispensing Area

Opioid agonist medications are typically administered to patients through a window that resembles a bank teller window. Many opioid treatment programs will administer medication from more than one window to facilitate a smoother flow of traffic and decrease waiting time. The dimensions and placement of the window can aid in reducing the risk of medication diversion. The window should be positioned to provide nursing staff with a clear and complete view of the patient as he or she ingests medication. The dimensions of the opened window should allow patients to be visible from the waist up. The ideal window is approximately three feet high and three feet wide.

Because the dispensing window is a large opening, a safety barrier such as bars or Plexiglas can be used to cover part of the space (although Plexiglas may impede the detection of breath alcohol, clear communication, and the use of breath alcohol tests). Although less aesthetically pleasing, bars provide a strong physical barrier that can decrease accessibility to the staff and to controlled substances. The windows must be capable of being secured with a locking mechanism that is approved by the DEA or other, non-U.S. regulatory agencies.

The area directly in front of medication windows should be relatively open so staff can have a full view of patients at all times. An unobstructed view by the nursing staff of patient activities is recommended to provide some regulation of patient movement within the clinic. If this is not possible because of preexisting features of the building design, security mirrors can be strategically placed to aid staff in observing patients as they wait in a dispensing line.

In addition, there should be a means for immediately alerting security personnel if a potential, or actual, problem arises. Some programs are staffed with security personnel who are present and visible throughout the clinic. It is not uncommon for dosing windows to be equipped with panic buttons to directly alert security officers or the local police department. These buttons should be easily accessible to nursing staff but not visible to the patient (e.g., under a ledge at the window).

Medical Area

The examination/treatment room should be well lit and provide privacy for the patient to discuss issues freely with medical staff. The room should be large enough to include an examination table and storage space for medical supplies, including equipment such as an electrocardiogram (ECG) machine, microscope, otoscope/opthalmoscope, thermometer, scale, and centrifuge. Although not essential, a phlebotomy chair can prove to be very valuable for blood draws. The room also should have adequate countertop space and a sink for hand washing. Materials contaminated with body fluids should be disposed according to exposure control plans set forth by the clinic to prevent transmission of blood-borne pathogens (i.e., standard precautions). Discarded needles and any other items that could cause injury ("sharps") should be disposed in leak-proof, puncture-resistant, labeled containers. Other waste contaminated with blood or body fluids should be placed in bags that are easily closed, designed to prevent leakage during transport, and labeled with a biohazard symbol.

Hours of Operation

The hours of operation for an OTP are an important aspect of the overall administration of the clinic and should be selected after allowing for several considerations, including the needs of the patient population, community concerns, the hours of operation of local transportation systems, and the level of personnel available to provide staffing of the clinic. The neighboring community should be considered when designing the OTP's hours of operation. For example, hours may be selected that do not conflict with local church services, or with school dismissal. If a program is considering a change in clinic hours, this offers the program an excellent opportunity to seek both community and patient input. The program should provide hours for medication and psychosocial services that permit all patients, including those who are employed, disabled, or caring for children at home, to receive the full complement of services provided by the program. Some state and accreditation agencies encourage opioid treatment programs to provide early morning and/or late evening hours to accommodate the maximum number and diversity of patients (JCAHO 2003).

Most programs make all treatment-related activities (e.g., counseling, case management, medical services) available during the same times medication is administered. Many clinics design periods when they are open (e.g., early morning), then closed (e.g., lunch), and then open again later in the same day (e.g., late afternoon and/or evening) to exert some control over patient flow; with this operating system, patients can then be given specific times when they should attend the clinic. Access to the earliest medication times is sometimes viewed as a privilege and may be selectively given to employed and/or drug-abstinent patients (Ball and Ross 1991). Closed hours allow staff to focus on record maintenance or to attend multidisciplinary team meetings without interruptions.

For programs carrying a large census, it may be necessary to give patients intervals to report to the clinic or limit the number of patients permitted in the clinic at a given time to minimize the large numbers of patients reporting for dosing at one time (which can become a strain on clinic staff). If employed patients are assigned a specified reporting time during the day, every effort should be made to schedule these patients according to their work hours. Some clinics with a large census and small facility may detain patients before they enter the building, if a large number of patients suddenly report to the clinic. If patients are held outside, for example, in a line at the door, security and other staff should be on-site monitoring patients and maintaining order. An outdoor line, although sometimes necessary, often provokes community concerns and generally should be avoided.

Staffing of the Opioid Treatment Program

Overview

Opioid treatment programs should take into account the needs of the patient population (e.g., age and ethnicity) when developing a team of staff. OTPs are typically staffed by a physician, a program director (who in some cases is the physician), nurses, counselors and support staff (Calsyn et al. 1990). This multidisciplinary group should operate as a team and provide expertise consistent with the wide variety of services that are delivered on-site.

Physician

Every OTP needs to have a physician who functions as the medical director for the clinic. Some areas, such as certain states in the United States, require that the medical director of an OTP demonstrate knowledge of addiction medicine through experience and certifications. The medical director should coordinate all medical aspects of care provided through the clinic, including medical evaluations of new patients, orders for medications (both methadone and other medications that may be prescribed through the clinic), assessments of patients who develop new medical problems, and referral and coordination with outside medical providers when patients are treated at other sites. In some clinics, day-to-day management of minor medical problems is provided by a nurse practitioner or physician's assistant.

Program Director

The program director provides overall administrative oversight for the clinic to ensure compliance with regulatory, funding, and accreditation/governmental requirements. The program director acts as the primary liaison with outside agencies, including accreditation and governmental organizations, professional groups, and the local community. The program director also has overall responsibility for the policies and procedures of the clinic, facility maintenance, budgetary matters, and personnel-related matters such as hiring staff, annual performance reviews, and disciplinary actions.

Nursing Staff

Nurses are necessary for the administration of medication, but they also provide a wide range of other services to the patients. Nurses are often the only clinic staff to interact with patients every day, because they provide daily medication administration. This interaction gives nurses an opportunity to assess a patient's health and emotional status on a daily basis and to evaluate the necessity for medical or counseling interventions. Patients may present with a variety of physical or emotional concerns, which must be evaluated on an individual basis. Nursing staff may be the first to notice even a slight behavioral or emotional change that may be pertinent to the patient's well-being.

In addition to these daily responsibilities, nurses are essential during the intake or admission process. Their responsibilities can include collecting blood for laboratory testing, obtaining electrocardiograms, completing a patient history, HIV counseling (which may include informing patients of their HIV results), obtaining vital signs, and administering intradermal skin tests for tuberculosis.

Finally, nursing staff can be instrumental in providing education in the opioid treatment clinic. Nurses should be well versed in teaching in group settings and in one-on-one instruction. Some examples of possible topics for nursing groups in OTPs are nutrition, tuberculosis, HIV, breast self-examination, gender-specific health issues, hepatitis, sexually transmitted diseases, and personal hygiene. In addition to patient education, nursing staff may provide staff training as needed.

Counselors

Counseling staff help to guide patients through the rehabilitative process by first engaging the patient in the treatment process, assessing the patient's strengths and weakness, developing a plan of action toward abstinence from illicit opiates, and then generalizing the abstinence plan to other substances of abuse (McCann et al. 1994). Therapeutic work between the counselor and the patient may occur through individual and/or group interactions, as well as with the involvement of family members and significant others (Hagman 1994).

Regulations and accreditation standards require that counselors be qualified and deemed competent to assess the background of the patient, develop an appropriate treatment plan, and monitor the patient's progress throughout treatment. In the United States, it is increasingly common for states to require that counselors obtain credentials such as the CAC (certified addiction counselor) and maintain these credentials through continuing education. These requirements are designed to move the counseling profession toward more standardized education and skills requirements.

Case Manager

Both clinical practice and empirical observations support the integration of case management services into addiction treatment programs, because those seeking treatment often present with significant psychosocial problems that can benefit from such services (Siegal 1998). An on-site case manager allows counselors to focus on clinical issues during the therapeutic encounter, whereas the case manager then is responsible for addressing the patient's additional psychosocial needs.

Support Staff

Support staff can include clerical, laboratory, financial, facilities management, security, technical, and administration members of the clinic staff. The size and complexity of the program dictates the size of the support staff. These staff, although often not directly involved in the treatment process, should be aware of the program's mission and goals, including identified competencies as noted later in this section.

All Staff

Because opioid dependence is a chronic condition and because it is not uncommon for treatment to include relapses and problems that reach beyond the actual drug use itself, it is important for staff to be aware of their own thoughts and feelings about drug use and addiction. All staff involved with the program must accept that drug addiction is a chronic problem that is not easily resolved. Progress in treatment can be slow and requires limited and realistic goals for patients and staff. Relapse to drug use is not uncommon, and staff that acknowledge and understand that relapse can occur are better prepared to manage patients during drug-using episodes and to deal with the resulting crises. All clinic staff need to maintain objectivity, patience, a rational perspective on drug addiction, and a firm understanding of what can reasonably be accomplished in treatment, especially when patients challenge staff and test limits. Understanding individual and family dynamics is important, because staff come to learn of arrangements between family members and the patient's role in his or her family's operations. The need for clear and frequent communication among staff is extremely important both in the day-to-day operation of the clinic and in the periodic assessments of the mission, goals, and objective of the clinic. For a new staff member at a clinic, supervision can be key to that member's success in working with the patient population. For all staff at an opioid treatment clinic, supervision is a valuable mechanism for addressing staff member's responses to a patient's behavior.

Staff Training

Staff training is an essential component of a treatment program. Training upon hiring is customary, but ongoing training of staff is essential to maintain an understanding of current guidelines in the field of substance abuse and opioid treatment. This training can be achieved through in-service instruction, seminars, workshops, and academic courses. Clinic personnel are from various disciplines, and training requirements may be mandated by either the program itself, governmental agencies, or professional organizations. Some staff may have more intensive and individualized training requirements to maintain licensure or professional certification (Brill 1991).

Assessing Patient Eligibility and Appropriateness for Treatment

Under most circumstances, individuals applying for treatment at an OTP must have a current diagnosis of opioid dependence based on accepted criteria such as those listed in the *Diagnostic and Statistical Manual of Mental Disorders* (DSM-IV-TR) (APA 2000) to be eligible for treatment. There can be exceptions under certain circumstances, as described in more detail below. In the United States, regulations stipulate the conditions under which a person can be admitted to an opioid treatment program.

Determining Opioid Dependence

Before discussing the determination that a person is currently opioid dependent, it is useful to consider the word dependence and how it can be used. Dependence is often applied in two different ways by clinicians and researchers. The first way is to speak of "physical" or "physiologic dependence," which is usually indicated by a person showing tolerance or a withdrawal syndrome when he or she stops using a psychoactive substance. Tolerance is present when the person needs more of the substance to achieve a previous type of effect or experiences a reduced effect with continued use of the same quantity of the substance. Withdrawal is a set of signs and symptoms that occur when the person stops, or markedly reduces, the amount of the substance they take. The second way is to speak of a "syndrome of dependence," using criteria such as those found in the DSM-IV-TR (APA 2000) (table 9.2). Probably a better term for this syndrome of dependence is addiction. Included in criteria such as those found in the DSM-IV-TR are features of physical dependence, such as evidence of withdrawal when a person stops using the substance.

Physical dependence is not the only feature of a syndrome of dependence; it is not the defining feature, and it is not even a necessary feature. For example, patients with terminal cancer can be prescribed opioids daily to help control their pain and thus be physically dependent on opioids (i.e., a withdrawal syndrome would be present if opioid medication were suddenly stopped). These patients would not fulfill the criteria for a syndrome of dependence, however (table 9.2). On the other hand, a person could use illicit opioids only on the weekends, develop problems because of such opioid use, but not show evidence of withdrawal—that person is not physically dependent.

In the United States, federal regulations require that an individual is currently dependent on opioids and present evidence of dependence for at

Table 9.2 **DSM-IV-TR Criteria for Substance Dependence**

A maladaptive pattern of substance use, leading to clinically significant impairment or distress, as manifested by three (or more) of the following, occurring at any time in the same 12-month period:

1. Tolerance, as defined by either of the following:
   a. A need for markedly increased amounts of the substance to achieve intoxication or desired effect
   b. Markedly diminished effect with continued use of the same amount of the substance
2. Withdrawal, as manifested by either of the following:
   a. The characteristic withdrawal syndrome for the substance (refer to criteria A and B of the criteria sets for withdrawal from the specific substances)
   b. The same (or a closely related) substance is taken to relieve or avoid withdrawal symptoms
3. The substance is often taken in larger amounts or over a longer period than was intended
4. There is a persistent desire or unsuccessful efforts to cut down or control substance use
5. A great deal of time is spent in activities necessary to obtain the substance (e.g., visiting multiple doctors or driving long distances), use the substance (e.g., chain-smoking), or recover from its effects
6. Important social, occupational, or recreational activities are given up or reduced because of substance use
7. The substance use is continued despite knowledge of having a persistent or recurrent physical or psychological problem that is likely to have been caused or exacerbated by the substance (e.g., current cocaine use despite recognition of cocaine-induced depression, or continued drinking despite recognition that an ulcer was made worse by alcohol consumption)

Source: Reprinted with permission from *Diagnostic and Statistical Manual of Mental Disorders,* copyright 2000. American Psychiatric Association.

least one year before admission to be eligible for *maintenance* treatment at an OTP. The physician can usually make a reasonable clinical judgment of dependence by using a combination of objective and self-report data without conducting a formal structured interview based on the DSM-IV-TR criteria. A self-report of daily opioid use is typically found in a person who is opioid dependent. It is often difficult to determine when a person became dependent on opioids, however, and a criminal history associated with opioid use and past treatment episodes may be used to validate a one-year history of dependence. Evidence on physical examination of drug use (e.g., needle tracking) and one or several opioid-positive urine samples may also help to substantiate the diagnosis of dependence. Additionally, persons under the age of 18 years must have written consent from a parent or legal guardian and demonstrate two unsuccessful attempts at short-term detoxification (as defined below) or drug-free treatment in the past 12 months to be eligible for maintenance (CFR 42 Part 8.12).

Opioid-dependent individuals also can be admitted to an opioid treatment program for *detoxification,* or what is also called medically supervised withdrawal. In the United States, federal regulations describe two forms of detoxification—short term (i.e., a withdrawal that lasts 30 days or less) and long term (i.e., a withdrawal that lasts more than 30 days but no more than 180 days). According to federal regulations, the program physician must refer for alternative long-term treatment patients with two or more unsuccessful medically supervised withdrawal episodes within a 12-month period. In addition, a program may not admit a person for a medically supervised withdrawal more than two times in one year.

Exceptions: Patients Who Are Not Currently Opioid Dependent

Under certain circumstances, a program physician may decide to admit a person who is not currently opioid dependent to an OTP. In the United States, federal regulations recognize three populations who may be admitted for maintenance treatment even though they are not currently opioid dependent. These exceptions make clinical sense and are not unique to treatment in the United States. In all three cases, patients must have evidence of previously being physically dependent on opioids, but the one-year history of addiction may be waived.

The first such population includes persons who have been released from incarceration within the past six months. Such patients must have documented evidence that they would have qualified for treatment prior to their incarceration, and a physician must believe maintenance treatment is now medically justified. The second group that can be admitted without a one-year history of opioid dependence is women who are pregnant and are at risk for relapse to opioid use. Again, a physician must determine that starting maintenance treatment is medically justified, and the physician must also certify the pregnancy. Finally, previously treated patients who have voluntarily withdrawn from maintenance can be readmitted for up to two years after their discharge from treatment, even if they are not currently dependent on opioids. Such readmission can occur only if there is medical justification.

Initial Assessment for Admission

In addition to the previously described determination of eligibility, persons being admitted for opioid treatment should undergo a thorough medical assessment to identify any medical problems that need to be addressed. This should include laboratory tests, a complete medical and substance abuse history and physical examination (including vital signs, skin test for tuberculosis, nutrition, and pain evaluation), a medical assessment by the program physician or their designee (e.g., a nurse practitioner), urine testing for drugs of abuse, an offer of HIV testing, and a breath check for evidence of recent alcohol use.

Patients entering opioid treatment are at high risk for tuberculosis, and the clinic is an excellent site for screening and coordinating treatment of patients who have a positive purified protein derivative (PPD). Patients with an initial negative skin test for tuberculosis should be retested on an annual basis. At any time during treatment, if patients report exposure to or develop symptoms of tuberculosis, they should be evaluated by program medical staff and may need to have a tuberculin skin test repeated. If the treatment program is unable to treat patients with a positive PPD, they should be referred to the local health department.

Poor nutrition is common for patients entering treatment. The nutritional status of each patient should be evaluated at the time of admission. Nursing staff utilizing a standard nutrition survey may do this. Unexpected weight loss or gain, vomiting, diarrhea, and constipation are symptoms that should be included in the evaluation. Nutritional status should be evaluated annually or on an as-needed basis. If intervention is needed that cannot be provided at the program, a referral should be made and follow-up is advised.

Patients also should be evaluated for pain upon admission. Chronic pain is very common among persons with opioid dependence; surveys in opioid treatment programs have found between one-third and two-thirds of patients report chronic pain (Jamison et al. 2000; Rosenblum et al. 2003). It is important for staff to differentiate between withdrawal-related pain (muscle aches, abdominal pain) and pain of another etiology. According to the Joint Commission on Accreditation of Healthcare Organizations (JCAHO 2003), a United States-based accreditation organization for hospitals and other health care programs, the pain evaluation must be appropriate for the age of the patient, with a rating of intensity and quality (e.g., location, frequency, duration). Additionally, the treatment program should have a mechanism to ensure that follow-up evaluations are completed on a regular basis.

During the initial assessment, the patient's readiness to learn must be assessed to assist with development of treatment goals. Results from all initial assessments (e.g., eligibility criteria, medical and psychosocial evaluation, determination of level of readiness to learn) should be utilized to guide both the treatment goals and plans. Procedures should be in place for a formal medical evaluation to be conducted annually. Typically, this could mirror the medical evaluation completed at admission. If on-site gynecological examinations are not provided, female patients should be referred for this service.

Admission to the Program

Once it has been determined the patient is eligible for treatment, an admission to the OTP may follow on the same day or within the next few days. In the United States, before receiving any medication, patients must sign the consent for treatment with an approved narcotic drug (Form FDA 2635) and undergo any remaining assessments that were not completed during the initial assessment period; then, they can receive their first dose of the opioid agonist medication. A full description of the procedure for methadone and buprenorphine dose induction can be found in chapters 5 and 11, respectively. In the United States, federal regulations stipulate the first dose of methadone cannot be greater than 30 mg, and the total dose the first day should not be greater than 40 mg (unless the treating physician documents that the 40 mg did not suppress opiate abstinence symptoms). Once the patient has entered an opioid treatment program, continuing evaluation and treatment for medical and other psychiatric disorders is necessary (see chaps. 18 and 19).

DAILY OPERATION OF AN OPIOID TREATMENT PROGRAM
Rules and Regulations

The rules and regulations for an OTP can provide a clear set of guidelines and expectations for patients, help staff reach agreement among themselves regarding the operation of their program, and also give staff a mechanism for confronting patients about problematic behaviors in the clinic. Properly thought out, communicated, and posted for patient review, the rules and regulations for a program can ensure a safe and effective treatment and work environment for patients and staff.

The primary means for communicating to patients the rules and regulations of the clinic is to give patients a written copy at the time of admission to the clinic or at the time of their application for admission. The rules-and-regulations document should be written in a clear, simple, and easily understandable format. When given to a patient, a member of the staff should *verbally* review the rules with the patient. Alternatively, this review could be done with an audio or videotape presentation. The importance of this introduction to the clinic rules and regulations cannot be emphasized too strongly. This review communicates several messages to the patient: that staff are serious about the rules, that staff care about the patients and their understanding of the rules, and that the clinic is a well-run operation that is a professional site for the delivery of treatment. This meeting can include topics such as the clinic's expectations regarding compliance with the medication-reporting schedule, dosing plans in the event of an emergency, attendance at individual and/or group counseling, payment of clinic fees, consequences of noncompliance with the urine sample submission schedule, maintenance of confidentiality, and an agreement to participate actively in the treatment process. In addition, rules regarding loitering, invalid urine samples, illicit drug and alcohol use, possession of drugs or weapons, drug transactions, verbal or physical aggression toward staff or other patients, and theft or destruction of staff, patient, or program property should be included (Deitch 1979; Elk et al. 1993).

The rules also should express the program's mission, the general goals of treatment, the mechanisms used by the clinic to achieve those goals, and the services available. Included in the rules and regulations should be an explanation of the patient's rights and responsibilities. The rules and regulations also should outline how patients can address grievances related to treatment. Patients should be given the opportunity to complain about a program policy or a program decision such as termination, and a clear and concise route for such a procedure should be provided. Typically, the patient's counselor will assist the patient through the grievance procedure unless the counselor is the source of the grievance (in which case the counselor's supervisor should manage the grievance).

Finally, while there is a tendency to focus on the clinic's expectations of the patient while engaged in treatment, it is also important to discuss with the patient what he or she can expect from the clinic. The clinic should provide treatment in a safe, clean environment; there should be strict maintenance of confidentiality; and the patient should expect to be treated with compassion and respect and without discrimination or prejudice. Accreditation standards outline additional items that may be appropriate for inclusion in the program rules and regulations.

Medication Procedures: Administration and Management

In opioid treatment programs in the United States, opioid agonist medications may only be administered or dispensed by a practitioner licensed under the appropriate state law and registered under this state law and federal laws to administer or dispense opioid drugs (*Federal Register* 66). Oral opioid medicine is commonly mixed with cherry juice or an orange-flavored drink to make it palatable. The dosage may be measured using a manual pipette pump. Alternately, treatment programs equipped with computers may use an automated dispensing pump controlled by dedicated software. Most of these systems are equipped with or can be adapted to maintain dosage records and large portions of the patient's medical record.

Opioid treatment programs should have strict policies regarding the procedures for administration of opioid agonist medications, as diversion is a major concern. Although the proper ingestion of medication at the window is the responsibility of the patient and the nursing staff, all staff members should be alert and aware of possible diversion. Simply observing the patient ingest the medication and requiring the patient to speak to the nurse prior to leaving, in most cases, can accomplish this. It is also helpful to have the patient drink water after the medication. The medication should not leave the nurse's line of vision. The patient should not have cups or other containers at the dosing window that might allow the methadone to be poured, stored, and taken out of the clinic. Distractions to the nursing staff should be at a minimum so they will not lose their focus while administering medication. Crowding at the dosing window by patients can occur at busier dosing times as the waiting lines grow. Preventing this undesirable situation may require assistance from security or other clinic staff to monitor lines.

It is important to have procedures for the proper identification of patients. Policies and procedures to ensure medication is given to the correct person should be in place and strictly enforced. Some OTPs require patients to provide picture identification such as a driver's license before receiving medication. Programs may issue their own individual picture identification cards, although there are liabilities with such a system (such as the cost, issues of confidentiality, and the risk that the patient will lose the card). It is also possible to take a photograph of a patient and then store it in a computer file with a hard-copy back-up (in case the computer is not accessible). Note that staff should obtain written consent from the patient before taking the photograph. Finally, many programs utilize a unique identifier number system so that a number instead of a name identifies a patient.

Take-Home Dosing Procedures

Early in treatment patients typically attend the OTP on a daily basis to receive supervised administration of medication. As patients stabilize, however, and achieve a significant period of sustained abstinence, it is reasonable to consider giving take-home doses of medication. A take-home dose is simply a prepared daily dose of medication that is given to the patient for self-administration on a subsequent day of treatment. In the United States, accreditation and regulatory standards outline criteria for determining a person's eligibility to receive take-home doses of medication. A take-home dose is often a highly desirous privilege, because it reduces the patient's visits to the clinic. It may also be used as an effective tool to promote behavior change to achieve treatment goals (see chap. 8).

Patients who are in maintenance treatment can be given several take-home doses if they have been doing well in treatment for a sustained period. In the United States, patients who are admitted to a short-term (30 days or less) opioid agonist withdrawal or interim maintenance treatment are required to attend the clinic each day. According to federal regulations, patients enrolled in maintenance treatment with an opioid agonist medication may receive a single take-home dose of medication for a day that the clinic is closed for business (e.g., Sunday). During the first 90 days in treatment, federal regulations allow patients to receive a single dose of medication to take at home beyond the take-home dose for business closure (table 9.3). Subsequently, patients may earn up to two and three take-home doses of medication beyond the dose for business closure during their second and third 90 days of treatment, respectively. Beyond the ninth month and up to the first year of treatment, a patient may be given a max-

Table 9.3 **Schedule of Allowed Take-Home Doses that an OTP Can Use in the United States**

Time in Treatment (months)	Number of THs Allowed if Meeting Performance Criteria	Number of THs Allowed Due to Closure (e.g., Sundays)	Total THs Allowed
0–3	1	1	2
4–6	2	1	3
7–9	3	1	4
10–12	5	1	6
13–24	—	—	14
25+	—	—	30

Note: Numbers shown are allowed but are not required to be provided. A program must also comply with state regulations regarding take-home doses of medication. TH, take-home dose of medication

imum six-day supply of take-home doses of medication, so long as the program's performance criteria are met. These criteria may include adherence to clinic rules, abstinence from drug and alcohol use, no evidence of criminal activity, and employment or other productive use of time. After the first year of continuous treatment, patients may earn a maximum two-week supply, and a maximum 30-day supply is available after two continuous years of treatment. Although take-home dosing may in general be based on the criteria outlined in the federal regulations, some state regulations are more stringent. In this case, the programs must follow the most stringent policy. Last, the earning of take-home doses is at the discretion of the clinic and may be contingent on other treatment achievements beyond those noted in the federal and state regulations.

Take home dosing can relieve pressures on staff associated with daily attendance (e.g., a high volume of patients at the dosing window) and reduce the number of interactions needed with patients (e.g., counseling visits). Thus, practical reasons may exist for a clinic to want to decrease patients' attendance to a less than daily schedule. It is probably best for treatment outcome, however, if take-home doses are only used with patients who are well engaged in treatment and for whom there is clear and objective evidence of success, such as urine samples that are negative for illicit drugs and documented evidence of employment or other socially appropriate use of time.

Take-Home Recall Policies

Diversion of medication while it is being administered at the dosing window, as discussed above, is a relatively rare occurrence. Diversion of take-home doses of medication is also of concern, because there is less direct control by staff when medication is given to patients to take at home. There are many procedures that can assist in ensuring take-home medications are handled appropriately by patients.

First, educating patients about the program's take-home policy and requirements is of utmost importance. It is helpful to have an instruction form available. The patients should sign the form, indicating that they understand their responsibilities when receiving take-home medication. Each patient should be given a copy of the signed take-home policy form.

Second, the take-home bottle should be secured in a way that minimizes the chance for tampering. Take-home medication bottles must have child-resistant lids and may also have foam-sealed, tamper-resistant lids. Bottles may be sealed in a variety of ways such as plastic shrink-wrapping over the entire bottle or a seal over the lid. Several products are commercially available to assist programs in their choice of method for sealing the bottle.

Another means for decreasing tampering, diversion, or abuse of take-home doses is to secure bottles when at home. Opioid agonist medication does not need to be refrigerated. Especially when the patient has small children at home, however, it is a good policy to require storage of medications in a lock box. Before receiving take-home medication, patients should bring the lock box to the clinic to be approved by their counselor. Some programs may offer the sale of the boxes at the clinic.

The return of empty take-home bottles to the clinic can decrease the likelihood of diversion of opioid agonist medication. When returning a take-home bottle, the bottle's label should be intact and all information on it should be easily read.

Finally, recall procedures are an excellent way to reduce diversion. In one system, for example, the patient can be asked to call a dedicated phone line that has a recorded message announcing identification numbers of those patients who are required to return their recalled medication that day. Patient names should not be used on a recording, as this violates confidentiality. Alternatively, staff may call patients at a predetermined time and phone number and inform the patient their medication has been recalled. The patient whose medication has been recalled must report to the clinic that same day or no later than the next day with their medication packaged in the same manner it was dispensed. Consequences can be implemented upon failure to comply, such as denying the next take-home dose (Elk et al. 1993; Lowinson and Millman 1979) or discharging the patient from treatment for repeated failures to comply with take-home dose rules.

Emergency Dosing Plan

It is extremely important to have a plan for providing doses of medication during an emergency. In the United States, federal, state, and accreditation standards require that an OTP evaluate the potential emergencies that a clinic may experience for its particular location. Emergencies may range from weather (e.g., blizzards, tornadoes, floods, and other natural disasters such as earthquakes and fires) to power outages and terrorism. Clinics must have a plan for managing services in the event of an emergency so that there is minimal impact on the patient population. Patients should be informed at admission and throughout treatment about how they may get information about the clinic services in the event of an emergency. It is recommended that clinics establish with local radio or television stations a mechanism for announcing changes. Additionally, the OTP may choose to have an identified phone line that provides recorded information about changes to clinic operations. Last, governmental and accreditation agencies may require a 24-hour contact line for verification of medication doses.

OTHER ISSUES IN THE TREATMENT OF OPIOID-DEPENDENT PATIENTS

Boundaries in Staff-Patient Interactions

Issues of boundaries in interactions among all levels of staff and patients often arise in opioid treatment programs. Patients interact with numerous staff and depend on them for different aspects of their treatment. Blurring of boundaries can be as subtle as accepting candy from a patient, which the patient may construe as a nicety to be repaid with a small favor. A boundary invasion also can take the form of a staff member disclosing personal information about themselves or other staff to the patient. Seemingly harmless information can be misconstrued and used as a detriment to staff. A good rule of thumb is to carefully consider the therapeutic value of each interaction with the patient. Staff should be encouraged to ask themselves how a statement or action would be helpful to the patient's successful treatment.

Many professional groups, such as the American Psychological Association and the American Psychiatric Association, strictly prohibit nonprofessional relationships with patients. Professionals may face legal ramifications both from the patient and the professional organization for violations of those codes of conduct. An awareness of these professional guidelines may aid new staff in appreciating the importance of maintaining appropriate boundaries in the clinic.

Confidentiality

In the United States, identifying information for individuals applying to or in treatment for a substance abuse problem is protected under the Code of Federal Regulations (CFR 42 Part 2) (Parrino 1993). These regulations prohibit disclosing any information that may identify an individual as having, at any time, a problem with drugs and/or alcohol and require that individual to give their permission, in writing, before the treatment provider shares any such information (e.g., with a police officer, outside physician, or family member). If the patient has released the information to someone, the regulations prohibit the recipient of that information from forwarding those records to someone else. The regulations also indicate how and when information may be disclosed, and also specify situations in which information may be disclosed without the patient's permission—such as medical emergencies or in the case of state or regulatory agency reviews. The regulations require staff to report any indication or acknowledgment of child abuse/neglect or the abuse/neglect of an elderly dependent. Violation of these regulations is punishable by fines and in some cases imprisonment.

In the United States, as of April 14, 2003, covered entities (defined as health care providers, health plans, and health care clearing houses) may not use or disclose protected health information (PHI) except as permitted or required by the Health Insurance Portability and Accountability Act (HIPAA) of 1996. HIPAA (CFR 42 Parts 160 and 164) regulations do not overturn the confidentiality rules in the Code of Federal Regulations but do change some of them. The intent of HIPAA is to establish federal guidelines to protect the privacy of medical records and other personal health information, and the HIPAA rules apply to transmission of this information electronically or in written form (Legal Action Center 2003).

Because the HIPAA and confidentiality regulations use complex and sometimes confusing verbiage, it is suggested that the OTP offer an abbreviated and more reader-friendly summary of the regulations for patients. Further, staff members need guidance as to the application of the regulation to determine whether HIPAA preempts or overrides state laws or where it may appear to contradict the Federal Confidentiality Rules.

The Legal Action Center (LAC) is the public organization in the United States that has been developed to address issues related to patients with drug and alcohol problems, HIV, AIDS, and persons involved with the criminal justice system. The LAC offers an excellent resource that can aid OTPs in complying with these confusing yet important regulations. The center's book, *Confidentiality and Communication* (2003), is designed to help drug and alcohol treatment and prevention programs and the organizations and agencies that work with these programs to understand the interplay between the federal laws governing Confidentiality of Alcohol and Drug Abuse Patient Records and the new Health Insurance Portability and Accountability Act, and to comply with both.

Provision of Care: Case Management, Counseling, and Group Therapy

Issues related to counseling and group therapy in the context of the opioid treatment program are addressed in detail in chapters 7 and 8. In the United States, federal regulations require programs to provide a range of services, including medical evaluations, counseling, and other treatments such as vocational and educational programs.

Each patient should be assigned a primary counselor who is responsible for conducting a psychosocial assessment and for generating an integrated summary and treatment plan based on this assessment. In addition, the counselor should meet regularly with the patient and coordinate other treatment services (e.g., vocational rehabilitation, social services). A clinic's caseload for each counselor will depend on the severity and number of presenting problems, counselor competency level, and existing caseload guidelines. No single counselor in a clinic should have all new patients or all highly stable patients, but rather a mix of types. Typical caseloads for counselors are between 30 and 50 patients, although a caseload of 50 can be excessive under some circumstances. The OTP should review state regulations that may outline caseload requirements more specifically.

Group therapy can be a cost- and treatment-effective means of providing services. In the OTP, group treatment can take several forms, including didactic sessions (e.g., related to health issues such as HIV infection), special subgroup issues (e.g., women's issues), topics related directly to achieving and maintaining abstinence (e.g., senior patients discussing with new patients how to avoid using drugs), and groups on issues related only indirectly to drug use (e.g., problems in familial interactions).

Staff Supervision and Training

For new staff at an OTP, the initial orientation and competency training can be key to that staff member's success in working with their patient caseload. The objective of the orientation program is to train the new employee to complete job-specific tasks and duties and to learn and understand program policies and procedures. This orientation and training increases the likelihood that the new employee will be competent to complete the duties of their job description (JCAHO 2003).

The need for clear and frequent communication among staff is extremely important in both the day-to-day operation of the clinic, and in the periodic assessments of the mission, goals, and objectives of the clinic. Further, for all staff at an OTP, supervision and training are valuable mechanisms for addressing staff members' responses to patient behavior. In-service instruction, self-learning packets, seminars, workshops, and academic courses can achieve training objectives. For supervisors to provide an appropriately individualized orientation and training, newly hired staff should complete a self-assessment of their knowledge that can form the basis for their individualized orientation and training plan. Further, training should be tailored to the job of the staff member. For example, it is imperative that nursing and counseling staff have training in how to identify and manage incidents involving opiate overdose. Some staff may have more intensive and individualized educational/training requirements to maintain licensure or professional certification (Brill 1991).

Although training upon hiring is customary, ongoing training of staff is essential to maintain an understanding of current updates in the field of substance abuse and opioid dependency treatment. Each program should determine and require mandatory updates on an annual basis for topics such as cardiopulmonary resuscitation (CPR), the treatment of pain, the acute management of an aggressive person, and fire and electrical safety. Training requirements may be mandated by the programs' policies, governmental regulatory agencies, accreditation agencies, and professional organizations.

Urinalysis Testing

In the United States, federal regulations require an OTP to provide adequate drug abuse testing; however, the OTP may choose the specific drugs to be tested depending on local patterns of abuse and compliance with state and accreditation standards. Historically, programs have used urine specimens for analysis, but the OTP may explore other alternatives to testing such as oral fluid (saliva) testing. Federal regulations require that patients receiving maintenance be tested at least eight times per year. Furthermore, regulations require only an initial drug screen for patients admitted to short-term (≤30 days) withdrawal programs and once-per-month testing for long-term withdrawal (>30 days but not exceeding 180 days). Samples for drug abuse are to be analyzed at a laboratory that meets federal and state requirements and should be collected in a way that minimizes personal invasiveness, loss of patient privacy, and the chance of falsification. Drug screen panels may include opiates, methadone, amphetamines, cocaine, barbiturates, benzodiazepines, marijuana, and other substances that may be prevalent in the clinic's locale.

While an OTP must adhere to governmental and accreditation standards, in actuality clinics may operate by using more stringent methods, such as increased frequency of collection with a more comprehensive testing panel of drugs. The method for collecting urine samples from patients can vary, but most programs utilize some type of monitored or observed specimen collection procedure with a same sexed staff member to ensure the authenticity of the specimen. Before providing urine samples, patients may be required to leave coats and bags outside the bathroom where the specimen is collected. Programs have developed alternate methods of detecting false samples, such as temperature monitoring and adulterant testing (e.g., specific gravity, pH, creatinine). As with oral fluid testing, adulterant testing enhances the services at the OTP by supporting the patient's privacy and respect.

Increasing the frequency of testing to greater than eight times per year improves the chance for detecting illicit drug use, but the cost associated with more frequent testing can make it difficult for clinics to conduct such as schedule. Some clinics enhance surveillance by collecting urine samples frequently, such as once a week, but only testing samples monthly. By not informing patients which week's samples are being tested, this procedure approximates a comprehensive random testing schedule.

Standard Precautions

In the United States, the Occupational Safety and Health Administration (OSHA) has set forth a standard requiring the implementation of provisions to protect all personnel who may come in contact with blood, urine, or other potentially infectious materials. In compliance with this standard, a clinic policy and procedure should be formulated and strictly enforced to minimize exposure to infectious materials. If an exposure does occur the policy should provide a plan of action. This plan should be reviewed and updated annually, or more often if necessary, in keeping with OSHA standards.

Practicing common sense is the basis for standard precautions. Staff should wash their hands regularly and directly after contact with blood or potentially infectious materials. The clinic must provide staff with specialized personal protective equipment that prevents exposure of skin, mucous membranes, and eyes to potentially infectious materials. The type of personal protective equipment worn should be appropriate to the nature of the anticipated contamination. Typical protective equipment found in an OTP are gloves, gowns, masks, eye protection, and face shields. The use of personal protective equipment is mandatory and should be enforced. These items should be easily accessible and the supply maintained.

Management of Behavioral Problems

The population of people with opioid dependence attending an OTP can represent a wide spectrum of patients, presenting with variable levels of motivation and needs for treatment of comorbid psychiatric and other medical disorders. Although it can be tempting to simply discharge from the clinic a patient who has shown problematic behavior, this may not be the optimal long-term solution for the patient, the community, or the clinic. It is also important, however, for clinics to clearly spell out specific circumstances that will lead to discharge (e.g., selling drugs, bringing a weapon on to the grounds, threatening to harm other patients or staff, diverting medication). This section reviews several of these specific behavioral problems and techniques that may be helpful in managing the patient who exhibits such problematic behaviors.

The Aggressive Patient

A patient may become aggressive for many different reasons, including enforcement of program policies or confrontations with other patients. Preparedness is the key component to diffuse the situation quickly and without incident. So how should staff react when a patient becomes hostile or threatening?

One member of the staff should become the spokesperson for the program. It may be the counselor, or a supervisor if the situation demands a staff member with more authority. The first consideration is the safety of the patient, the staff, and other patients. Staff should maintain a safe distance from the patient and remove any articles of clothing or jewelry from around their necks. The staff member should try to calm the patient (without engaging in physical contact). Attempts should be made to move the patient to a less public area that provides an easy exit for the spokesperson or patient. If that is not possible, other patients should be removed from the immediate area for their safety.

Staff who are not involved in the actual confrontation should contact security personnel (if available) and make themselves visible to the patient. Security officers should also make their presence known and remain nearby as long as lead staff member is in control. There should never be any physical contact with the patient unless they physically threaten to harm someone. It is important to quickly assess the patient's level of intoxication and, if possible, the substance involved. For example, alcohol can produce angry and aggressive behavior; PCP can trigger aggression and at times psychotic behavior, whereas cocaine can produce paranoia or agitation. Police and ambulance escort assistance may be necessary if deescalation is not achieved.

Drug Dealing in the Vicinity of the Clinic

The potential for drug transactions is generally increased in the vicinity of the clinic. This risk is lower in programs composed of long-term patients who may have less need to supplement an insufficient methadone dose, who may have higher rates of employment, school, or involvement in other constructive and rewarding activities, and who may have less contact with individuals new to the treatment process who may still be using illicit drugs.

Suspicions of drug dealing may arise when there is a change in the frequency of drug-positive urine tests. Increased loitering in and around the program may be indicative of active drug dealing. Exchanges of money between patients or conflicts between patients may suggest that drug dealing is occurring. Program policy should clearly detail what actions may be taken. Some programs warn that a search of person and property is permitted for cause, with illicit drugs being confiscated and destroyed and the patient discharged from the clinic.

Patients Who Present at the Clinic Impaired

It is inevitable that staff will encounter patients impaired because of the use of alcohol or drugs. A thorough knowledge of the physiologic and behavioral indications of intoxication is crucial for the safety of the patient and staff. Staff should be well trained to assess and intervene in the case of an impaired patient, in particular, because the intoxicated patient may present a risk to himself or herself, other patients, and staff. Depending on the substance used, the patient's behavior may include aggression, requiring intervention by security. If the patient is driving, then there is danger of injury to the patient or others on the road. If indicated, the staff should attempt to call a cab or family member to pick up the patient. If a patient is unwilling to accept this assistance and leaves the clinic area, the police may be called and given information describing the patient's impaired status, vehicle, and license tag number without stating that the patient is in substance abuse treatment (i.e., complying with the regulations regarding confidentiality).

A combination of medications and drugs may precipitate serious medical complications, and a program should have specific guidelines and policies for alternate dosing (e.g., reduced or placebo dosing) for patients who are impaired. Determination of the need for alternative dosing is facilitated by use of objective data such as the breath alcohol level, which is easily ascertained with commercially available equipment. It is important to remember that a patient may have a very low breath alcohol level but appear extremely intoxicated; therefore, policies should allow for clinical judgment.

Loitering in the Vicinity of the Clinic

The issue of loitering is often a source of significant contention between the community and the program (Genevie et al. 1988). A program may prohibit loitering in a variety of ways, usually through the rules and regulations that specifically indicate when and for how long a patient may be in or around the program. Some programs access local zoning laws that legally prohibit loitering within a specific distance of the program. Enforcement of a no loitering policy often falls to program staff or hired security.

SUMMARY

A well-operating opioid treatment program recognizes the importance of the facility's location, its internal design and organization, and its role in the surrounding community. The OTP must operate under governmental and accreditation guidelines, and ensure that staff are competent to provide care within theses guidelines. In addition, the OTP itself should establish its mission, vision, and values with its own set of policies and procedures that are well known to both staff and patients. These policies and procedures aid in the smooth and professional operation of the clinic, by making clear expectations and consequences of behavior for patients who attend the clinic. Despite the best efforts and organization of an OTP, however, patients can present with behavior problems such as loitering, drug dealing, and diversion of medication. The optimal operation of a clinic occurs when these special behavior problems have been anticipated and a plan for response to them is in place as a part of the organization of the program.

References

APA (2000). Diagnostic and Statistical Manual of Mental Disorders, 4th ed. Text Revision. Washington, DC: American Psychiatric Association.

Ball JC, Levine BK, Demaree RG, Neman JF (1975). Pretreatment criminality of male and female drug abuse patients in the United States. *Addict Dis* 1: 481–9.

Ball JC, Ross A (1991). *The Effectiveness of Methadone Maintenance Treatment.* New York: Springer-Verlag.

Besteman KJ, Brady JV (1994). Implementing mobile drug abuse treatment: problems, procedures, and perspectives. In: Fletcher BW, Inciardi JA, Horton AM, eds. *Drug Abuse Treatment: The Implementation of Innovative Approaches.* Westport, CT: Greenwood Press, 33–42.

Brady JV (1993). Enhancing Drug Abuse Treatment by Mobile Health Services. In: Inciardi JA, Tims FM, Fletcher BW, eds. *Innovative Approaches in the Treatment of Drug Abuse: Program Models and Strategies.* Westport, CT: Greenwood Press, 35–42.

Brill L (1991). *The Clinical Treatment of Substance Abusers.* New York: Free Press.

Calsyn DA, Saxon AJ, Blaes P, Lee-Meyer S (1990). Staffing patterns of American methadone maintenance programs. *J Subst Abuse Treat* 7: 255–9.

Deitch DA (1979). Program management: magical expectations and harsh realities. In: DuPont RL, Goldstein A, O'Donnell J, eds. *Handbook on Drug Abuse.* Washington, DC: U.S. Government Printing Office.

Elk R, Grabowski J, Rhoades H, McLellan AT (1993). A substance-abuse research-treatment clinic: effective procedures and systems. *J Subst Abuse Treat* 10: 459–71.

Federal Register 66, no.11:4097. January 17, 2001.

Genevie L, Struening EL, Kallos JE, Geiler I, Muhlin GL, Kaplan S (1988). Urban community reaction to health facilities in residential areas: lessons from the placement of methadone facilities in New York City. *Int J Addict* 23: 603–16.

Hagman G (1994). Methadone maintenance counseling. Definition, principles, components. *J Subst Abuse Treat* 11: 405–13.

Jamison RN, Kauffman J, Katz NP (2000). Characteristics of methadone maintenance patients with chronic pain. *J Pain Symptom Manage* 19: 53–62.

JCAHO (2003). Standards for behavioral health care. Accreditation policies standards intent statement. Oak Brook, IL: Joint Commission Resources, Inc.

Legal Action Center (2003). Confidentiality and Communication: A Guide to Federal Drug and Alcohol Confidentiality Law and HIPAA, 5th ed. New York: Legal Action Center.

Lowinson JH, Millman RB (1979). Clinical aspects of methadone maintenance treatment. In: DuPont RL, Goldstein A, O'Donnell J, eds. *Handbook on Drug Abuse.* Washington, DC: U.S. Government Printing Office.

McCann MJ, Rawson RA, Obert JL, Hasson AJ (1994). Treatment of Opiate Addiction with Methadone: A Counselor Manual. Washington, DC: Substance Abuse and Mental Health Services Administration.

Nurco DN, Shaffer JW, Ball JC, Kinlock TW (1984). Trends in the commission of crime among narcotic addicts over successive periods of addiction and nonaddiction. *Am J Drug Alcohol Abuse* 10: 481–9.

Parrino MW (1993). State Methadone Treatment Guidelines. Washington, DC: Substance Abuse and Mental Health Services Administration, U.S. Department of Health and Human Services.

Powell DJ (1993). *Clinical Supervision in Alcohol and Drug Abuse Counseling. Principles, Models, Methods.* San Francisco, CA: Jossey Bass Publishers.

Rosenblum A, Joseph H, Fong C, Kipnis S, Cleland C, Portenoy RK (2003). Prevalence and characteristics of chronic pain among chemically dependent patients in methadone maintenance and residential treatment facilities. *JAMA* 289: 2370–8.

Siegal HA (1998). Comprehensive Case Management for Substance Abuse Treatment. Washington, DC: Substance Abuse and Mental Health Services Administration.

Stancliff S, Myers JE, Steiner S, Drucker E (2002). Beliefs about methadone in an inner-city methadone clinic. *J Urban Health* 79: 571–8.

Wiebe J, Huebert KM (1996). Community mobile treatment. What it is and how it works. *J Subst Abuse Treat* 13: 23–31.

III

OTHER MEDICATION
APPROACHES

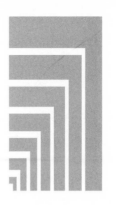

IO

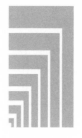

Pharmacology of Buprenorphine

Eric C. Strain, M.D.

Buprenorphine is a mixed agonist-antagonist opioid. Several other mixed agonist-antagonist opioids have been marketed as analgesics in humans, including butorphanol (Stadol), dezocine (Dalgan), nalbuphine (Nubain), and pentazocine (Talwin). Each has a somewhat unusual profile of opioid receptor effects, and this group of medications has been developed, in part, with the hope that abuse would be less than that seen with full agonist opioids such as morphine.

Buprenorphine was initially developed as an analgesic and is still marketed for this indication under the names Buprenex and Temgesic. The sublingual form of buprenorphine is marketed primarily for the indication of opioid dependence treatment (although a sublingual analgesic form is available in some countries), as Subutex or Suboxone. The latter form also contains naloxone.

The characterization of buprenorphine's pharmacologic profile produced an early interest in its potential use for the treatment of opioid dependence (Jasinski et al. 1978). This chapter provides a review of the pharmacology of buprenorphine, including its actions at different opioid receptors, its absorption, metabolism, and excretion, and the pharmacologic rationale for combining buprenorphine with naloxone.

BUPRENORPHINE'S OPIOID RECEPTOR PROPERTIES

Buprenorphine is an opioid mixed agonist-antagonist; that is, it exerts effects at both the mu opioid receptor, where it acts as a partial agonist, and at the kappa opioid receptor, where it acts as an antagonist (hence, the characterization as an "agonist-antagonist"). It has high affinity for both of these receptors types. A brief review of agonists, partial agonists, and antagonists is given here to provide some background for understanding the pharmacologic effects of buprenorphine.

A *full agonist* is a compound that occupies a receptor and activates that receptor; increasing the dose of an agonist produces greater and greater effects until a maximal (and sometimes toxic) effect is achieved. In contrast, a *partial agonist* occupies a receptor and activates that receptor but can produce only a limited maximal effect, which is not as great as the maximal effect of a full agonist for that receptor. At low doses, partial agonists can produce effects that are very similar or identical to that seen with similar low doses of a full agonist. However, at higher doses the partial agonist has a "ceiling" on the size of the effect it can produce. An *antagonist* is a compound that occupies a receptor but does not activate it (e.g., naltrexone, naloxone). These relationships are shown in figure 10.1, which provides illustrative dose-response curves for a full agonist, partial agonist, and antagonist.

These features of partial agonists result in a unique profile of effects. When a partial agonist opioid is given to someone who is not physically dependent on opioids, it produces agonist effects (such as mild euphoria, analgesia, or constipation); however, when given to someone who is physically dependent on opioids and has a high level of tolerance to opioids, a partial agonist could act like an antagonist (because it does not activate the receptor as much as the full agonist does). Thus, under these circumstances a partial agonist could precipitate withdrawal. (Note that if a partial agonist medication regularly precipitated withdrawal, it would not be realistic to try to use it for the treatment of opioid dependence.)

Although, in general, buprenorphine does not precipitate withdrawal when given to opioid-dependent persons, there is evidence it can produce antagonist-like effects under certain circumstances. For example, a study of subjects maintained on 100 mg per day of oral methadone found that acute, single doses of sublingual buprenorphine/naloxone given 20 hours after a dose of methadone could precipitate withdrawal (Rosado et al. 2004). The sensitivity of different subjects varied widely in that study, however, with some persons having withdrawal after receiving 4 mg of buprenorphine and others having no withdrawal despite receiving 32 mg. Further discussion of the clinical implications of buprenorphine's potential for precipitation of withdrawal can be found in chapter 11.

In addition to buprenorphine's partial agonist effects at the mu opioid receptor, it is also a kappa receptor antagonist. It has been suggested

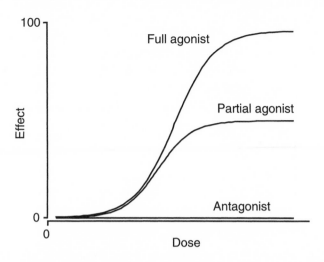

Figure 10.1. Dose-response curves for a full agonist, partial agonist, and antagonist medication. The dose is shown along the x axis, and an effect (such as respiratory depression or gastrointestinal motility) is shown along the y axis. As the dose of an antagonist increases, no change in the measured effect is seen. As the dose of a full agonist increases, a greater effect is produced until a maximal effect is achieved. As the dose of a partial agonist increases, it initially produces effects that are similar to those seen with a full agonist. However, the two curves then begin to diverge, and a lesser maximal effect is seen with the partial agonist. Buprenorphine is an example of a partial agonist at the mu opioid receptor.

that the kappa antagonist effects of buprenorphine at higher doses may offset the partial mu agonist effects (this has been called "noncompetitive autoinhibition") (Cowan et al. 1977). Noncompetitive autoinhibition has been used to explain the observation that buprenorphine has a bell-shaped dose-response curve; that is, as the dose of buprenorphine increases, measured effects (such as decreased gastrointestinal motility, respiratory depression, or analgesia) first increase but then decrease in magnitude as the dose is further increased (fig. 10.2). Note that, because buprenorphine is a partial opioid agonist, the peak for this bell-shaped curve falls below the maximal effect that is seen for full agonist opioids (fig. 10.1).

PHARMACOLOGY OF BUPRENORPHINE

The Structure of Buprenorphine

Buprenorphine is a thebaine derivative that was first synthesized in 1973 by Alan Cowan and John Lewis. Its chemical structure is shown in figure 10.3. It has high lipid solubility, and the parent compound appears to ex-

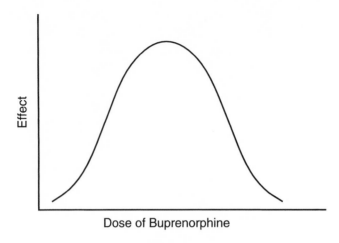

Figure 10.2. Buprenorphine's bell-shaped dose-response curve. Buprenorphine produces increasing effects as its dose increases up to a certain point, but then its effects diminish (the right side of this curve). Because buprenorphine is a partial agonist, the peak of this curve is less than the maximal effect that would be seen with a full opioid agonist. Thus, the maximal effects seen for this curve correspond to a point below the maximal effect seen for a full agonist opioid in figure 10.1.

ert the primary pharmacologic effects in the central nervous system, although its primary metabolite, norbuprenorphine, may exert some opioid agonist effects outside the central nervous system.

Absorption, Metabolism, and Excretion

When used as an analgesic, buprenorphine is typically given by injection. Buprenorphine has poor bioavailability when swallowed, because it is degraded in the intestine and liver (i.e., it is metabolized in the gastrointestinal tract and undergoes extensive hepatic first-pass effects). For this reason, doses used for analgesia or opioid dependence treatment are not effective if swallowed. When delivered as a sublingual solution, however, buprenorphine has relatively good absorption, with about 50 percent bioavailability (Kuhlman et al. 1996). Absorption of buprenorphine into the buccal mucosa is relatively rapid, and this may then serve as a reservoir that provides a slow and steady supply of medication over several hours. The marketed products for opioid dependence treatment are sublingual tablets.

Many of the early clinical trials testing the efficacy and safety of buprenorphine for the treatment of opioid dependence used a sublingual

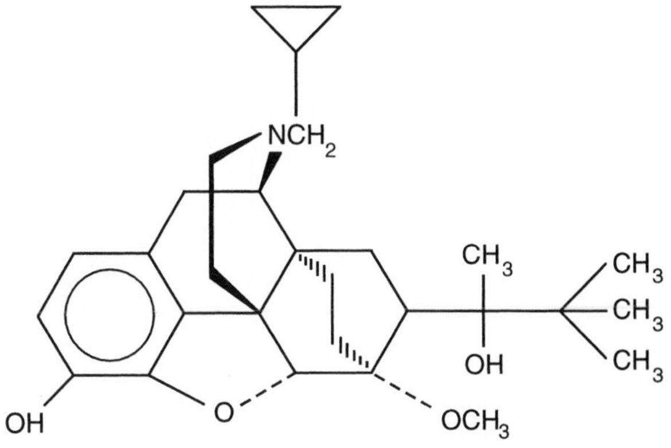

Buprenorphine

Figure 10.3. The structure of buprenorphine.

solution form rather than tablets. When administered as a sublingual solution, buprenorphine must be held under the tongue for 3–5 minutes to ensure adequate absorption (Mendelson et al. 1997; Weinberg et al. 1988). Buprenorphine sublingual tablets are held under the tongue until they dissolve (i.e., 3–10 minutes). Comparisons of relative bioavailability of buprenorphine solution versus tablets show that tablets deliver less buprenorphine than the solution (Chawarski et al. 1998; Nath et al. 1999; Schuh and Johanson 1999), but these differences in the relative bioavailability of tablets containing buprenorphine (and tablets containing buprenorphine combined with naloxone) versus buprenorphine solution decrease over days of regular buprenorphine dosing and are not significantly different after two weeks of stabilization on either type of formulation (Strain et al. 2004).

In general, when reviewing clinical studies that used sublingual buprenorphine, some allowance for dose differences between solution versus tablets should be made. Specifically, a higher dose of buprenorphine tablet would be needed to achieve the same relative dose of buprenorphine solution, but primarily for the first weeks of treatment.

Perhaps of more significance for the clinical use of sublingual buprenorphine is that plasma levels of buprenorphine can differ considerably between different persons maintained on the same dose of buprenorphine (when taken as either tablets or solution). Studies have shown that buprenorphine and norbuprenorphine blood levels (the latter is the primary ac-

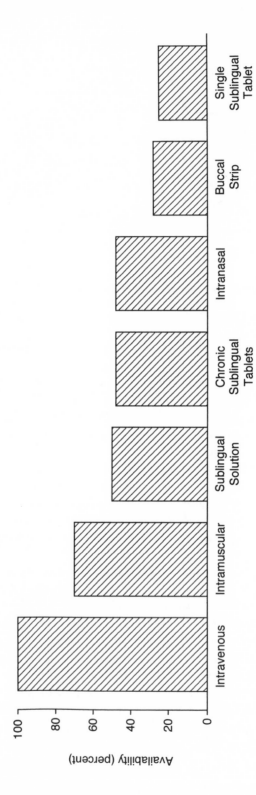

Figure 10.4.   The relative bioavailability of buprenorphine when taken by different routes of administration.

tive metabolite of buprenorphine) can vary more than twofold between subjects who receive the same dose of buprenorphine (Chawarski et al. 1999; Schuh and Johanson 1999; Strain et al. 2004).

Several other novel delivery systems in addition to the sublingual form of buprenorphine have been considered for this medication, including intranasal spray and a transdermal patch. These systems can also provide good delivery of buprenorphine. Figure 10.4 shows the relative bioavailability of buprenorphine given by different routes of administration.

Buprenorphine is highly lipid soluble. Once absorbed, a high percentage of it is bound to plasma protein (96%) and undergoes enterohepatic circulation. Buprenorphine readily crosses the blood-brain barrier; but it appears that only buprenorphine (i.e., not its metabolites) can cross the blood-brain barrier and enter the central nervous system (Marquet 2002).

Sublingual buprenorphine is metabolized into norbuprenorphine and other products in the liver (and metabolized in the gastrointestinal tract wall when taken orally). Buprenorphine is transformed by dealkylation in the liver by the cytochrome P450 3A4 enzyme into norbuprenorphine, which is an active metabolite with analgesic activity one-fourth to one-fiftieth as potent at that of buprenorphine (Ohtani et al. 1995). Norbuprenorphine's effects appear to be exerted primarily outside the central nervous system, however, and norbuprenorphine is not typically found in the brain (Ohtani et al. 1997). Buprenorphine and norbuprenorphine then undergo further transformation into nonactive metabolites. Buprenorphine is also a weak inhibitor of the P450 3A4 system.

Buprenorphine and its metabolites are primarily excreted in the bile as inactive forms (glucuronides). They then undergo enterohepatic circulation. Excretion of active and inactive forms of buprenorphine also occurs through urine. A commercial urine test for buprenorphine is available.

Buprenorphine's Half-life and Duration of Effects

When a single dose of buprenorphine is administered intravenously, the drug shows rapid redistribution consistent with its high lipophilicity; the terminal half-life for a single dose is estimated to be two to three hours (Bullingham et al. 1980). When sublingual doses are administered chronically and then abruptly discontinued, decay kinetics show an initial half-life of about three to four hours, followed by a second longer decay component of 45 hours (McQuay and Moore 1995). Buprenorphine has slow dissociation from opioid receptors, and its duration of effects can be prolonged (Boas and Villiger 1985). Consistent with this long duration of action, clinical studies have shown that buprenorphine can be provided on a less than daily basis, and in some cases can be dosed as infrequently as every four days (Gross et al. 2001; Petry et al. 1999, 2000).

Pharmacology of Buprenorphine: Clinical Features

Analgesic Effects

Buprenorphine is an effective injectable analgesic (Dobkin 1977; Dobkin et al. 1977; Hanks 1987; Kamel and Geddes 1978) that is 25 times more potent than morphine (Wallenstein et al. 1986). However, note that this relative potency is only valid for lower comparison doses of morphine, which is a full agonist opioid. Because buprenorphine is a partial agonist opioid (fig. 10.1), increasing the dose of buprenorphine will produce a relative plateau in analgesic effects, whereas increasing the dose of morphine can continue to produce greater analgesic effects. (However, increasing the dose of a full agonist opioid such as morphine can also produce greater adverse effects, such as respiratory depression.) The duration of buprenorphine's analgesic effects may vary depending on the degree of pain and can last six hours or more (Lewis 1995). In the United States, the Food and Drug Administration (FDA)-approved labeling for buprenorphine recommends a usual analgesic dose of 0.3 mg given by injection (intravenous or intramuscular) every six hours.

Respiratory Depression

An important pharmacologic feature of buprenorphine with clinical implications is that its respiratory depressant effects differ from those seen with full opioid agonists. A study of acute, high sublingual doses of buprenorphine (up to 32 mg of the solution form) administered to persons without current physical dependence on opioids found that buprenorphine produced mild decreases in respiratory rate (the maximum decrease was four breaths per minute) and correspondingly small decreases in oxygen saturation (to 95–96%) that did not require medical intervention (Walsh et al. 1994). Furthermore, it appears there is a relative plateau in these effects as dose increases, suggesting a lowered risk of fatality may be associated with buprenorphine overdose. Preclinical studies have also shown that buprenorphine appears to produce a more limited degree of respiratory depression when compared with full agonist opioids (Doxey et al. 1982; Liguori et al. 1996).

Clinically significant respiratory depressant effects can occur when acute, high doses of buprenorphine are combined with a sedative medication such as a benzodiazepine. In France, where buprenorphine is widely used in the treatment of opioid dependence, buprenorphine-related overdose fatalities have been reported (Reynaud et al. 1998; Tracqui et al. 1998). In virtually all these cases, it appears that persons dissolved and injected several buprenorphine tablets along with the injection of an intravenous benzodiazepine (typically, flunitrazepam). Caution regarding the use of benzodiazepines in persons with a history of opioid dependence is warranted (as a general clinical recommendation), given the potential for abuse of this class of compounds. On the other hand, sublingual buprenorphine has been tested extensively in several large outpatient clinical trials in which there was concurrent benzodiazepine use (typically oral abuse of benzodiazepines), and adverse respiratory effects were not noted (Johnson et al. 2000; Strain et al. 1994).

Opioid Blockade or Cross-tolerance

An important pharmacologic feature of medications for the treatment of opioid dependence is that they provide cross-tolerance blockade to the effects of other administered opioids. Central to buprenorphine's development were results from several clinical pharmacology studies examining buprenorphine's capacity to block the effects of other opioid agonists. For example, an early and important study tested buprenorphine's efficacy with respect to heroin self-administration and found that maintenance on daily subcutaneous buprenorphine produced substantial and significant reductions in heroin self-administration (Mello and Mendelson 1980). A more recent study of heroin self-administration also found sublingual buprenorphine was effective (i.e., that it decreased self-administration), although doses as high as 16 mg per day of buprenorphine tablets did not completely suppress heroin use (Comer et al. 2001).

Other laboratory studies with humans have administered challenges of mu agonist opioids to persons maintained on different doses of buprenorphine and have shown that the reported effects of these challenges are significantly decreased when persons are maintained on buprenorphine (Bickel et al. 1988; Jasinski et al. 1978; Strain et al. 1997; Walsh et al. 1995). These effects appear to be dose-related (i.e., there is more attenuation of injected opioid effects as the maintenance dose of buprenorphine is increased). However, this blockade appears to be incomplete with buprenorphine doses of about 8 mg per day or less of solution, and doses as high as 32 mg per day of solution may be needed to achieve marked and clinically significant blockade of the positive effects of mu agonist opioids.

Buprenorphine has a long duration of action, and some studies have examined the duration of its blockade efficacy. In one study, subjects maintained on different daily doses of sublingual buprenorphine solution (up to 12 mg per day) had significant decreases in response to hydromorphone challenges for up to three days after the last dose of active buprenorphine (Rosen et al. 1994). Similar results (significant attenuation of hydromorphone effects that lasted for three days) were found in another study of subjects maintained on 8 mg per day of buprenorphine solution, although the blockade then began to dissipate on the fifth day after active buprenorphine dosing (Schuh et al. 1999).

These studies of the blockade efficacy of buprenorphine suggest that daily doses of 8 mg may provide only incomplete blockade of effects when a short-acting opioid agonist such as heroin is administered. However, an 8 mg per day dose may be sufficient to suppress self-administration (i.e., a person may experience the reinforcing effects of an opioid agonist while maintained on 8 mg per day of buprenorphine, but such effects may be sufficiently mild because of the blockade to make further self-administration of that agonist no longer attractive). In general, daily buprenorphine doses greater than 8 mg will probably be needed to maximize cross-tolerance, and dose increases should be strongly considered for the person who reports feeling significant effects from an opioid agonist while maintained on buprenorphine.

Withdrawal Suppression

Although buprenorphine's blockade efficacy has been evaluated extensively in several human clinical pharmacology studies, relatively little systematic work has tested its use in suppressing the signs and symptoms of opioid withdrawal. Such research may have been considered unnecessary because it is clear from clinical use that buprenorphine is able to effectively suppress opioid withdrawal.

An older study conducted at the National Institute on Drug Abuse Addiction Research Center (NIDA ARC) examined the efficacy of buprenorphine in suppressing spontaneous withdrawal in subjects maintained on daily subcutaneous morphine (Jasinski et al. 1984). This is a procedure that was well established at the ARC and commonly used to test novel medications for their capacity to suppress spontaneous opioid withdrawal. Participants would be maintained on morphine given four times per day, then have a double-blind switch to the test medication (buprenorphine in this case). In this report, buprenorphine was effective in diminishing opioid withdrawal, although some mild opioid withdrawal symptoms were noted during the first week of the change from morphine to buprenorphine.

Other studies have reported on transitioning persons from methadone to buprenorphine and, in general, have found that buprenorphine appears to decrease the opioid withdrawal symptoms that would otherwise have been seen (Banys et al. 1994; Jasinski et al. 1983; Jasinski and Preston 1995; Levin et al. 1997). However, some of these studies did not contain a control comparison condition (either placebo or an active medication such as methadone), making it difficult to judge the relative efficacy of buprenorphine. And, as noted earlier, investigators have occasionally noted isolated cases in which persons receiving methadone have experienced what appears to be buprenorphine-related precipitated withdrawal rather than suppression of methadone spontaneous withdrawal (Banys et al. 1994).

Physiologic, Subjective, and Cognitive/Psychomotor Performance Effects of Buprenorphine

In persons who are not dependent on opioids, buprenorphine can produce acute physiologic and psychological effects that are similar to other mu agonist opioids. That is, it can produce pupillary constriction, decreases in respiratory rate, and increased tolerance to pain. In persons with a history of opioid abuse, but not physically dependent on opioids, acute sublingual doses of buprenorphine produce pupillary constriction that begins within an hour and can last for three to four days, depending on the dose of buprenorphine taken (Walsh et al. 1994). Although the types of physiologic effects seen with buprenorphine are similar to those seen with other full mu agonist opioids, the maximal effect produced by buprenorphine is less than that seen with full agonist opioids. Chronic dosing with buprenorphine does not appear to be associated with clinically significant changes on the electrocardiogram. Specifically, this medication does not appear to significantly increase the QTc interval (Wedam et al. 2004).

The subjective effects of buprenorphine can vary as a function of the type of person ingesting the dose (for example, physically dependent on opioids versus nondependent), the route of administration (sublingual versus injected), and the dose received. Acute doses of buprenorphine produce a profile of subjective effects that is similar to other mu agonist opioids, such as feelings of high or good effects (Pickworth et al. 1993). For sublingual doses of buprenorphine, subjective effects generally have a slower onset and a lower peak than parenteral injection (Stoller et al. 2001).

Anecdotal reports have revealed that buprenorphine may have anti-depressant-like effects beyond its ability to relieve opioid withdrawal symptoms (Bodkin et al. 1995; Emrich et al. 1982). The possible anti-depressant effect of opioids is not restricted to buprenorphine; similar reports have been made for other opioids as well, including methadone. Although such effects may occur, the clinical utility of buprenorphine's antidepressant effects is likely limited, especially for persons without opioid dependence.

Acute, high doses of buprenorphine can produce mild impairments in certain performance tasks for persons who are not physically dependent on opioids. However, tolerance develops and chronic dosing with buprenorphine appears to produce few effects on psychomotor performance or cognitive functioning (Mintzer et al. 2004; Soyka et al. 2001). This supports the clinical observation that it is possible for persons maintained on buprenorphine to drive, and perform other such tasks, without a problem.

Pharmacology of Buprenorphine Combined with Naloxone

Because buprenorphine has poor oral bioavailability, sublingual administration has been the primary route used in studies of clinical efficacy for treating opioid dependence, and the approved product for opioid dependence treatment is a sublingual tablet. In the course of developing a marketable form of sublingual buprenorphine, it was recognized that a water-soluble tablet containing buprenorphine could be abused. Buprenorphine abuse has been reported in a wide variety of countries where it is available (Chowdhury and Chowdhury 1990; Gray et al. 1989; Morrison 1989; O'Connor et al. 1988; Obadia et al. 2001; Robinson et al. 1993; Sakol et al. 1989; Singh et al. 1992; Strang 1985), and it is possible a buprenorphine tablet could be dissolved and then injected. Indeed, this has happened in France, where buprenorphine tablets have been widely prescribed and diversion and abuse of these tablets has occurred (Deveaux and Vignau 2002; Obadia et al. 2001; Strain et al. 2003; Thirion et al. 2002).

To decrease the abuse liability of the tablet, a combination buprenorphine/naloxone formulation was created. This buprenorphine/naloxone tablet capitalizes on the differential absorption of naloxone by the sublingual versus parenteral (i.e., injection) routes. Naloxone, a pure opioid antagonist, has poor sublingual absorption (Preston et al. 1990; Strain et al. 2004). Thus, a tablet taken by the therapeutic route (sublingual) will produce a predominantly buprenorphine effect, but a tablet dissolved and abused by injection will produce a predominantly naloxone effect, because naloxone has good parenteral bioavailability. Thus, a person who is dependent on opioids other than buprenorphine will experience a precipitated withdrawal syndrome from injecting the buprenorphine/naloxone mixture and this should act as a major deterrent to abuse of the medication by this route. Studies testing the effects of various combinations of buprenorphine with naloxone concluded that a combination ratio of 4:1 for buprenorphine/naloxone would produce the desired balance of effect (Fudala et al. 1998; Mendelson et al. 1999), and two buprenorphine/naloxone combination tablets (2/0.5 and 8/2 mg) are marketed in the United States. As predicted, persons maintained on short-acting opioids experience precipitated withdrawal when buprenorphine/naloxone is injected, but not when it is taken sublingually (Stoller et al. 2001).

There are four groups of persons who might try to abuse buprenorphine/naloxone tablets. One of these groups consists of persons physically dependent on short-acting opioids (for example, heroin or oxycodone) and another of persons dependent on long-acting opioids such as methadone. In each of these two cases, dissolving and injecting buprenorphine/naloxone tablets should precipitate withdrawal (Stoller et al. 2001). A third group comprises persons who are not physically dependent on opioids, such as sporadic users who may be early in their experimentation with opioid abuse. For this group, dissolving and injecting a buprenorphine/naloxone tablet would not precipitate withdrawal, because they are not physically dependent on opioids (Strain et al. 2000). Last, the fourth group consists of persons maintained on prescribed sublingual buprenorphine/naloxone who may try to inject additional buprenorphine on top of their maintenance dose. Members of this group may be at particular risk for dissolving and injecting buprenorphine tablets, because they have a ready supply. Furthermore, because buprenorphine has high affinity for the mu opioid receptor, the dose of naloxone is probably insufficient to precipitate withdrawal (Eissenberg et al. 1996). Thus, while the addition of naloxone decreases the risk that buprenorphine tablets will be dissolved and injected, it does not eliminate this potential entirely.

Summary

A better understanding of buprenorphine's clinical use can be achieved through familiarity with the novel pharmacologic features of this opioid medication. Buprenorphine is a mixed agonist-antagonist opioid that exerts partial agonist effects at the mu receptor and antagonist effects at the kappa receptor. It has relatively poor availability when swallowed but reasonable sublingual bioavailability. Although the delivery system for this medication (a sublingual tablet) is novel compared with other well-known medications for the treatment of opioid dependence, there are several pharmacologic characteristics that make the medication unique and attractive. These include its long duration of action, the ceiling on its dose-response curve that improves safety, and its low abuse potential. The addition of naloxone to buprenorphine is a useful strategy that should further reduce the likelihood that this medication will be diverted and abused.

References

Banys P, Clark HW, Tusel DJ, Sees K, Stewart P, Mongan L, Delucchi K, Callaway E (1994). An open trial of low dose buprenorphine in treating methadone withdrawal. *J Subst Abuse Treat* 11: 9–15.

Bickel WK, Stitzer ML, Bigelow GE, Liebson IA, Jasinski DR, Johnson RE (1988). Buprenorphine: dose-related blockade of opioid challenge effects in opioid dependent humans. *J Pharmacol Exp Ther* 247: 47–53.

Boas RA, Villiger JW (1985). Clinical actions of fentanyl and buprenorphine. The significance of receptor binding. *Br J Anaesth* 57: 192–6.

Bodkin JA, Zornberg GL, Lukas SE, Cole JO (1995). Buprenorphine treatment of refractory depression. *J Clin Psychopharmacol* 15: 49–57.

Bullingham RE, McQuay HJ, Moore A, Bennett MR (1980). Buprenorphine kinetics. *Clin Pharmacol Ther* 28: 667–72.

Chawarski MC, Schottenfeld RS, O'Connor PG, Pakes J (1999). Plasma concentrations of buprenorphine 24 to 72 hours after dosing. *Drug Alcohol Depend* 55: 157–63.

Chawarski MC, Schottenfeld RS, Pakes J, O'Connor PG (1998). Bioequivalence of liquid and tablet formulations of buprenorphine. In: Harris LS, ed. *Proceedings of the 60th Annual Scientific Meeting of The College on Problems of Drug Dependence, Inc.* NIDA Res Monogr 179.

Chowdhury AN, Chowdhury S (1990). Buprenorphine abuse: report from India. *Br J Addict* 85: 1349–50.

Comer SD, Collins ED, Fischman MW (2001). Buprenorphine sublingual tablets: effects on IV heroin self-administration by humans. *Psychopharmacology (Berl)* 154: 28–37.

Cowan A, Lewis JW, Macfarlane IR (1977). Agonist and antagonist properties of buprenorphine, a new antinociceptive agent. *Br J Pharmacol* 60: 537–45.

Deveaux M, Vignau J (2002). Buprenorphine maintenance treatment in primary care: an overview of the French experience and insight into the prison setting. In: Kintz P, Marquet P, eds. *Buprenorphine Therapy of Opiate Addiction (Forensic Science and Medicine)*, 69–81. Totowa, NJ: Humana Press, Inc.

Dobkin AB (1977). Buprenorphine hydrochloride: determination of analgesic potency. *Can Anaesth Soc J* 24: 186–93.

Dobkin AB, Esposito B, Philbin C (1977). Double-blind evaluation of buprenorphine hydrochloride for post-operative pain. *Can Anaesth Soc J* 24: 195–202.

Doxey JC, Everitt JE, Frank LW, MacKenzie JE (1982). A comparison of the effects of buprenorphine and morphine on the blood gases of conscious rats. *Br J Pharmacol* 75: 118P.

Eissenberg T, Greenwald MK, Johnson RE, Liebson IA, Bigelow GE, Stitzer ML (1996). Buprenorphine's physical dependence potential: antagonist-precipitated withdrawal in humans. *J Pharmacol Exp Ther* 276: 449–59.

Emrich HM, Vogt P, Herz A (1982). Possible antidepressive effects of opioids: action of buprenorphine. *Ann N Y Acad Sci* 398: 108–12.

Fudala PJ, Yu E, Macfadden W, Boardman C, Chiang CN (1998). Effects of buprenorphine and naloxone in morphine-stabilized opioid addicts. *Drug Alcohol Depend* 50: 1–8.

Gray RF, Ferry A, Jauhar P (1989). Emergence of buprenorphine dependence. *Br J Addict* 84: 1373–4.

Gross A, Jacobs EA, Petry NM, Badger GJ, Bickel WK (2001). Limits to buprenorphine dosing: a comparison between quintuple and sextuple the maintenance dose every 5 days. *Drug Alcohol Depend* 64: 111–6.

Hanks GW (1987). The clinical usefulness of agonist-antagonistic opioid analgesics in chronic pain. *Drug Alcohol Depend* 20: 339–46.

Jasinski DR, Boren JJ, Henningfield JE, Johnson RE, Lange WR, Lukas SE (1984). Progress Report from the NIDA Addiction Research Center, Baltimore, Maryland. *NIDA Res Monogr* 49: 69–76.

Jasinski DR, Henningfield JE, Hickey JE, Johnson RE (1983). Progress Report of the NIDA Addiction Research Center, Baltimore, Maryland, 1982. *NIDA Res Monogr* 43: 92–98.

Jasinski DR, Pevnick JS, Griffith JD (1978). Human pharmacology and abuse potential of the analgesic buprenorphine: a potential agent for treating narcotic addiction. *Arch Gen Psychiatry* 35: 501–16.

Jasinski DR, Preston KL (1995). Laboratory studies of buprenorphine in opioid abusers. In: Cowan A, Lewis JW, eds. *Buprenorphine: Combatting Drug Abuse with a Unique Opioid*, 189–211. New York: Wiley-Liss, Inc.

Johnson RE, Chutuape MA, Strain EC, Walsh SL, Stitzer ML, Bigelow GE (2000). A comparison of levomethadyl acetate, buprenorphine, and methadone for opioid dependence. *N Engl J Med* 343: 1290–7.

Kamel MM, Geddes IC (1978). A comparison of buprenorphine and pethidine for immediate postoperative pain relief by the i.v. route. *Br J Anaesth* 50: 599–603.

Kuhlman JJ, Lalani S, Magluilo J, Levine B, Darwin WD (1996). Human pharmacokinetics of intravenous, sublingual, and buccal buprenorphine. *J Anal Toxicol* 20: 369–78.

Levin FR, Fischman MW, Connerney I, Foltin RW (1997). A protocol to switch high-dose, methadone-maintained subjects to buprenorphine. *Am J Addict* 6: 105–16.

Lewis JW (1995). Clinical pharmacology of buprenorphine in relation to its use as an analgesic. In: Cowan A, Lewis JW, eds. *Buprenorphine: Combatting Drug Abuse with a Unique Opioid*, 151–163. New York: Wiley-Liss, Inc.

Liguori A, Morse WH, Bergman J (1996). Respiratory effects of opioid full and partial agonists in rhesus monkeys. *J Pharmacol Exp Ther* 277: 462–72.

Marquet P (2002). Pharmacology of high-dose buprenorphine. In: Kintz P, Marquet P, eds. *Buprenorphine Therapy of Opiate Addiction*, 1–11. Totowa, NJ: Humana Press.

McQuay HJ, Moore RA (1995). Buprenorphine kinetics in humans. In: Cowan A, Lewis JW, eds. *Buprenorphine: Combatting Drug Abuse with a Unique Opioid*, 137–47. New York, Wiley-Liss, Inc.

Mello NK, Mendelson JH (1980). Buprenorphine suppresses heroin use by heroin addicts. *Science* 207: 657–9.

Mendelson J, Jones RT, Welm S, Baggott M, Fernandez I, Melby AK, Nath RP (1999). Buprenorphine and naloxone combinations: the effects of three dose ratios in morphine-stabilized, opiate-dependent volunteers. *Psychopharmacology (Berl)* 141: 37–46.

Mendelson J, Upton RA, Everhart ET, Jacob P, III, Jones RT (1997). Bioavailability of sublingual buprenorphine. *J Clin Pharmacol* 37: 31–37.

Mintzer MZ, Correia CJ, Strain EC (2004). A dose-effect study of repeated administration of buprenorphine/naloxone on performance in opioid-dependent volunteers. *Drug Alcohol Depend* 74: 205–9.

Morrison V (1989). Psychoactive substance use and related behaviours of 135 regular illicit drug users in Scotland. *Drug Alcohol Depend* 23: 95–101.

Nath RP, Upton RA, Everhart ET, Cheung P, Shwonek P, Jones RT, Mendelson JE (1999). Buprenorphine pharmacokinetics: relative bioavailability of sublingual tablet and liquid formulations. *J Clin Pharmacol* 39: 619–23.

O'Connor JJ, Moloney E, Travers R, Campbell A (1988). Buprenorphine abuse among opiate addicts. *Br J Addict* 83: 1085–7.

Obadia Y, Perrin V, Feroni I, Vlahov D, Moatti JP (2001). Injecting misuse of buprenorphine among French drug users. *Addiction* 96: 267–72.

Ohtani M, Kotaki H, Nishitateno K, Sawada Y, Iga T (1997). Kinetics of respiratory depression in rats induced by buprenorphine and its metabolite, norbuprenorphine. *J Pharmacol Exp Ther* 281: 428–33.

Ohtani M, Kotaki H, Sawada Y, Iga T (1995). Comparative analysis of buprenorphine- and norbuprenorphine-induced analgesic effects based on pharmacokinetic-pharmacodynamic modeling. *J Pharmacol Exp Ther* 272: 505–10

Petry NM, Bickel WK, Badger GJ (1999). A comparison of four buprenorphine dosing regimens in the treatment of opioid dependence. *Clin Pharmacol Ther* 66: 306–14.

Petry NM, Bickel WK, Badger GJ (2000). A comparison of four buprenorphine dosing regimens using open-dosing procedures: is twice-weekly dosing possible? *Addiction* 95: 1069–77.

Pickworth WB, Johnson RE, Holicky BA, Cone EJ (1993). Subjective and physiologic effects of intravenous buprenorphine in humans. *Clin Pharmacol Ther* 53: 570–6.

Preston KL, Bigelow GE, Liebson IA (1990). Effects of sublingually given naloxone in opioid-dependent human volunteers. *Drug Alcohol Depend* 25: 27–34.

Reynaud M, Petit G, Potard D, Courty P (1998). Six deaths linked to concomitant use of buprenorphine and benzodiazepines. *Addiction* 93: 1385–92.

Robinson GM, Dukes PD, Robinson BJ, Cooke RR, Mahoney GN (1993). The misuse of buprenorphine and a buprenorphine-naloxone combination in Wellington, New Zealand. *Drug Alcohol Depend* 33: 81–86.

Rosado J, Strain EC, Walsh SL, Bigelow GE (2004). *Assessing Buprenorphine/Naloxone's Withdrawal Precipitation Potential in Methadone-Maintained Volunteers*. San Juan, PR: College on Problems of Drug Dependence.

Rosen MI, Wallace EA, McMahon TJ, Pearsall HR, Woods SW, Price LH, Kosten TR (1994). Buprenorphine: duration of blockade of effects of intramuscular hydromorphone. *Drug Alcohol Depend* 35: 141–9.

Sakol MS, Stark C, Sykes R (1989). Buprenorphine and temazepam abuse by drug takers in Glasgow—an increase. *Br J Addict* 84: 439–41.

Schuh KJ, Johanson CE (1999). Pharmacokinetic comparison of the buprenorphine sublingual liquid and tablet. *Drug Alcohol Depend* 56: 55–60.

Schuh KJ, Walsh SL, Stitzer ML (1999). Onset, magnitude and duration of opioid blockade produced by buprenorphine and naltrexone in humans. *Psychopharmacology (Berl)* 145: 162–74.

Singh RA, Mattoo SK, Malhotra A, Varma VK (1992). Cases of buprenorphine abuse in India. *Acta Psychiatr Scand* 86: 46–48.

Soyka M, Horak M, Dittert S, Kagerer S (2001). Less driving impairment on buprenorphine than methadone in drug-dependent patients? *J Neuropsychiatry Clin Neurosci* 13: 527–8.

Stoller KB, Bigelow GE, Walsh SL, Strain EC (2001). Effects of buprenorphine/naloxone in opioid-dependent humans. *Psychopharmacology (Berl)* 154: 230–42.

Strain EC, Clarke HW, Auriacombe M, Lagier G, Mallaret M, Thirion X (2003). French experience with buprenorphine. *NIDA Res Monogr* 183: 134–41.

Strain EC, Moody DE, Stoller KB, Walsh SL, Bigelow GE (2004). Relative bioavailability of different buprenorphine formulations under chronic dosing conditions. *Drug Alcohol Depend* 74: 37–43.

Strain EC, Stitzer ML, Liebson IA, Bigelow GE (1994). Comparison of buprenorphine and methadone in the treatment of opioid dependence. *Am J Psychiatry* 151: 1025–30.

Strain EC, Stoller K, Walsh SL, Bigelow GE (2000). Effects of buprenorphine versus buprenorphine/naloxone tablets in non-dependent opioid abusers. *Psychopharmacology (Berl)* 148: 374–83.

Strain EC, Walsh SL, Preston KL, Liebson IA, Bigelow GE (1997). The effects of buprenorphine in buprenorphine-maintained volunteers. *Psychopharmacology (Berl)* 129: 329–38.

Strang J (1985). Abuse of buprenorphine. *Lancet* 2: 725.

Thirion X, Lapierre V, Micallef J, Ronfle E, Masut A, Pradel V, Coudert C, Mabriez JC, Sanmarco JL (2002). Buprenorphine prescription by general practitioners in a French region. *Drug Alcohol Depend* 65: 197–204.

Tracqui A, Kintz P, Ludes B (1998). Buprenorphine-related deaths among drug addicts in France: a report on 20 fatalities. *J Anal Toxicol* 22: 430–4.

Wallenstein SL, Kaiko RF, Rogers AG, Houde RW (1986). Crossover trials in clinical analgesic assays: studies of buprenorphine and morphine. *Pharmacotherapy* 6: 228–35

Walsh SL, Preston KL, Bigelow GE, Stitzer ML (1995). Acute administration of buprenorphine in humans: partial agonist and blockade effects. *J Pharmacol Exp Ther* 274: 361–72.

Walsh SL, Preston KL, Stitzer ML, Cone EJ, Bigelow GE (1994). Clinical pharmacology of buprenorphine: ceiling effects at high doses. *Clin Pharmacol Ther* 55: 569–80.

Wedam EF, Haigney MCP, Bigelow GE, Johnson RE (2004). *EKG QT-prolongation effects of methadone, LAAM and buprenorphine in a randomized trial*. San Juan, PR: College on Problems of Drug Dependence.

Weinberg DS, Inturrisi CE, Reidenberg B, Moulin DE, Nip TJ, Wallenstein S, Houde RW, Foley KM (1988). Sublingual absorption of selected opioid analgesics. *Clin Pharmacol Ther* 44:335–42.

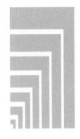

I I

Clinical Use of Buprenorphine

Eric C. Strain, M.D.

Buprenorphine is an opioid mixed agonist-antagonist that was initially developed and marketed as an analgesic. Early interest was expressed, however, in the possible use of buprenorphine for the treatment of opioid dependence (Jasinski et al. 1978; Mello and Mendelson 1980). Several clinical trials were conducted starting in the mid-1980s and especially in the 1990s that compared the efficacy and safety of buprenorphine with methadone and placebo. Many of these trials were conducted in the United States under the sponsorship of the National Institute on Drug Abuse (NIDA), which set up a special division (the Medications Development Division, or MDD); the purpose of MDD was to develop new medications for the treatment of substance abuse disorders. NIDA/MDD and the owner of buprenorphine (which then was Reckitt and Colman and presently is Reckitt Benckiser) diligently pursued the development of buprenorphine for the United States market during the 1990s. Buprenorphine's initial approval and use for the treatment of opioid dependence was in France, however, and occurred six years before its availability in the United States (i.e., in 1996). With the unavailability of LAAM and the limited use of naltrexone as treatment options for opioid dependence, the possibility exists that buprenorphine will have the largest impact on the treatment of opioid dependence since the introduction of methadone 40 years ago.

The final success of buprenorphine will depend on the extent of its use by the health care field. In this respect, buprenorphine's success is closely linked to its availability in office-based treatment settings, and this topic is addressed in chapter 12. The pharmacologic properties of buprenorphine are reviewed in chapter 10. The purpose of this chapter is to discuss the efficacy and safety of buprenorphine when used for the treatment of opioid dependence and to review its clinical use for this indication.

THE EFFICACY OF BUPRENORPHINE

Most studies of buprenorphine's efficacy have compared its use with methadone's use in the short-term (i.e., less than one year) outpatient treatment of opioid dependence. Four studies have compared buprenorphine with placebo, and several other studies have investigated the use of buprenorphine on a less-than-daily basis. Finally, although the focus of clinical trials has been on the use of sublingual buprenorphine for the outpatient treatment of opioid dependence, buprenorphine has also been used by both the sublingual and parenteral routes of administration for the short-term (e.g., three to five day) detoxification of opioid dependence. Each of these topics is addressed here.

Buprenorphine Compared with Methadone

Numerous clinical trials have compared sublingual buprenorphine solution with methadone in the outpatient treatment of opioid dependence (for reviews of these studies, see Ling and Wesson 2003; Mattick et al. 2002; Strain 2002). In general, these studies have found that the two medications are equally effective for primary outcome measures, such as treatment retention and rates of opioid-positive urine samples, as well as secondary outcome measures, such as amount of money spent on drugs and reports of dose adequacy.

In reviewing these clinical trials, it is important to recognize that the methodology of studies such as these is significantly different from the clinical practice under which a medication is used. For example, well-conducted studies use double-blind dosing—neither patients nor staff who come into contact with patients know what dose and which medication the patient is taking. Patient awareness of doses may enhance treatment compliance, so this double-blind dosing could contribute to poorer outcomes in a clinical trial than those achieved with routine practice. Similarly, most clinical trials have used an intensive urine-testing schedule (e.g., collecting and testing urine samples three times per week). Such a schedule is dramatically different from most routine clinical practice; it is designed to detect *any* drug use but is poorer at detecting *changes* in drug use. Thus, rates of drug-positive urine samples can be quite high in these studies. Finally, the doses of buprenorphine and methadone selected should be roughly equivalent in efficacy. If they are not, a study difference may simply reflect a dose difference (e.g., comparing a high, effective dose of methadone with a low, ineffective dose of buprenorphine), rather than a true medication difference.

A summary of studies comparing buprenorphine with methadone is presented in table 11.1. With respect to treatment retention, results from these studies suggest that methadone produces outcomes that are equal to (Bickel et al. 1988; Mattick et al. 1999; Oliveto et al. 1999; Schottenfeld et al. 1997; Strain et al. 1994a, 1994b) or better than (Ahmadi et al. 2003; Fischer et al. 1999; Mattick et al. 2003; Pani et al. 2000; Petitjean et al. 2001) buprenorphine, although two studies have found buprenorphine produces significantly better treatment retention than low doses of methadone (Johnson et al. 1992, 2000b). Although the evidence may seem to lean toward an advantage of methadone over buprenorphine with respect to treatment retention, methadone's superiority in these studies may be related to dose; that is, comparisons of higher doses of methadone with lower doses of buprenorphine may reflect dose differences rather than medication difference, and studies that have used multiple doses of methadone support this possibility. For example, one study showed that 80 mg per day of methadone produced better retention than 8 mg per day of buprenorphine, but that 8 mg per day of buprenorphine was equally as effective as 30 mg per day of methadone (Ling et al. 1996).

Another outcome measure of particular interest is illicit opioid use. Methadone may have a slight advantage over buprenorphine with respect to treatment retention, but it would appear that the two medications produce generally similar results when compared on rates of opioid-positive urine samples (table 11.1). In almost all studies shown in table 11.1, buprenorphine and methadone did not significantly differ in rates of opioid-positive urine samples. This discrepancy between treatment retention (where methadone may have a slight advantage) and urinalysis results (where there is no significant difference between medications) may reflect buprenorphine's partial opioid agonist effect. A lower agonist effect may translate to lower treatment retention (i.e., a lower rate of reinforcement manifests as a higher rate of treatment dropout), but there may be sufficient receptor occupancy to provide the needed blockade when illicit opioids are ingested.

Finally, when comparing across these studies, the different forms of buprenorphine used (solution versus tablets) must be factored into the conclusions made. (See the section on absorption, metabolism, and excretion in chap. 10 for a review and discussion of the relative bioavail-

Table 11.1 Studies Comparing Buprenorphine with Methadone for the Treatment of Opioid Dependence

Reference	No. of Participants	Study Duration (weeks)	Buprenorphine Form*	Buprenorphine Dose(s)	Methadone Dose	Outcomes Retention	Outcomes Opioid Urinalysis
Bickel et al. 1988 DB	45	13	Solution	2	M30	B = M	B = M
Johnson et al. 1992 DB	162	17	Solution	8	M20 + M60	B > M20	B, M60 > M20
Kosten et al. 1993 DB	125	24	Solution	2 + 6	M35 + M65	M > B	M > B
Strain et al. 1994b DB	164	26	Solution	8–16	M50–90	B = M	B = M
Strain et al. 1994a DB	51	26	Solution	8–16	M50–90	B = M	B = M
Ling et al. 1996 DB	225	52	Solution	8	M30 + M80	M80 > B, M30	M80 > B, M30
Schottenfeld et al. 1997 DB	116	24	Solution	4 + 12	M20 + M65	No difference between groups	B12, M65 > B4, M20
Oliveto et al. 1999 DB	180	13	Solution	12	M65	B = M	M > B
Fischer et al. 1999	60	24	Tablets	2–8	Up to M80	M > B	B > M
Pani et al. 2000 DB	72	26	Tablets	8	M60	M > B (trend)	B = M
Johnson et al. 2000† DB	220	17	Solution	16–32 mg	M20 + M60–100	B, M60–100 > M20	B, M60–100 > M20
Petitjean et al. 2001 DB	58	6	Tablets	4–16	M30–120	M > B	B = M
Mattick et al. 2003 DB	405	13	Tablets	Flexible	Flexible	M > B	B = M
Ahmadi et al. 2003‡ DB	204	24	Tablets	5	50	M > B	Not reported

Note: DB in the reference column indicates dosing was double-blind; references without DB were open label; all doses shown are in milligrams (mg). B, buprenorphine; M, methadone

*All studies administered buprenorphine sublingually.

†This study also included a group of participants who received LAAM medication; buprenorphine doses were given three times per week rather than daily.

‡This study also included a group of participants who received naltrexone medication; although the study is described as double-blind, it is not clear if it was double-dummy.

ability for different forms of buprenorphine.) As seen in table 11.1, until 1999–2000, clinical trials used the solution form of buprenorphine. Since 2000, however, all studies have used the tablet form. The dose of buprenorphine delivered in the earlier solution studies was probably higher than doses used in later tablet studies.

Overall, it appears that sublingual doses of buprenorphine tablets in the range of 8–12 mg per day can produce treatment outcomes similar to those seen with moderate (50–60 mg per day) doses of methadone. Higher doses of methadone, such as 80 mg per day, however, may be more effective than doses of buprenorphine typically used in these clinical trials. Efficacy greater than that produced by 65 mg of methadone has not been demonstrated with buprenorphine doses of up to 12 mg of solution (which would probably be approximately 16 mg of buprenorphine in the tablet form). Studies utilizing higher daily doses of buprenorphine, such as 32 mg or more in a tablet form, however, need to be conducted to determine whether these are medication- or dose-related limits (especially for treatment retention). The available evidence suggests that neither buprenorphine nor methadone are clearly and overwhelmingly superior to the other, and an equally important question is whether buprenorphine is superior to placebo. This is addressed in the next section.

Buprenorphine Compared with Placebo

Although studies comparing buprenorphine with methadone are useful, clinical trials comparing a medication with placebo are especially valuable in gaining approval by government regulatory bodies for clinical use. Four outpatient studies have examined the efficacy of buprenorphine compared with placebo. The first was a U.S. study that compared buprenorphine (doses of 2 and 8 mg per day of sublingual solution) with placebo (0 mg per day of sublingual solution) (Johnson et al. 1995b). This study enrolled 150 patients who were dependent on opioids and used a novel design that lasted only two weeks. Results showed that active buprenorphine was preferred and had better efficacy than placebo.

The second study was technically not a placebo-controlled trial (Ling et al. 1998). This was a large multicenter clinical trial $(N = 736)$ conducted in the United States. The study design compared four different daily doses of buprenorphine solution (1, 4, 8, and 16 mg). The 1-mg dose in this study was conceptualized as an active placebo condition. The study found 8 mg was superior to 1 mg on measures of treatment effectiveness. There was no difference in outcomes for the 8- versus 16-mg doses.

The third placebo-controlled study was also a multicenter study conducted in the United States that enrolled a large number of participants ($N = 326$). This study had three groups and compared two forms of buprenorphine tablets that both contained 16 mg—one tablet form contained buprenorphine only, and the other contained buprenorphine combined with 4 mg of naloxone—and placebo (Fudala et al. 2003). The study lasted four weeks and was conducted in office-based settings rather than the more traditional opioid treatment program sites utilized in most other outpatient clinical trials with buprenorphine. The study was ended early because the two active conditions were superior to placebo on a number of outcome measures.

The final placebo-controlled study was conducted in Sweden and enrolled a smaller number of participants ($N = 40$), who were randomly assigned to either 16 mg per day of sublingual buprenorphine tablets or a six-day buprenorphine taper followed by placebo dosing (Kakko et al. 2003). The initial six days of the study were conducted on an inpatient unit, followed by one year of outpatient treatment. No subjects in the placebo group remained in treatment at the end of the year, compared with 75 percent of the participants receiving 16 mg per day of buprenorphine. Of note, four of the 20 patients treated with placebo had died during the year of the study, versus none of the patients treated with active maintenance buprenorphine.

These studies show that buprenorphine is clearly more effective than placebo. This occurs despite, in some cases, participants receiving relatively rich concurrent nonpharmacologic treatments (Kakko et al. 2003). Although differences in the efficacy of buprenorphine versus methadone are relatively minimal, there is a clear and large difference between buprenorphine and placebo.

Alternate-Day Buprenorphine Dosing

Buprenorphine has been abused in several countries, and one means to decrease the risk of such abuse is to add naloxone to buprenorphine, as discussed in chapter 10. The addition of naloxone should decrease the potential for abuse by dissolving and injecting tablets. Another means to decrease the diversion and abuse of buprenorphine is to administer buprenorphine on a less-than-daily basis. There has been considerable interest in using buprenorphine on an alternate-day basis, and several studies provide data supporting this use. This approach capitalizes on buprenorphine's long duration of action and allows patients to receive doses every other day, every third day, or perhaps over even longer intervals (although efficacy for longer intervals is less well established).

Although some early studies of alternate-day buprenorphine dosing simply gave placebo on nonmedication days without a compensatory increase in buprenorphine dose on active medication days (Fudala et al. 1990; Johnson et al. 1995a), corresponding increases of the dose on active medication days result in improved outcomes. Thus, a patient maintained on 8 mg per day of sublingual buprenorphine would be switched to 16 mg of every-other-day sublingual buprenorphine, or 24 mg if the dosing interval were 72 hours (e.g., a Friday dose before a weekend with no medication).

Some patients can probably tolerate 72–96 hours between doses of buprenorphine, if the active dose has been increased accordingly for the longer interval (Bickel et al. 1999; Petry et al. 1999, 2000a). Attempts to extend the time interval to 120 hours by increasing the dose six-fold have met less success (Gross et al. 2001; Petry et al. 2001). However, these studies have simply increased the amount of buprenorphine by the number of doses to be skipped (e.g., an 8 mg per day dose is given as 16 mg for a 48-hour interval, 24 mg for a 72-hour interval, 32 mg for a 96-hour interval, and 40 mg for a 120-hour interval). It would be valuable to know if outcomes can be improved by giving more than a simple multiple of the daily dose to compensate for the longer interval (e.g., an 8 mg per day dose is given as 48 or 56 mg for a 120-hour interval).

Perhaps of most relevance is the use of thrice-weekly buprenorphine, which might be administered through an opioid treatment program with supervised dose administration. Studies of thrice-weekly dosing show that it is preferred over daily dosing by patients (Amass et al. 1998, 2001), although outcomes for such a dosing schedule are equivocal, with one study showing it is as effective as daily dosing (Schottenfeld et al. 2000) and another showing it is associated with higher rates of opioid-positive urine results (Perez de los Cobos et al. 2000).

Less-than-daily buprenorphine dosing may have advantages, especially if buprenorphine is used in an opioid treatment program setting. As noted, it decreases the chance of diversion of take-home doses. It also may improve patient cooperation, because it reduces the frequency of clinic visits. Finally, less-than-daily dosing provides greater flexibility to clinicians. If a patient needs to be switched from a daily schedule to an intermittent schedule, or vice versa, this is relatively easy to accomplish once the patient is treated with buprenorphine.

Buprenorphine for Opioid Withdrawal

The clinical trials reviewed in previous sections have examined the efficacy of buprenorphine as a medication used in the maintenance treatment of opioid dependence. However, several studies have also examined buprenorphine's efficacy when used for the treatment of opioid withdrawal. Most of these studies use withdrawals lasting a few days, and they appear to be primarily conducted in inpatient settings. Early studies often used the marketed analgesic product and delivered doses by injection (rather than sublingual solution or tablets). These parameters may differ from the more current use of buprenorphine for the treatment of opioid withdrawal, but the results from these clinical trials provide data that can inform a decision regarding the efficacy of buprenorphine for medically supervised withdrawal.

When buprenorphine has been used for relatively brief withdrawals, it has been given intramuscularly one to three times per day or sublingually one to four times per day. In general, the doses used are lower than doses used in the clinical trials comparing buprenorphine with methadone—thus, for example, intramuscular dosing may be 0.3–0.6 mg three times for the first day, 0.15–0.3 mg three times for the second day, and then a single 0.15- to 0.3-mg dose on the third day (table 11.2). Because sublingual tablets of buprenorphine are now available in many countries, however, it is more appropriate to use this form than the injectable analgesic form for withdrawals. A high-dose or low-dose schedule may be used, depending on the patient's level of physical dependence (table 11.2).

Several reports have been published on clinical experience using buprenorphine for relatively short periods for the treatment of opioid withdrawal (DiPaula et al. 2002; Fingerhood et al. 2001; Gandhi et al. 2003; Parran et al. 1994; Resnick et al. 2001; Tamaskar et al. 2003; Vignau 1998; White et al. 2001). These are not controlled trials, however, so fac-

Table 11.2 **Buprenorphine for Opioid Withdrawal**

Time of Administration	Buprenorphine Dose Schedule		
	High Dose*	Low Dose*	Injectable†
First dose	4 mg (2 × 2 mg tablets)	2.0 mg (1 × 2 mg tablets)	1.5 mg
24 hours	8 mg (4 × 2 mg tablets)	1.6 mg (4 × 0.4 mg tablets)	1.2 mg
48 hours	8 mg (4 × 2 mg tablets)	1.2 mg (3 × 0.4 mg tablets)	0.9 mg
72 hours	8 mg (4 × 2 mg tablets)	0.8 mg (2 × 0.4 mg tablets)	0.45 mg

*This schedule is based on the use of buprenorphine tablets.
†This schedule is based on the use of the injectable form of buprenorphine.

tors such as expectancy effects may influence the treatment outcomes observed. Fortunately, several controlled studies have also examined the efficacy of buprenorphine for such brief withdrawals (Cheskin et al. 1994; Janiri et al. 1994; Kakko et al. 2003; Nigam et al. 1993; Seifert et al. 2002; Umbricht et al. 2003). In general, results from these controlled studies show that buprenorphine is more effective than clonidine in relieving opioid withdrawal symptoms, but controlled clinical trials of buprenorphine's efficacy compared with other medications such as methadone is less clear.

Two other aspects of buprenorphine's use in opioid withdrawal should be briefly addressed here. First is work that has examined the efficacy of a single dose of buprenorphine that is used to treat withdrawal. This idea capitalizes on buprenorphine's long duration of action; the underlying idea is that a single, larger dose of buprenorphine will provide a taper over time simply through the gradual decline in buprenorphine's effects. A variant on this approach is to provide multiple doses, as if "loading" the patient, in a single day of pharmacologic treatment. There have been a few reports on buprenorphine used in this way (Assadi et al. 2004; Kutz and Reznik 2001, 2002). Doses have ranged between 12 mg given by injection and 32 mg given as sublingual solution, and outcomes appear to be good with respect to suppression of withdrawal symptoms and safety. This is an interesting procedure that has the potential to be clinically helpful, but further research is needed to establish appropriate dosing procedures and to determine longer-term outcomes.

The second topic relevant to the utilization of buprenorphine in the treatment of opioid withdrawal relates to buprenorphine's use as a transition agent to treatment with naltrexone. Starting an opioid-dependent patient on naltrexone can be problematic and often may involve an inpatient or residential stay for the person to achieve a sufficient period of abstinence before the first dose of naltrexone (see chap. 14). It may be possible to use buprenorphine as a transition medication, so that an opioid-dependent person is initially treated with buprenorphine but then is switched to naltrexone without the naltrexone precipitating withdrawal. A few reports have described efforts in this regard (Johnson et al. 2000a; Kosten et al. 1992; Umbricht et al. 1999; Umbricht-Schneiter et al. 1996). In these studies, participants have received low doses of oral naltrexone (e.g., 1–12.5 mg per day) while still being maintained on buprenorphine and have tolerated the naltrexone, although it appears the likelihood of precipitated withdrawal increases with larger doses. Apparently, however, there is also variability among patients in the response to naltrexone when they are maintained on buprenorphine, and more controlled studies are needed to determine the optimal mechanisms for using buprenorphine to transition patients to naltrexone—especially on an outpatient basis.

Buprenorphine for Cocaine Use Disorders

Several preclinical studies have found evidence that self-administration of cocaine decreases in animals maintained on buprenorphine (Mello et al. 1989, 1990). This intriguing finding suggests that buprenorphine might have efficacy for cocaine use disorders, in addition to its efficacy for opioid dependence. Initial clinical studies, in general, failed to find an anticocaine effect for buprenorphine (Compton et al. 1995; Schottenfeld et al. 1997; Strain et al. 1994a), but there has been some renewed interest and evidence that there may be such an effect (Montoya et al. 2004).

SAFETY AND SIDE EFFECTS OF BUPRENORPHINE

The relative safety of buprenorphine was initially established when it was being reviewed and approved for use as an analgesic. The enhanced safety profile of buprenorphine is thought to be due to its being a partial agonist opioid. Buprenorphine (including the buprenorphine/naloxone combination) is a very safe medication, especially when administered without other medications. With the availability and increasing clinical use of buprenorphine for the treatment of opioid dependence, there are two areas of primary concern with this medication's safety: respiratory depression and potential liver damage. Each will be briefly reviewed here.

Buprenorphine and Respiratory Depression

Buprenorphine has been used extensively in France, where it has been available since 1996 for the treatment of opioid dependence, and it is estimated that more than 70,000 persons are treated with buprenorphine (Strain et al. 2003). There have been several reports from France on cases of fatal overdoses with buprenorphine, which appear to have occurred when buprenorphine tablets were dissolved and injected in combination with an injected benzodiazepine (Reynaud et al. 1998; Tracqui et al. 1998). (Prescribing benzodiazepines for patients treated with buprenorphine appears to be quite common in France, with one study reporting that 43% of buprenorphine-treated patients also receive a concurrent prescription for a benzodiazepine—and most commonly flunitrazepam, an injectable benzodiazepine [Thirion et al. 2002].) The observation that combining buprenorphine with a benzodiazepine could produce significant respiratory depression is not new (Faroqui et al. 1983), but the more extensive use of buprenorphine has made this a more pertinent issue.

Although caution should be exercised in prescribing a benzodiazepine with buprenorphine, it is also useful to keep an appropriate perspective on this concern. Apparently, most cases of fatal respiratory depression occurred when buprenorphine and a benzodiazepine (typically flunitrazepam) were both injected. For many patients, such as those in the United States, injectable benzodiazepines are essentially not available. Furthermore, numerous outpatient clinical trials were conducted in the United States with buprenorphine in which the medication was used with no reported fatalities, and there was a subgroup of patients with concurrent benzodiazepine use in these studies. Finally, buprenorphine's partial agonism suggests that high and even very high acute doses when taken alone are unlikely to produce respiratory depression (Walsh et al. 1994).

As with other opiates, buprenorphine should be administered with caution in patients with compromised respiratory function. If a patient has respiratory depression because of excessive buprenorphine dosing, naloxone (greater than 3 mg per 70 kg) or doxapram (Dopram) (a central respiratory stimulant) may be effective.

Buprenorphine and Liver Function

Very high doses of buprenorphine, especially if delivered intravenously and in a person with a history of hepatitis, can produce significant increases in liver function test results such as transaminase levels (Berson et al. 2001). A retrospective chart review of patients treated with buprenorphine found a statistically significant but clinically small increase in transaminase levels for patients treated with buprenorphine who had a history of hepatitis C (Petry et al. 2000b).

Patients should be screened for hepatitis and elevated liver functions before starting to receive buprenorphine and monitored in the initial weeks and months of treatment, depending on the baseline (pre-buprenorphine) results. Buprenorphine is not contraindicated in patients with elevated liver function test results. No clear guidelines exist regarding the frequency of liver function testing. If the patient has high baseline liver function test results (greater than three times the upper limit of normal), then consultation with a hepatologist should be considered, and retesting within one to two weeks of the onset of buprenorphine treatment should occur (depending on how high the baseline levels were). If the patient has normal or mildly elevated baseline liver function tests (i.e., less than three times the upper limit of normal), repeat testing should occur within the first four to six weeks of buprenorphine treatment.

Other Side Effects with Buprenorphine

Increased central nervous system (CNS) depression might occur in patients receiving buprenorphine along with other medications (in addition to the interaction with benzodiazepines as described above), such as opioid analgesics, general anesthetics, phenothiazines, other tranquilizers, sedative/hypnotics, or other CNS depressants (including alcohol). Adverse effects observed with buprenorphine are similar to other opioids (Lofwall et al. Forthcoming) and, in general, include effects due to under- or overmedication. The most common adverse related events reported in a one-year clinical trial (ranked in order of frequency) were withdrawal, insomnia, sweating, asthenia (lack of strength or energy), rhinitis (inflammation of the nasal mucosa), headache, nausea, constipation, generalized pain, abdominal pain, anxiety, chills, somnolence, nervousness, diarrhea, watery eyes, back pain, vomiting, dizziness, depression, and flu-like syndrome (Ling et al. 1998). Maintenance on buprenorphine does not appear to be associated with significant impairment in cognitive processing or performance (Mintzer et al. 2004).

CLINICAL USE OF BUPRENORPHINE

When buprenorphine is used for the treatment of opioid dependence, it is typically prescribed as a sublingual tablet. In general, two tablet sizes are marketed: a small tablet containing 2 mg of buprenorphine and a large tablet containing 8 mg of buprenorphine. In addition to these two sizes, there are two forms of buprenorphine tablets: those that contain only buprenorphine (sometimes called monotherapy tablets and marketed as "Subutex") and those containing buprenorphine combined with naloxone (sometimes called combination tablets and marketed as "Suboxone"). The latter contain a dose ratio of 4:1 for buprenorphine/naloxone (i.e., tablets of 2/0.5 mg and 8/2 mg). The tablets are not scored and are not meant to be broken. Although early clinical trials used a sublingual solution of buprenorphine, it is not marketed for clinical use.

In general, if combination tablets are available they should be used. There are very limited circumstances under which monotherapy tablets might be indicated (e.g., a person who has an allergy to naloxone, a woman who is pregnant). For purposes of the following discussion, the reader should assume that the term "buprenorphine" means the combination tablet unless otherwise specified.

Several issues pertinent to the clinical use of buprenorphine for the treatment of opioid dependence are discussed next.

Starting the Patient on Buprenorphine

The Person Not Physically Dependent on Opioids

Under certain circumstances, a person not physically dependent on opioids may be started on buprenorphine. For example, a person who was maintained successfully on buprenorphine but was incarcerated may wish to resume buprenorphine treatment after release from jail. Under this circumstance, the nondependent person should be started on the lowest possible dose of buprenorphine (2 mg) and have the dose gradually increased over subsequent days and weeks. The goal should be to resume the previous stabilization dose or to ensure that no craving for opioids is present.

The Person Physically Dependent on Opioids

As a partial mu agonist opioid, it is possible that starting a patient on buprenorphine could precipitate opioid withdrawal under the appropriate conditions (i.e., buprenorphine dose, level of physical dependence, and length of time since last use of the abused opioid), as explained in detail in chapter 10. To minimize this risk, it is generally recommended that the patient exhibit a mild degree of opioid withdrawal before the first dose of buprenorphine (table 11.3) (McNicholas 2004). Opioid withdrawal can be assessed by using standardized instruments such as the Wang scale (Wang et al. 1974), the Clinical Institute Narcotic Assessment (CINA; table 11.4) (Peachey and Lei 1988), or the Weak Opioid Withdrawal scale (WOW; table 11.5) (Haertzen 1974). The patient can be reassured that the first dose of buprenorphine will alleviate the withdrawal symptoms they have at the time of dosing, and it should also be explained that there is a risk of precipitated withdrawal if they ingest an opioid shortly before the first dose of buprenorphine.

The first sublingual dose of buprenorphine can be 4 mg (McNicholas 2004). If the combination product is available (buprenorphine/naloxone), the patient can be started directly on this form of the medication (i.e., a first dose of 4/1 mg). If clinically indicated, a repeat dose of 4 mg of buprenorphine (4/1 mg of buprenorphine/naloxone) can be given after two or

Table 11.3 Signs and Symptoms of Opioid Withdrawal

Signs	Symptoms
Diarrhea	Anorexia
Lacrimation (runny eyes)	Dysphoria
Mydriasis (pupillary dilation)	Fatigue
Perspiration	Irritability
Piloerection (goose flesh)	Muscle aches
Restlessness	Nausea
Rhinnorhea (runny nose)	Poor sleep
Vomiting	
Yawning	

more hours on the first day, for a total first-day dose of 8 mg of buprenorphine (Johnson et al. 2003).

Dosing over subsequent days should be increased as clinically indicated, with dose increases occurring on a daily basis. In an outpatient clinical trial with buprenorphine solution conducted several years ago, an induction schedule for the first four days utilized doses of 2, 4, 8, and 16 mg and was tolerated (Ling et al. 1998). Thus, it is not unreasonable to use tablet doses of 8/2 and 16/4 mg on the first and second days of treatment (McNicholas 2004). The goal of this initial period of treatment should be the alleviation of spontaneous withdrawal symptoms and craving to use opioids. In addition, the dose of buprenorphine should block the effects of other opioids. Considerable variability exists between persons in the blood levels produced by the same dose of buprenorphine (Schuh and Johanson 1999; Strain et al. 2004), so the eventual dose on which different patients stabilize may differ considerably. The daily dose of buprenorphine will probably be between 8 and 32 mg per day (i.e., 8/2 and 32/8 mg of buprenorphine/naloxone).

Maintaining the Patient on Buprenorphine

Studies of buprenorphine for the treatment of opioid dependence have used maintenance doses as low as 1 mg per day of solution and as high as 32 mg per day of tablets (table 11.1). Most clinical trials comparing buprenorphine with methadone used maintenance doses of about 8 mg per day of solution (which is approximately equal to 8–12 mg of bupre-

Table 11.4 Clinical Institute Narcotic Assessment (CINA)

NAUSEA AND VOMITING: Ask, "Do you feel sick to your stomach? Have you vomited?"—Observation

  0 = No nausea, no vomiting

  2 = Mild nausea with no retching or vomiting

  4 = Intermittent nausea with dry heaves

  6 = Constant nausea, frequent heaves and/or vomiting

GOOSE FLESH: Observation

  0 = No goose flesh visible

  1 = Occasional goose flesh but not elicited by touch, not prominent

  2 = Prominent goose flesh, in waves and elicited by touch

  3 = Constant goose flesh over chest and arms

SWEATING: Observation

  0 = No sweat visible

  1 = Barely perceptible sweating, palms moist

  2 = Beads of sweat obvious on forehead

  3 = Drenching sweat over face and chest

RESTLESSNESS: Observation

  0 = Normal activity

  1 = Somewhat more than normal activity (may move legs up and down, shift position occasionally)

  2 = Moderately fidgety and restless, shifting position frequently

  3 = Gross movements most of the time or constantly thrashes about

TREMOR: Arms extended and fingers spread apart—Observation

  0 = No tremor

  1 = Not visible but can be felt finger tip to finger tip

  2 = Moderate, with patient's arm extended

  3 = Severe even if arms not extended

LACRIMATION: Observation

  0 = No lacrimation

  1 = Eyes watering, tears at corners of eyes

  2 = Profuse tearing from eyes over face

NASAL CONGESTION: Observation

  0 = No nasal congestion, sniffling

  1 = Frequent sniffling

  2 = Constant sniffling with watery discharge

YAWNING: Observation

  0 = No yawning

  1 = Frequent yawning

  2 = Constant, uncontrolled yawning

(continued)

Table 11.4 **Continued**

ABDOMINAL CHANGES: Ask, "Do you have any pains in your lower abdomen?"

   0 = No abdominal complaints, normal bowel sounds

   1 = Reports waves of abdominal crampy pain, active bowel sounds

   2 = Reports crampy abdominal pain, diarrheal movements, active bowel sounds

CHANGES IN TEMPERATURE: Ask, "Do you feel hot or cold?"

   0 = No report of temperature change

   1 = Reports feeling hot or cold, hands cold and clammy

   2 = Uncontrollable shivering

MUSCLE ACHES: Ask, "Do you have any muscle cramps?"

   0 = No muscle aches reported, e.g., arm and neck muscle soft at rest

   1 = Mild muscle pains

   2 = Reports severe muscle pains, muscles of legs, arms, and neck in constant state of contraction

HEART RATE: _____

SYSTOLIC BLOOD PRESSURE (Supine): _____

Scores are derived by summing items. For heart rate and systolic blood pressure, values are first divided by 10 and then added to the remaining eleven items.

Source: Peachy, J. E., and Lei, H. (1988). Assessment of opioid dependence with naloxone. *Br J Addict* 83:193–201. Reproduced with permission of Carfax Publishing, Ltd., P.O. Box 25, Abingdon, Oxfordshire OX14 3UE, United Kingdom.

norphine tablets), and this dose appears to provide efficacy equivalent to about 50–60 mg per day of methadone. Some patients may require higher daily doses of buprenorphine, however, and as noted, the maintenance daily dose will probably be between 8 and 32 mg per day of buprenorphine for most patients.

The goal of treatment is to move from induction (i.e., dose stabilization) to maintenance treatment. A key indicator of maintenance is a marked decrease in illicit opioid use with active progression by the patient to abstinence from illicit opioid use. Continued illicit drug use may occur during maintenance (especially early in the maintenance phase), and appropriate treatment steps should be taken based on the type and frequency of this use. If illicit opioid use is occurring, then further dose increases of buprenorphine may be indicated. In addition, the maintenance phase of treatment is a time during which other issues are addressed (e.g., comorbid disorders that are untreated, the sequelae of the person's use of illicit drugs). An important component of treatment during the maintenance

Table 11.5 **Weak Opioid Withdrawal (WOW) Scale**

1. I am not as active as usual. (T)
2. I have had very peculiar and strange experiences. (T)
3. My sex drive is decreased. (T)
4. I have a pleasant feeling in my stomach. (F)
5. My face feels hot. (T)
6. I have felt my body drift away from me. (T)
7. The way I feel right now, I would rather be guided by someone I trust than to follow my own judgment. (T)
8. I feel as if I would be more popular with people today. (F)
9. I feel sluggish. (T)
10. I have often been frightened in the middle of the night. (T)
11. Something is making me break out in goose bumps. (T)
12. I seem to be able to see the comical side of things more than usual. (F)
13. I often feel that I must get up and walk around. (T)
14. I have spells of feeling hot and cold. (T)
15. I am often troubled by constipation. (T)
16. I would like to listen to music all day. (F)
17. People might say that I am a little dull today. (T)
18. My eyes are watering more than usual. (T)
19. I am afraid of losing my mind. (T)
20. My memory seems sharper to me than usual. (F)
21. Once in a while I notice my muscles jerking. (T)

Note: Also known as ARCI scale no. 194. The patient responds as either true or false for each item. Those items followed by a "T" are scored with 1 point if the patient responds true, and those items followed by an "F" are scored with 1 point if the patient responds false. A total score is then derived by summing the responses.

phase for many patients is nonpharmacologic interventions (e.g., individual and group therapies, family counseling, vocational and educational programs; see chap. 7). Although dose induction and stabilization provide a significant first step in the treatment process, these other nonpharmacologic services are important for the overall treatment of the patient.

The maintenance phase of treatment may last indefinitely, and the goals of this phase may evolve as the patient achieves stability in his or her life. Maintenance should not be viewed as a period of only a few months, however, or even one or two years. For many patients, the stability provided by maintenance treatment should result in an indefinite period with medication.

Using Buprenorphine for Medically Supervised Withdrawal

The efficacy of buprenorphine in rapid withdrawals from opioids has been discussed (table 11.2). Although there have been studies and reports on the clinical use of buprenorphine for such rapid withdrawals (i.e., in general, lasting just a few days), controlled clinical trials examining the use of buprenorphine for longer withdrawals (e.g., three or six months) have not been reported.

Some reports have suggested that abrupt discontinuation of chronic buprenorphine dosing results in a very mild withdrawal syndrome (Jasinski et al. 1978). Evidence from the disengagement phase of some of the methadone/buprenorphine comparison clinical trials (table 11.1) suggests, however, that patients on buprenorphine relapse to opioid use and drop out of treatment at rates similar to those seen for patients receiving methadone.

Although studies of buprenorphine for longer-term opioid withdrawal are lacking, general recommendations that have been derived from methadone studies may also apply to the use of buprenorphine (see also chap. 5). Thus, withdrawals with gradual decreases in dose should be optimal. Dose changes should be made only after patients have achieved stabilization on their current dose, and patient awareness of the dose schedule and advance warning of dose changes may lead to better outcomes. Unlike methadone, where very small dose changes can be made, buprenorphine dose changes can only occur in increments of 2 mg because tablets are not scored. (Some countries do have a 0.4-mg sublingual tablet available.)

Summary and Conclusions Regarding the Clinical Use of Buprenorphine

Buprenorphine is a safe and effective medication that can be useful for the treatment of opioid dependence. There is more than nine years of community experience with buprenorphine's use in the treatment of opioid dependence, and this medication is maturing into a useful component of the substance abuse treatment system in several countries. Although it has a novel pharmacologic profile, it probably should no longer be considered a novelty medication. Its availability for use in office-based treatment (see chap. 12) gives it a particular niche that contributes to its usefulness.

The clinical use of buprenorphine is relatively straightforward. In the United States, the Substance Abuse and Mental Health Services Administration's (SAMHSA) Center for Substance Abuse Treatment (CSAT) has published a book of guidelines on buprenorphine's use for the treatment of opioid dependence (McNicholas 2004). A copy of this resource can be obtained at no charge by contacting the National Clearinghouse for Alcohol and Drug Information (800-729-6686 or www.kap.samhsa.gov/

products/manuals/index.htm). The clinician interested in using buprenorphine may want to seek out this reference and other resources that can be of value in learning more about the clinical use of buprenorphine for the treatment of opioid dependence.

References

Ahmadi J, Ahmadi K, Ohaeri J (2003). Controlled, randomized trial in maintenance treatment of intravenous buprenorphine dependence with naltrexone, methadone or buprenorphine: a novel study. *Eur J Clin Invest* 33: 824–9.

Amass L, Bickel WK, Crean JP, Blake J, Higgins ST (1998). Alternate-day buprenorphine dosing is preferred to daily dosing by opioid-dependent humans. *Psychopharmacology (Berl)* 136: 217–25.

Amass L, Kamien JB, Mikulich SK (2001). Thrice-weekly supervised dosing with the combination buprenorphine-naloxone tablet is preferred to daily supervised dosing by opioid-dependent humans. *Drug Alcohol Depend* 61: 173–81.

Assadi SM, Hafezi M, Mokri A, Razzaghi EM, Ghaeli P (2004). Opioid detoxification using high doses of buprenorphine in 24 hours: a randomized, double blind, controlled clinical trial. *J Subst Abuse Treat* 27: 75–82.

Berson A, Gervais A, Cazals D, Boyer N, Durand F, Bernuau J, Marcellin P, Degott C, Valla D, Pessayre D (2001). Hepatitis after intravenous buprenorphine misuse in heroin addicts. *J Hepatol* 34: 346–50.

Bickel WK, Amass L, Crean JP, Badger GJ (1999). Buprenorphine dosing every 1, 2, or 3 days in opioid-dependent patients. *Psychopharmacology (Berl)* 146: 111–8.

Bickel WK, Stitzer ML, Bigelow GE, Liebson IA, Jasinski DR, Johnson RE (1988). A clinical trial of buprenorphine: comparison with methadone in the detoxification of heroin addicts. *Clin Pharmacol Ther* 43: 72–78.

Cheskin LJ, Fudala PJ, Johnson RE (1994). A controlled comparison of buprenorphine and clonidine for acute detoxification from opioids. *Drug Alcohol Depend* 36: 115–21.

Compton PA, Ling W, Charuvastra VC, Wesson DR (1995). Buprenorphine as a pharmacotherapy for cocaine abuse: a review of the evidence. *J Addict Dis* 14: 97–114.

DiPaula BA, Schwartz R, Montoya ID, Barrett D, Tang C (2002). Heroin detoxification with buprenorphine on an inpatient psychiatric unit. *J Subst Abuse Treat* 23: 163–9.

Faroqui MH, Cole M, Curran J (1983). Buprenorphine, benzodiazepines and respiratory depression. *Anaesthesia* 38: 1002–3.

Fingerhood MI, Thompson MR, Jasinski DR (2001). A comparison of clonidine and buprenorphine in the outpatient treatment of opiate withdrawal. *Subst Abuse* 22: 193–9.

Fischer G, Gombas W, Eder H, Jagsch R, Peternell A, Stuhlinger G, Pezawas L, Aschauer HN, Kasper S (1999). Buprenorphine versus methadone maintenance for the treatment of opioid dependence. *Addiction* 94: 1337–47.

Fudala PJ, Bridge TP, Herbert S, Williford WO, Chiang CN, Jones K, Collins J, Raisch D, Casadonte P, Goldsmith RJ, Ling W, Malkerneker U, McNicholas L, Renner J, Stine S, Tusel D (2003). Office-based treatment of opiate addiction with a sublingual-tablet formulation of buprenorphine and naloxone. *N Engl J Med* 349: 949–58.

Fudala PJ, Jaffe JH, Dax EM, Johnson RE (1990). Use of buprenorphine in the treatment of opioid addiction. II. Physiologic and behavioral effects of daily and alternate-day administration and abrupt withdrawal. *Clin Pharmacol Ther* 47: 525–34.

Gandhi DH, Jaffe JH, McNary S, Kavanagh GJ, Hayes M, Currens M (2003). Short-term outcomes after brief ambulatory opioid detoxification with buprenorphine in young heroin users. *Addiction* 98: 453–62.

Gross A, Jacobs EA, Petry NM, Badger GJ, Bickel WK (2001). Limits to buprenorphine dosing: a comparison between quintuple and sextuple the maintenance dose every 5 days. *Drug Alcohol Depend* 64: 111–6.

Haertzen CA (1974). An Overview of Addiction Research Center Inventory Scales (ARCI): An Appendix and Manual of Scales. DHEW Pub. No. (ADM) 74-92. Rockville, MD: National Institute on Drug Abuse.

Janiri L, Mannelli P, Persico AM, Serretti A, Tempesta E (1994). Opiate detoxification of methadone maintenance patients using lefetamine, clonidine and buprenorphine. *Drug Alcohol Depend* 36: 139–45.

Jasinski DR, Pevnick JS, Griffith JD (1978). Human pharmacology and abuse potential of the analgesic buprenorphine: a potential agent for treating narcotic addiction. *Arch Gen Psychiatry* 35: 501–16.

Johnson RE, Becker AB, Jones HE, Strain EC, Bigelow GE (2000a). How fast can patients be transitioned from buprenorphine to naltrexone and can opioid blockade be maintained? A pilot study. *Drug Alcohol Depend* 60: S101.

Johnson RE, Chutuape MA, Strain EC, Walsh SL, Stitzer ML, Bigelow GE (2000b). A comparison of levomethadyl acetate, buprenorphine, and methadone for opioid dependence. *N Engl J Med* 343: 1290–7.

Johnson RE, Eissenberg T, Stitzer ML, Strain EC, Liebson IA, Bigelow GE (1995a). Buprenorphine treatment of opioid dependence: clinical trial of daily versus alternate-day dosing. *Drug Alcohol Depend* 40: 27–35.

Johnson RE, Eissenberg T, Stitzer ML, Strain EC, Liebson IA, Bigelow GE (1995b). A placebo controlled clinical trial of buprenorphine as a treatment for opioid dependence. *Drug Alcohol Depend* 40: 17–25.

Johnson RE, Jaffe JH, Fudala PJ (1992). A controlled trial of buprenorphine treatment for opioid dependence [see comments]. *JAMA* 267: 2750–5.

Johnson RE, Strain EC, Amass L (2003). Buprenorphine: how to use it right. *Drug Alcohol Depend* 70: S59–S77.

Kakko J, Svanborg KD, Kreek MJ, Heilig M (2003). 1-year retention and social function after buprenorphine-assisted relapse prevention treatment for heroin dependence in Sweden: a randomised, placebo-controlled trial. *Lancet* 361: 662–8.

Kosten TR, Morgan C, Kleber HD (1992). Phase II clinical trials of buprenorphine: detoxification and induction onto naltrexone. *NIDA Res Monogr* 121: 101–19.

Kutz I, Reznik V (2001). Rapid heroin detoxification using a single high dose of buprenorphine. *J Psychoactive Drugs* 33: 191–3.

Kutz I, Reznik V (2002). Heroin detoxification with a single high dose of buprenorphine. *Isr J Psychiatry Relat Sci* 39: 113–9.

Ling W, Charuvastra C, Collins JF, Batki S, Brown LS, Jr., Kintaudi P, Wesson DR, McNicholas L, Tusel DJ, Malkerneker U, Renner JA, Jr., Santos E, Casadonte P, Fye C, Stine S, Wang RI, Segal D (1998). Buprenorphine maintenance treatment of opiate dependence: a multicenter, randomized clinical trial. *Addiction* 93: 475–86.

Ling W, Wesson DR (2003). Clinical efficacy of buprenorphine: comparisons to methadone and placebo. *Drug Alcohol Depend* 70: S49–S57.

Ling W, Wesson DR, Charuvastra C, Klett CJ (1996). A controlled trial comparing buprenorphine and methadone maintenance in opioid dependence. *Arch Gen Psychiatry* 53: 401–7.

Lofwall MR, Stitzer ML, Bigelow GE, Strain EC (Forthcoming). Comparative Safety and Side Effect Profiles of Buprenorphine and Methadone in the Outpatient Treatment of Opioid Dependence. *Addict Disord Their Treat.*

Mattick RP, Ali R, White J, O'Brien S, Wolk S, Danz C (1999). A randomised double-blind trial of buprenorphine tablets versus methadone syrup for maintenance therapy: efficacy and cost-effectiveness. *NIDA Research Monograph* 180: 77.

Mattick RP, Ali R, White JM, O'Brien S, Wolk S, Danz C (2003). Buprenorphine versus methadone maintenance therapy: a randomized double-blind trial with 405 opioid-dependent patients. *Addiction* 98: 441–52.

Mattick RP, Kimber J, Breen C, Davoli M (2002). Buprenorphine maintenance versus placebo or methadone maintenance for opioid dependence. *Cochrane Database Syst Rev* CD002207.

McNicholas L (2004). Clinical Guidelines for the Use of Buprenorphine in the Treatment of Opioid Addiction. Rockville, MD: U.S. Department of Health and Human Services.

Mello NK, Mendelson JH (1980). Buprenorphine suppresses heroin use by heroin addicts. *Science* 207: 657–9.

Mello NK, Mendelson JH, Bree MP, Lukas SE (1989). Buprenorphine suppresses cocaine self-administration by rhesus monkeys. *Science* 245: 859–62.

Mello NK, Mendelson JH, Bree MP, Lukas SE (1990). Buprenorphine and naltrexone effects on cocaine self-administration by rhesus monkeys. *J Pharmacol Exp Ther* 254: 926–39.

Mintzer MZ, Correia CJ, Strain EC (2004). A dose-effect study of repeated administration of buprenorphine/naloxone on performance in opioid-dependent volunteers. *Drug Alcohol Depend* 74: 205–9.

Montoya ID, Gorelick DA, Preston KL, Schroeder JR, Umbricht A, Cheskin LJ, Lange WR, Contoreggi C, Johnson RE, Fudala PJ (2004). Randomized trial of buprenorphine for treatment of concurrent opiate and cocaine dependence. *Clin Pharmacol Ther* 75: 34–48.

Nigam AK, Ray R, Tripathi BM (1993). Buprenorphine in opiate withdrawal: a comparison with clonidine. *J Subst Abuse Treat* 10: 391–4.

Oliveto AH, Feingold A, Schottenfeld R, Jatlow P, Kosten TR (1999). Desipramine in opioid-dependent cocaine abusers maintained on buprenorphine vs methadone. *Arch Gen Psychiatry* 56: 812–20.

Pani PP, Maremmani I, Pirastu R, Tagliamonte A, Gessa GL (2000). Buprenorphine: a controlled clinical trial in the treatment of opioid dependence. *Drug Alcohol Depend* 60: 39–50.

Parran TV, Adelman CL, Jasinski DR (1994). A buprenorphine stabilization and rapid-taper protocol for the detoxification of opioid-dependent patients. *Am J Addict* 3: 306–13.

Peachey JE, Lei H (1988). Assessment of opioid dependence with naloxone. *Br J Addict* 83: 193–201.

Perez de los Cobos J, Martin S, Etcheberrigaray A, Trujols J, Batlle F, Tejero A, Queralto JM, Casas M (2000). A controlled trial of daily versus thrice-weekly buprenorphine administration for the treatment of opioid dependence. *Drug Alcohol Depend* 59: 223–33.

Petitjean S, Stohler R, Deglon JJ, Livoti S, Waldvogel D, Uehlinger C, Ladewig D (2001). Double-blind randomized trial of buprenorphine and methadone in opiate dependence. *Drug Alcohol Depend* 62: 97–104.

Petry NM, Bickel WK, Badger GJ (1999). A comparison of four buprenorphine dosing regimens in the treatment of opioid dependence. *Clin Pharmacol Ther* 66: 306–14.

Petry NM, Bickel WK, Badger GJ (2000a). A comparison of four buprenorphine dosing regimens using open-dosing procedures: is twice-weekly dosing possible? *Addiction* 95: 1069–77.

Petry NM, Bickel WK, Badger GJ (2001). Examining the limits of the buprenorphine interdosing interval: daily, every-third-day and every-fifth-day dosing regimens. *Addiction* 96: 823–34.

Petry NM, Bickel WK, Piasecki D, Marsch LA, Badger GJ (2000b). Elevated liver enzyme levels in opioid-dependent patients with hepatitis treated with buprenorphine. *Am J Addict* 9: 265–9.

Resnick RB, Galanter M, Resnick E, Pycha C (2001). Buprenorphine treatment of heroin dependence (detoxification and maintenance) in a private practice setting. *J Addict Dis* 20: 75–83.

Reynaud M, Petit G, Potard D, Courty P (1998). Six deaths linked to concomitant use of buprenorphine and benzodiazepines. *Addiction* 93: 1385–92.

Schottenfeld RS, Pakes J, O'Connor P, Chawarski M, Oliveto A, Kosten TR (2000). Thrice-weekly versus daily buprenorphine maintenance. *Biol Psychiatry* 47: 1072–9.

Schottenfeld RS, Pakes JR, Oliveto A, Ziedonis D, Kosten TR (1997). Buprenorphine vs methadone maintenance treatment for concurrent opioid dependence and cocaine abuse [see comments]. *Arch Gen Psychiatry* 54: 713–20.

Schuh KJ, Johanson CE (1999). Pharmacokinetic comparison of the buprenorphine sublingual liquid and tablet. *Drug Alcohol Depend* 56: 55–60.

Seifert J, Metzner C, Paetzold W, Borsutzky M, Passie T, Rollnik J, Wiese B, Emrich HM, Schneider U (2002). Detoxification of opiate addicts with multiple drug abuse: a comparison of buprenorphine vs. methadone. *Pharmacopsychiatry* 35: 159–64.

Strain EC (2002). High dose buprenorphine for the treatment of opioid dependence. In: Marquet P, ed. *Buprenorphine Therapy of Opiate Addiction*, 29–49. Totowa, NJ: Humana Press.

Strain EC, Clarke HW, Auriacombe M, Lagier G, Mallaret M, Thirion X (2003). French experience with buprenorphine. *NIDA Res Monogr* 183: 134–41.

Strain EC, Moody DE, Stoller KB, Walsh SL, Bigelow GE (2004). Relative bioavailability of different buprenorphine formulations under chronic dosing conditions. *Drug Alcohol Depend* 74: 37–43.

Strain EC, Stitzer ML, Liebson IA, Bigelow GE (1994a). Buprenorphine versus methadone in the treatment of opioid-dependent cocaine users. *Psychopharmacology (Berl)* 116: 401–6.

Strain EC, Stitzer ML, Liebson IA, Bigelow GE (1994b). Comparison of buprenorphine and methadone in the treatment of opioid dependence. *Am J Psychiatry* 151: 1025–30.

Tamaskar R, Parran TV, Jr., Heggi A, Brateanu A, Rabb M, Yu J (2003). Tramadol versus buprenorphine for the treatment of opiate withdrawal: a retrospective cohort control study. *J Addict Dis* 22: 5–12.

Thirion X, Lapierre V, Micallef J, Ronfle E, Masut A, Pradel V, Coudert C, Mabriez JC, Sanmarco JL (2002). Buprenorphine prescription by general practitioners in a French region. *Drug Alcohol Depend* 65: 197–204.

Tracqui A, Kintz P, Ludes B (1998). Buprenorphine-related deaths among drug addicts in France: a report on 20 fatalities. *J Anal Toxicol* 22: 430–4.

Umbricht A, Hoover DR, Tucker MJ, Leslie JM, Chaisson RE, Preston KL (2003). Opioid detoxification with buprenorphine, clonidine, or methadone in hospitalized heroin-dependent patients with HIV infection. *Drug Alcohol Depend* 69: 263–72.

Umbricht A, Montoya ID, Hoover DR, Demuth KL, Chiang CT, Preston KL (1999). Naltrexone shortened opioid detoxification with buprenorphine. *Drug Alcohol Depend* 56: 181–90.

Umbricht-Schneiter A, Montoya ID, Demuth KL, Preston KL (1996). Opioid detoxification with buprenorphine alone or in combination with naltrexone. In: Harris LS, ed. Problems of Drug Dependence, 1995: Proceedings of the 57th Annual Scientific Meeting, The College on Problems of Drug Dependence, Inc., pp. 117. Rockville, MD: U.S. Department of Health and Human Services, National Institutes of Health.

Vignau J (1998). Preliminary assessment of a 10-day rapid detoxification programme using high dosage buprenorphine. *Eur Addict Res* 4: 29–31.

Walsh SL, Preston KL, Stitzer ML, Cone EJ, Bigelow GE (1994). Clinical pharmacology of buprenorphine: ceiling effects at high doses. *Clin Pharmacol Ther* 55: 569–80.

Wang RI, Wiesen RL, Lamid S, Roh BL (1974). Rating the presence and severity of opiate dependence. *Clin Pharmacol Ther* 16: 653–8.

White R, Alcorn R, Feinmann C (2001). Two methods of community detoxification from opiates: an open-label comparison of lofexidine and buprenorphine. *Drug Alcohol Depend* 65: 77–83.

12

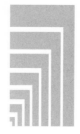

Office-Based Treatment with Buprenorphine and Other Medications

David Fiellin, M.D., and Eric C. Strain, M.D.

It is almost easier to define office-based opioid treatment (OBOT) by what it is not. Office-based treatment of opioid dependence is not treatment provided through a specialized outpatient clinic (i.e., it is not a methadone treatment program). However, this definition of OBOT leaves a large variety of modalities that can be included as office-based treatment, ranging from a solo practitioner's office to a large multispecialty clinic or group practice, and a variety of approaches ranging from pharmacologic withdrawal to maintenance treatment. Office-based opioid treatment almost uniformly refers to treatment of opioid dependence using a partial or full agonist opioid pharmacotherapy. In general, these medications are made available by physician prescription and dispensed in either an observed or unobserved manner via a pharmacy. OBOT is not restricted to a particular medical specialty; but certain types of physicians may be more likely to practice OBOT, such as general practitioners, internists, family physicians, and psychiatrists; virtually all types of generalists or specialists could provide OBOT under the proper circumstances.

Office-based opioid treatment has been gaining popularity in recent years for three reasons. First, it is believed that providing treatment for opioid dependence in an office setting mainstreams the treatment of addictions. One hope is that the treatment of patients with addictive disorders will be seen as similar to the treatment of other medical conditions and that the stigma associated with these disorders and the patients with these conditions will be reduced substantially. Second, OBOT should allow treatment services to be better integrated with other medical care. Patients with substance abuse disorders have high rates of comorbid conditions (both psychiatric and somatic) (Brooner et al. 1997; Sullivan and Fiellin 2004), and providing addictions and other services in a single setting has been shown to improve compliance with recommended treatments for at least some of these comorbid disorders (Umbricht-Schneiter et al. 1994). Finally, it is hoped that OBOT will expand treatment capacity. The most common form of non-OBOT service is methadone clinics, and in some countries (most notably the United States), it has been quite difficult to expand the capacity of the methadone clinic system.

Although office-based treatment of opioid dependence was not uncommon 100 years ago, declining social acceptability and governmental interventions made OBOT exceedingly rare in many parts of the world for much of the twentieth century. This has changed in recent years. Perhaps the most rapid and largest expansion of OBOT has been in France, where buprenorphine is extensively prescribed and used in office settings for the treatment of opioid dependence (Auriacombe et al. 2001, 2004; Strain et al. 2003). OBOT, however, is a treatment modality that is relatively new, especially as it relates to systematic study in which its safety and efficacy are compared with the more common treatment, methadone delivered by a specialty clinic.

This chapter provides an overview of OBOT; it begins by reviewing studies that have examined office-based opioid treatment. These studies have been conducted with patients maintained on either buprenorphine or methadone; each medication is considered separately. The next section provides a review of some of the practical issues associated with OBOT. The chapter ends with a section that provides a summary of this topic, including future directions for the study of OBOT.

Studies and Reports on Office-Based Treatment for Opioid Dependence

Office-Based Treatment with Methadone

There has long been interest in the idea that methadone treatment for opioid dependence could be provided by a physician in an office setting, and early plans for this type of treatment were provided by Vincent Dole (Dole, 1971). Practically, this treatment might be initiated in one of two ways: first, a patient is treated in a special clinic (e.g., a methadone clinic) and stabilized before being transitioned to OBOT; second, a patient with problematic opioid use directly enters treatment provided by an office-based physician (i.e., is not stabilized in a methadone treatment clinic initially). The first means has been described in a few reports from the United States and an article from Australia (Ritter et al. 2003). The second means, entering office-based methadone treatment directly, has been described in reports from Europe (primarily the United Kingdom). Each of these experiences is summarized here.

OBOT with Methadone in the United Kingdom

Several reports have described the experience in the United Kingdom with office-based treatment of opioid dependence. Historically, individual practitioners prescribed opioids (usually injectable forms) to a small number of patients in office-based settings until the 1960s; however, a rise in the number of patients dependent on opioids led to the establishment of treatment clinics in 1968 (Strang and Gossop 1994). These clinics prescribed injectable opioids (primarily heroin and methadone) and were typically associated with hospitals. Patients previously treated by individual physicians transferred to these clinics during the 1970s, and the role of individual practitioners diminished during this period.

In the 1980s, however, there was a shift back to general practitioner-based treatment of addictions in the United Kingdom. In part, this appears to have been a reaction to the liabilities of the clinic system, but it also was a means for expanding treatment capacity and mainstreaming addictions care (similar to arguments invoked with the use of office-based buprenorphine treatment in the United States). Surveys of opioid-dependent patients in the United Kingdom reported a preference to receive treatment from general practitioners (Bennett and Wright 1986; Hindler et al. 1995), although not all patients thought general practitioners would look favorably on treating them (Telfer and Clulow 1990), and not all general practitioners felt that they were well equipped for this type of practice (Davies and Huxley 1997; Preston and Campion-Smith 1997).

Although the clinic system initially provided primarily injectable forms of opioids, these clinics began switching to oral forms of opioids during the 1970s. By the 1980s there was a clear switch from injectable forms of heroin and methadone to the oral form of methadone (Mitcheson 1994). This change in route of administration carried through to the individual practitioner. At the time of a survey in 1995, methadone was the most common opioid prescribed for opioid dependence (96% of such prescriptions), and although 9 percent of these prescriptions were still for an injectable form, the most common route of administration was oral (80% for an oral liquid form and 11% for tablets) (Strang et al. 1996).

Although individual practitioners prescribed opioids, medications were and are typically administered under the supervision of a pharmacist, whose role in the provision of medical care is more extensive in the United Kingdom than in the United States (McBride et al. 1994; Scott and McNulty 1996; Scott et al. 1994). Pharmacy distribution is often done on a daily basis (in 65% of cases in one survey), based on the physician's instruction (Matheson et al. 1999).

As the treatment of drug abuse in the United Kingdom shifted back to individual practitioners working in office settings in the 1980s and 1990s, a series of evaluations were conducted to determine the relative efficacy and safety of this form of treatment. In general, these studies have shown that office-based methadone treatment produces good outcomes (Keen et al. 2000, 2003) that are similar to those seen with clinic-based treatment (Gossop et al. 1999); that office-based methadone treatment does not appear to produce increases in methadone-related deaths (Keen et al. 2002); and that these services can achieve good penetration into the general practitioner community when support is provided (i.e., 30–59% participation by practitioners in one survey) (Weinrich and Stuart 2000). One notable observation on this practice in the United Kingdom relates the extent to which office-based physicians adhere to established guidelines for this type of care. Studies have documented low adherence to national guideline recommendations and high rates of practice variability (Strang and Sheridan 1998). Making guidelines readily available to practitioners, however, has been demonstrated to improve adherence to these procedures (Strang and Sheridan 2003; Weinrich and Stuart 2000).

The current use of office-based methadone treatment in the United Kingdom reflects, in part, unique historical aspects of the British system. These include a long history of little illicit opioid use, a history of successful office-based treatment, a willingness to experiment with clinic-based treatment using injectable forms of drugs (such as heroin), and the migration back to an emphasis on office-based services (but now primarily with oral methadone). Underlying these changes is a thread of pragmatism—a problem is identified, a means for addressing it is tried, if it works it is kept (e.g., oral methadone), but if it does not succeed then something else is tried (e.g., office-based treatment). With proper support to individual physicians, this appears to be a system that works and works relatively well.

OBOT with Methadone in the United States

There have been fewer reports on office-based methadone treatment (or what is called "medical methadone maintenance") in the United States. Reports on the evaluation of such programs have originated from four cities: Baltimore, Maryland (two different programs), Chicago, Illinois (a pilot study), Waterbury, Connecticut (a randomized clinical trial), and New York, New York (the most extensively reported such program). Assessments associated with each of these programs have been published and are reviewed here.

The first report from Baltimore was of 21 patients treated under an Investigational New Drug (IND) application obtained by Dr. Michael Hayes in the early 1980s (Schwartz et al. 1999). This was not a controlled study but rather a report on the naturalistic outcomes for patients treated in a private physician's office. Those recruited into the program were highly stable (e.g., they were required to have at least five years abstinence from illicit drug use and, in actuality, had an average of 9.7 years of continuous abstinence before transfer to OBOT), and participants were seen every four weeks and received a 28-day supply of methadone in the form of diskettes. After 12 years, 12 patients (57%) remained in the program and continued to do well. Six patients returned to the methadone clinic, two patients died, and one successfully withdrew off methadone. This may be viewed best as a small pilot project with an extremely long follow-up assessment (12 years), and it showed that approximately one-half of highly stable patients at methadone clinics can successfully transition to an office setting.

The second report from Baltimore was a randomized, controlled trial of methadone medical maintenance (King et al. 2002). In this study, patients needed to fulfill criteria for stability over the previous 12-month period (rather than the five years noted in the previous report), and participants were randomly assigned to one of three conditions: routine methadone treatment at their clinic, medical maintenance at a physician's office, or medical maintenance at their methadone clinic. A total of 73 patients participated in the study and results showed that there were few differences between the three forms of care (e.g., in rates of illicit drug use). However, patients in the medical maintenance conditions were more satisfied with their treatment (especially those in the office-based condition). This randomized trial provides further evidence that office-based methadone treatment can be provided to stable patients without significant increases in drug use, that this modality is well liked by patients, and that outcomes are similar to those seen with more traditional clinic-based methadone treatment.

A pilot study of methadone medical maintenance was conducted in Chicago (Senay et al. 1993). This was also a random assignment study and enrolled 130 patients who had at least one year of methadone maintenance treatment and six months of stability in treatment. Participants were randomly assigned either to continue in routine treatment for six months and then have the option of entering medical maintenance or to directly enter medical maintenance. Unlike other studies, however, visits occurred twice per month rather than once per month (with take-home doses for 13 days), and medical maintenance involved more intensive services than other studies (e.g., both a monthly physician visit and a monthly counseling session, and both scheduled and random urine testing). These services, though slightly more intensive than in other medical maintenance programs, may be viewed as appropriate given that participants were required to have only six months of treatment stability. Results across a number of domains of interest, including urine testing and Addiction Severity Index (ASI) scores, showed that the medical maintenance and control condition had similar outcomes. Like other studies, patient satisfaction for medical maintenance was high and because of the program's success it was continued after the study was completed. This study may be most important for showing that the window defining treatment stability can be relatively short (six months).

A third randomized study of medical maintenance was conducted in Waterbury, Connecticut, and used primary care physicians to deliver treatment to patients (Fiellin et al. 2001). Like the Chicago study, stable methadone-maintained patients were randomly assigned to either medical maintenance (22 participants) or usual care at their methadone clinic (24 participants). In this study patients needed to have at least one year of treatment without evidence of illicit drug use to qualify for the project, and office visits occurred once per week with six days of take-home doses of liquid methadone provided. Although no significant difference occurred in rates of illicit drug use between the two groups, an interesting outcome from this study was the high rate of illicit drug use found for both study groups (38–50% of patients had evidence of illicit opioid use during the six months of the study). This may reflect the high frequency of urine testing in this study versus other studies of medical maintenance, as well as the use of hair testing during the study (which may have also increased the validity of self-reported drug use by participants). The physicians providing OBOT in this study reported high satisfaction with this treatment, which is especially notable given that a substantial proportion of their patients did have some evidence of continued illicit drug use.

Finally, there have been a series of reports from New York on the use of methadone medical maintenance (Des Jarlais et al. 1985; Novick and Joseph 1991; Novick et al. 1988, 1994; Salsitz et al. 2000). This body of work represents the most extensive and sustained literature on the use of methadone medical maintenance in the United States. Although not a randomized clinical trial, this informative series of papers documents the success of a form of methadone treatment that was first initiated by Drs. Marie Nyswander and Vincent Dole in 1983.

In the most recent update of this ongoing project, 158 patients had been referred to medical maintenance as of August 1998. As of 1996, patients were required to have at least four years of methadone treatment with stability in treatment (e.g., no illicit drug or excessive alcohol use, stable prosocial involvement in daily activities such as employment or education, emotional and somatically healthy, or in appropriate treatment) for the previous three years (Salsitz et al. 2000). Participants are seen once per month and receive a monthly supply of methadone diskettes. Most patients referred to medical maintenance have been compliant (84%), and among those who were discharged the most common reason was cocaine use (58% of the 26 discharged patients). Twenty of the compliant patients had died while in treatment, and the three most frequent causes of death were smoking-related illness (40% of deaths), hepatitis C (20% of deaths), and AIDS (15% of deaths). Among active patients, 10% were on methadone doses of between 5 and 25 mg per day, and 42% were on doses of between 80 and 120 mg per day. This work emphasizes the stigma associated with traditional clinic-based methadone treatment and how OBOT can both reduce stigma and provide a physician advocate for the patient that informs and teaches other health care providers about methadone treatment.

Summary of Office-Based Treatment with Methadone

Although the core feature of OBOT is consistent across these reports—that is, the provision of methadone medication in an office setting through individual contact with a physician and with a substantial number of take-home doses—there is considerable variety in how this is accomplished. These differences fall into two general categories: the criteria used to enter medical methadone treatment and the operational aspects of treatment delivery once a person has been accepted into this modality. For the former, in general, stability has been defined in terms of time and has ranged from as little as six months to as much as five years. Various other criteria have been used as well, such as involvement in some form of meaningful pastime such as work or school. Operational aspects have also differed considerably—for example, in the form of methadone provided (diskettes versus liquid), the number of doses provided (13 days versus a month), the frequency of office visits, and the amount of nonpharmacologic treatment provided concurrently.

Although these differences between reports are important, there are several general conclusions that can be made about OBOT with methadone. First, it works for a substantial proportion of select patients (probably at least 50% and perhaps in excess of 80%). Second, patients clearly like it and benefit from it. Finally, though not clearly addressed in these reports, the implication exists that it should be less costly.

Several areas still need to be addressed when considering OBOT with methadone. First, it remains to be determined whether this is only an option for a small proportion of patients or if it would be effective on a larger scale. The stability criteria used in the existent literature would restrict this practice to a minority of patients currently receiving treatment with methadone in opioid treatment programs. It would be helpful to determine whether methadone OBOT could be initiated as a routine aspect of treatment, perhaps as part of an integrated set of services revolving around a methadone clinic. Recent changes in methadone regulations in the United States that allow methadone OBOT in association with a methadone clinic should allow this to occur (Fiellin and O'Connor 2002; Kreek and Vocci 2002). Second, it would be extremely valuable to compare the cost of methadone OBOT with typical methadone clinic fees. If methadone OBOT is less costly, this might lead to heightened interest and motivation by third-party payers and governmental agencies for expansion of methadone OBOT. Finally, the optimal parameters for methadone OBOT remain to be determined. That is, how much time in stable treatment should elapse before a patient is transferred to OBOT, what is the optimal frequency of physician visits, and what are the optimal nonpharmacologic services that should be provided to patients? Methadone OBOT should be viewed with the same enthusiasm as a new medication for the treatment of opioid dependence would be viewed, because it is an exciting and novel form of treatment that offers an opportunity to expand capacity, provide integrated care, and improve patient satisfaction with the services provided.

Office-Based Treatment with Buprenorphine

Most reports regarding methadone OBOT have originated from the United States and United Kingdom, but the greatest experience with buprenorphine OBOT has been in France. There have been some reports from other countries on the use of buprenorphine in primary care settings, including pilot studies showing that this medication could be effective and safely provided from an office setting (Fiellin et al. 2002; Galanter et al. 2003; O'Connor et al. 1996; Resnick et al. 2001). Three studies on buprenorphine use outside France will be briefly reviewed before discussing in more detail the French experience with office-based buprenorphine treatment.

OBOT *with Buprenorphine in Countries Other than France*

The first of these studies was conducted in Australia and compared outcomes for 115 patients dependent on opioids randomly assigned to a buprenorphine withdrawal performed either in office settings or a clinic (Gibson et al. 2003). The withdrawal was conducted over five days, and outcomes for the two groups were nearly identical across several outcome measures, including treatment retention and drug use. The study included a cost analysis showing that the office-based treatment was slightly more expensive, although this may have reflected the need to use clinic services on the weekend when primary care offices were closed.

The other two studies were conducted in the United States and examined the efficacy of maintenance treatment with sublingual buprenorphine delivered in an office setting. The first of these studies used buprenorphine solution rather than tablets, and doses were administered under supervision three times weekly (i.e., there were no take-home doses provided) (O'Connor et al. 1998). The study compared this treatment with the same buprenorphine-dosing schedule but provided in a traditional methadone clinic and found that patients treated in the primary care setting ($N = 23$) had significantly better treatment retention and less illicit opioid use than patients treated at the clinic ($N = 23$). The second study was a large, multisite, double-blind clinical trial that used daily doses of buprenorphine (16 mg) and buprenorphine/naloxone (16/4 mg) tablets and compared these conditions with placebo (Fudala et al. 2003). Although this was an office-based study, participants were seen daily and received take-home doses only for weekends and holidays. Both active conditions were superior to placebo, and the study was terminated early because of the clear superiority of buprenorphine and buprenorphine/

naloxone. After the double-blind clinical trial patients could enter an open-label safety study during which up to ten days of take-home doses of buprenorphine could be provided. The information reported about the operational aspects of and treatment outcomes for this office-based practice is limited.

Although these are two studies of buprenorphine OBOT, the methodological aspects of each are substantially different from what might be expected in the day-to-day clinical practice of OBOT. In this respect, reports describing the French experience with office-based buprenorphine treatment provide meaningful information about real-world experience in using buprenorphine.

OBOT *with Buprenorphine in France*

Buprenorphine was approved for use in France in February 1996. At that time the country had a very small methadone treatment system in place, so there was potentially high demand for opioid substitution treatment. Indeed, there was a rapid increase in use of buprenorphine; in 1996 it was estimated there were already 25,000 patients being treated with buprenorphine in France (Auriacombe et al. 2001). By the late 1990s this number had increased to 65,000 patients being treated with buprenorphine, and by March 2001 it was estimated that there were 74,300 patients being treated with buprenorphine (Auriacombe et al. 2004; Strain et al. 2003).

In part, the rapid increase in the number of patients treated with buprenorphine in France may be related to the lack of ready availability of methadone treatment. Other important reasons buprenorphine has been extensively used in France include: (1) the virtual lack of restrictions on physicians who wish to prescribe buprenorphine for the treatment of opioid dependence (i.e., it is readily available for use in office-based settings); (2) a single-payer health care system in France that does not provide a disincentive to treat addictions (as is the case in the United States); and (3) the methadone treatment system remains relatively small and restricted in access (although it has expanded in recent years).

For the purposes of this review, our primary interest is in what is known about buprenorphine OBOT in France and what are the relative strengths and limitations of this program. Knowing this would be especially useful given that office-based buprenorphine treatment is now available in other countries.

An important feature of buprenorphine's use in France is that the only form available is the monotherapy product—that is, the buprenorphine/

naloxone combination product is not marketed in France (as of 2004). In addition, as in the United Kingdom, dispensing by pharmacists is readily available and utilized. A third important factor is that in France, in general, there are high rates of benzodiazepine prescribing by practitioners. When reviewing the use of buprenorphine in France, the high rate of concurrent benzodiazepine use by buprenorphine-maintained patients occurs in a setting where use of this class of medication is quite common—even among patients who are not maintained on buprenorphine. These three aspects of buprenorphine's use in France help to understand some of the consequences of buprenorphine's use in that country, especially when considering its diversion and abuse.

Regarding the specifics of buprenorphine use in France, general practitioners can prescribe the medication for up to 28 days at a time, and a pharmacy can dispense up to seven days at a time. Pharmacists have the capability of dispensing daily doses under supervision and commonly do so during the induction phase (71% of patients), although this decreases during maintenance dosing (to 23% of patients) (Vignau et al. 2001). Although it is recommended that daily doses not exceed 16 mg per day, one survey found that 15 percent of patients were maintained on daily doses of 20 mg or greater (Thirion et al. 2002). The same survey found that most buprenorphine was prescribed by general practitioners; in the region where the survey was conducted, 85 percent of prescriptions were written by general practitioners. Another report indicated that 95 percent of physicians prescribing buprenorphine are general practitioners and that 20 percent of general practitioners had prescribed buprenorphine (Strain et al. 2003). Although most buprenorphine is provided through general practitioners in France, one survey found 73 percent of them had ten or fewer patients treated with buprenorphine and 43% of these had fewer than five buprenorphine patients (Bouchez and Vignau 1998), and a second survey found the mean number of patients followed by each general practitioner was 4.1, with 61% of general practitioners monitoring only one or two buprenorphine-maintained patients (Thirion et al. 2002).

Surveys of French physicians suggest that there is a willingness to prescribe buprenorphine, especially among those physicians with previous experience in treating patients with injecting drug use; furthermore, relations with patients improve and buprenorphine is perceived as having good efficacy when prescribed to patients with opioid dependence (Bouchez and Vignau 1998; Moatti et al. 1998). Similarly, pharmacists report improved relationships with patients who are opioid dependent and treated with buprenorphine (Bouchez and Vignau 1998). The wide use of buprenorphine, most commonly for a few patients by each physician, suggests that use of the medication has become a normal part of mainstream medical treatment in France and that it is accepted as such.

This ready availability of buprenorphine through office-based treatment has clearly expanded treatment capacity in France. In a setting where there are essentially no restrictions in its use by physicians, however, both abuse of prescribed buprenorphine and diversion can and does occur. For example, one early survey found that 8 percent of patients prescribed buprenorphine admitted they injected their doses intravenously (Bouchez and Vignau 1998). A paper published five years later reported that nearly one-half of patients (47%) maintained on buprenorphine had injected this medication at some point (Vidal-Trecan et al. 2003). Another survey found that during a four-month period most patients treated with buprenorphine had seen a single physician (66%), but 22 percent of patients had seen two physicians, 11 percent had seen between three and five physicians, and 1 percent had attended treatment with more than five physicians (Thirion et al. 2002). Finally, a survey of persons seeking new needles at various sites assessed the extent of buprenorphine misuse and found that more than one-half of respondents (58%) had injected buprenorphine at some point in the previous six months (Obadia et al. 2001). Nearly one-quarter (24%) had injected only buprenorphine in that six-month period (i.e., they had not used heroin or other illicit opioids). In that same survey, one-third of the subjects were in buprenorphine maintenance treatment, and of these patients, 71% had injected buprenorphine at some point in the previous six months. Results such as these highlight the potential for diversion and abuse of buprenorphine when it is readily available, but they should be weighed against the benefits of this treatment such as decreases in opioid overdose mortality associated with buprenorphine's availability (Auriacombe et al. 2004).

As mentioned earlier, a special feature of medical care in France is the high rate of prescribing benzodiazepines by general practitioners (which is not restricted to patients treated with buprenorphine). For example, one study found that benzodiazepines were prescribed occasionally or on a regular basis to 37 percent of patients treated with buprenorphine (Vignau et al. 2001), a second report indicated that benzodiazepines are the medication most commonly prescribed with buprenorphine and that 21 percent of patients in treatment and 33 percent of patients out of treatment who took buprenorphine also ingested benzodiazepines (Strain et al. 2003), and a third study found that 28% of general practitioners had prescribed buprenorphine and flunitrazepam together on the same form (Thirion et al. 2002). These rates of benzodiazepine use are particularly worrisome given the risk of death associated with the combination of buprenorphine with benzodiazepines (when both are injected), and this rate of use highlights how office-based treatment may involve a standard of care that can differ from that seen in more controlled clinical trials of OBOT.

Summary of OBOT with Buprenorphine in France

The French experience with buprenorphine is extremely helpful in drawing attention to both the strengths and potential weaknesses of OBOT. Most importantly, it shows how this modality of care can substantially increase access to care. In addition, it suggests that OBOT can mainstream addictions treatment into routine medical care. It does not require the development of new programs or services, but capitalizes upon an existing and well-established health care system. It appears that buprenorphine office-based treatment has become accepted by a sizable proportion of French general practitioners—it is not limited to a small or select group of trained specialists.

This system of care comes at some cost, however, most notably because diversion and abuse of the medication has occurred. Apparently, there is a small but significant number of patients who use prescribed buprenorphine intravenously, who sell or give away their tablets, or who obtain tablets from multiple physicians. OBOT with buprenorphine has multiple benefits, but a system that allows easy access to treatment and medication with few restrictions to care is not without potential liabilities. The medical and social benefits would appear to outweigh these costs, but the French experience shows how OBOT is not with liabilities, especially depending on the details of its design and execution.

PRACTICAL ISSUES ASSOCIATED WITH OFFICE-BASED TREATMENT OF OPIOID DEPENDENCE

The use of opioid medications in office-based treatment of opioid dependence raises several practical and logistical considerations. The uniqueness of this practice requires attention and forethought as the basic components of addiction treatment are incorporated into the routine clinical practice environment. There is little empiric data on which to base recommendations for the implementation of these components of care. Luckily, however, only a few structural changes need to be made in general office-based medical practice when care is expanded to include treatment for patients dependent on opioids, and many of the components of care are analogous to standard procedures used in the treatment of other chronic medical conditions. In addition, guidelines have been produced that can provide guidance to the practice in the process of adapting to office-based treatment with buprenorphine or methadone (see, for example, the Federation of State Medical Boards policy on opioid addiction treatment in the office, available at www.fsmb.org; Fiellin and Barthwell 2003; McNicholas 2004). When planning to provide office-based treatment for opioid dependence, the practical issues that need to be considered include selecting the appropriate patient, making provision for psychosocial counseling, conducting monitoring through urine toxicology analysis, educating office staff, identifying referral resources for medical and psychiatric comorbidities, and ensuring reimbursement for the necessary components of care. Each of these topics will be considered here.

Selecting the Patient for OBOT

As discussed earlier, patients dependent on opioids treated in an office setting will generally either be in another form of addictions treatment, such as a methadone clinic, or not in treatment and seeking to enter OBOT directly. In the former case, the physician should obtain the patient's permission and then communicate with the methadone program directly for details on the patient's treatment history. Although talking with the methadone program physician is a logical step, in many programs the patient's counselor will have a greater familiarity with the patient's performance in treatment and is a good resource to contact. Specific questions should be asked about the frequency of urine testing, types of drugs that have been tested, and results; adherence to counseling; current methadone dose; and outstanding issues in the patient's treatment plan (table 12.1).

For the patient entering OBOT directly, information from other professionals may not be readily available. In this case it is important to confirm that the patient has a diagnosis of opioid dependence (see chap. 9 for criteria used to make a diagnosis of opioid dependence). For patients currently in treatment with the physician for other conditions (e.g., a patient who has been in treatment for months or years because of hypertension), the physician may have a good comfort level with individual patients, their psychosocial situation, and their suitability for OBOT. If such a history of working together with a patient does not exist, it may be useful to seek out other information about the patient—from a family member or close friend and/or past treatment providers (including past episodes in methadone treatment) to help gauge the suitability of a new patient seeking OBOT.

Table 12.1 **Patient Factors to Consider When Planning Possible Office-Based Opioid Treatment**

For a patient transferring from a methadone treatment program
  Continuously enrolled in the methadone maintenance treatment program for one to five years
  Clinically stable as evidenced by
    Past 12 months with no illicit drug use based on urine toxicology results
    Confirmation of good treatment performance by program staff familiar with the patient

For all patients (transfers from methadone treatment programs and patients not currently in opioid dependence treatment)
  No evidence of dependence on cocaine, alcohol, or drugs other than nicotine
  No untreated major psychiatric conditions
  Stable source of financial support for living (e.g., employed, spouse/significant other employed)
  Stable source of payment for medication and office visits
  Without active legal concerns
  Compliant with other treatment regimens
  No history of multiple treatment relapses in higher level of care

Provision of Psychosocial Counseling

Treatment outcomes for patients dependent on opioids receiving opioid agonist medication are improved when psychosocial services are provided along with medication (Fiellin et al. 2002; McLellan et al. 1993). The range of psychosocial treatments and the goals of this type of treatment have been reviewed in chapters 7 and 8. In brief, these treatments are designed to (1) address patients' motivation for treatment and abstinence, (2) assist patients in developing skills to cope with triggers to relapse, (3) change the contingencies under which patients experience reinforcement, (4) help patients manage painful affective states (e.g., grief, anger, dysthymia, demoralization), (5) help patients improve their relationships and interpersonal functioning, and (6) increase adherence to medication.

Psychosocial counseling for patients receiving office-based treatment may be provided either in the office (on-site) or via referral (off-site). In the United States, the Drug Addiction Treatment Act of 2000 (the legislation that creates the provision for office-based treatment of opioid dependence in that country), requires that physicians have the capacity to refer patients for ancillary services, but not that these services be provided within the physician's office. Models of care can range from recommendations that patients attend off-site self-help groups (e.g., Narcotics Anonymous or Alcoholics Anonymous) to the provision of group therapy or individual drug counseling within the office setting. Off-site services also vary based on the local availability of resources.

Psychosocial services can be provided by individuals from a variety of training backgrounds, including nursing, social work, psychology, medicine and psychiatry, and addiction counseling (Fiellin et al. 2002; Fudala et al. 2003). The clinician attempting to identify resources in the local community is advised to investigate services covered by an individual patient's insurance (if applicable for that country), communicate with local colleagues who have training in addiction medicine and/or psychiatry, contact the local health department, and determine services provided by local and federal governments. In the United States, a federal substance abuse treatment facility locator is provided by the Substance Abuse and Mental Health Services Administration (http://csat.samhsa.gov). Other ways to obtain information about locally available treatment resources include contacting the local or regional chapter of an addiction medicine society, such as the American Academy of Addiction Psychiatry (www .aaap.org) or the American Society of Addiction Medicine (which has chapters in other countries besides the United States; www.asam.org). Other professional organizations that can be useful resources include the American Association for the Treatment of Opioid Dependence (www .aatod.org) and The Association for Addiction Professionals (formerly an addictions counselors professional organization; www.naadac.org). Organizations that can provide information about referral resources for counseling and therapy include the American Psychiatric Association (www .psych.org), the American Psychological Association (www.apa.org), and the National Association of State Alcohol/Drug Abuse Directors (www .nasadad.org). Although these organizations are located in the United States, clinicians in other countries can contact them to determine whether they have international members residing in their own country (the case for several of these societies), or if they can provide contact information for analogous organizations in their own country.

When possible, the physician providing OBOT should seek out specific training in addictions when making a counseling referral for patients in OBOT. The approach to patients with addictive disorders can differ from other types of mental health treatment, and some locations may have a limited number of counseling service providers with experience caring for patients dependent on opioids receiving buprenorphine or methadone. The lack of counselors or therapists who are experienced in the treatment of patients with addictions, however, should not prevent the clinician from providing OBOT, and the physician may develop experience with a local counselor or therapist in the treatment of opioid dependence.

Monitoring through Urine Toxicology Analysis

Urine toxicology monitoring, in addition to patient self-report of illicit drug use, is considered routine practice for patients receiving treatment for opioid dependence. Urine toxicology monitoring has been shown to be a valuable component of treatment for patients with addictive disorders (McCarthy 1994). The use of urine testing as a marker for assessing abstinence is similar to other areas of medicine where surrogate markers are used to assess the status of a chronic medical condition. In this way, urine toxicology assessments in the treatment of opioid dependence are akin to monitoring the disease process and tailoring treatment interventions in diabetes (periodic hemoglobin A1C assessment), cardiovascular diseases (lipid profile monitoring), cerebrovascular disease (blood pressure monitoring), and reactive airway disease (peak flow monitoring). Rather than being viewed as punitive, intermittent assessment of treatment response status through urine toxicology analysis should be considered a routine part of clinical care in patients with opioid dependence. As with psychosocial services, the clinician can collect the samples on-site or off-site. Samples collected on-site may be evaluated on-site through rapid assessment procedures or sent to an off-site laboratory for analysis (see chap. 17 for a discussion of urine testing). In one study of office-based treatment, the ability to receive timely and accurate results from urine toxicology testing was noted to be a particular challenge and required additional attention to ensure clinician responses (Fiellin et al. 2004).

A range of substances can be detected in urine toxicology testing. Routine testing for patients dependent on opioids receiving treatment in an office-based setting should include screening for naturally occurring opioids (e.g., codeine, morphine), as well as synthetic or semisynthetic opioids (e.g., oxycodone, methadone). In addition to opioids, the physician may decide to test for other substances commonly abused, such as benzodiazepines, cocaine (the latter test is actually for benzoylecgonine, the metabolite of cocaine found in urine), marijuana, or other drugs regularly found in the local community.

On-site testing can be performed by using special urine containers that incorporate chemical reagents and can assess urine temperature in an effort to determine validity (see chap. 17 for a description). As an alternative to on-site testing, clinicians can make arrangements with commercial vendors to have urine samples picked up at their office and transported to a laboratory for analysis or to have both the collection of the urine specimen and analysis occur at a remote laboratory.

The physician will need to decide whether to have testing conducted on a scheduled basis (i.e., known to the patient, such as at their monthly doctor's visit), or randomly. In the latter case, patients can be required to call the office at a scheduled time (e.g., each Monday, Wednesday, and Friday morning between 7:00 and 8:00 a.m.) to find out if they need to provide a urine sample that day. The disadvantage of scheduled testing is that patients can more easily avoid detection of drug use. The disadvantage of random testing is that it is inconvenient and time consuming for the patient and the office staff. Episodic random urine testing can provide the clinician with a method to validate patient self-report and to detect episodes of illicit drug use that a patient may not report.

The frequency of testing will vary based on the stage of treatment, results of prior urine toxicology analyses, the clinician's concern over ongoing illicit drug use, and the patient's desire for monitoring. However, in the first year of treatment urine testing should rarely occur less than once per month.

Educating Office Staff

The extent of the need to educate office staff regarding the treatment of patients dependent on opioids will vary based on the level of training of the staff, their prior experience caring for patients with addictive disorders and/or patients receiving opioid agonist medications, and the extent of involvement they will have in the care of these patients. In general, office-based physicians should take the time to educate their staff regarding the rationale and logistics of office-based treatment before the introduction of this treatment model in their office. Items that should be addressed include information on the nature of dependence, medical disorders commonly co-occurring with the disorder, the role and duration of pharmacotherapy in the treatment of opioid dependence, the importance of maintaining patient's confidentiality, patient and provider expectations in the treatment plan, and the role of psychosocial counseling treatments. Contrary to expectations, office staff generally react favorably to the provision of care to patients dependent on opioids once they have had the chance to interact with these patients. It is useful to involve clinical personnel (e.g., nurses, nurse practitioners, physician assistants, pharmacists) in the training process if they will be involved in the care of patients dependent on opioids to ensure that the team has a similar level of understanding regarding treatment strategies.

Identifying Referral Resources for Medical and Psychiatric Comorbidities

As discussed elsewhere in this chapter, patients dependent on opioids have a high prevalence of comorbid medical (Sullivan and Fiellin 2004) and psychiatric (Brooner et al. 1997) conditions. Because of this, opioid treatment programs often provide on-site medical or psychiatric service, although these services are often limited because of fiscal and time constraints. Office-based treatment offers the opportunity for physicians to provide integrated care for substance use disorders and comorbid conditions. However, patients may manifest comorbidities that are beyond the expertise of their office-based provider and require referral for specialist care. Therefore, it is useful for office-based physicians to establish and maintain a list of physicians with expertise in the areas of hepatitis C, HIV, pain management, and psychiatry. Because these medical comorbidities often have distinctive presentations and interactions with opioid dependence it is desirable, although not imperative, that these consultants have experience in treating patients with substance use disorders.

Assuring Reimbursement for the Necessary Components of Care

Payment for substance abuse treatment services can vary considerably from one country to the next. Services may be covered by governmental agencies or private insurance companies, require the patient to pay themselves, or have some combination of these sources. For office-based treatment of opioid dependence, the range of services that must be covered by some form of payment includes physician office visits, medication, laboratory analyses, urine toxicology tests, and psychosocial counseling services. The extent to which these services are covered by insurance depends on the insurance type (public versus private) and the comprehensiveness of the plan. For instance, although some insurance plans will provide reimbursement for physician office visits and medication, there may be a limit on the duration of care that is covered, a ceiling or limitation on the medication dose, or no reimbursement for additional counseling services. Finally, reimbursements and policies may vary based on the training of the provider (e.g., primary care versus psychiatry versus addiction specialist), the billing codes that are used, and the location of care.

Paying for substance abuse treatment makes sense (see chap. 2 for a more extensive discussion of the costs and benefits of substance abuse treatment). Cost-benefit projections were made with the introduction of buprenorphine for treatment of opioid dependence (Barnett et al. 2001).

Allowing for the prevalence of HIV in the community in which buprenorphine is used, the possible cost for the medication, and the potential impact of buprenorphine on methadone treatment, this model found buprenorphine was cost effective. Similarly, an assessment of buprenorphine's economic impact when used in office-based treatment for opioid dependence found that it would be cost effective, especially if it was able to attract into treatment patients with high costs to society (e.g., multiple detoxifications, criminal activity) (Rosenheck and Kosten 2001).

Whereas payment for substance abuse treatment, and OBOT specifically, may vary between countries and even within countries, the multiple benefits associated with treatment suggest that providing payment for these services makes good economic and especially clinical sense. In certain parts of the world (e.g., France), payment for OBOT is readily available and utilized. In other parts of the world (e.g., the United States), a more patchwork system exists, and better reimbursement systems must be developed. In other parts of the world (e.g., certain third-world countries), health care systems provide essentially no coverage for addictions treatment. Advocating for expansion of services and equitable financing of care for the treatment of substance abuse disorders, including those provided in office-based treatment, is imperative.

Summary and Conclusions

Office-based treatment for opioid dependence provides a unique opportunity to increase treatment access for a large number of patients dependent on opioids who may otherwise not receive care. Office-based treatment can be provided with methadone (e.g., in the United Kingdom and, under special regulations, in the United States) or buprenorphine (in many countries). The advent of this treatment modality provides an opportunity to mainstream the treatment of addictive disorders into routine medical practice, appears to have been met with general acceptance and a level of service that is parallel to other forms of medical treatment, and has significant public health benefits.

Implementation of office-based practice requires attention to a limited number of standard components of care that closely parallel services provided for other chronic medical conditions, including ongoing monitoring, attention to behavioral components of treatment, specialized staff training, referral for comorbid conditions, and negotiation for appropriate reimbursement. The use of office-based treatment for opioid dependence is an important component in the practice of medicine, and its utilization should enable practicing physicians to improve the lives of a large number of deserving patients.

References

Auriacombe M, Fatseas M, Dubernet J, Daulouede JP, Tignol J (2004). French field experience with buprenorphine. *Am J Addict* 13 Suppl 1: S17–S28

Auriacombe M, Franques P, Tignol J (2001). Deaths attributable to methadone vs buprenorphine in France. *JAMA* 285: 45.

Barnett PG, Zaric GS, Brandeau ML (2001). The cost-effectiveness of buprenorphine maintenance therapy for opiate addiction in the United States. *Addiction* 96: 1267–78.

Bennett T, Wright R (1986). Opioid users' attitudes towards and use of NHS clinics, general practitioners and private doctors. *Br J Addict* 81: 757–63.

Bouchez J, Vignau J (1998). The French experience—the pharmacist, general practitioner and patient perspective. *Eur Addict Res* 4: 19–23.

Brooner RK, King VL, Kidorf M, Schmidt CW, Jr., Bigelow GE (1997). Psychiatric and substance use comorbidity among treatment-seeking opioid abusers. *Arch Gen Psychiatry* 54: 71–80.

Davies A, Huxley P (1997). Survey of general practitioners' opinions on treatment of opiate users. *BMJ* 314: 1173–4.

Des Jarlais DC, Joseph H, Dole VP, Nyswander ME (1985). Medical maintenance feasibility study. *NIDA Res Monogr* 58: 101–10.

Dole, V. P. (1971). Methadone maintenance treatment for 25,000 heroin addicts. *JAMA* 215: 1131–4.

Fiellin DA, Barthwell AG (2003). Guideline development for office-based pharmacotherapies for opioid dependence. *J Addict Dis* 22: 109–20.

Fiellin DA, O'Connor PG (2002). New federal initiatives to enhance the medical treatment of opioid dependence. *Ann Intern Med* 137: 688–92.

Fiellin DA, O'Connor PG, Chawarski M, Pakes JP, Pantalon MV, Schottenfeld RS (2001). Methadone maintenance in primary care: a randomized controlled trial. *JAMA* 286: 1724–31.

Fiellin DA, O'Connor PG, Chawarski M, Schottenfeld RS (2004). Processes of care during a randomized trial of office-based treatment of opioid dependence in primary care. *Am J Addict* 13 Suppl 1: S67–S78.

Fiellin DA, Pantalon MV, Pakes JP, O'Connor PG, Chawarski M, Schottenfeld RS (2002). Treatment of heroin dependence with buprenorphine in primary care. *Am J Drug Alcohol Abuse* 28: 231–41.

Fudala PJ, Bridge TP, Herbert S, Williford WO, Chiang CN, Jones K, Collins J, Raisch D, Casadonte P, Goldsmith RJ, Ling W, Malkerneker U, McNicholas L, Renner J, Stine S, Tusel D (2003). Office-based treatment of opiate addiction with a sublingual-tablet formulation of buprenorphine and naloxone. *N Engl J Med* 349: 949–58.

Galanter M, Dermatis H, Resnick R, Maslansky R, Neumann E (2003). Short-term buprenorphine maintenance: treatment outcome. *J Addict Dis* 22: 39–49.

Gibson AE, Doran CM, Bell JR, Ryan A, Lintzeris N (2003). A comparison of buprenorphine treatment in clinic and primary care settings: a randomised trial. *Med J Aust* 179: 38–42.

Gossop M, Marsden J, Stewart D, Lehmann P, Strang J (1999). Methadone treatment practices and outcome for opiate addicts treated in drug clinics and in general practice: results from the National Treatment Outcome Research Study. *Br J Gen Pract* 49: 31–4.

Hindler C, Nazareth I, King M, Cohen J, Farmer R, Gerada C (1995). Drug users' views on general practitioners. *BMJ* 310: 302.

Keen J, Oliver P, Mathers N (2002). Methadone maintenance treatment can be provided in a primary care setting without increasing methadone-related mortality: the Sheffield experience 1997–2000. *Br J Gen Pract* 52: 387–9.

Keen J, Oliver P, Rowse G, Mathers N (2003). Does methadone maintenance treatment based on the new national guidelines work in a primary care setting? *Br J Gen Pract* 53: 461–7.

Keen J, Rowse G, Mathers N, Campbell M, Seivewright N (2000). Can methadone maintenance for heroin-dependent patients retained in general practice reduce criminal conviction rates and time spent in prison? *Br J Gen Pract* 50: 48–9.

King VL, Stoller KB, Hayes M, Umbricht A, Currens M, Kidorf MS, Carter JA, Schwartz R, Brooner RK (2002). A multicenter randomized evaluation of methadone medical maintenance. *Drug Alcohol Depend* 65: 137–48.

Kreek MJ, Vocci FJ (2002). History and current status of opioid maintenance treatments: blending conference session. *J Subst Abuse Treat* 23: 93–105.

Matheson C, Bond CM, Hickey F (1999). Prescribing and dispensing for drug misusers in primary care: current practice in Scotland. *Fam Pract* 16: 375–9.

McBride AJ, Mali I, Atkinson R (1994). Supervised administration of methadone by pharmacists. *BMJ* 309: 1234.

McCarthy J (1994). Quantitative urine drug monitoring in methadone programs: potential clinical uses. *J Psychoactive Drugs* 26: 199–206.

McLellan AT, Arndt IO, Metzger DS, Woody GE, O'Brien CP (1993). The effects of psychosocial services in substance abuse treatment. *JAMA* 269: 1953–9.

McNicholas L (2004). Clinical guidelines for the use of buprenorphine in the treatment of opioid addiction. Rockville, MD: U.S. Department of Health and Human Services.

Mitcheson M (1994). Drug clinics in the 1970s. In: Strang J, Gossop M, eds. *Heroin Addiction and Drug Policy: The British System*, 178–91. Oxford: Oxford University Press.

Moatti JP, Souville M, Escaffre N, Obadia Y (1998). French general practitioners' attitudes toward maintenance drug abuse treatment with buprenorphine. *Addiction* 93: 1567–75.

Novick DM, Joseph H (1991). Medical maintenance: the treatment of chronic opiate dependence in general medical practice. *J Subst Abuse Treat* 8: 233–9.

Novick DM, Joseph H, Salsitz EA, Kalin MF, Keefe JB, Miller EL, Richman BL (1994). Outcomes of treatment of socially rehabilitated methadone maintenance patients in physicians' offices (medical maintenance): follow-up at three and a half to nine and a fourth years. *J Gen Intern Med* 9: 127–30.

Novick DM, Pascarelli EF, Joseph H, Salsitz EA, Richman BL, Des Jarlais DC, Anderson M, Dole VP, Nyswander ME (1988). Methadone maintenance patients in general medical practice. A preliminary report. *JAMA* 259: 3299–3302.

O'Connor PG, Oliveto AH, Shi JM, Triffleman E, Carroll KM, Kosten TR, Rounsaville BJ (1996). A pilot study of primary-care-based buprenorphine maintenance for heroin dependence. *Am J Drug Alcohol Abuse* 22: 523–31.

O'Connor PG, Oliveto AH, Shi JM, Triffleman EG, Carroll KM, Kosten TR, Rounsaville BJ, Pakes JA, Schottenfeld RS (1998). A randomized trial of buprenorphine maintenance for heroin dependence in a primary care clinic for substance users versus a methadone clinic. *Am J Med* 105: 100–5.

Obadia Y, Perrin V, Feroni I, Vlahov D, Moatti JP (2001). Injecting misuse of buprenorphine among French drug users. *Addiction* 96: 267–72.

Preston A, Campion-Smith C (1997). General practitioners' attitudes towards treatment of opiate misusers. Education may make general practitioners feel more confident [letter; comment]. *BMJ* 315: 601–2.

Resnick RB, Galanter M, Resnick E, Pycha C (2001). Buprenorphine treatment of heroin dependence (detoxification and maintenance) in a private practice setting. *J Addict Dis* 20: 75–83.

Ritter AJ, Lintzeris N, Clark N, Kutin JJ, Bammer G, Panjari M (2003). A randomized trial comparing levo-alpha acetylmethadol with methadone maintenance for patients in primary care settings in Australia. *Addiction* 98: 1605–13.

Rosenheck R, Kosten T (2001). Buprenorphine for opiate addiction: potential economic impact. *Drug Alcohol Depend* 63: 253–62.

Salsitz EA, Joseph H, Frank B, Perez J, Richman BL, Salomon N, Kalin MF, Novick DM (2000). Methadone medical maintenance (MMM): treating chronic opioid dependence in private medical practice—a summary report (1983–1998). *Mt Sinai J Med* 67: 388–97.

Schwartz RP, Brooner RK, Montoya ID, Currens M, Hayes M (1999). A 12-year follow-up of a methadone medical maintenance program. *Am J Addict* 8: 293–9.

Scott R, McNulty H (1996). Community pharmacists are increasingly supervising treatments. *BMJ* 313: 945.

Scott RT, Burnett SJ, McNutty H (1994). Supervised administration of methadone by pharmacists. *BMJ* 308: 1438.

Senay EC, Barthwell AG, Marks R, Bokos P, Gillman D, White R (1993). Medical maintenance: a pilot study. *J Addict Dis* 12: 59–76.

Strain EC, Clarke HW, Auriacombe M, Lagier G, Mallaret M, Thirion X (2003). French experience with buprenorphine. *NIDA Res Monogr* 183: 134–41.

Strang J, Gossop M (1994). *Heroin Addiction and Drug Policy: the British System.* Oxford: Oxford University Press.

Strang J, Sheridan J (1998). Effect of government recommendations on methadone prescribing in South East England: comparison of 1995 and 1997 surveys. *BMJ* 317: 1489–90.

Strang J, Sheridan J (2003). Effect of national guidelines on prescription of methadone: analysis of NHS prescription data, England 1990–2001. *BMJ* 327: 321–2.

Strang J, Sheridan J, Barber N (1996). Prescribing injectable and oral methadone to opiate addicts: results from the 1995 national postal survey of community pharmacies in England and Wales. *BMJ* 313: 270–2.

Sullivan LE, Fiellin DA (2004). Hepatitis C and HIV infections: implications for clinical care in injection drug users. *Am J Addict* 13: 1–20.

Telfer I, Clulow C (1990). Heroin misusers: what they think of their general practitioners. *Br J Addict* 85: 137–40.

Thirion X, Lapierre V, Micallef J, Ronfle E, Masut A, Pradel V, Coudert C, Mabriez JC, Sanmarco JL (2002). Buprenorphine prescription by general practitioners in a French region. *Drug Alcohol Depend* 65: 197–204.

Umbricht-Schneiter A, Ginn DH, Pabst KM, Bigelow GE (1994). Providing medical care to methadone clinic patients: referral vs on-site care. *Am J Public Health* 84: 207–10.

Vidal-Trecan G, Varescon I, Nabet N, Boissonnas A (2003). Intravenous use of prescribed sublingual buprenorphine tablets by drug users receiving maintenance therapy in France. *Drug Alcohol Depend* 69: 175–81.

Vignau J, Duhamel A, Catteau J, Legal G, Pho AH, Grailles I, Beauvillain J, Petit P, Beauvillain P, Parquet PJ (2001). Practice-based buprenorphine maintenance treatment (BMT): how do French healthcare providers manage the opiate-addicted patients? *J Subst Abuse Treat* 21: 135–44.

Weinrich M, Stuart M (2000). Provision of methadone treatment in primary care medical practices: review of the Scottish experience and implications for US policy. *JAMA* 283: 1343–8.

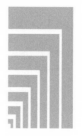

I3

Pharmacology and Clinical Use of LAAM, Clonidine, and Lofexidine

Eric C. Strain, M.D.

Although three medications are generally available and approved by various governmental agencies for the treatment of opioid dependence (methadone, buprenorphine, and naltrexone), three other medications have been shown to have utility in some aspect of the treatment of this disorder. The first of these, levomethadyl acetate (also called L-alpha-acetyl-methadol or LAAM), is not marketed for the treatment of opioid dependence at the time of this writing. However, it is possible that a pharmaceutical company could resume sales of LAAM, and information about it is provided here for both historical purposes and in case it does become available again. The other two medications are clonidine and lofexidine, two alpha$_2$-adrenergic agonists that are used for the acute treatment of opioid withdrawal. Clonidine is approved and used primarily for the treatment of hypertension but has also been studied extensively for symptomatic treatment during opioid detoxification, although it is not approved for this indication. Lofexidine, a compound related to clonidine, is approved for the use of opioid withdrawal in some European countries. This chapter reviews each of these three medications, providing an overview of their pharmacologic characteristics and summaries of their safety, efficacy, and guidelines for clinical use.

L-Alpha-acetylmethadol (LAAM)

Initial interest in the development of LAAM for the treatment of opioid dependence occurred during the 1970s—a time when methadone treatment was rapidly expanding in the United States and being launched in several other countries. As methadone treatment became widely used, concerns arose that diversion of prescription methadone was leading to street trade of methadone take-home doses within the drug-abusing community. In addition, daily clinic attendance for methadone treatment was inconvenient for many patients, and it was hoped that a medication administered on a less-than-daily basis, such as LAAM, would help decrease the need for frequent clinic visits without increasing the risk of diversion of take-home doses. Even though considerable research on the safety and efficacy of LAAM was conducted in the 1970s, the approval process for LAAM languished during the 1980s. However, in the late 1980s there was renewed interest in gaining approval for the use of LAAM, and in 1993 LAAM was approved by the U.S. Food and Drug Administration (FDA) for the treatment of opioid dependence.

Use of LAAM was quite limited after its approval. In the United States, it was available only in the regulated methadone clinic system. Although precise numbers are not known, it is generally believed that there were less than 10,000 patients treated with LAAM at any given time in the United States and that use of LAAM had not had an impact on the expansion of treatment capacity.

In 1997, LAAM was approved for opioid dependence treatment in Europe. In March 2001, however, it was withdrawn from the European market following reports of ten cases of cardiac disorders observed in patients treated with LAAM. Seven of the patients had prolongation of the QTc interval, and three of the ten had a cardiac arrest associated with arrhythmia. In the United States, the FDA announced a label change for LAAM based on the risk of arrhythmias (Schwetz 2001) but did not withdraw the medication from the market. However, LAAM was subsequently withdrawn by the manufacturer in the first half of 2004 and became unavailable for use in treatment.

Pharmacology of LAAM

LAAM is a mu agonist opioid like methadone and, like other opioids, acute doses produce sedation and analgesia. The effects of LAAM last longer than those of methadone, however. In general, this longer duration has been attributed to the active metabolites nor-LAAM and dinor-LAAM

(Finkle et al. 1982; McMahon et al. 1965). It was originally reported that the onset of effects for intravenous LAAM is slower than for oral LAAM. It was believed that this delay was due to the time required for the active metabolites nor- and dinor-LAAM to be formed by the liver. However, other evidence suggests intravenous LAAM exerts direct bioactive effects with a much quicker onset than effects attributable solely to active metabolites (Walsh et al. 1998).

LAAM's Absorption, Distribution, and Excretion

LAAM has good oral bioavailability and is rapidly absorbed from the gastrointestinal tract. Considerable variability exists among individuals in the subsequent pharmacokinetics of LAAM, so generalizations regarding some effects may not reflect the profile of effects produced in a particular individual patient. After acute oral dosing, peak plasma concentrations of LAAM typically occur within 3 hours, and conversion of LAAM to nor-LAAM and dinor-LAAM begins rapidly after absorption of LAAM, with peak concentrations of nor-LAAM metabolites within 1 to 2 hours and of dinor-LAAM within 20 to 30 hours after peak blood levels of the parent compound are reached. LAAM is not converted directly to dinor-LAAM; rather, dinor-LAAM is converted from nor-LAAM (i.e., there is a sequential series of demethylations of the parent compound). The half-life for oral LAAM after an acute dose is about 0.5 to 1 day, for nor-LAAM it is about 1 to 2 days, and for dinor-LAAM it is about 3 to 4 days (although considerable individual variability in these half-lives can occur). The half-life for oral LAAM after chronic dosing is about 2.6 days, for nor-LAAM, about 2 days, and for dinor-LAAM, about 4 days (although, again, there can be considerable individual variability in these half-lives). Thus, the drug and its active metabolites remain in the body for prolonged periods. LAAM is excreted in both urine and feces, with a greater proportion via feces.

Efficacy of LAAM

The effects of LAAM were studied in both humans and animals during the 1950s and 1960s (Fraser and Isbell 1952; Keats and Beecher 1952; McMahon et al. 1965), but studies of LAAM for the treatment of opioid dependence were only begun in the early 1970s. Some of these studies were nonblind clinical trials (Freedman and Czertko 1981; Marcovici et al. 1981; Resnick et al. 1976; Senay et al. 1977; Taintor et al. 1975; Trueblood et al. 1978; Wilson et al. 1976; Zaks et al. 1972), whereas others were double-blind trials with small samples (Jaffe et al. 1970, 1972; Jaffe and Senay 1971; Karp-Gelernter et al. 1982; Savage et al. 1976). These studies demonstrated that, in general, LAAM was tolerated and similar to methadone in treatment efficacy.

In the mid-1970s, two large sample outpatient clinical trials of LAAM efficacy were conducted. The first of these was a double-blind, multisite veterans cooperative study comparing outcomes for patients maintained on LAAM (80 mg three times per week) with patients maintained on either 50 or 100 mg per day of methadone (Ling et al. 1976). The second study was an open (nonblind) multisite cooperative study that enrolled 636 patients receiving methadone maintenance who were randomly assigned to either continue on their methadone or switch to LAAM (Ling et al. 1978). Overall, these two studies demonstrated that LAAM and methadone were similar in terms of safety and efficacy.

Two more contemporary double-blind outpatient clinical trials have also demonstrated LAAM's efficacy. The first of these examined the relative efficacy of three different LAAM doses (Monday/Wednesday/Friday doses of 25/25/35, 50/50/70, or 100/100/140 mg) in the treatment of 180 opioid-dependent volunteers (Eissenberg et al. 1997). Results from the study showed dose-related differences in use of illicit opioids, with patients receiving higher LAAM doses having better outcomes. The second study compared four groups: (1) daily low-dose methadone, 2) daily high-dose methadone (both with take-home doses of methadone given four times per week to match clinic reporting frequency across all test medications), (3) thrice-weekly buprenorphine, and (4) thrice-weekly LAAM (Johnson et al. 2000). The study included a double-blind flexible dosing procedure so that doses were increased if clinically indicated, and an escape mechanism for participants who were doing poorly in their assigned condition. Compared to the low-dose methadone condition, volunteers in the other three groups had significantly better treatment retention and lower rates of opioid-positive urine samples. However, there were minimal differences between LAAM and the other two conditions (thrice-weekly buprenorphine and high-dose methadone).

These multiple clinical trials with LAAM show that it is an effective medication that can produce outcomes similar to methadone when comparable doses are used. Some of these early clinical studies also noted anecdotal patient reports that LAAM provides a more even subjective effect than methadone, but this possible medication difference has never been systematically investigated.

Safety and Side Effects of LAAM

LAAM is a full agonist at the mu opioid receptor, and side effects seen with LAAM are similar to those seen with other mu agonists. The multisite veterans cooperative study described previously included an extensive evaluation of LAAM's safety (Ling et al. 1976). No significant adverse events (e.g., deaths) occurred, and side effects were of low frequency and mild. In a study of 623 patients who received LAAM, the most commonly reported side effects were difficulty sleeping, constipation, sweating, and nervousness (Fudala et al. 1997). The frequency of serious adverse events reported in that study was quite low (41 in total), and the only one definitely related to LAAM resulted from a staff dosing error.

In a person who is not physically dependent on opioids, an acute dose of LAAM can produce the characteristic features of an opioid overdose, including respiratory depression and death if a high dose is ingested. Because LAAM's active metabolites remain in the body a long time, consumption of LAAM by a person who is not tolerant to the effects of opioids should be considered a medical emergency and monitoring should be continued for at least one to two days. If the administration of an opioid antagonist such as naloxone is required, repeat dosing may be necessary given the long duration of effect (i.e., respiratory depression) produced by LAAM's metabolites.

As noted previously, reports that LAAM was associated with prolongation of the QTc interval and potentially fatal arrhythmias led to its withdrawal from the European market and a change in the FDA label for the U.S. market. LAAM's effects on cardiac conduction are probably not unique to this opioid; there have been case reports of arrhythmias associated with high-dose methadone (Krantz et al. 2002). However, it is possible that LAAM has a greater propensity than other opioids for cardiac conduction abnormalities. If LAAM becomes available again for the treatment of opioid dependence, then electrocardiogram monitoring before and during LAAM maintenance would be indicated and is recommended on the U.S. approved label. Use of LAAM would be contraindicated if other medications that can prolong the QTc interval were being prescribed to a patient (e.g., certain psychotropics).

Clinical Use of LAAM

Induction

Few studies have directly examined the optimal schedule for starting a patient on LAAM. A clinical report of experience with a slow schedule

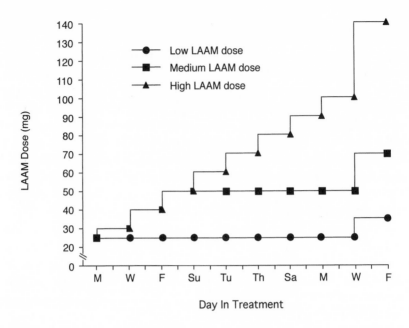

Figure 13.1. Examples of induction schedules for low-, medium-, and high-dose LAAM.

(doses of 20, 20, 30, 30, 40, 40, 50, 50, 60, 60, 70, 70, and 75 mg on each successive day of treatment with clinic visits occurring on Mondays, Wednesdays, and Fridays) versus a rapid schedule (doses of 20, 30, 40, 40, and 50 mg on successive days, again using a Monday, Wednesday, Friday schedule) concluded the rapid schedule was safe, well-tolerated, and preferred by patients (Judson and Goldstein 1979). Another report assessed the effectiveness and safety of LAAM during the first 28 days of induction after patients were assigned to one of three different fixed doses (fig. 13.1) (Jones et al. 1998). Dose assignments were 25 (low, $N = 62$), 50 (medium, $N = 59$), and 100 mg (high, $N = 59$) of LAAM. All patients were dependent on illicit opioids and received an initial 25-mg dose of LAAM. The patients assigned to the 50- and 100-mg LAAM groups received 30 mg of LAAM as their second dose, and then their dose was increased by 10 mg every other day until a dose of 50 or 100 mg was achieved. All doses of LAAM were well tolerated by most patients. The greatest number of dropouts, however, was in the high-dose group ($N = 15$ versus 8 and 8 in the medium- and low-dose groups, respectively), and half of these patients dropped out because of side effects that suggested overmedication. Illicit drug use decreased in all groups; however, patients in the high-dose induction group who remained in the study used illicit opiates less than patients in the low- and medium-dose groups. Patients in the high-dose group also reported less craving for heroin. Thus, high-dose LAAM induction is recommended for patients who can tolerate this level, but doses may need to be lower for patients who experience signs of overmedication.

For patients currently in methadone treatment, LAAM can provide a means to decrease the frequency of clinic visits without the risk of diversion of methadone take-home doses. When converting a patient from methadone to LAAM, it is recommended that the methadone dose be multiplied by a factor of 1.2 to 1.3 to determine the LAAM dose. Thus, a patient maintained on 50 mg per day of methadone would be given 60–65 mg of LAAM, with a compensatory increase on Fridays to allow for the longer interval between Friday and Monday doses (as described below). The transition from methadone to LAAM can be done on consecutive days—there is no need to taper the dose of methadone and gradually increase the dose of LAAM.

In summary, when scheduling LAAM induction, it is recommended that patients entering LAAM treatment directly from use of illicit opioids start at a dose of 30–40 mg. Based on clinical response, the dose can be increased 10 mg every other day during the induction period with little difficulty. It appears prudent, however, to increase the dose more slowly after a dose of 65–75 mg is achieved. For patients in methadone treatment, a direct transition to LAAM can be accomplished by using a LAAM dose that is 1.2–1.3 times the daily dose of methadone.

Maintenance on LAAM

Most research on maintenance dosing with LAAM has been conducted by using a thrice-weekly schedule—Monday/Wednesday/Friday—with a higher dose administered on Fridays to allow for the longer interdose interval between Friday and Monday. Typically, Friday doses are 20–40 percent greater than Monday/Wednesday doses. During the time the Friday dose is being adjusted for adequate coverage over the 72-hour period, it may be useful to use a small supplementary dose of methadone on Sunday to avoid opioid withdrawal symptoms. Nevertheless, some patients may continue to complain of withdrawal symptoms during the 72-hour dose omission period. For these patients, the LAAM dose may need to be administered on an every-other-day schedule, if possible. If this scheduling is impossible (i.e., the clinic is closed on weekends) the maximally recommended 40 percent increase in the Friday dose should be used. Chronic use of supplemental methadone is not recommended.

Patients maintained on LAAM should not receive a dose of LAAM every day; it is important to stress that LAAM is a medication that should be taken only every 48–72 hours. Dosing daily will result in a buildup of active metabolites of LAAM, and the person who consumes LAAM daily will experience a LAAM overdose.

Most patients can be maintained on a dose of 75 and 115 mg for the 48- and 72-hour dosing periods, respectively. Dosing of LAAM is complicated for patients who fail to take the medication as scheduled because of the long-acting metabolites. If one dosing day is missed, patients can receive their next regularly scheduled dose. If two consecutive dosing days are missed, patients may receive 50 percent of their maintenance dose upon returning to the clinic and then resume taking their regular dose at the next scheduled visit. If more than two dosing days are missed, however, patients can be reinducted onto their maintenance dose by receiving a dose that is approximately 50 percent of their scheduled dose and then increasing the dose by 10 mg at each subsequent clinic visit. If patients miss a dose, return to the clinic on a nonscheduled dosing day, and the clinician wishes to return them to their regular clinic attendance schedule, the clinician may give them a dose of methadone and resume their LAAM dosing the next day.

Discontinuation of LAAM

Few reports have been published on the optimal schedule for withdrawing a patient from LAAM. One double-blind study examined gradual versus abrupt LAAM detoxification (Judson et al. 1983). Patients in the study were randomly assigned either to an abrupt detoxification group that had their LAAM dose (50/50/65 mg on a Monday/Wednesday/Friday schedule) abruptly switched to placebo or to a gradual detoxification group that had their LAAM dose (also 50/50/65 mg on a Monday/Wednesday/Friday schedule) decreased over a 15-week period. The study results suggest that the abrupt discontinuation was no worse than the gradual detoxification and, depending on the approach used in the data summarization and analysis, could even be better. For example, total scores for self-reported opioid withdrawal and total opioid use based on urine tests both were greater for patients in the gradual detoxification group. The efficacy of rapid LAAM withdrawal may be due to the presence of the long-acting metabolites. The results from this study suggest that rapid withdrawal of LAAM can be clinically useful.

Summary of LAAM

LAAM is an effective medication for the treatment of opioid dependence, but its safety was questioned relatively early after its launch in Europe. In the United States, there are probably two reasons that it has not been used extensively: its limited availability through the methadone clinic system and the concerns about cardiac side effects (reinforced by its withdrawal from the European market and the change in the FDA label). Although the risk of cardiac conduction effects associated with using LAAM may be greater than that seen with methadone or buprenorphine, many other medications are used in medicine that can have significant side effects but are still available and helpful in relieving the suffering of patients. It is unfortunate that the field of addictions, with a very limited number of effective medications available, does not have LAAM as an option for the treatment of opioid dependence at this time.

CLONIDINE

Clonidine is a nonopioid medication that can be used for the treatment of opioid withdrawal symptoms. It is an alpha$_2$-adrenergic agonist agent that is available in several countries as an antihypertensive medication. In the United States its use in the treatment of opioid withdrawal is "off-label" (i.e., opioid withdrawal is not an FDA-approved indication). It seems that clonidine was more commonly used for the treatment of opioid withdrawal in the 1980s and 1990s, and this relatively common use was related, in part, to the belief (and some evidence) that it has a low abuse potential (Preston et al. 1985). This may not be a valid assumption, however, because there have also been several reports of clonidine abuse (Anderson et al. 1997; Beuger et al. 1998; Dennison 2001; Schaut and Schnoll 1983).

Pharmacology of Clonidine

There is a significant adrenergic/noradrenergic component to opioid withdrawal symptoms, which include increased heart rate and blood pressure, heightened reactivity to environmental stimuli, restlessness, and agitation. Furthermore, opioid withdrawal is accompanied by hyperactivity in the locus coeruleus, a site in the central nervous system that controls nora-drenergic function. Alpha$_2$-adrenergic agonist agents act on these central nervous system receptors to cause a decrease or dampening of noradren-ergic hyperactivity, which, in turn, results in a decrease in certain opioid withdrawal signs and symptoms.

Absorption, Distribution, and Excretion

Clonidine has good oral bioavailability, with a peak effect occurring 3–5 hours after oral ingestion and a half-life of 12–16 hours. It is primarily metabolized in the liver, although there is some renal clearance (and thus caution should be exercised when it is used in patients with impaired re-nal functioning). Clonidine is also available in transdermal patches, a highly convenient form of administration that greatly reduces the possi-bility of abuse.

Efficacy of Clonidine

Several reports and studies have examined the use of clonidine in the treat-ment of opioid withdrawal, especially as a bridging medication that might allow an opioid-dependent patient to detoxify and remain drug free for a sufficient time to be started on naltrexone without precipitating a with-drawal syndrome. In general, these studies have demonstrated that cloni-dine can effectively diminish signs of opioid withdrawal in a patient un-dergoing abrupt discontinuation of daily opioid use (Cami et al. 1985; Charney et al. 1981; Gold et al. 1978; Gossop 1988; Gowing et al. 2003). For example, Jasinski and colleagues (1985) stabilized opioid dependence in research volunteers living on a residential research unit by giving in-jections of morphine four times each day. When the injections were tem-porarily stopped, the volunteers experienced withdrawal symptoms. The study showed that clonidine was effective in decreasing signs and symp-toms of this spontaneous opioid withdrawal compared with placebo. Clonidine was more effective than morphine in suppressing autonomic signs of withdrawal (such as rhinorrhea and lacrimation), but morphine was more effective than clonidine in suppressing the subjective symptoms associated with withdrawal.

Another inpatient study compared buprenorphine with clonidine and showed that the two medications generally had similar efficacy during an inpatient withdrawal procedure, but that buprenorphine relieved with-drawal symptoms better early in treatment (Cheskin et al. 1994). Other studies have reported on the outpatient use of clonidine for the treatment of opioid withdrawal, including use in the form of patches, and found that clonidine can be effective even though success rates appear to be lower than those achieved when it is used on an inpatient basis (Fingerhood et al. 2001; Rounsaville et al. 1985; Spencer and Gregory 1989; Washton and Resnick 1980).

Safety and Side Effects of Clonidine

The primary concern associated with the use of clonidine in the treatment of opioid withdrawal is that patients may become hypotensive; patients treated with clonidine for opioid withdrawal frequently have significant decreases in both systolic and diastolic blood pressures (Cheskin et al. 1994; Gossop 1988). This is consistent with clonidine's primary use as an antihypertensive. In addition, some clinical trials using clonidine in the treatment of opioid withdrawal have reported sedation (Charney et al. 1981), whereas others have noted that patients have problems falling and staying asleep when receiving clonidine (Kleber et al. 1980). Dry mouth and constipation are two other side effects reportedly associated with clonidine use. Several of these side effects may be related to opioid withdrawal rather than clonidine use. Overall, the primary concern associated with clonidine use is the possibility of changes in blood pressure.

Clinical Use of Clonidine

For patients being treated on an outpatient basis, 0.1 mg of clonidine can be given orally as a first test dose on the first day, with close monitoring of blood pressure following this dose. If the first 0.1-mg dose is tolerated (i.e., no hypotension or other adverse effect, such as excessive sedation), then patients should receive this same dose of clonidine (0.1 mg) every 4–6 hours while awake, with the frequency of dosing based on withdrawal suppression and toleration of the medication. Typical dosing of clonidine is three times per day (i.e., a total of 0.3 mg on the first day for outpatients).

During the second day of outpatient treatment the dose of clonidine may be increased up to 0.2 mg, three times per day, depending on the balance between withdrawal suppression and hypotension. If needed, doses can be raised further on the third and fourth days, up to 0.3–0.4 mg, three times per day. Thus, after three to four days of clonidine treatment on an outpatient basis, a stable total daily dose of 0.6–1.2 mg per day should be achieved. This dose can be maintained for several days, if needed, or a dose reduction procedure can then be instituted. Doses should be decreased 0.1–0.2 mg per day, as tolerated. If the patient is experiencing sedation associated with clonidine, dose reductions should initially be for the daytime doses rather than the bedtime dose. Outpatients should be cautioned regarding the possibility of sedation associated with clonidine and should avoid activities such as driving if they experience such sedation.

If detoxification is being conducted on an outpatient basis, then under optimal circumstances supplies or prescriptions of clonidine should be given to a responsible, non-drug-abusing family member or friend of the patient (given the potential abuse of clonidine and the potential for hypotension if the patient inappropriately ingests extra clonidine). If an outpatient is given a supply of clonidine to manage him or herself, then limited amounts (e.g., enough for one to two days) should be given.

If detoxification is occurring on an inpatient unit, a more aggressive dosing schedule may be used, with doses increased over the first one to two days and withdrawal off clonidine accomplished within a week. Finally, if a patient is being concurrently treated for high blood pressure with other antihypertensives, clonidine should be used with particular caution because there may be an increased likelihood of hypotension.

LOFEXIDINE

Like clonidine, lofexidine is an alpha$_2$-adrenergic agonist. Although there was interest and considerable research on lofexidine's use as an antihypertensive during the 1980s, development of lofexidine for hypertension was eventually dropped because it was not as effective for this purpose as was clonidine. Renewed interest in the development of lofexidine for the treatment of opioid withdrawal was motivated, in part, by its lower side-effect profile when compared with clonidine. Lofexidine is not currently available in many countries, but it is available as "BritLofex" in the United Kingdom where it is approved for the treatment of opioid withdrawal.

Pharmacology of Lofexidine

The neurochemical rationale for use of lofexidine is essentially the same as that described for clonidine, and the pharmacology of lofexidine is very similar to clonidine's pharmacology.

Absorption, Distribution, and Excretion

Lofexidine also has good oral bioavailability, and peak plasma concentrations occur two to five hours after an oral dose. Elimination is primarily mediated through the renal system, and there appears to be considerable variability among people in the extent of the biotransformation of lofexidine prior to its excretion.

Efficacy of Lofexidine

Since the latter half of the 1990s, the number of studies testing the efficacy and safety of lofexidine for the treatment of opioid withdrawal has been a growing. Most of this work has been done in the United Kingdom, where lofexidine was approved for use in 1992. Use of it has grown steadily in the United Kingdom; for example, it is estimated that there were about 3,000 episodes of treatment with lofexidine in 1993, compared to more than 21,000 in 1999 (Strang et al. 1999).

There have been several reports of nonblind studies examining the efficacy of lofexidine (Akhurst 1999; Bearn et al. 1998; Brown and Fleming 1998; Gold et al. 1981; White et al. 2001), and seven double-blind, controlled studies involving lofexidine (table 13.1). Most of these studies have compared lofexidine with clonidine, although two have compared it with methadone. No double-blind studies comparing lofexidine to buprenorphine have been reported.

In general, these studies show that lofexidine is equally effective or perhaps even slightly more effective than clonidine for suppression of opioid withdrawal symptoms (table 13.1). Lofexidine also appears to produce outcomes similar to methadone when used for brief (ten-day) inpatient withdrawals, although only two studies have addressed these relative efficacies. Lofexidine produces fewer adverse effects than clonidine, however—especially less hypotension. This feature makes lofexidine a more attractive medication than clonidine for the treatment of opioid withdrawal.

Safety and Side Effects of Lofexidine

Although lofexidine produces less hypotension than clonidine at doses equally effective for withdrawal suppression, it is not devoid of hypotensive effects. Controlled studies of lofexidine have noted the need to withhold some doses of this medication because of low blood pressure. In a survey of lofexidine use for 1,074 opioid detoxifications conducted both on an inpatient and outpatient basis, the three most commonly reported

Table 13.1 Summary of Double-Blind Studies Comparing Lofexidine with an Active Control Condition

Study	Control Condition	Total Number of Patients	Study Design	Outcome
Bearn et al. 1996	M	86	Ten-day inpatient taper; maximum L dose: 2 mg/day	No difference in retention; slightly more withdrawal symptoms for L (especially days 3–7)
Kahn et al. 1997	C	28	Inpatient treatment up to 17 days; maximum daily dose: L, 1.8 mg; C, 0.9 mg	No difference in withdrawal symptoms between the two groups; less hypotension with L
Lin et al. 1997	C	80	Inpatient treatment up to 7 days; maximum daily dose: L, 1.6 mg; C, 0.6 mg	No difference in withdrawal symptoms between the two groups; significantly less hypotension with L
Carnwath and Hardman 1998	C	50	Outpatient treatment for 12 days; maximum daily dose: L, 1.6 mg; C, 0.8 mg	Nonsignificantly better treatment completion for L; C with more hypotension (requiring home visits)
Gerra et al. 2001	C	40	Three-day outpatient withdrawal with concurrent NTX induction	Lower withdrawal symptoms and less sedation, hypotension, and mood problems with L
Howells et al. 2001	M	74	Men in prison; 10-day taper; maximum daily dose: L, 2 mg; M, 30 mg	No difference in withdrawal symptoms between the two groups
Walsh et al. 2003	C	8	Within-subject laboratory study; examined attenuation of N-precipitated withdrawal	Neither C or L significantly altered N-precipitated withdrawal

Abbreviations: B, buprenorphine; C, clonidine; L, lofexidine; M, methadone; N, naloxone; NTX, naltrexone adverse events were dizziness (8.5%), hypotension (7.5%), and dry mouth (5.3%) (Akhurst 1999). Slightly more than one percent (1.4%) of these patients had lofexidine discontinued because of decreased blood pressure or heart rate. However, there was no comparison group in this report, so it is not possible to determine the specificity of these events for lofexidine.

Clinical Use

Lofexidine treatment can be initiated with an oral dose of 0.2 mg (given either two or three times per day, for a total daily dose of 0.4–0.6 mg on the first day). Doses of lofexidine can be increased over subsequent days, with a maximum total daily dose generally about 1.6 mg per day (i.e., 0.4 mg, four times per day). In the United Kingdom, total daily doses as high as 2.4 mg may be given. Dose reductions of 0.2 mg per day can then be made every day, as tolerated by the patient. A more rapid withdrawal (e.g., over five days) may be more effective than a longer withdrawal (e.g., ten days), although this has only been examined on an inpatient basis (Bearn et al. 1998).

Conclusions Regarding the Efficacy of Clonidine and Lofexidine

Research has shown that clonidine is clearly more effective than placebo in the treatment of opioid withdrawal and that it is at least as useful as opioid agonists for some outcome measures. In general, however, it seems that clonidine is better at suppressing the physiologic *signs* of opioid withdrawal than the subjective *symptoms* of withdrawal. At the clinical level, patients do not appear to be in withdrawal, but they may still complain they feel like they are in withdrawal. Lofexidine appears to be as effective as clonidine for the treatment of opioid withdrawal and to produce fewer adverse events. If available, it should be considered a useful option that supersedes clonidine for the treatment of opioid withdrawal. Several important areas need to be addressed regarding lofexidine, however, including its relative efficacy compared with other treatment medications and especially buprenorphine.

Summary

Each of the three medications reviewed in this chapter have attractive and unique features that make them useful in the treatment of opioid dependence. LAAM can be dosed intermittently, clonidine and lofexidine do not have the abuse potential of opioid agonists, and lofexidine is associated with a lower rate of hypotension than clonidine. Each also has liabilities, however. LAAM is not currently available because of the concern that it may have cardiotoxic effects. Clonidine can produce hypotension in some patients. Lofexidine is not available in most countries and has been studied on a limited basis, especially compared with other opioid medications. Despite these liabilities, it would be valuable if clinicians had each of these medications available for use, because treatment providers and patients would benefit from having a choice of medications that would allow for clinical tailoring to patient characteristics and needs.

References

Akhurst JS (1999). The use of lofexidine by drug dependency units in the United Kingdom. *Eur Addict Res* 5: 43–49.

Anderson F, Paluzzi P, Lee J, Huggins G, Svikis D (1997). Illicit use of clonidine in opiate-abusing pregnant women. *Obstet Gynecol* 90: 790–4.

Bearn J, Gossop M, Strang J (1998). Accelerated lofexidine treatment regimen compared with conventional lofexidine and methadone treatment for in-patient opiate detoxification. *Drug Alcohol Depend* 50: 227–32.

Beuger M, Tommasello A, Schwartz R, Clinton M (1998). Clonidine use and abuse among methadone program applicants and patients. *J Subst Abuse Treat* 15: 589–93.

Brown AS, Fleming PM (1998). A naturalistic study of home detoxification from opiates using lofexidine. *J Psychopharmacol* 12: 93–96.

Cami J, de Torres S, San L, Sole A, Guerra D, Ugena B (1985). Efficacy of clonidine and of methadone in the rapid detoxification of patients dependent on heroin. *Clin Pharmacol Ther* 38: 336–41.

Charney DS, Sternberg DE, Kleber HD, Heninger GR, Redmond DE, Jr. (1981). The clinical use of clonidine in abrupt withdrawal from methadone. Effects on blood pressure and specific signs and symptoms. *Arch Gen Psychiatry* 38: 1273–7.

Cheskin LJ, Fudala PJ, Johnson RE (1994). A controlled comparison of buprenorphine and clonidine for acute detoxification from opioids. *Drug Alcohol Depend* 36: 115–21.

Dennison SJ (2001). Clonidine abuse among opiate addicts. *Psychiatr Q* 72: 191–5.

Eissenberg T, Bigelow GE, Strain EC, Walsh SL, Brooner RK, Stitzer ML, Johnson RE (1997). Dose-related efficacy of levomethadyl acetate for treatment of opioid dependence. A randomized clinical trial. *JAMA* 277: 1945–51.

Fingerhood MI, Thompson MR, Jasinski DR (2001). A comparison of clonidine and buprenorphine in the outpatient treatment of opiate withdrawal. *Subst Abus* 22: 193–99.

Finkle BS, Jennison TA, Chinn DM, Ling W, Holmes ED (1982). Plasma and urine disposition of 1-alpha-acetylmethadol and its principal metabolites in man. *J Anal Toxicol* 6: 100–5.

Fraser HF, Isbell H (1952). Actions and addiction liabilities of alpha-acetyl-methadols in man. *J Pharmacol Exp Ther* 105: 458–65.

Freedman RR, Czertko G (1981). A comparison of thrice weekly LAAM and daily methadone in employed heroin addicts. *Drug Alcohol Depend* 8: 215–22.

Fudala PJ, Vocci F, Montgomery A, Trachtenberg AI (1997). Levomethadyl acetate (LAAM) for the treatment of opioid dependence: a multisite, open-label study of LAAM safety and an evaluation of the product labeling and treatment regulations. *J Maintenance Addict* 1: 9–39.

Gold MS, Pottash AC, Sweeney DR, Extein I, Annitto WJ (1981). Opiate detoxification with lofexidine. *Drug Alcohol Depend* 8: 307–15.

Gold MS, Redmond DE, Jr., Kleber HD (1978). Clonidine blocks acute opiate-withdrawal symptoms. *Lancet* 2: 599–602.

Gossop M (1988). Clonidine and the treatment of the opiate withdrawal syndrome. *Drug Alcohol Depend* 21: 253–9.

Gowing L, Farrell M, Ali R, White J (2003). Alpha$_2$ adrenergic agonists for the management of opioid withdrawal. *Cochrane Database Syst Rev* 2: CD002024.

Jaffe JH, Schuster CR, Smith BB, Blachley PH (1970). Comparison of acetylmethadol and methadone in the treatment of long-term heroin users. A pilot study. *JAMA* 211: 1834–6.

Jaffe JH, Senay EC (1971). Methadone and l-methadyl acetate. Use in management of narcotics addicts. *JAMA* 216: 1303–5.

Jaffe JH, Senay EC, Schuster CR, Renault PR, Smith B, DiMenza S (1972). Methadyl acetate vs methadone. A double-blind study in heroin users. *JAMA* 222: 437–42.

Jasinski DR, Johnson RE, Kocher TR (1985). Clonidine in morphine withdrawal. Differential effects on signs and symptoms. *Arch Gen Psychiatry* 42: 1063–6.

Johnson RE, Chutuape MA, Strain EC, Walsh SL, Stitzer ML, Bigelow GE (2000). A comparison of levomethadyl acetate, buprenorphine, and methadone for opioid dependence. *N Engl J Med* 343: 1290–7.

Jones HE, Strain EC, Bigelow GE, Walsh SL, Stitzer ML, Eissenberg T, Johnson RE (1998). Induction with levomethadyl acetate: safety and efficacy. *Arch Gen Psychiatry* 55: 729–36.

Judson BA, Goldstein A (1979). Levo-alpha-acetylmethadol (LAAM) in the treatment of heroin addicts. I. Dosage schedule for induction and stabilization. *Drug Alcohol Depend* 4: 461–6.

Judson BA, Goldstein A, Inturrisi CE (1983). Methadyl acetate (LAAM) in the treatment of heroin addicts. II. Double-blind comparison of gradual and abrupt detoxification. *Arch Gen Psychiatry* 40: 834–40.

Karp-Gelernter E, Savage C, McCabe OL (1982). Evaluation of clinic attendance schedules for LAAM and methadone: a controlled study. *Int J Addict* 17: 805–13.

Keats AS, Beecher HK (1952). Analgesic activity and toxic effects of acetylmethadol isomers in man. *J Pharmacol Exp Ther* 105: 210–5.

Kleber HD, Gold MS, Riordan CE (1980). The use of clonidine in detoxification from opiates. *Bull Narc* 32: 1–10.

Krantz MJ, Lewkowiez L, Hays H, Woodroffe MA, Robertson AD, Mehler PS (2002). Torsade de pointes associated with very-high-dose methadone. *Ann Intern Med* 137: 501–4.

Ling W, Charuvastra C, Kaim SC, Klett CJ (1976). Methadyl acetate and methadone as maintenance treatments for heroin addicts. A veterans administration cooperative study. *Arch Gen Psychiatry* 33: 709–20.

Ling W, Klett CJ, Gillis RD (1978). A cooperative clinical study of methadyl acetate. I. Three-times-a-week regimen. *Arch Gen Psychiatry* 35: 345–53.

Marcovici M, O'Brien CP, McLellan AT, Kacian J (1981). A clinical, controlled study of l-alpha-acetylmethadol in the treatment of narcotic addiction. *Am J Psychiatry* 138: 234–6.

McMahon RE, Culp HW, Marshall FJ (1965). The metabolism of alpha-dl-acetylmethadol in the rat: the identification of the probable active metabolite. *J Pharmacol Exp Ther* 149: 436–45.

Preston KL, Bigelow GE, Liebson IA (1985). Self-administration of clonidine, oxazepam, and hydromorphone by patients undergoing methadone detoxification. *Clin Pharmacol Ther* 38: 219–27.

Resnick RB, Orlin L, Geyer G, Schuyten-Resnick E, Kestenbaum RS, Freedman AM (1976). l-Alpha-acetylmethadol (LAAM): prognostic considerations. *Am J Psychiatry* 133: 814–9.

Rounsaville BJ, Kosten T, Kleber H (1985). Success and failure at outpatient opioid detoxification. Evaluating the process of clonidine- and methadone-assisted withdrawal. *J Nerv Ment Dis* 173: 103–10.

Savage C, Karp EG, Curran SF, Hanlon TE, McCabe OL (1976). Methadone/LAAM maintenance: a comparison study. *Compr Psychiatry* 17: 415–24.

Schaut J, Schnoll SH (1983). Four cases of clonidine abuse. *Am J Psychiatry* 140: 1625–7.

Schwetz BA (2001). From the Food and Drug Administration. *JAMA* 285: 2705.

Senay EC, Dorus W, Renault PF (1977). Methadyl acetate and methadone. An open comparison. *JAMA* 237: 138–42.

Spencer L, Gregory M (1989). Clonidine transdermal patches for use in outpatient opiate withdrawal. *J Subst Abuse Treat* 6: 113–7.

Strang J, Bearn J, Gossop M (1999). Lofexidine for opiate detoxification: review of recent randomised and open controlled trials. *Am J Addict* 8: 337–48.

Taintor Z, Hough G, Plumb M, Murphy BF (1975). l-alpha-acetylmethadol and methadone in Buffalo: safety and efficacy. *Am J Drug Alcohol Abuse* 2: 317–30.

Trueblood B, Judson BA, Goldstein A (1978). Acceptability of methadyl acetate (LAAM) as compared with methadone in a treatment program for heroin addicts. *Drug Alcohol Depend* 3: 125–32.

Walsh SL, Johnson RE, Cone EJ, Bigelow GE (1998). Intravenous and oral l-alpha-acetylmethadol: pharmacodynamics and pharmacokinetics in humans. *J Pharmacol Exp Ther* 285: 71–82.

Walsh SL, Strain EC, Bigelow GE (2003). Evaluation of the effects of lofexidine and clonidine on naloxone-precipitated withdrawal in opioid-dependent humans. *Addiction* 98: 427–39.

Washton AM, Resnick RB (1980). Clonidine for opiate detoxification: outpatient clinical trials. *Am J Psychiatry* 137: 1121–2.

White R, Alcorn R, Feinmann C (2001). Two methods of community detoxification from opiates: an open-label comparison of lofexidine and buprenorphine. *Drug Alcohol Depend* 65: 77–83.

Wilson BK, Spannagel V, Thomson CP (1976). The use of l-alpha-acetylmethadol in treatment of heroin addiction: an open study. *Int J Addict* 11: 1091–1100.

Zaks A, Fink M, Freedman AM (1972). Levomethadyl in maintenance treatment of opiate dependence. *JAMA* 220: 811–3.

I4

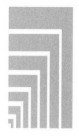

Pharmacology and Clinical Use of Naltrexone

Maria A. Sullivan, M.D., Ph.D., Sandra D. Comer, Ph.D., and Edward V. Nunes, M.D.

Naltrexone, an orally bioavailable antagonist at opiate receptors, is indicated for the treatment of opiate dependence. In recent years, it has shown efficacy and has been approved for the treatment of alcohol dependence as well. Conceptually, naltrexone is an ideal pharmacotherapy for opiate dependence because it blocks the effects of opiates but is not a controlled substance and has no euphoric agonist effects. As a clinical treatment, however, it has had only limited usefulness because of poor compliance, including high treatment dropout rates. Use of the medication has been applied most successfully in narrow populations of highly motivated patients, such as professionals at risk of losing their professional licenses or probationers at risk of returning to jail.

Naltrexone has been cited as an example of a treatment with strong theoretical potential but limited practical effectiveness in clinical use. However, renewed efforts in the past decade to improve the clinical effectiveness and usefulness of naltrexone have begun to bear fruit. These include adapting contemporary behavioral therapy methods to improve compliance with oral naltrexone and the development of long-acting depot injections of naltrexone, which circumvents the problem of patients stopping the oral medication and relapsing to heroin use. In view of these efforts, naltrexone remains an important part of the therapeutic armamentarium and an important alternative to agonist maintenance or drug-free methods for the treatment of opiate dependence. It is likely to find application in a more broad population of patients dependent on opioids in the future.

PHARMACOLOGY

Pharmacologic Effects

Naltrexone was one of many compounds synthesized after World War II in an effort to produce safer and more effective opiate analgesics. It consists of several simple modifications of the basic morphine molecular structure, similar to modifications that have been used to produce other partial agonists or mixed agonist-antagonist drugs including buprenorphine and naloxone. Naltrexone itself produces little or no psychoactive effect in normal research volunteers even at high doses, which is remarkable given that the endogenous opioid system is important in normal hedonic functioning. Because endogenous opioids are involved in the brain reward system, it would be reasonable to hypothesize that naltrexone might produce anhedonic or dysphoric effects. Although some evidence from small, early trials suggested that patients with a history of opiate dependence might be susceptible to dysphoric effects in response to naltrexone (Crowley et al. 1985; Hollister et al. 1981), reports of such effects have been inconsistent. Most large clinical studies of recovering opioid-dependent individuals have not found naltrexone to have an adverse effect on mood (Greenstein et al. 1984; Malcolm et al. 1987; Miotto et al. 2002; Shufman et al. 1994). Some studies have actually found improvements in mood during the course of treatment with naltrexone (Miotto et al. 1997; Rawlins and Randall 1976).

Naltrexone functions as a competitive antagonist at all three major opioid receptor types: mu, delta, and kappa (Gutstein and Akil 2001), and precipitates withdrawal in patients dependent on opioids because it competes with opiate agonists for receptor sites and produces a sudden net reduction in opiate agonist effect. The risk of naltrexone-precipitated withdrawal has implications for patient eligibility and induction methods, topics that are covered later in the chapter.

The major therapeutic feature of naltrexone pharmacology that makes it useful for the treatment of opiate dependence is that when occupying receptors, it completely blocks the effects of opiate agonists that might be taken. Because the interaction at opioid receptors is competitive, it is possible to override the blockade. For example, patients needing acute pain relief who are taking naltrexone can be treated with high doses of a short-acting opiate analgesic to override the competitive antagonism produced by naltrexone (O'Brien and Kampman 2004). Attempts by opiate-abusing patients to override the blockade, though a theoretical concern, have not emerged as a common problem clinically (see Behavioral Pharmacology section).

Pharmacokinetics

Naltrexone, taken orally, is rapidly absorbed from the gut and reaches peak blood levels after about one hour. It is metabolized by both liver and kidney, and the parent compound has a half-life of approximately four hours. The major active metabolite is 6-beta-naltrexol, which is also an active opiate antagonist and has approximately a 13-hour half-life in plasma. A single 50-mg dose produces a peak blood level of approximately 10 ng/ml, and blood levels can be expected to fall below 2 ng/ml by 24 hours (Meyer et al. 1984; Wall et al. 1981). Both acute and chronic administration of 100 mg of oral naltrexone produce peak plasma levels of approximately 45 ng/ml at one hour, which declines to 2 ng/ml at 24 hours, suggesting that naltrexone does not accumulate in plasma after chronic treatment (Verebey et al. 1976). Note, however, that disappearance of the drug from blood plasma does not mean that the effects are gone, because the drug may still be present at receptors after blood levels have declined.

Behavioral Pharmacology

Blockade of the effects of opiate agonists after a single dose of 50 mg of naltrexone lasts for approximately 24 hours. If a 100- or 150-mg dose is given, evidence shows that the blockade will last 48–72 hours or longer (Navaratnam et al. 1994; Schuh et al. 1999; Verebey et al. 1976). These data support the clinical use of naltrexone in three weekly visits using doses of 100–150 mg. The dose of heroin needed to override the blockade produced by standard clinical doses of naltrexone is unknown. Yet one recent report showed that heroin doses as high as 500 mg were blocked by a naltrexone implant that produced plasma levels of 2.8 ng/ml naltrexone and 9.0 ng/ml 6-beta-naltrexol (Brewer 2002). Given that a typical $10 street bag of heroin in the United States contains roughly 20 mg of heroin, it appears that the doses of oral naltrexone currently used in clinical practice will provide more than adequate blockade of commonly used street doses of heroin. Also, doses a low as 12.5 mg can provide very good blockade under some circumstances (Schuh et al. 1999).

Several preclinical studies have demonstrated that blockade of opioid receptors for as little as 8 days produces an increase in the density of opioid-binding sites (Unterwald et al. 1995; Yoburn et al. 1986; Zernig et al. 1994). Consistent with the increased binding, both the analgesic potency and toxicity of morphine were increased in rodents who had been implanted with naltrexone pellets for 8 days (Yoburn et al. 1986). These data have implications for individuals maintained on naltrexone in that they may be at increased risk of heroin overdose after discontinuing treatment if they choose to use opioids again (Miotto et al. 1997). Overdoses have been reported after discontinuing naltrexone (discussed in detail below), but one laboratory study designed to examine whether changes in sensitivity to opioid effects occur after discontinuation of naltrexone administration observed no increases (Cornish et al. 1993).

Maintenance Treatment of Patients Dependent on Opioids: Early Clinical Trials

Effectiveness

Early clinical trials of naltrexone in general populations of patients dependent on opioids were relatively discouraging. Dropout rates were very high, and few patients completed more than 30–60 days of treatment (Azatian et al. 1994; Callahan et al. 1980; Kosten and Kleber 1984). These poor results can be attributed to the fact that oral naltrexone maintenance requires rigid compliance to daily ingestion of the medication, and naltrexone treatment is "a one-way street," in that once the medication is stopped and a patient resumes regular opiate use, it is usually not possible to restart the naltrexone without precipitating withdrawal. A more recent randomized clinical trial conducted in Iran (Ahmadi et al. 2003) provides more contemporary evidence for poorer treatment outcome of naltrexone than agonist maintenance in a 24-week comparison between naltrexone (50 mg per day), sublingual buprenorphine (5 mg per day), and methadone (50 mg per day). The study enrolled 204 patients dependent on illicit intravenous buprenorphine. The rate of treatment completion was 21 percent in the group assigned to naltrexone compared with 59 percent for those assigned to buprenorphine and 84 percent for those assigned to methadone. In an extensive review of 707 participants in naltrexone treatment trials, Kirchmayer and colleagues found insufficient evidence to justify the use of naltrexone as a maintenance treatment for opioid addicts (Kirchmayer et al. 2002).

Earlier clinical experience and trials did suggest greater compliance and effectiveness in highly motivated patients, such as professionals in jeopardy of losing their licenses (Washton et al. 1984) or patients in the parole and criminal justice systems at risk of returning to jail (Cornish et al. 1997). Another early study examined using voucher incentives to increase motivation for compliance with naltrexone (Grabowski et al. 1979). These studies did suggest considerable potential promise for naltrexone depending on appropriate environmental circumstances or behavioral interventions.

Safety

One major safety concern is the risk of precipitating opiate withdrawal by administering naltrexone to a patient who is already dependent on opiate agonists. Such precipitated withdrawal can be quite severe and unpleasant. Like other forms of opiate withdrawal, it is not usually dangerous in the medical sense, although dehydration may be substantial and vomiting may lead to aspiration. Delirium has occasionally been described anecdotally (Amraoui et al. 1999; Bell et al. 1999).

Another concern is the complication introduced if pain treatment is needed. Patients being treated with naltrexone should carry an identification card in their wallet indicating their medication status, or wear a medical alert bracelet. In the event of serious injury, or the need for treatment of severe acute pain or surgery, treating physicians will need to be aware that higher doses of opioid analgesics may be needed initially.

The third safety issue is liver toxicity. This issue has warranted close attention in light of the high rate of hepatitis in intravenous drug users and the possibility of hepatocellular injury caused by the medication. Several studies to date, however, have demonstrated that liver enzyme (transaminase) levels do not change significantly, even after daily administration of high doses of naltrexone (100–350 mg) (Brahen et al. 1988; Marrazzi et al. 1997; Sax et al. 1994) or during use of depot naltrexone (Comer et al. 2002). Alcoholics treated with naltrexone have actually shown liver enzyme decreases, presumably because they are drinking less alcohol (Kranzler et al. 1998; Volpicelli et al. 1997). Elevated liver enzymes typically occur only at doses greater than 300 mg per day when naltrexone is administered for several weeks; the elevation is a dose- and time-related phenomenon. It is reversible if the dose is lowered or if the medication is discontinued. As a result, liver enzyme monitoring is prudent during treatment with naltrexone and guidelines generally suggest that naltrexone should not be administered in patients with advanced liver disease (O'Brien and Cornish 1999). In a recent review of the literature, however, Brewer and Wong found no evidence that naltrexone, even at high doses, causes clinically significant liver disease or exacerbates preexisting liver disease such as hepatitis B or C (Brewer and Wong 2004). They conclude that even marked liver dysfunction does not represent an absolute contraindication to using naltrexone.

A final major safety concern is risk of overdose when patients discontinue a naltrexone regimen. Patients who take naltrexone are protected from a fatal opiate overdose because naltrexone blocks the respiratory depressant effects of opiates. Once naltrexone is discontinued, patients are not protected by the blockade. At this time, however, they also have lost the tolerance to opiates that they had before taking naltrexone. Thus, if such patients take their previously accustomed doses of heroin or other opiates, in the absence of tolerance, they indeed may be at risk for respiratory depression and fatal overdose. There is also a theoretical risk that antagonist maintenance might render opiate receptors supersensitive to agonist effects once the antagonist is discontinued. This concern was raised by preclinical animal studies (Ayesta et al. 1992; Yoburn et al. 1985; Zukin et al. 1982), although other studies have failed to confirm such an effect (Cornish et al. 1993; Jenab et al. 1995).

Concern about the safety of naltrexone maintenance was raised by a report in which 81 opiate-dependent patients had been treated with naltrexone maintenance (Miotto et al. 1997). The incidence of overdoses (13) and deaths (4) was high during the subsequent year, although a number of the overdoses were suicide attempts or their relationship to naltrexone treatment itself was otherwise unclear. For the most part, the deaths occurred well after naltrexone had been discontinued. The incidence of death in untreated opiate-dependent patients is known to be common; one report suggested the rate could be as high as 2–4 percent per year (Joe and Simpson 1987). In a 24-year follow-up study of California narcotics addicts, Hser and colleagues found that 27.7 percent of the 581 addicts they monitored had died and that death was strongly correlated with disability, protracted heavy alcohol use, heavy criminal involvement, and tobacco use (Hser et al. 1993). Several other contemporary trials also have reported occasional deaths (for example, Carroll et al. 2001 had one death; Carroll et al. 2002 had two deaths due to suspected overdose; Rothenberg et al. 2002a had one death; and Rothenberg et al. 2002b had one death). Thus, although the death rate in opiate-dependent patients is known to be high in general, these data do raise concern as to whether naltrexone may increase the risk of death. Recent reviews of clinical trials have noted that individuals leaving naltrexone treatment experience up to eight times the rate of overdoses recorded among those leaving agonist treatment (Digiusto et al. 2004; Ritter 2002). Mortality rates following naltrexone treatment are equivalent to or higher than those for un-treated heroin users (Ritter 2002).

In summary, more research is needed to understand the risks of opi-oid overdose after discontinuation of naltrexone. In view of the high mortality rates in chronically heroin-dependent patients, it is not clear whether the deaths observed represent an increase over what would be expected from the natural course of the illness. Patients dependent on opi-oids treated with naltrexone need to be warned, however, that if they dis-continue the medication they will not be in a tolerant state, and doses of opioids that they would previously have taken routinely when in a de-pendent, tolerant state, could be lethal. Future human laboratory and brain-imaging research should further examine the issue of supersensitiv-ity of opioid receptors in response to chronic naltrexone treatment. Fu-ture clinical trials of both naltrexone and agonist maintenance agents should include careful long-term follow-up, especially among treatment dropouts, in an effort to detect and describe all serious adverse outcomes.

APPLICATIONS OF BEHAVIORAL THERAPY TO ENHANCE THE EFFECTIVENESS OF NALTREXONE

As previously discussed, naltrexone is potentially a highly efficacious medi-cation, providing complete and long-lasting blockade of the euphoric ef-fects of short-acting opiates such as heroin. Medication compliance has been a serious stumbling block in effective use of the medication for drug abuse treatment, however. In the past decade, a series of clinical trials have tested the effectiveness of naltrexone when used in combination with be-havioral therapy aimed at improving compliance (table 14.1). These tri-als, which are described below, have yielded promising results.

Recent Clinical Trials

The efficacy of a voucher-based incentive program for improving compli-ance with naltrexone was demonstrated by Preston and colleagues (1999) who randomly assigned 58 recently detoxified individuals to one of three 12-week treatment conditions. A contingent group could earn vouchers for ingesting naltrexone; an escalating schedule was used in which voucher values increased over time so long as the patient continued to ingest his or her naltrexone regularly. Members of a noncontingent control group were linked to a patient in the contingent group and received vouchers matched in frequency and value that were not contingent on

Table 14.1 Clinical Trials Combining Behavioral Therapies with Naltrexone

Study	Sample Size (N)	Method	Retention Rate	Serious Adverse Events
Preston et al. 1999	58	12-week study Three groups (randomly assigned): (1) contingent vouchers, (2) noncontingent vouchers, (3) no vouchers	Contingent vouchers: 50% at 12 weeks; mean, 7.4 weeks (significantly greater than no-voucher group; $p = .002$). Noncontingent vouchers: 30% at 12 weeks; mean, 5.0 weeks No vouchers: 5% at 12 weeks; mean, 2.3 weeks	None
Carroll et al. 2001	127	12-week study Three groups (randomly assigned): (1) standard NTX, (2) CM + NTX, (3) SO involvement + CM + NTX	At 12 weeks SO + CM + NTX: 47% CM + NTX: 42.9% Standard NTX: 25.6%	One minor adverse event; one death due to over-dose after a subject stopped naltrexone in the follow-up phase
Carroll et al. 2002	55	12-week study Three groups (randomly assigned): (1) standard NTX, (2) NTX + low-value CM (maximum total reinforce-ment value, $561), (3) NTX + high-value CM (maximum value, $1,152)	At 12 weeks Overall retention: 41.8% Low-value CM + NTX: 8.9 weeks High-value CM + NTX: 7.3 weeks Standard NTX: 6.2 weeks CM contrast did not yield a significant difference ($p = .17$)	Three participants died during the 6-month follow-up: one due to complications related to a head injury from a fall and two of sus-pected drug overdoses.
Rothenberg et al. 2002a	47	24-week study Single group trial of BNT—involved individual and network sessions—and	Overall retention 4 weeks: 55% 8 weeks: 40% 24 weeks: 19%	One death due to over-dose 2 weeks after sub-ject discontinued NTX and dropped out of

Study	N	Method	Results	Adverse events
		monitoring of NTX compliance by SO	Subjects using heroin only (no methadone at baseline). 4 weeks: 65% 8 weeks: 55% 24 weeks: 31%	study; one nonfatal accidental overdose resulting in ER visit; one ER visit for gastrointestinal distress.
Rothenberg et al. 2002b	69	24-week study Two groups (randomly assigned: (1) BNT with individual and network sessions and monitoring by other, (2) CE with individual sessions and unmonitored NTX	BNT group retention at 24 weeks: 27% CE group retention at 24 weeks: 9% ($p = .05$)	One rehospitalized for derandomized patient who became suicidal, one death due to accidental heroin overdose in patient noncompliant with NTX
Fals-Stewart and Farrell 2003	124 (all men)	24-week study Two groups (randomly assigned): (1) BFC plus monitored NTX, (2) IBT plus nonmonitored NTX	BFC patients: mean of 34.2 treatment sessions attended IBT patients: mean of 26.5 treatment sessions ($p < .01$) BFC patients had longer continuous abstinence from opioids at one-year follow-up ($p < .05$)	None reported
Krupitsky et al. 2004	52	24-week study Two groups (randomly assigned: (1) biweekly visits + active NTX, or (2) biweekly visits + placebo NTX	NTX-maintained patients retained at 24 weeks: 44.4% Control group retained at 24 weeks: 16% ($p < .05$)	One patient receiving placebo died of a drug overdose after dropping out of study; one NTX patient attempted suicide by heroin overdose but survived because of blockade

Note: CM, contingency management; SO, significant other; NTX, naltrexone; BNT, behavioral NTX therapy; CE, compliance enhancement; BFC, behavioral family counseling; IBT, individual-based treatment. All participants had a history of opioid dependence, and all studies included maintenance NTX except Krupitsky et al. 2004 (which had a placebo control condition as noted).

their ingestion of naltrexone. A no-voucher control group received only encouragement from staff to ingest naltrexone. The difference between contingent voucher and control groups was dramatic, with approximately 50 percent versus 5 percent staying in treatment and taking naltrexone for the full 12-week trial (fig. 14.1). This study clearly showed that contingency management could effectively enhance retention and adherence to a naltrexone treatment regimen.

Carroll and colleagues (2001) examined the effectiveness of two different strategies for enhancing naltrexone compliance. A contingency management (CM) intervention was tested alone and in combination with a significant-other (SO) intervention, and both were compared with a usual-care control group. Participants ($N = 127$) were randomly assigned to one of the three conditions and outcomes were evaluated for 12 weeks. Rates of retention were similar in the SO plus CM group (47%) and the CM alone group (43%) and were noticeably lower in the standard-care group offered naltrexone (26%). Detected opiate use was also lower in the CM groups. The researchers conclude that behavioral therapies such as CM can be effective for addressing naltrexone noncompliance.

A subsequent randomized clinical trial ($N = 55$) sought to address the optimal magnitude of reinforcement in contingency management (CM) (Carroll et al. 2002). Individuals were assigned to one of three treatment conditions: standard naltrexone, standard naltrexone plus low-value CM (a maximum of $561 could be earned), and standard naltrexone plus high-value CM (a maximum of $1,152 could be earned). The investigators replicated their previous findings in that treatment retention and number of naltrexone doses ingested were both higher for the CM groups than for the standard-treatment group. Higher- versus lower-value incentives made no difference under conditions studied in this population.

Evidence suggesting the potential importance of the family network in securing compliance with naltrexone comes from a double-blind trial of naltrexone in St. Petersburg, Russia. Krupitsky and colleagues examined abstinence and retention in patients randomly assigned to naltrexone plus biweekly drug counseling ($N = 27$) or naltrexone placebo plus biweekly counseling ($N = 25$) (Krupitsky et al. 2004). At the end of this 6-month study, 44 percent of the patients receiving naltrexone remained in the study and had not relapsed, as compared with 16 percent in the control group ($p < 0.05$). Randomization to naltrexone thus resulted in significantly better retention and less relapse to heroin dependence than placebo. The authors attribute the relatively high compliance seen in this study to the fact that patients' families, typically their parents, were involved in supervising medication dosing.

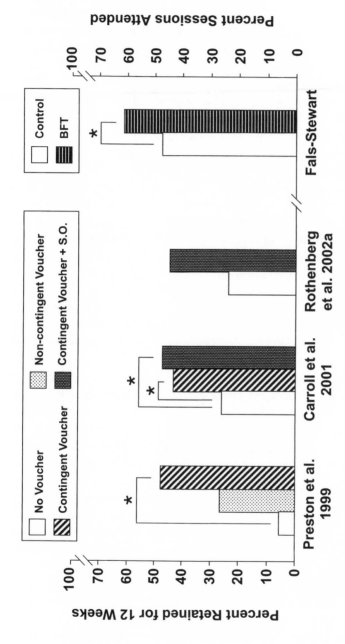

Figure 14.1. **Results from clinical trials testing the efficacy of naltrexone when combined with behavioral interventions.** The left three sections show results for treatment retention, and the right section shows results for sessions attended (with the maximum number possible being 56). BFT, behavioral family therapy; S.O., significant other. Significant differences on pairwise comparison analyses are indicated with an asterisk (*); $p < .05$.

Other investigators have tried to examine family or partner interventions more systematically. Rothenberg and colleagues developed and piloted a new therapy called behavioral naltrexone therapy (BNT) (Rothenberg et al. 2002a). This is an intensive behavioral therapy involving both individual and network sessions (i.e., sessions with partners or relatives), who are instructed in how to monitor naltrexone compliance by their significant other. As in the Carroll et al. studies described above, patients assigned to BNT also earned vouchers for taking naltrexone and providing opiate-negative urine specimens. The same investigators (Rothenberg et al. 2002b) then conducted a controlled trial ($N = 69$) that showed better treatment retention in patients assigned to receive BNT as compared with compliance enhancement (CE), a standard medication encouragement and support condition.

At 12 weeks, 44.4 percent of BNT participants remained in treatment compared with 23.5 percent of CE patients (Rothenberg et al. 2002b). Although these results seem very promising, the between-group comparison did not reach statistical significance. Furthermore, the low overall retention rates suggest that more work needs to be done to improve naltrexone compliance interventions involving CM and/or significant others.

In a recent trial examining the effects of behavioral family counseling on naltrexone maintenance, Fals-Stewart and O'Farrell assigned men ($N = 124$) living with a non-drug-abusing family member to one of two 24-week treatments following detoxification (Fals-Stewart and O'Farrell 2003). In behavioral family counseling (BFC), patients had both individual and family sessions and took naltrexone in the presence of a family member. In individual-based treatment (IBT), patients had individual sessions and took prescribed naltrexone on their own without family monitoring. BFC patients compared with those receiving IBT had higher retention in treatment during the 24-week treatment period, as demonstrated by more scheduled treatment sessions attended. BFC patients also ingested more doses of naltrexone and had more days abstinent from opioids and other drugs during treatment. Finally, patients in the BFC condition also had longer periods of continuous abstinence from opioids in the year after the 24-week treatment period than patients in the IBT condition.

Overall, the studies described above show relatively good 12-week treatment retention rates ranging from 40 to 50 percent when naltrexone is combined with contingency management and/or family or partner involvement. They provide support for continued development of these interventions as strategies to enhance naltrexone compliance and treatment efficacy.

Clinical Guidelines for Naltrexone in Maintenance Treatment of Opioid Dependence

Overview: Advantages and Disadvantages

The advantages of naltrexone maintenance as a treatment alternative for opiate-dependent patients include: (1) it is not a controlled substance and, therefore, can be prescribed flexibly in a wide variety of settings and by a wide variety of practitioners; (2) it is effective if compliance with the oral medication is good, in particular, in the setting of behavioral therapy; and (3) because many opiate-dependent patients avoid treatment and specifically avoid methadone or other agonist treatment, the availability of naltrexone may encourage a previously unreached subpopulation to access treatment.

Disadvantages of oral naltrexone include: (1) it appears to be less effective than agonist maintenance, such as methadone or buprenorphine, at clinically relevant doses. The latter produce lower dropout rates and better compliance than naltrexone maintenance. (2) It does not protect against opiate overdose if the patient stops the medication, which is an important safety concern that needs to be considered at the outset of any treatment plan.

Selection of Patients

Evidence from previous research suggests that indications for naltrexone maintenance treatment include a less severe degree of opiate dependence, high motivation, the presence of significant sanctions for relapse to opiates, strong social support, and/or prior success with naltrexone or drug-free treatment. More recent evidence from research in the author's group supports dependence on a long-acting opiate agonist, such as methadone, or dependence on larger quantities of a short-acting agonist, such as heroin (i.e., five or more bags per day), as poor prognostic indicators for naltrexone maintenance (Rothenberg et al. 2002a; Sullivan et al. 2000). Other contraindications would include a history of previous drug overdoses, advanced liver disease, or prior failure in a course of naltrexone maintenance. Questioning of patients regarding their history of overdoses and impulsive drug taking is an important safety consideration given evidence for risk of opiate overdose after discontinuing naltrexone. Because naltrexone produces dose-dependent liver irritation, liver function should be carefully assessed before embarking on a trial of naltrexone. If a patient has early-stage alcoholism or viral hepatitis with relatively intact liver functioning, naltrexone is probably safe as long as liver enzymes are carefully monitored during treatment. Among patients with advanced liver damage and low reserves of functional liver tissue due to cirrhosis, methadone or other treatment options are probably more prudent.

Naltrexone Induction

Clinical guidelines suggest that a patient must be opiate free for at least 10 days before they can safely begin taking naltrexone without risk of precipitating opiate withdrawal (O'Brien and Cornish 1999). Outpatient opiate detoxification can be attempted, although inpatient detoxification is more often successful because of the high risk of relapse on an outpatient basis (see chap. 16). However, in the current fiscal climate, most inpatient detoxifications last for only four to five days and often involve decreasing doses of long-acting opiate agonists. Therefore, the patient discharged from such a detoxification must remain abstinent for a subsequent period of at least five to ten days. Naltrexone readiness is sometimes determined by administering a naloxone challenge. This test consists of an escalating series of small naloxone doses ranging from 0.2 to 0.8 mg (Judson et al. 1980; Zilm and Sellers 1978). If the challenge produces no withdrawal symptoms, the patient may be considered ready to start naltrexone. The early period after hospital discharge is a time of high risk for relapse, and patients who can successfully remain abstinent for a week or more after discharge from the inpatient detoxification program have a relatively good prognosis. Thus, the extended abstinence requirement combined with short detoxification durations tends to limit even the possibility of starting on naltrexone to a relatively narrow population of patients with a better prognosis.

Several methods have been developed in an effort to expand naltrexone eligibility by speeding the induction of patients onto naltrexone and compressing the process into a period of one week or less. One method that has been developed is to begin naltrexone within a few days after discontinuing opiates but suppress the withdrawal symptoms using aggressive treatment with adjuvant medications that may include clonidine, which suppresses the sympathetic hyperarousal of withdrawal; benzodiazepines, such as clonazepam, which reduce the anxiety and insomnia; and ondansetron, which reduces the nausea and stomach upset (Kleber et al. 1980; O'Connor et al. 1995; Washton and Resnick 1981). A more recent variation on this has been to begin a detoxification by administering one or two doses of the partial opiate agonist buprenorphine, followed by several days of no opiate medication, during which clonidine, clonazepam, and other adjuvants are administered, followed by initiation of naltrexone (Fingerhood et al. 2001; Kutz and Reznik 2001; O'Connor et al. 1997; Umbricht et al. 1999). In either of these methods, naltrexone is best started on the first day at a low dose in the range of 6 to 12 mg and then gradually increased to 25 mg and 50 mg over the next few days, as tolerated. The authors have successfully used these methods to induct patients onto naltrexone (Rothenberg et al. 2002a; Sullivan et al. 2000).

Very few clinical trials have been carried out to date to assess these rapid induction methods. Trials that have been conducted suggest that the addition of buprenorphine results in significantly lower mean withdrawal scores than with clonidine alone (O'Connor et al. 1997), and thus higher rates of successfully completed detoxification (Fingerhood et al. 2001; O'Connor et al. 1997). Not surprisingly, these complex detoxification methods can be challenging to administer clinically. Small initial doses of naltrexone are important, as is aggressive preloading with the adjuvant medications. The difficulty of suppressing symptoms may be related to the degree of opiate dependency before detoxification. The clinician must be prepared to treat precipitated withdrawal, including its more serious manifestations, such as dehydration, which can lead to fainting and injury. It is also important to be alert for atypical withdrawal symptoms, particularly changes in sensorium or delirium, which do occasionally occur with precipitated withdrawal (Bell et al. 1999; Golden and Sakhrani 2004).

In recent years, "ultrarapid" methods of detoxifying patients and beginning naltrexone have been widely publicized (for review, see Albanese et al. 2000; O'Connor and Kosten 1998; Streel and Verbanck 2003, and chapter 5). These methods use general anesthesia, during which the patient's system is loaded with antagonist medication and cannot be recommended at this time, because there is no evidence from clinical trials to support their efficacy or any advantages relative to standard detoxification methods. Furthermore, deaths have been reported, raising serious safety concerns regarding this method.

Outpatient Management

Once a patient is detoxified and stabilized on naltrexone, the major issue becomes noncompliance with the medication and relapse to opiates. At the point of relapse, the patient generally becomes readdicted, even after just a few doses of opiate agonist, at which point the patient cannot restart naltrexone and needs to be referred back to either inpatient detoxification or agonist maintenance.

Stabilization: First Month

The first month after induction onto naltrexone is an especially high-risk period for noncompliance and relapse. Clinical experience and results from recent clinical trials suggest that clinic-based, clinic-observed administration of naltrexone is recommended during this period. This can be accomplished by having the patient come to the office or the clinic three times per week with two or three days elapsing between visits. The typical dosing schedule is 100 mg on Monday and Wednesday and 150 mg on Friday. Enlisting a significant other to monitor the ingestion of medication is also an option, but direct clinic-observed ingestion is preferred at the onset. Urine should be monitored for opiates at each clinic or office visit; rapid on-site tests that are now available (see chap. 17) can be used in office-based settings. It is recommended to give the patient a few spare doses to take at home, preferably supervised by the significant other, in case of missed visits. Disputed results (i.e., when the test is positive, but the patient says that he or she did not use opiates) can be confirmed by retest or follow-up urine testing at commercial laboratories.

Clinical trials reviewed previously suggest that behavioral therapy is important for improving the prognosis of naltrexone maintenance, and one of these methods (voucher incentives, cognitive behavioral relapse prevention, or family or couples therapy) should be strongly considered as part of the treatment plan. It is important to assess patients for concurrent psychopathology, especially depression, and to treat the patient accordingly (e.g., with antidepressant medications). Subacute withdrawal symptoms, including insomnia and anxiety, are particularly troubling to patients and should be monitored carefully. Difficulties with sleep can be treated with a sedating antidepressant, such as trazodone, or a sedating tricyclic antidepressant, but a history of abuse of these medications is a contraindication to their use. Anxiety can be treated with tapering doses of longer-acting benzodiazepines, such as clonazepam or chlordiazepoxide. This may be particularly appropriate if benzodiazepines have been used during the naltrexone induction procedure. There is significant concern about the potential to abuse benzodiazepines in opiate-dependent patients (see chap. 17), and a history of benzodiazepine dependence in the past would be a relative contraindication to this approach. Antidepressant medications or mild doses of antihistamines are alternatives that may provide relief from anxiety.

Maintenance: Second and Subsequent Months

Once a patient succeeds in complying with naltrexone for the first month, the risk of relapse continues, but at a lower probability. One approach is to stay with clinic-based administration if it is feasible for the patient to attend the office or clinic at least three times per week. It is prudent to supply the patient and/or significant others with emergency supplies of naltrexone in case the patient is not able to get to the clinic, because it is paramount for the patient not to miss any doses of naltrexone. An alternative is to switch to home-based administration of naltrexone at 50 mg per day. For home-based administration, it is best if there is a significant other who can be trained to monitor the medication, presuming that the patient is abstinent and urine samples are negative for opiates.

Significant others involved in naltrexone maintenance treatment should be individuals who (1) are not struggling with substance abuse themselves and (2) are supportive and invested in the identified patient being well. The therapist describes to the significant other, or "monitor," that he or she will function as an additional set of eyes and ears in the treatment process, not as a babysitter or police officer but as a supportive sounding board to reinforce relapse-prevention strategies discussed in counseling sessions. It is best for the monitor and patient to establish a set time of day that will be designated to take naltrexone. This time should fit naturally into the patient's schedule. The patient and monitor are advised that it is during this time—regardless of what else may be going on in their lives—that they have an opportunity to celebrate the individual's abstinence. The monitor should provide ample positive reinforcement for the patient's adherence to naltrexone and treatment gains. To secure this plan, daily monitoring logs should be kept to document the time and date of the naltrexone ingestion. Monitors are encouraged to call the primary clinician if the monitoring process is disrupted or if relapse is suspected. If a lapse occurs while a patient has been compliant with naltrexone, our experience suggests that a return to clinic-based administration of naltrexone is advisable until the patient can provide at least two consecutive opioid-negative urine specimens. If, on the other hand, the patient both lapses and becomes noncompliant with naltrexone, a naloxone challenge is in order to determine whether the patient has again become dependent on opioids.

During the second and subsequent months of naltrexone maintenance, it is important to continue behavioral therapy to bolster motivation, anticipate situations that produce high risk for relapse, and address family and couples issues that may promote or protect against relapse.

Voucher incentives have been found to be effective, particularly reinforcement schedules in which the voucher value increases on a regular basis with consecutive negative urine specimens or consecutive compliance with clinic-based medication dosing (Jones et al. 2001; Preston et al. 2001; Silverman et al. 1996). Vouchers may be especially powerful for patients of low socioeconomic status (SES), for whom the monetary value is a significant benefit. For high SES patients with more financial resources, our experience suggests the vouchers may have less impact in the sense that those patients derive less motivation from them.

Naltrexone has been found modestly effective for the treatment of alcohol dependence (Kranzler et al. 2004; O'Malley 1996; Volpicelli et al. 1995) and may also have some role in the treatment of nicotine dependence (Brauer et al. 1999; Covey et al. 1999; Krishnan-Sarin et al. 2003). Thus, it is possible that concurrent abuse of these substances may improve during naltrexone treatment. In general, it is important to set abstinence from all substances as a goal, because use of chemical substances is likely to be an important trigger for relapse to opiates. Some data suggest that marijuana use is not immediately detrimental to treatment outcomes (Church et al. 2001; Epstein and Preston 2003), however. Thus, the top priority for such patients remains that of maintaining abstinence from opiates, with abstinence from other substances as a secondary goal.

Management of Noncompliance, Lapse, and Relapse

Three possible scenarios are associated with noncompliance, lapse, and relapse, and each of these has specific implications and presents particular difficulties.

1. The Patient Stops Naltrexone But Remains Abstinent from Opiates

Patients in this category may complain of side effects from naltrexone or simply desire to get off medications. It is best to work with patients in a motivational framework and to make an effort to understand their wishes to discontinue medication, rather than to take a dogmatic approach. Behavioral therapy and urine monitoring should be continued, and contingency plans (e.g., rehospitalization for detoxification or initiation of agonist maintenance) should be made in anticipation of potential relapse.

2. The Patient Continues to be Compliant with Naltrexone but Also Is Using Opioids

This is a higher-risk situation because if the patient stops taking the naltrexone at this point, he or she will rapidly reestablish dependence on opiates. Thus, the first priority is to maintain compliance with naltrexone. Clinic-based naltrexone administration should be continued or reinstituted if the patient has been taking the medication at home. This clinical intervention not only provides for more reliable monitoring of naltrexone but also sends a message to the patient that naltrexone compliance is of paramount importance. If a patient in this situation continues to take the naltrexone reliably, then opiate effects should be blocked, and opiate-seeking behavior should eventually be extinguished. Watchful waiting in conjunction with vigilance around naltrexone compliance and monitoring sometimes pays off, such that the patient eventually becomes abstinent. It is important to be aware, however, that if patients discontinue naltrexone, they may be motivated to hide this fact from the clinicians. Patients in this situation may harbor the irrational belief that they can resume naltrexone despite use of opiates. They may also feel embarrassed about admitting failure to their clinicians. Thus, a reliable objective method to detect compliance versus noncompliance is desirable.

Packaging naltrexone pills into gelatin capsules together with riboflavin is the best method currently available for conveniently monitoring whether medication has been taken (Anton et al. 1999; Del Boca et al. 1996; Oncken et al. 2001). Riboflavin is excreted in the urine, and examination of the urine under a black light should reveal vivid fluorescence if the medication has been taken in the previous 12 to 24 hours. The riboflavin method is far from foolproof; for example, vitamin pills containing riboflavin can produce fluorescence. Nonetheless, it provides some objective feedback on compliance. If the urine is negative for fluorescence, the clinician should discuss this finding with the patient in a motivational framework and review the medication procedures and barriers to compliance.

3. The Patient Stops Using Naltrexone and Continues to Use Opiates

This relatively dangerous scenario requires careful clinical management. First, as previously discussed, a patient who has stopped naltrexone has little or no tolerance for opiates and is at risk for a fatal overdose. Thus, at minimum, close monitoring and adequate warnings are warranted. Second, opiate dependence may be reestablished relatively quickly, even within a few days, depending on the amount and spacing of opiate exposure. At this point, the patient may be unable to resume oral naltrexone without experiencing precipitated withdrawal. Successful resumption of naltrexone in this scenario is very rare in our experience, despite the fact that patients may appear determined and motivated to resume naltrexone. The best clinical course of action in this situation would be to move such a patient as quickly as possible to buprenorphine maintenance, methadone maintenance, or inpatient detoxification. Buprenorphine maintenance is an attractive option in this scenario because it may be more acceptable to patients than methadone and can be prescribed flexibly in a variety of office- and clinic-based settings, if these are available (see chap. 12). Thus, "buprenorphine rescue" should be seriously considered for patients who have stopped naltrexone and are using opioids. Naltrexone could be reconsidered as an option in the future, although the history of failure in a prior naltrexone trial might indicate a poor prognosis for a future trial of naltrexone as well.

New Directions in Naltrexone Treatment for Opioid Dependence

Depot and Implanted Naltrexone

The concept underlying depot naltrexone is that compliance problems with oral medication can be circumvented by a dosing method that provides blockade of opiate effects for prolonged periods. Currently at least three manufacturers in the United States have developed injectable depot naltrexone formulations and are testing these in clinical trials. The presence of significant blockade of intravenous heroin effects has been demonstrated in the human laboratory for up to four weeks after injections (Comer et al. 2002).

Depot naltrexone formulations could be a powerful solution to the problem of impulsive noncompliance with oral naltrexone and consequent relapse. With this product available, efforts could shift to engendering compliance with a monthly injection, rather than daily pill ingestion. A 60-day clinical trial testing the effectiveness of depot naltrexone for long-term maintenance of opiate dependence and the tolerability of chronic injections shows promising results (Comer et al. Forthcoming), but trials of longer duration are needed.

Naltrexone implant is a method that involves a minor operation to implant a subdermal reservoir that slowly releases naltrexone for 6 to 12 months. This prolonged delivery would have the same advantages as depot naltrexone but an even longer duration of action. The most active development of naltrexone implants has occurred in Australia, where several products have been developed and tested (Hulse and O'Neill 2002; Hulse and Tait 2003). However, rigorous testing in the human laboratory to confirm the strength and duration of blockade and clinical trials to determine clinical efficacy for treatment of opiate dependence have yet to be conducted, and are needed.

Depot and implant formulations of naltrexone seem ideal solutions to the problem of improving compliance and effectiveness, but these are as yet unproven, especially as long-term treatments. Therefore, efforts are still needed to improve the effectiveness of oral naltrexone. Further, in a situation analogous to the use of depot neuroleptics for treatment of chronic psychotic disorders, combinations or oral and depot medication may be advantageous in certain clinical situations. Efforts to improve the effectiveness of oral naltrexone should include continued research with behavioral therapies to enhance compliance. Offering adequate concurrent treatment of other co-occurring psychiatric problems and behavioral deficits could also enhance naltrexone compliance.

Conclusions

A decade ago the outlook on naltrexone as a treatment for opiate dependence by most practitioners and specialists was pessimistic, except with regard to special patient populations, such as probationers or medical professionals. Recent research and clinical work, however, have opened new and more promising avenues. Naltrexone has been shown to be an effective adjunct to the treatment of alcoholism and has been investigated for the treatment of other drug dependencies, such as nicotine dependence. For opiate dependence, behavioral therapies have been found to enhance the compliance and effectiveness of naltrexone maintenance, although antagonist therapy is not yet able to equal the effectiveness of adequately dosed agonist maintenance. Nonetheless, clinical researchers have revealed ways of rendering naltrexone useful for a broader population of opiate-dependent patients. These trials have also helped to clarify the risks, including the risk of overdose death, once patients have stopped taking naltrexone. Finally, depot injections and/or naltrexone implants hold substantial promise to improve the effectiveness and safety of naltrexone. Through these long-acting delivery techniques, naltrexone may ultimately rival agonist maintenance in its effectiveness for the long-term maintenance treatment of opiate dependence.

References

Ahmadi J, Ahmadi K, Ohaeri J (2003). Controlled, randomized trial in maintenance treatment of intravenous buprenorphine dependence with naltrexone, methadone or buprenorphine: a novel study. *Eur J Clin Invest* 33: 824–9.

Albanese AP, Gevirtz C, Oppenheim B, Field JM, Abels I, Eustace JC (2000). Outcome and six month follow up of patients after Ultra Rapid Opiate Detoxification (UROD). *J Addict Dis* 19: 11–28.

Amraoui A, Burgos V, Baron P, Alexandre JY (1999). [Acute delirium psychosis induced by naltrexone chlorhydrate]. *Presse Med* 28: 1361–2.

Anton RF, Moak DH, Waid LR, Latham PK, Malcolm RJ, Dias JK (1999). Naltrexone and cognitive behavioral therapy for the treatment of outpatient alcoholics: results of a placebo-controlled trial. *Am J Psychiatry* 156: 1758–64.

Ayesta FJ, Ableitner A, Emmett-Oglesby MW, Herz A, Shippenberg TS (1992). Paradoxical effect of chronic fentanyl treatment on naltrexone-induced supersensitivity and upregulation. *J Pharmacol Exp Ther* 260: 168–74.

Azatian A, Papiasvilli A, Joseph H (1994). A study of the use of clonidine and naltrexone in the treatment of opioid addiction in the former USSR. *J Addict Dis* 13: 35–52.

Bell JR, Young MR, Masterman SC, Morris A, Mattick RP, Bammer G (1999). A pilot study of naltrexone-accelerated detoxification in opioid dependence. *Med J Aust* 171: 26–30.

Brahen LS, Capone TJ, Capone DM (1988). Naltrexone: lack of effect on hepatic enzymes. *J Clin Pharmacol* 28: 64–70.

Brauer LH, Behm FM, Westman EC, Patel P, Rose JE (1999). Naltrexone blockade of nicotine effects in cigarette smokers. *Psychopharmacology (Berl)* 143: 339–46.

Brewer C (2002). Serum naltrexone and 6-beta-naltrexol levels from naltrexone implants can block very large amounts of heroin: a report of two cases. *Addict Biol* 7: 321–3.

Brewer C, Wong VS (2004). Naltrexone: report of lack of hepatotoxicity in acute viral hepatitis, with a review of the literature. *Addict Biol* 9: 81–87.

Callahan EJ, Rawson RA, McCleave B, Arias R, Glazer M, Liberman RP (1980). The treatment of heroin addiction: naltrexone alone and with behavior therapy. *Int J Addict* 15: 795–807.

Carroll KM, Ball SA, Nich C, O'Connor PG, Eagan DA, Frankforter TL, Triffleman EG, Shi J, Rounsaville BJ (2001). Targeting behavioral therapies to enhance naltrexone treatment of opioid dependence: efficacy of contingency management and significant other involvement. *Arch Gen Psychiatry* 58: 755–61.

Carroll KM, Sinha R, Nich C, Babuscio T, Rounsaville BJ (2002). Contingency management to enhance naltrexone treatment of opioid dependence: a randomized clinical trial of reinforcement magnitude. *Exp Clin Psychopharmacol* 10: 54–63.

Church SH, Rothenberg JL, Sullivan MA, Bornstein G, Nunes EV (2001). Concurrent substance use and outcome in combined behavioral and naltrexone therapy for opiate dependence. *Am J Drug Alcohol Abuse* 27: 441–52.

Comer SD, Collins ED, Kleber HD, Nuwayser ES, Kerrigan JH, Fischman MW (2002). Depot naltrexone: long-lasting antagonism of the effects of heroin in humans. *Psychopharmacology (Berl)* 159: 351–60.

Comer SD, Sullivan MA, Rothenberg JL, Yu E, Kleber HD, O'Brien CP, Hawks R, Chiang N (Forthcoming). *Multi-site, double-blind, placebo-controlled clinical trial of a 30-day sustained release depot formulation of naltrexone in the treatment of opioid dependence.*

Cornish JW, Henson D, Levine S, Volpicelli J, Inturrisi CE, Yoburn BC, O'Brien CP (1993). Naltrexone maintenance: effect on morphine sensitivity in normal volunteers. *Am J Addict* 2: 34–38.

Cornish JW, Metzger D, Woody GE, Wilson D, McLellan AT, Vandergrift B, O'Brien CP (1997). Naltrexone pharmacotherapy for opioid dependent federal probationers. *J Subst Abuse Treat* 14: 529–34.

Covey LS, Glassman AH, Stetner F (1999). Naltrexone effects on short-term and long-term smoking cessation. *J Addict Dis* 18: 31–40.

Crowley TJ, Wagner JE, Zerbe G, Macdonald M (1985). Naltrexone-induced dysphoria in former opioid addicts. *Am J Psychiatry* 142: 1081–4.

Del Boca FK, Kranzler HR, Brown J, Korner PF (1996). Assessment of medication compliance in alcoholics through UV light detection of a riboflavin tracer. *Alcohol Clin Exp Res* 20: 1412–7.

Digiusto E, Shakeshaft A, Ritter A, O'Brien S, Mattick RP (2004). Serious adverse events in the Australian National Evaluation of Pharmacotherapies for Opioid Dependence (NEPOD). *Addiction* 99: 450–60.

Epstein DH, Preston KL (2003). Does cannabis use predict poor outcome for heroin-dependent patients on maintenance treatment? Past findings and more evidence against. *Addiction* 98: 269–79.

Fals-Stewart W, O'Farrell TJ (2003). Behavioral family counseling and naltrexone for male opioid-dependent patients. *J Consult Clin Psychol* 71: 432–42.

Fingerhood MI, Thompson MR, Jasinski DR (2001). A comparison of clonidine and buprenorphine in the outpatient treatment of opiate withdrawal. *Subst Abus* 22: 193–9.

Golden SA, Sakhrani DL (2004). Unexpected delirium during rapid opioid detoxification (ROD). *J Addict Dis* 23: 65–75.

Grabowski J, O'Brien CP, Greenstein R, Ternes J, Long M, Steinberg-Donato S (1979). Effects of contingent payment on compliance with a naltrexone regimen. *Am J Drug Alcohol Abuse* 6: 355–65.

Greenstein RA, Arndt IC, McLellan AT, O'Brien CP, Evans B (1984). Naltrexone: a clinical perspective. *J Clin Psychiatry* 45: 25–28.

Gutstein HB, Akil H (2001). Opioid analgesics. In: Hardman JG, Limbird LE, eds *Goodman and Gilman's The Pharmacologic Basis of Therapeutics,* 569–619. New York: McGraw Hill.

Hollister LE, Johnson K, Boukhabza D, Gillespie HK (1981). Aversive effects of naltrexone in subjects not dependent on opiates. *Drug Alcohol Depend* 8: 37–41.

Hser YI, Anglin D, Powers K (1993). A 24-year follow-up of California narcotics addicts. *Arch Gen Psychiatry* 50: 577–84.

Hulse GK, O'Neill G (2002). A possible role for implantable naltrexone in the management of the high-risk pregnant heroin user. *Aust N Z J Obstet Gynaecol* 42: 93–94.

Hulse GK, Tait RJ (2003). A pilot study to assess the impact of naltrexone implant on accidental opiate overdose in 'high-risk' adolescent heroin users. *Addict Biol* 8: 337–42.

Jenab S, Kest B, Inturrisi CE (1995). Assessment of delta opioid antinociception and receptor mRNA levels in mouse after chronic naltrexone treatment. *Brain Res* 691: 69–75.

Joe GW, Simpson DD (1987). Mortality rates among opioid addicts in a longitudinal study. *Am J Public Health* 77: 347–8.

Jones HE, Haug N, Silverman K, Stitzer M, Svikis D (2001). The effectiveness of incentives in enhancing treatment attendance and drug abstinence in methadone-maintained pregnant women. *Drug Alcohol Depend* 61: 297–306.

Judson BA, Himmelberger DU, Goldstein A (1980). The naloxone test for opiate dependence. *Clin Pharmacol Ther* 27: 492–501.

Kirchmayer U, Davoli M, Verster AD, Amato L, Ferri A, Perucci CA (2002). A systematic review on the efficacy of naltrexone maintenance treatment in opioid dependence. *Addiction* 97: 1241–9.

Kleber HD, Gold MS, Riordan CE (1980). The use of clonidine in detoxification from opiates. *Bull Narc* 32: 1–10.

Kosten TR, Kleber HD (1984). Strategies to improve compliance with narcotic antagonists. *Am J Drug Alcohol Abuse* 10: 249–66.

Kranzler HR, Armeli S, Feinn R, Tennen H (2004). Targeted naltrexone treatment moderates the relations between mood and drinking behavior among problem drinkers. *J Consult Clin Psychol* 72: 317–27.

Kranzler HR, Modesto-Lowe V, Nuwayser ES (1998). Sustained-release naltrexone for alcoholism treatment: a preliminary study. *Alcohol Clin Exp Res* 22: 1074–9.

Krishnan-Sarin S, Meandzija B, O'Malley S (2003). Naltrexone and nicotine patch smoking cessation: a preliminary study. *Nicotine Tob Res* 5: 851–7.

Krupitsky EM, Zvartau EE, Masalov DV, Tsoi MV, Burakov AM, Egorova VY, Didenko TY, Romanova TN, Ivanova EB, Bespalov AY, Verbitskaya EV, Neznanov NG, Grinenko AY, O'Brien CP, Woody GE (2004). Naltrexone for heroin dependence treatment in St. Petersburg, Russia. *J Subst Abuse Treat* 26: 285–94.

Kutz I, Reznik V (2001). Rapid heroin detoxification using a single high dose of buprenorphine. *J Psychoactive Drugs* 33: 191–3.

Malcolm R, O'Neil PM, Von JM, Dickerson PC (1987). Naltrexone and dysphoria: a double-blind placebo controlled trial. *Biol Psychiatry* 22: 710–6.

Marrazzi MA, Wroblewski JM, Kinzie J, Luby ED (1997). High-dose naltrexone and liver function safety. *Am J Addict* 6: 21–29.

Meyer MC, Straughn AB, Lo MW, Schary WL, Whitney CC (1984). Bioequivalence, dose-proportionality, and pharmacokinetics of naltrexone after oral administration. *J Clin Psychiatry* 45: 15–19.

Miotto K, McCann M, Basch J, Rawson R, Ling W (2002). Naltrexone and dysphoria: fact or myth? *Am J Addict* 11: 151–60.

Miotto K, McCann MJ, Rawson RA, Frosch D, Ling W (1997). Overdose, suicide attempts and death among a cohort of naltrexone-treated opioid addicts. *Drug Alcohol Depend* 45: 131–4.

Navaratnam V, Jamaludin A, Raman N, Mohamed M, Mansor SM (1994). Determination of naltrexone dosage for narcotic agonist blockade in detoxified Asian addicts. *Drug Alcohol Depend* 34: 231–6.

O'Brien CP, Cornish JW (1999). Opioids: antagonists and partial agonists. In: Galanter M, Kleber HD, eds. *Textbook of Substance Abuse Treatment*, 281–94. Washington, DC: American Psychiatric Press.

O'Brien CP, Kampman KM (2004). Opioids: antagonists and partial agonists. In: Galanter M, Kleber HD, eds. *Textbook of Substance Abuse Treatment*. Washington, DC: American Psychiatric Press.

O'Connor PG, Carroll KM, Shi JM, Schottenfeld RS, Kosten TR, Rounsaville BJ (1997). Three methods of opioid detoxification in a primary care setting. A randomized trial. *Ann Intern Med* 127: 526–30.

O'Connor PG, Kosten TR (1998). Rapid and ultrarapid opioid detoxification techniques. *JAMA* 279: 229–34.

O'Connor PG, Waugh ME, Carroll KM, Rounsaville BJ, Diagkogiannis IA, Schottenfeld RS (1995). Primary care-based ambulatory opioid detoxification: the results of a clinical trial. *J Gen Intern Med* 10: 255–60.

O'Malley SS (1996). Opioid antagonists in the treatment of alcohol dependence: clinical efficacy and prevention of relapse. *Alcohol Alcohol Suppl* 1: 77–81.

Oncken C, Van Kirk J, Kranzler HR (2001). Adverse effects of oral naltrexone: analysis of data from two clinical trials. *Psychopharmacology (Berl)* 154: 397–402.

Preston KL, Silverman K, Umbricht A, DeJesus A, Montoya ID, Schuster CR (1999). Improvement in naltrexone treatment compliance with contingency management. *Drug Alcohol Depend* 54: 127–35.

Preston KL, Umbricht A, Wong CJ, Epstein DH (2001). Shaping cocaine abstinence by successive approximation. *J Consult Clin Psychol* 69: 643–54.

Rawlins M, Randall M (1976). Aftercare on narcotic antagonists: prospects and problems. *Int J Addict* 11: 501–11.

Ritter AJ (2002). Naltrexone in the treatment of heroin dependence: relationship with depression and risk of overdose. *Aust N Z J Psychiatry* 36: 224–8.

Rothenberg JL, Sullivan MA, Bornstein G, Epstein E, Nunes EV (2002a). Behavioral naltrexone therapy (BNT): efficacy of a new behavioral treatment for heroin dependence and future directions, presented at the Sixty-fourth Annual Scientific Meeting of the College on Problems of Drug Dependence, Quebec, Canada, June 8–13, 2002.

Rothenberg JL, Sullivan MA, Church SH, Seracini A, Collins E, Kleber HD, Nunes EV (2002b). Behavioral naltrexone therapy: an integrated treatment for opiate dependence. *J Subst Abuse Treat* 23: 351–60.

Sax DS, Kornetsky C, Kim A (1994). Lack of hepatotoxicity with naltrexone treatment. *J Clin Pharmacol* 34: 898–901.

Schuh KJ, Walsh SL, Stitzer ML (1999). Onset, magnitude and duration of opioid blockade produced by buprenorphine and naltrexone in humans. *Psychopharmacology (Berl)* 145: 162–74.

Shufman EN, Porat S, Witztum E, Gandacu D, Bar-Hamburger R, Ginath Y (1994). The efficacy of naltrexone in preventing reabuse of heroin after detoxification. *Biol Psychiatry* 35: 935–45.

Silverman K, Wong CJ, Higgins ST, Brooner RK, Montoya ID, Contoreggi C, Umbricht-Schneiter A, Schuster CR, Preston KL (1996). Increasing opiate abstinence through voucher-based reinforcement therapy. *Drug Alcohol Depend* 41: 157–65.

Streel E, Verbanck P (2003). Ultra-rapid opiate detoxification: from clinical applications to basic science. *Addict Biol* 8: 141–6.

Sullivan MA, Rothenberg JL, Church SH, Nunes EV (2000). Predictors of retention in behavioral naltrexone therapy (BNT), presented at the Sixty-second Annual Scientific Meeting of the College on Problems of Drug Dependence, San Juan, Puerto Rico, June 17–22, 2000.

Umbricht A, Montoya ID, Hoover DR, Demuth KL, Chiang CT, Preston KL (1999). Naltrexone shortened opioid detoxification with buprenorphine. *Drug Alcohol Depend* 56: 181–90.

Unterwald EM, Rubenfeld JM, Imai Y, Wang JB, Uhl GR, Kreek MJ (1995). Chronic opioid antagonist administration upregulates mu opioid receptor binding without altering mu opioid receptor mRNA levels. *Brain Res Mol Brain Res* 33: 351–5.

Verebey K, Volavka J, Mule SJ, Resnick RB (1976). Naltrexone: disposition, metabolism, and effects after acute and chronic dosing. *Clin Pharmacol Ther* 20: 315–28.

Volpicelli JR, Rhines KC, Rhines JS, Volpicelli LA, Alterman AI, O'Brien CP (1997). Naltrexone and alcohol dependence. Role of subject compliance. *Arch Gen Psychiatry* 54: 737–42.

Volpicelli JR, Volpicelli LA, O'Brien CP (1995). Medical management of alcohol dependence: clinical use and limitations of naltrexone treatment. *Alcohol Alcohol* 30: 789–98.

Wall ME, Brine DR, Perez-Reyes M (1981). Metabolism and disposition of naltrexone in man after oral and intravenous administration. *Drug Metab Dispos* 9: 369–75.

Washton AM, Gold MS, Pottash AC (1984). Successful use of naltrexone in addicted physicians and business executives. *Adv Alcohol Subst Abuse* 4: 89–96.

Washton AM, Resnick RB (1981). Clonidine in opiate withdrawal: review and appraisal of clinical findings. *Pharmacotherapy* 1: 140–6.

Yoburn BC, Goodman RR, Cohen AH, Pasternak GW, Inturrisi CE (1985). Increased analgesic potency of morphine and increased brain opioid binding sites in the rat following chronic naltrexone treatment. *Life Sci* 36: 2325–32.

Yoburn BC, Nunes FA, Adler B, Pasternak GW, Inturrisi CE (1986). Pharmacodynamic supersensitivity and opioid receptor upregulation in the mouse. *J Pharmacol Exp Ther* 239: 132–5.

Zernig G, Butelman ER, Lewis JW, Walker EA, Woods JH (1994). In vivo determination of mu opioid receptor turnover in rhesus monkeys after irreversible blockade with clocinnamox. *J Pharmacol Exp Ther* 269: 57–65.

Zilm DH, Sellers EM (1978). The quantitative assessment of physical dependence on opiates. *Drug Alcohol Depend* 3: 419–28.

Zukin RS, Sugarman JR, Fitz-Syage ML, Gardner EL, Zukin SR, Gintzler AR (1982). Naltrexone-induced opiate receptor supersensitivity. *Brain Res* 245: 285–92.

IV

OTHER TREATMENT APPROACHES

15

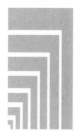

Medication-Free Treatment of Opioid Dependence

George De Leon, Ph.D., Hendrée E. Jones, Ph.D.,
and Maxine L. Stitzer, Ph.D.

A substantial number of opioid-dependent persons may receive care with opioid medications in opioid treatment programs (OTPs) and physicians' offices, but another important and valuable component of the substance abuse treatment system is drug-free programs of care. Although traditionally called "drug free," such services might more appropriately be named "medication-free" or "opioid agonist-free" programs. Given the familiarity of the term drug free, however, this chapter will refer to these programs using this name to capture the different types of treatment provided without the concurrent use of prescribed medications.

Perhaps the most well known and extensively studied form of drug-free treatment is the therapeutic community (TC). This chapter begins by reviewing what is known about TCs, including the salient features of these programs, their use in treating patients dependent on opioids, and the outcomes achieved. In addition, new and innovative approaches within the TC model are discussed, such as TCs that incorporate forms of methadone treatment into their programming.

The second half of this chapter reviews issues associated with other forms of drug-free treatment for opioid dependence. Considerably less research has been done on these programs than on TCs. Included in this section is a discussion of reinforcement-based therapy (RBT), which is a novel form of drug-free treatment that includes incentives integrated into a relatively rich set of treatment services.

These two types of treatment—TCs and other drug-free treatment programs—are important parts of the substance abuse treatment system. They provide services to a substantial number of patients and are valuable alternatives to the OTP system. For the many patients dependent on opioids who do not want to be maintained on opioid agonist medications (e.g., methadone, buprenorphine), drug-free treatment provides a means for maintaining abstinence and improving the quality of their lives.

THE THERAPEUTIC COMMUNITY MODALITY OF TREATMENT

Contemporary therapeutic communities (TCs) for addictions and related disorders are sophisticated human services agencies. Today, the term *therapeutic community* is generic, describing a variety of short- and long-term residential programs, as well as day treatment and ambulatory programs that serve a wide spectrum of drug- and alcohol-abusing patients. These utilize the essential elements of the TC approach and may be implemented in a variety of community and institutional settings.

Information based on membership data from Therapeutic Communities of America (TCA), the national organization of TC programs, yields a picture of the TC modality in community settings. More than 500 TC-oriented facilities are serving thousands of admissions and their families in every region of the United States. According to a 2003 survey of the membership of TCA, TC programs had a capacity of nearly 20,000 beds, and more than 55,000 persons were treated in residential TC programs in 2002 (information available at www.therapeuticcommunitiesofamerica.org). TC programs are located primarily in urban centers, with occasional facilities in rural settings. With a few exceptions, TC programs are publicly funded, primarily through state and, to a lesser extent, federal and local allocations (Etheridge et al. 1997). Fee-for-service clients represent a relatively small percentage of the residential treatment population in TC programs.

A report by Pompi includes results from a survey of 45 members of TCA that was conducted in late 1988 and early 1989 (Pompi 1994). That survey found that the population in community-based residential treatment exceeded 41,000 persons, of whom 19.1 percent were adolescents (<21 years of age). The mean age of this population was 25.8 years, and the number of persons treated by the 45 agencies ranged from as few as 40 persons to as many as 5,276.

Description of the Clientele That Access the TC System

TCs for addictions emerged in the 1960s as drug-free treatment primarily for heroin abusers. In these early years the large majority of admissions to TCs claimed heroin as their primary drug of abuse, although use and abuse of alcohol and other substances was also very common (De Leon and Schwartz 1984; Simpson and Sells 1982). During the past three decades the percentage of primary heroin users in TCs has declined such that most persons who enter contemporary TCs are multiple drug abusers who frequently have some combination of opioid, marijuana, alcohol, and cocaine or crack use. As will be reported below, however, evaluation research consistently documents a positive treatment impact on opioid and other illicit drug use.

Clients in long-term residential TC programs are mainly Caucasian, male, and 30 years old, although race-ethnic proportions differ by geographic regions, specific programs, and study samples. Most community-based TCs are integrated across gender, race, and ethnicity, but not age, with separate facilities for adolescent (<18 years) the rule. In general, Hispanics, Native Americans, and clients younger than 21 years represent smaller proportions of admissions to TCs.

A significant number of patients treated in TCs are from broken homes or have ineffective families and poor work histories and have engaged in criminal activities. Among adult admissions to TCs, fewer than one-third are employed full-time in the year before treatment, more than two-thirds have been arrested, and 30 to 40 percent have histories of drug treatment (De Leon 1999, 2004; Hubbard et al. 1997; Simpson and Sells 1982).

Psychological Profiles

Although TC clients differ with respect to demographic variables, socioeconomic background, and drug use patterns, psychological profiles obtained with the use of standard instruments demonstrate a common pattern, as has been shown in many TC studies (Jainchill 1994). This psychological profile mirrors features of both psychiatric and criminal populations. For example, the character-disorder elements and poor self-concept found in delinquent and repeat offenders are present, as are the elements of dysphoria and confused thinking of emotionally unstable or psychiatric populations. Thus, in addition to their substance abuse, patients in TCs have considerable degrees of psychological disability.

In studies in which the Diagnostic Interview Schedule (DIS) was used to assess for psychiatric disorders, more than 70 percent of patients admitted to TCs had a lifetime history of non-drug-related psychiatric disorders in addition to substance abuse problems. The most frequent non-drug-related diagnoses were phobias, generalized anxiety disorder, psychosexual dysfunction, and antisocial personality disorder. There were few cases of schizophrenia, but lifetime affective disorders occurred in more than one-third of those studied (De Leon 1993; Jainchill 1994).

Results from the Drug Abuse Treatment Outcome Study (DATOS), a national survey of substance abuse treatment in the United States, confirm the general conclusion that long-term residential TCs serve substance abusers with severe social and psychological problems in addition to multiple drug use disorders. Compared with other treatment modalities, for example, DATOS found that TC clients have higher criminal involvement, poorer employment histories, and higher rates of sexual risk behavior and suicidality (Hubbard et al. 1997).

Description of the Program Elements

Contact and Referral

Voluntary contacts with TCs occur through self-referral, recommendations made by social agencies and treatment providers, and active recruitment by TCs. Outreach teams (usually trained graduates of TCs and selected human services staff) will recruit patients from hospitals, jails, courtrooms, social agencies, and on the street, conducting brief orientations or face-to-face interviews to determine a person's receptivity to the idea of treatment in a TC.

Approximately one-third of adult admissions enter community-based TCs under legal pressure (probation, parole, court diverted) (De Leon 1988, 2004; Etheridge et al. 1997). Although most adult admissions to TCs are technically voluntary entries, many (particularly opioid abusers) report other forms of perceived pressures to seek treatment (e.g., family, work, health, housing, financial, and fears of arrest) (De Leon 1988). Notably, compared with adults, most adolescents admitted have been referred to treatment under some form of legal pressure (Jainchill et al. 1997; Pompi and Resnick 1987).

Medically Supervised Withdrawal

With some exceptions, admission to residential treatment does not require medically supervised withdrawal. Thus, traditional TCs do not usually provide this service on the premises. Most individuals whose primary

drugs of abuse are opioids, cocaine, alcohol, barbiturates, and/or amphetamines have undergone self- or medical withdrawal before seeking
admission to the TC. A small proportion may still require medically supervised withdrawal during the admission evaluation. For opioid abusers
this withdrawal can usually be managed without pharmacologic assistance during the initial days of residence. Abusers of other drugs usually
are offered the option of a medically supervised withdrawal at a nearby
hospital. Individuals who use barbiturates are routinely referred for medically supervised withdrawal, after which they are reassessed for admission. A small percentage of patients admitted to TCs have been primarily
involved with hallucinogens or phencyclidine (PCP). For those who appear compromised from the use of such substances, a referral is made for
psychiatric services, after which the individuals can return for residential
treatment.

TC Perspective and Treatment Approach

The TC approach to treating substance abuse is grounded in a theoretical perspective of the disorder and recovery detailed in other writings (De
Leon 2000). This perspective emerged primarily from the personal recovery experiences of the first generation of participants in TCs, who were
primarily opioid abusers. In brief, the TC views substance abuse as a disorder of the whole person. Although individuals differ in the substance of
choice, abuse involves some or all areas of functioning. Cognitive, behavioral, and mood disturbances appear, as do medical and mental health
problems. Thinking may be unrealistic or disorganized. Values are confused, nonexistent, or antisocial. Deficits frequently exist in verbal, reading, writing, and marketable skills and, whether couched in existential or
psychological terms, moral issues are apparent. Thus, the multidimen-
sional problems of the substance abuser require a multi-interventional
approach such as that provided by a residential TC.

In the TC perspective physiologic factors may be important contributors to ongoing drug use, but these remain minor relative to the social
and psychological problems that precede them and the behavioral deficits
that accumulate with continued substance abuse. Thus, addiction is a
symptom, not the essence of the disorder. The problem is the person, not
the drug. Recovery is a developmental process of incremental learning toward a stable change in behavior, attitudes, and values of "right living"
associated with maintaining a drug-free lifestyle.

The developmental recovery process itself can be understood as a passage through stages of incremental learning. The learning that occurs at

each stage facilitates change at the next, and each change reflects movement toward the goals associated with recovery. The planned duration of treatment is generally 18 months, which comprises twelve months in a structured residential TC, followed by six months of aftercare delivered in a step-down sequence provided in a TC-oriented halfway house and outpatient settings.

The quintessential ingredient of the TC approach may be termed "community as method" (De Leon 1997, 2000). What distinguishes the TC from other treatment approaches (and other communities) is the *purposive use of the peer-staff community to facilitate social and psychological change in individuals*. Thus, in a therapeutic community all activities are designed to produce therapeutic and educational change in individual participants, and all participants are mediators of these therapeutic and educational changes. Table 15.1 outlines the key components and activities of a generic TC-oriented program.

TC Evaluation Research

The effectiveness of the TC approach for treating substance abuse is documented in a substantial literature that has developed over the past three decades and is based on both single-program studies and large-scale multimodality, multiprogram evaluations such as the Drug Abuse Reporting Program (DARP), Treatment Outcome Prospective Study (TOPS), Drug Abuse Treatment Outcome Study (DATOS), and the National Treatment Improvement Evaluation Study (NTIES). Reviews of this literature are contained in a NIDA Monograph Report on TCs (NIDA 2002) and in numerous other publications (De Leon 1984, 1985; Gerstein 2004; Hubbard et al. 1989; Simpson and Sells 1982; Simpson et al. 1997; Tims et al. 1994).

The findings regarding short- and long-term posttreatment outcomes for TCs are consistent and can be briefly summarized. Significant clinical improvements are noted on separate outcome variables (i.e., drug use, criminality, and employment) and on composite indices for measuring individual success. Maximally to moderately favorable outcomes (in terms of reductions in drug use, arrest rates, retreatment, and increased employment) occur in more than half of the sample followed. In studies that investigated psychological outcomes, findings also showed marked improvement at follow-up, particularly for primary opioid abusers (De Leon 1984; Holland 1983; Hubbard et al. 1997). For example, among primary opioid abusers, a direct relationship has been demonstrated between posttreatment behavioral success (drug use, crime, and employment) and psy-

Table 15.1   **Components of a Generic TC Program Model**

Community Separateness

TC-oriented programs have their own names, often innovated by the clients, and are housed in a space or locale that is separate from other agency or institutional programs or units or, in general, from the drug-related environment. In the residential settings, clients remain away from outside influences 24 hours a day for several months before earning short-term day-out privileges. In the nonresidential "day-treatment" settings, the individual is in the TC environment for 4–8 hours and then monitored by peers and family. Even in the least restrictive outpatient settings, TC-oriented programs and components are in place. Members gradually detach from old networks and relate to the drug-free peers in the program.

A Community Environment

The inner environment of a TC facility contains communal space to promote a sense of commonalty and collective activities (e.g., groups, meetings). The walls display signs that state in simple terms the philosophy of the program, the messages of right living and recovery. Corkboards and black boards identify all participants by name, seniority level, and job function in the program, and daily schedules are posted. These visuals display an organizational picture of the program that the individual can relate to and comprehend, factors that promote affiliation.

Community Activities

To be utilized effectively, treatment or educational services must be provided within a context of the peer community. Thus, with the exception of individual counseling, all activities are programmed in collective formats. These include at least one daily meal prepared, served, and shared by all members; a daily schedule of groups, meetings and seminars, team job functions, and organized recreational/leisure time; ceremony and rituals (e.g., birthdays, phase/progress graduations, etc.)

Staff Roles and Functions

The staff are a mix of self-help, recovered professionals and other traditional professionals (e.g., medical, legal, mental health, and educational) who must be integrated through cross training that is grounded in the basic concepts of the TC perspective and community approach. Professional skills define the function of staff (e.g., nurse, physician, lawyer, teacher, administrator, case worker, clinical counselor). Regardless of professional discipline or function, however, the generic *role of* all staff is that of community member who, rather than providers and treaters, are rational authorities, facilitators, and guides in the self-help community method.

Peers as Role Models

Members who demonstrate the expected behaviors and reflect the values and teachings of the community are viewed as role models. Indeed, the strength of the community as a context for social learning relates to the number and quality of its role models. All members of the community are expected to be role models—roommates; older and younger residents; and junior, senior, and directorial staff. TCs require these multiple role models to maintain the integrity of the community and assure the spread of social-learning effects.

(continued)

Table 15.1   Continued

A Structured Day

The structure of the program relates to the TC perspective, in particular, the view of the client and recovery. Ordered, routine activities counter the characteristically disordered lives of these clients and distract from negative thinking and boredom, factors that predispose to drug use. And, structured activities of the community facilitate learning self-structure for the individual, in time management, planning, setting and meeting goals, and, in general, accountability. Thus, regardless of its length, the day has a formal schedule of varied therapeutic and educational activities with prescribed formats, fixed times, and routine procedures.

Work as Therapy and Education

Consistent with the TC's self-help approach, all clients are responsible for the daily management of the facility (e.g., cleaning, activities, meal preparation and service, maintenance, purchasing, security, coordinating schedules, preparatory chores for groups, meetings, seminars activities, etc.). In the TC, the various work roles mediate essential educational and therapeutic effects. Job functions strengthen affiliation with the program through participation, provide opportunities for skill development, and foster self-examination and personal growth through performance challenge and program responsibility. The scope and depth of client work functions depend on the program setting (e.g., institutional versus free-standing facilities) and client resources (levels of psychological function, social and life skills).

Phase Format

The treatment protocol, or plan of therapeutic and educational activities, is organized into phases that reflect a developmental view of the change process. Emphasis is on incremental learning at each phase, which moves the individual to the next stage of recovery.

TC Concepts

A formal and informal curriculum focuses on teaching the TC perspective, particularly its self-help recovery concepts and view of right living. The concepts, messages, and lessons of the curriculum are repeated in the various groups, meetings, seminars, and peer conversations, as well as in readings, signs, and personal writings.

Peer Encounter Groups

The main community or therapeutic group is the encounter, although other forms of therapeutic, educational, and support groups are utilized as needed. The minimal objective of the peer encounter is similar in TC-oriented programs—to heighten individual awareness of specific attitudes or behavioral patterns that should be modified. The encounter process may differ in degree of staff direction and intensity, depending on the client subgroups (e.g., adolescents, prison inmates, the dually disordered).

Awareness Training

All therapeutic and educational interventions involve raising the individual's consciousness of the impact of their conduct/attitudes on themselves and the social environment and, conversely, the impact of the behaviors and attitudes of others on themselves and the social environment.

(*continued*)

Table 15.1 **Continued**

Emotional Growth Training

Achieving the goals of personal growth and socialization involves teaching individuals how to identify feelings, express feelings appropriately, and manage feelings constructively through the interpersonal and social demands of communal life.

Planned Duration of Treatment

The optimal length of time for full program involvement must be consistent with TC goals of recovery and its developmental view of the change process. How long the individual must be involved in the program depends on their phase of recovery, although a minimum period of intensive involvement is required to ensure internalization of the TC teachings.

Continuity of Care

Completion of primary treatment is a stage in the recovery process. Aftercare services are an essential component in the TC model. Whether implemented within the boundaries of the main program or separately as in residential or nonresidential halfway houses, or in ambulatory settings, the perspective and approach guiding aftercare programming must be *continuous* with that of primary treatment in the TC. Thus, the views of right living and self-help recovery and the use of a peer network are essential to enhance the appropriate use of vocational, educational, mental health, social and other typical aftercare or reentry services.

Source: De Leon, The Therapeutic Community: Theory, Model, and Method; reproduced from chapter 25, copyright 2000. Used with permission of Springer Publishing Company, Inc., New York 10036.

chological adjustment at two- and five-year follow-up evaluations (De Leon 1984; De Leon and Jainchill 1981).

The preceding intent-to-treat studies also uniformly report a consistent positive relationship between time spent in residential treatment and posttreatment outcome. For example, in long-term TC programs, success rates for primary opioid abusers (on composite indices of no drug use and no criminality) at two years after completion of treatment are approximately 90, 50, and 25 percent for graduates or completers, dropouts who remain in residential treatment for more than one year, and dropouts who remain in residential treatment for less than one year, respectively (De Leon 1984).

Though impressive, the research evidence supporting the impact of TC treatment for opioid (and other) abusers is mainly based on field effectiveness studies. Randomized clinical trials involving complex treatment models such as TCs in residential settings are difficult to implement (De Leon et al. 1995a). One evaluation based upon the TOPS survey included a comparison between TC and other residential programs that were not TC programs (Condelli and Hubbard 1994). The sociodemographic and drug use profiles of admissions to both conditions were similar (including 30% daily users of opioids). Findings showed that there was no relationship between retention and outcomes in the non-TC residential programs, whereas such a relationship was found for the TC residential programs. This comparison further supported conclusions about the effectiveness of the TC for opioid and nonopioid abusers, with the exception of primary alcohol abusers.

Within the past decade controlled, comparative, intent-to-treat studies of drug treatment in prison-based settings have further confirmed the effectiveness of the TC for substance abuse (Inciardi et al. 1997; Knight et al. 1999; Wexler et al. 1999). A meta-analysis of the prison TC research has also reproduced findings on the relationship between length of stay and outcomes (Lipton et al. 2002).

In summary, some 30 years of extensive field effectiveness studies and more recent controlled investigations support the conclusion that TC-oriented treatment is effective for substance abusers, particularly primary opioid abusers. Much of the recent research on TCs has focused on clarifying and maximizing retention in treatment. A growing body of evidence underscores the importance of client motivational and readiness factors in both seeking and completing treatment in the TC (De Leon et al. 2000).

Pharmacotherapy and the TC Approach

The use of medically prescribed drugs for substance abuse withdrawal or psychotropic medications for psychological symptoms is inconsistent with the TC perspective of the substance abuse disorder and recovery. The strategic need for such medications is recognized and accepted by TCs, as in cases of medically managed withdrawals and pharmacologic interventions for psychiatric emergencies. As a rule, however, these cases are managed in referred settings. The only medications that are dispensed in standard TC programs are those required for routine health care and for residents with chronic health conditions, such as diabetes, hypertension, HIV infection and AIDS, and hepatitis C infection.

However, TC policies and practices with respect to the use of pharmacotherapy have been undergoing modifications. Three examples from field observation reports and limited research studies illustrate how TCs are modifying these practices for some substance abusers, including opioid-dependent clients.

Pharmacotherapy in Long-Term Residential TC

Some TC agencies incorporate psychotropic medication for selected cases, reflecting the increasing number of admissions with serious psychological symptoms that are both drug- and non-drug-related. For example, programs recognize the special psychopharmacologic properties of cocaine/crack dependence (e.g., craving, severe mood alterations, violence, energy shifts) and how these affect the course of recovery in residential treatment as well as relapse rates after treatment. Thus, they accept the limited use of psychopharmacologic adjuncts to help ameliorate the depression and anxiety associated with the after-effects of these drugs.

Some agencies also manage methadone tapering in outpatient clinics as a stand-alone service, but methadone is also used to initiate client commitment to longer-term residential treatment. More recently, TC programs have been involved in clinical trials on the utility and efficacy of buprenorphine to facilitate withdrawal from illegal opioids, as a first step in the recovery process in the TC.

Residential TC: Methadone to Abstinence

Several TC agencies have provided special residential "methadone-to-abstinence" programs (M-to-A) for opioid abusers. A goal of these programs is to facilitate client involvement in the drug-free regimen of the TC through a gradual (3–6 months) withdrawal from methadone. The effectiveness of M-to-A programs has not been adequately evaluated, although clinical impression suggests that positive outcomes are seen in those patients who complete their methadone withdrawal and their full residential tenure in the TC. Nevertheless, only a small percentage of patients receiving methadone voluntarily enter these programs, limiting the utility of M-to-A programs for the larger population of opioid abusers seeking or in opioid treatment programs.

Modified TC: Methadone-Maintained Patients

In the past decade a rapprochement between pharmacotherapy and the "drug-free TC" was facilitated by the development of an intensive outpatient model serving methadone-maintained clients. This adaptation of the TC approach for patients receiving methadone in a day-treatment setting required some modifications in assumptions and program components as illustrated in a demonstration model called Passages (De Leon et al. 1995b). A significant change is in treatment philosophy, which accepts the validity and importance of methadone as a pharmacologic tool to be utilized in recovery and rehabilitation. Thus, the major goals of Passages are abstinence from all *nonprescribed* substances and acquisition of prosocial behaviors and attitudes.

The Passages program retains what is central to TC-oriented approaches, that is, the peer community method, with modifications for the methadone patient in a day-treatment modality. These modifications include greater emphasis on outreach and advocacy; increased flexibility in a phase format; reduction in the intensity of interpersonal interactions; guided implementation of all new behavioral expectations; and greater responsiveness to individual differences. Key innovations in this program include integration of an individual Client Action Plan (a weekly goal attainment tool) within the group context and creation of an extended program or Fellowship. It also includes the trainee stipend group, designed to develop a cadre of methadone clients with recovery experience in Passages and training in modified TC methods.

Passages has been evaluated in an open clinical trial (De Leon et al. 1995b), the main findings of which are summarized here. Multivariate analyses of the intent-to-treat sample revealed significantly better reductions in cocaine and heroin use among Passages than non-Passages participants. Those who remain in the Passages program show consistently better longitudinal improvement at six and twelve months postbaseline than dropouts from the program and a non-Passages comparison group.

The findings of this study provide the empirical basis for a large-scale controlled clinical trial of the Passages model. In addition, these results illustrate the potential for integrating complex psychosocial interventions using modified TC methods with methadone maintenance to facilitate recovery in opioid clients with serious substance abuse and related disorders. Finally, they also show how TCs continue to evolve and innovate in an effort to find the optimal mechanisms for improving the lives of patients with substance abuse disorders.

Non-TC Drug-free Treatment

Structure of the US Drug-free Treatment System

In the United States, 75 percent of treatment facilities are so-called outpatient drug-free clinics that offer primarily counseling services without medication support. The intensity of these services can vary from counseling once per week to intensive programs offering several hours per day of therapy, although group counseling two to three times per week is probably the most common offering within this modality. Methadone clinics comprise 8 percent of treatment facilities in the United States, outpatient rehabilitation programs that can include outpatient detoxification comprise 74 percent, residential or hospital-based inpatient detoxification programs comprise 15 percent, and long-term residential programs (in-

Table 15.2 **Distribution of Treatment Admissions by Primary Drug of Abuse**

Treatment Modality	Admissions* (%)		Completed Treatment (%)		Transferred to Further Treatment (%)	
	Opioid	Alcohol	Opioid	Alcohol	Opioid	Alcohol
IOP (N = 52,248)	6.9	47.1	23.5	51.8	14.5	7.9
Detoxification[†] (N = 73,564)	34.9	46.7	49.3	54.4	2.1	9.6
Short-term residential (N = 36,375)	9.9	47.2	58.7	67.0	7.4	11.2
Long-term residential (N = 26,603)	14.8	38.8	28.6	37.4	3.6	8.8
Hospital inpatient (N = 7,794)	4.5	58.0	53.7	58.8	16.8	25.1

Note: Data shown are for the United States, 2000, based on records submitted from 18 states. IOP, intensive outpatient program.

*The percent of admissions is shown for just the two substances of interest (alcohol and opioids). These do not total 100% for a treatment modality, because there were other primary substances prompting an admission (e.g., marijuana, sedatives).

[†]Detoxification includes both inpatient and outpatient settings.

cluding therapeutic communities) comprise the remaining 3 percent of treatment facilities (SAMHSA 2003b).

Table 15.2 shows the distribution of treatment admissions in the United States by modality of service for primary opioid and alcohol abusers in the year 2000 and the percent completing treatment within each modality (SAMHSA 2003a, 2004a, 2004b, 2004c, 2004d). Note that most opioid addicts entering treatment enroll in methadone maintenance and that patients dependent on opioids comprise a small percentage of the patient admissions to all treatment modalities except detoxification. In contrast, alcohol-dependent patients comprise a relatively large proportion of entries to all treatment modalities shown. The remaining admissions to the modalities listed in table 15.2 are primarily patients who are dependent on stimulants, sedatives, marijuana, or mixed patterns of drug abuse. Regarding treatment completion, and considering that the data for opioid versus alcohol abusers may come from different types of clinics within a modality of service, it appears that treatment completion is similar for opioid and alcohol abusers in most modalities, except for intensive outpatient programs (IOP), where opioid abusers have poorer treatment completion (23%) than alcoholics (52%).

Medically Supervised Withdrawal as a Precursor to Outpatient Aftercare Treatment

Because opioid abusers typically are physically dependent on opioids before treatment entry, medically supervised withdrawal is generally the first step in the treatment process. Evidence shows that a brief inpatient medically supervised withdrawal for a person dependent on illicit opioids can help reduce subsequent drug use and criminal activity following discharge (Chutuape et al. 2001a). However, because most patients relapse to opioid use within a month after completing their withdrawal (Broers et al. 2000; Gossop et al. 1989), this form of treatment is best viewed as one component of a continuum of services for substance abuse and a gateway to outpatient aftercare services. Medically supervised withdrawal usually includes the administration of medications designed to alleviate withdrawal discomfort. Tapering and then discontinuing medications allows patients to complete the withdrawal in a substance-free state and ready for the aftercare component of the treatment process.

Patients dependent on opioids may enter medically supervised withdrawal rather than methadone maintenance because of the lack of available methadone treatment slots, the negative attitudes and stigma associated with methadone maintenance that exists among many opioid-addicted individuals, or a desire to live without the constraints associated with involvement in an opioid treatment program (Gilman et al. 2001; Kipnis et al. 2001; Zule and Desmond 1998). One study compared the characteristics of opioid addicts voluntarily electing to enter either methadone maintenance or short-term (a 3- to 7-day) medically supervised withdrawal treatment. The study found that those patients seeking medically supervised withdrawal had more previous medically supervised withdrawal treatments, had been treated with methadone for less time in their life, and had higher Addiction Severity Index composite scores (i.e., more problems) for measures of alcohol, legal, employment, family/social, medical, and psychiatric issues than patients treated with methadone (Cumberbatch et al. 2004). This suggests that persons who preferentially select medically supervised withdrawal over methadone maintenance treatment may have a particularly difficult time remaining abstinent.

Transition into Aftercare Treatment

The higher problem severity levels detected in medically supervised withdrawal patients suggest an urgent need for continuation of care after the withdrawal. Aftercare services may not be available at the same programs that offer medically supervised withdrawal, however. Furthermore, compliance with entry into aftercare treatment is often very poor, even when aftercare is readily available. For example, evaluations of patients given instructions for treatment referral found that the average rate of admission into aftercare ranged from 10 to 40 percent (Lash 1998; McCusker et al. 1995; Sheffet et al. 1976).

Certain procedures have been found to improve aftercare treatment entry. One of the most effective methods identified is having the patient sample the aftercare provided during the medically supervised withdrawal program (i.e., before completion). For example, a study with alcoholic inpatients given the opportunity to attend aftercare groups in an aftercare facility while still inpatients found that the patients were significantly more likely to attend aftercare when given this chance than a control group that was not given the opportunity to sample aftercare (Verinis and Taylor 1994). In contrast, the same report found that continuing with the same counselor versus changing counselors from the inpatient medically supervised withdrawal phase to outpatient aftercare treatment had no impact on compliance with aftercare treatment. Other forms of familiarizing patients with aftercare (e.g., attendance orientation, contracts, reminders, and social reinforcement by the counselor) can also improve aftercare attendance (Lash et al. 2001, 2004). Programming telephone contact with medically supervised withdrawal patients during the first week or two after discharge from medically supervised withdrawal can also be an effective method. Finally, a study showed that combining a transportation service with a small ($13) incentive payment was highly effective for transitioning patients dependent on opioids completing a withdrawal to an aftercare program (Chutuape et al. 2001b). Seventy-six percent of patients attended the aftercare program in the escort plus incentive program compared with 44 percent of patients who only received the incentives and 24 percent who were provided neither transition intervention. Furthermore, these impressive results were obtained even though the aftercare program was located several miles from the medically supervised withdrawal program. Thus, the generally poor compliance rates seen for aftercare treatment entry can be countered by relatively simple transition interventions.

Outcomes for Opioid Abusers in Outpatient Drug-free Treatment

Few studies have reported treatment outcomes for opioid abusers enrolled in drug-free outpatient treatment, in part, because of the very small numbers of such patients that enter this treatment modality, as described earlier. One randomized clinical trial reported data from heroin abusers entering outpatient treatment (Katz et al. 2004). The use of a single role induction session was compared with standard group orientation; outcomes were three-month treatment retention and drug use. Role induction participants had greater treatment retention and were more satisfied with the treatment program than standard group orientation participants.

The lack of reports on treatment outcome for opiate abusers in outpatient treatment, however, is a significant gap in the treatment evaluation literature and one that should be addressed to characterize this treatment service and to determine which aspects of outpatient, drug-free treatment are effective. The need for such research is especially pressing because of the rise in prescription opioid abuse, and the subsequent appearance of this group of patients dependent on opioids seeking treatment in outpatient drug-free programs.

Reinforcement-Based Therapy

Recently, outcomes have been reported for an outpatient program especially designed for heroin abusers exiting short-term medically supervised withdrawal. The program, called reinforcement-based therapy (RBT), is interesting because it attempts to combine elements of residential treatment with intensive outpatient care by utilizing community recovery housing as a treatment option and incentive. Recovery houses are homes located in local neighborhoods that are near the treatment program. They are privately owned and operated as boarding houses, and they provide sleeping quarters and shared bathing, cooking, laundry, and lounging (i.e., family room with TV/VCR or CD player) facilities. Residents live in a structured environment under the watchful guidance of a house manager. Curfews are imposed, Narcotics Anonymous meeting attendance is required, chores are assigned, visitors are restricted, and use of drugs or alcohol is strictly prohibited. The RBT treatment program offers to pay rent for patients in these houses on an abstinence-contingent basis during the first three months of treatment. For those willing to take advantage of the recovery house option, the treatment program provides comprehensive services very similar to those that may be found in a residential program with the advantage that patients can gain experience with living in a natural environment while remaining drug-free. The program also has flexibility in that patients unwilling to take advantage of the recovery housing services can still be provided with relatively intensive day-treatment services that may be beneficial in themselves.

RBT Program Elements

To facilitate treatment entry, participants assigned to RBT are escorted from the medically supervised withdrawal unit to the RBT program. Patients are introduced to their assigned counselor and then immediately begin participating in the intensive day-treatment program described next. At the end of the treatment day, participants are escorted to a recovery house by treatment staff if they are willing to engage in this option. The next morning, participants are escorted from the recovery house back to the treatment program by a staff member to facilitate their treatment participation.

Schedule of Treatment

Participants are expected to attend the program seven days a week during the first three weeks, four days per week during weeks 4 to 12, and to regularly provide urine samples collected under observation by a same-gender research assistant. In the final three months of treatment, contact is reduced to twice a week for all RBT participants and incentives for housing, food, and recreation are no longer offered.

Each time a participant attends the clinic they provide a urine sample tested for heroin and cocaine. Expectations for clinic attendance are the same regardless of whether the urine sample is positive or negative for opioids and cocaine. The difference in programming for those who test positive and those who test negative is the duration and content of the counseling contact and activities. Participants testing negative for opiates and cocaine on a given day participate in the full range of counseling activities, including individual therapy sessions. Those testing positive meet with their counselor for an individual session focused on strategies for regaining abstinence. Transportation aid in the form of bus tokens or parking passes for each session attended is provided during the first three months independent of urine test results.

Elements of Counseling in RBT

On weekdays (Monday through Thursday), the RBT program includes one group-counseling session that focuses on relapse prevention skill building, lunch in the hospital cafeteria, employment search skills building (Job Club), and recreational activities. Relapse prevention skills building includes manualized sessions on topics such as relapse triggers, coping with drug availability, drug thoughts, dysphoric emotions, and environmental triggers. The content of these skills-building sessions is derived from existing manualized treatments (Budney and Higgins 1998; Carroll 1998). The format of the Job Club is based on a behavioral approach to vocational counseling that has been described previously (Azrin and Besalel 1980), in which the focus is to identify jobs compatible with the participant's current skill level and provide the patient with the skills necessary for obtaining and maintaining employment (e.g., locating and pursuing job leads, developing a resume, interviewing, being punctual and demonstrating the responsibility to retain a job). Patients participate in Job Club activities until they secure employment. Recreational activities include outings in the community such as attending movies and going to a local gymnasium. On Fridays, group skills building and a Social Club are held. During the Social Club, patients receive lunch and have the opportunity to interact with non-drug-using peers. Patients can attend Social Club throughout treatment, if they are drug negative. Individual counseling sessions are scheduled two to three times a week. Topics for drug-negative patients include reviewing urine test results, reviewing the day plan, discussing difficulties related to cravings or temptations, providing reinforcement of successes, monitoring job search activities, and setting new short and longer goals as needed.

RBT Outcome Evaluations

The outcomes of RBT have been evaluated in three studies. First, in a short-term evaluation of RBT (Gruber et al. 2000), 61 percent of RBT subjects versus 17 percent of controls receiving referrals for aftercare were enrolled in a treatment program at one month after withdrawal. Furthermore, 50 percent of RBT versus 21 percent of control subjects were abstinent from both heroin and cocaine at one month after withdrawal. The removal of abstinence-based incentives from the RBT group resulted in a dramatic decline in retention.

In the second study, the RBT model was again examined but with additional abstinence-based voucher reinforcers provided (Katz et al. 2001). In this study, 43 percent of the subjects completed ten or more weeks of treatment while submitting 92 percent opiate- and cocaine-free urine samples, and 32 percent became employed during the program.

The most recent evaluation of RBT was conducted in a large sample ($N = 130$) of opiate abusers invited into an aftercare research program after completing a brief (3- to 7-day) inpatient medically supervised withdrawal (Jones et al. Forthcoming). Participants were randomly assigned to RBT or usual care (referral to community outpatient treatment programs), and outcomes were tracked for twelve months to determine the extent and duration of any beneficial effects associated with the intensive aftercare program. The RBT group retained 60, 46, and 37 percent of participants for one, three, and six months, respectively. When compared at follow-up time points, the RBT-treated group had significantly higher urinalysis-confirmed rates of abstinence from opiates and cocaine than usual-care participants at one (54% versus 24%) and three (46% versus 25%) months. No significant differences in opioid or cocaine abstinence rates were observed between the RBT and usual-care groups at six (43% versus 31%) or twelve months (35% versus 32%), respectively. The improvement in the usual-care group appeared to be due to participants enrolling in methadone maintenance. The Addiction Severity Index results show significant increases in the number of days worked and the amount of legal income earned by the RBT group relative to usual care at three, six, and twelve months. The results of this randomized study suggest that an intensive reinforcement therapy that includes abstinence-based recovery housing may be a useful initial approach to postwithdrawal treatment. An additional study is underway to further determine the role of treatment intensity and the specific efficacy that RBT components have in drug treatment outcomes.

Summary and Conclusions

Opioid treatment programs have limited capacity, and the two forms of drug-free treatment reviewed here are important and often-overlooked components of the substance abuse treatment system. Drug-free treatment programs are relatively plentiful—they are not rare or unusual services. Although TCs have received attention and systematic research, outpatient drug-free programs that treat patients dependent on opioids are often overlooked and forgotten in the context of new medications (e.g., buprenorphine) and new modes of treatment (e.g., office-based treatment). This oversight is unfortunate.

Given that many opioid-dependent persons do not care to enter an opioid treatment program (i.e., methadone treatment), TCs and outpatient drug-free treatment programs should be considered viable and integral options for the treatment of opioid abusers. Whereas patients may need to undergo medically supervised withdrawal before drug-free treatment to address their physical dependence on opioids, this is a relatively simple step in the treatment process. Physical dependence on opioids should not limit the use of these forms of treatment.

Continued evolution of drug-free treatment occurs. For TCs, this includes its extension into new settings such as prisons, and its incorporation of new pharmacotherapies such as buprenorphine. These changes reflect the dynamic features of a treatment modality that is willing to experiment in its continued desire to improve the lives of its target patients. Similarly, studies with outpatient drug-free treatment show how innovation can improve treatment results, especially for patients undergoing a more traditional inpatient medically supervised withdrawal from opioids. The use of new incentive programs to improve drug-free treatment outcomes is a methodology that appears promising and useful. Continued evolution and evaluation of all forms of drug-free treatment is needed to better understand the optimal means for helping patients dependent on opioids improve their lives.

References

Azrin NH, Besalel VA (1980). *A Behavioral Approach to Vocational Counseling.* Baltimore: University Park Press

Broers B, Giner F, Dumont P, Mino A (2000). Inpatient opiate detoxification in Geneva: follow-up at 1 and 6 months. *Drug Alcohol Depend* 58: 85–92.

Budney AJ, Higgins ST (1998). A Community Reinforcement Plus Vouchers Approach: Treating Cocaine Addiction. DHHS Pub. No. 98-4309. Rockville, MD: U.S. Department of Health and Human Services.

Carroll KM (1998). A Cognitive-Behavioral Approach: Treating Cocaine Addiction. DHHS Pub. No. 98-4308. Rockville, MD: U.S. Department of Health and Human Services.

Chutuape MA, Jasinski DR, Fingerhood MI, Stitzer ML (2001a). One-, three-, and six-month outcomes after brief inpatient opioid detoxification. *Am J Drug Alcohol Abuse* 27: 19–44.

Chutuape MA, Katz EC, Stitzer ML (2001b). Methods for enhancing transition of substance dependent patients from inpatient to outpatient treatment. *Drug Alcohol Depend* 61: 137–43.

Condelli WS, Hubbard RL (1994). Client outcomes from therapeutic communities. In: Tims FM, De Leon G, Jainchill N, eds. Therapeutic Communities: Advances in Research and Application (NIDA Research Monograph), 80–98. Bethesda, MD: National Institute on Drug Abuse.

Cumberbatch Z, Copersino M, Stitzer M, Jones H (2004). Comparative drug use and psychosocial profiles of opioid dependents applying for medication versus medication-free treatment. *Am J Drug Alcohol Abuse* 30: 237–49.

De Leon G (1984). The Therapeutic Community: Study of Effectiveness. DHHS Pub. No. ADM 84-1286. Bethesda, MD: National Institute on Drug Abuse.

De Leon G (1985). The therapeutic community: status and evolution. *Int J Addict* 20: 823–44.

De Leon G (1988). Legal pressure in therapeutic communities. In: Leukefeld CG, Tims FM, eds. Compulsory Treatment of Drug Abuse: Research and Clinical Practice (NIDA Research Monograph), 160–77. Bethesda, MD: National Institute on Drug Abuse.

De Leon G (1993). Cocaine abusers in therapeutic community treatment. In: Tims FM, ed. Cocaine Treatment: Research and Clinical Perspectives (NIDA Research Monograph), 163–89. Washington, DC: U.S. Government Printing Office.

De Leon G (1997). *Community as Method: Therapeutic Communities for Special Populations and Special Settings.* Westport, CT: Greenwood Publishing Group.

De Leon G (1999). Therapeutic communities: research and applications. In: Glantz MD, Hartel CR, eds. *Drug Abuse: Origins and Interventions.* Washington, DC: American Psychological Association.

De Leon G (2000). *The Therapeutic Community: Theory, Model, and Method.* New York: Springer Publishing Company.

De Leon G (2004). Therapeutic Communities. In: Galanter M, Kleber HD, eds. *The American Psychiatric Press Textbook of Substance Abuse Treatment,* 485–501. Washington, DC: American Psychiatric Press.

De Leon G, Inciardi JA, Martin SS (1995a). Residential drug abuse treatment research: are conventional control designs appropriate for assessing treatment effectiveness? *J Psychoactive Drugs* 27: 85–91.

De Leon G, Jainchill N (1981). Male and female drug abusers: social and psychological status 2 years after treatment in a therapeutic community. *Am J Drug Alcohol Abuse* 8: 465–97.

De Leon G, Melnick G, Hawke J (2000). The motivation-readiness factor in drug treatment: implications for research and policy. In: Levy J, Stephens R, McBride D, eds. *Emergent Issues in the Field of Drug Abuse (Advance in Medical Sociology),* 103–129. Stamford, CT: JAI Press.

De Leon G, Schwartz S (1984). Therapeutic communities: what are the retention rates? *Am J Drug Alcohol Abuse* 10: 267–84.

De Leon G, Staines GL, Perlis TE, Sacks S, McKendrick K, Hilton R, Brady R (1995b). Therapeutic community methods in methadone maintenance (Passages): an open clinical trial. *Drug Alcohol Depend* 37: 45–57.

Etheridge RM, Hubbard RL, Anderson J, Craddock SG, Flynn PM (1997). Treatment structure and program services in the Drug Abuse Treatment Outcome Study (DATOS). *Psychol Addict Behav* 11: 244–60.

Gerstein DR (2004). Outcome Research: Drug Abuse. In: Galanter M, Kleber HD, eds. *The American Psychiatric Publishing Textbook of Substance Abuse Treatment,* 137–47. Washington, DC: American Psychiatric Publishing.

Gilman SM, Galanter M, Dermatis H (2001). Methadone anonymous: a 12-step program for methadone maintained heroin addicts. *Subst Abus* 22: 247–56.

Gossop M, Green L, Phillips G, Bradley B (1989). Lapse, relapse and survival among opiate addicts after treatment. A prospective follow-up study. *Br J Psychiatry* 154: 348–53.

Gruber K, Chutuape MA, Stitzer ML (2000). Reinforcement-based intensive outpatient treatment for inner city opiate abusers: a short-term evaluation. *Drug Alcohol Depend* 57: 211–23.

Holland S (1983). Evaluating community based treatment programs: a model for strengthening inferences about effectiveness. *Int J Ther Communities* 4: 285–306.

Hubbard RL, Craddock SG, Flynn PM, Anderson J, Etheridge RM (1997). Overview of 1-year follow-up outcomes in the Drug Abuse Treatment Outcome Study (DATOS). *Psychol Addict Behav* 11: 261–78.

Hubbard RL, Marsden ME, Rachal JV, Harwood HJ, Cavanaugh ER, Ginzburg HM (1989). *Drug Abuse Treatment: A National Study of Effectiveness.* Chapel Hill, NC: The University of North Carolina Press.

Inciardi JA, Martin SS, Butzin CA, Hooper RM, Harrison LD (1997). An effective model of prison-based treatment for drug-involved offenders. *J Drug Issues* 2: 261–278

Jainchill N (1994). Co-morbidity and therapeutic community treatment. In: Tims FM, De Leon G, Jainchill N, eds. Therapeutic Community: Advances in Research and Application (NIDA Research Monograph), 209–31. Bethesda, MD: National Institute on Drug Abuse.

Jainchill N, De Leon G, Yagelka J (1997). Ethnic differences in psychiatric disorders among adolescent substance abusers in treatment. *J Psychopathol Behav Assess* 19: 133–47.

Jones HE, Wong CJ, Tuten M, Stitzer ML (Forthcoming). Reinforcement Based Therapy: 12-Month evaluation of an outpatient drug-free treatment for heroin abusers. *Drug Alcohol Depend.*

Katz EC, Brown BS, Schwartz RP, Weintraub E, Barksdale W, Robinson R (2004). Role induction: a method for enhancing early retention in outpatient drug-free treatment. *J Consult Clin Psychol* 72: 227–34.

Katz EC, Gruber K, Chutuape MA, Stitzer ML (2001). Reinforcement-based outpatient treatment for opiate and cocaine abusers. *J Subst Abuse Treat* 20: 93–98.

Kipnis SS, Herron A, Perez J, Joseph H (2001). Integrating the methadone patient in the traditional addiction inpatient rehabilitation program—problems and solutions. *Mt Sinai J Med* 68: 28–32.

Knight K, Simpson DD, Hiller ML (1999). Three-year reincarceration outcomes for in-prison therapeutic community treatment in Texas. *Prison J* 79: 337–51.

Lash SJ (1998). Increasing participation in substance abuse aftercare treatment. *Am J Drug Alcohol Abuse* 24: 31–36.

Lash SJ, Burden JL, Monteleone BR, Lehmann LP (2004). Social reinforcement of substance abuse treatment aftercare participation: Impact on outcome. *Addict Behav* 29: 337–42.

Lash SJ, Petersen GE, O'Connor EA, Lehmann LP (2001). Social reinforcement of substance abuse aftercare group therapy attendance. *J Subst Abuse Treat* 20: 3–8.

Lipton DS, Pearson FS, Cleland CM, Yee D (2002). The effects of therapeutic communities and milieu therapy on recidivism: meta-analytic findings from the Correctional Drug Abuse Treatment Effectiveness (CDATE) Study. In: McGuire J, ed. *Offender Rehabilitation and Treatment: Effective Programmes and Policies to Reduce Re-offending.* West Sussex, England: John Wiley and Sons.

McCusker J, Bigelow C, Luippold R, Zorn M, Lewis BF (1995). Outcomes of a 21-day drug detoxification program: retention, transfer to further treatment, and HIV risk reduction. *Am J Drug Alcohol Abuse* 21: 1–16.

NIDA (2002). Therapeutic Community: What is a Therapeutic Community? NIH Pub. No. 02-4877. Bethesda, MD: National Institute on Drug Abuse.

Pompi KF (1994). Adolescents in therapeutic communities: retention and posttreatment outcome. In: Tims FM, De Leon G, Jainchill N, eds. Therapeutic Community: Advances in Research and Application (NIDA Research Monograph), 128–61. Bethesda, MD: National Institute on Drug Abuse.

Pompi KF, Resnick J (1987). Retention of court-referred adolescents and young adults in the therapeutic community. *Am J Drug Alcohol Abuse* 13: 309–25.

SAMHSA (2003a). The DASIS Report: Discharges from Intensive Outpatient Treatment: 2000. Arlington, VA, and Research Triangle Park, NC: Substance Abuse and Mental Health Services Administration, Office of Applied Studies.

SAMHSA (2003b). National Survey of Substance Abuse Treatment Services (N-SSATS): 2002. Data on Substance Abuse Treatment Facilities. DHHS Publication No. (SMA) 03-3777. Rockville, MD: Substance Abuse and Mental Health Services Administration, Office of Applied Studies.

SAMHSA (2004a). The DASIS Report: Discharges from Detoxification: 2000. Arlington, VA, and Research Triangle Park, NC: Substance Abuse and Mental Health Services Administration, Office of Applied Studies.

SAMHSA (2004b). The DASIS Report: Discharges from Hospital Inpatient Treatment: 2000. Arlington, VA, and Research Triangle Park, NC: Substance Abuse and Mental Health Services Administration, Office of Applied Studies.

SAMHSA (2004c). The DASIS Report: Discharges from Long-term Residential Treatment: 2000. Arlington, VA, and Research Triangle Park, NC: Substance Abuse and Mental Health Services Administration, Office of Applied Studies.

SAMHSA (2004d). The DASIS Report: Discharges from Short-term Residential Treatment: 2000. Arlington, VA, and Research Triangle Park, NC: Substance Abuse and Mental Health Services Administration, Office of Applied Studies.

Sheffet A, Quinones M, Lavenhar MA, Doyle K, Prager H (1976). An evaluation of detoxification as an initial step in the treatment of heroin addiction. *Am J Psychiatry* 133: 337–40.

Simpson D, Sells S (1982). Effectiveness for treatment of drug abuse: an overview of the DARP research programme. *Adv Alcohol Subst Abuse* 2: 7–29.

Simpson DD, Joe GW, Brown BS (1997). Treatment retention and follow-up outcomes in the Drug Abuse Treatment Outcome Study (DATOS). *Psychol Addict Behav* 11: 294–307.

Tims FM, De Leon G, Jainchill N (1994). Therapeutic Community: Advances in Research and Application. NIH Pub. No. 94-3633. Bethesda, MD: National Institute on Drug Abuse.

Verinis JS, Taylor J (1994). Increasing alcoholic patients' aftercare attendance. *Int J Addict* 29: 1487–94.

Wexler HK, De Leon G, Thomas G, Kressel D, Peters J (1999). The Amity prison TC evaluation: reincarceration outcomes. *Crim Justice Behavior* 26: 144–67.

Zule WA, Desmond DP (1998). Attitudes toward methadone maintenance: implications for HIV prevention. *J Psychoactive Drugs* 30: 89–97.

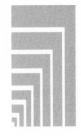

16

Medically Supervised Withdrawal as Stand-Alone Treatment

Michael Gossop, Ph.D.

For dependent opiate users, an intermediate treatment goal, and a preliminary phase of treatments that are aimed at abstinence, involves withdrawal from drugs or detoxification. Within U.S. federally funded treatment programs, more than 40 percent of those who were treated for heroin dependence during the early 1980s received treatment in a detoxification program (Lipton 1983). About a quarter of patients were admitted to methadone maintenance programs and about a third were admitted to drug-free treatment during the same period, in contrast. A more recent estimate suggested that 50 percent, or about 116,000 admissions per year in the United States, were for detoxification as a primary form of treatment (SAMHSA 1999).

THE PROBLEM OF WITHDRAWAL

Early formulations of drug dependence emphasized the importance of tolerance and withdrawal. DSM-III, for example, stated, "the diagnosis requires the presence of physiologic dependence." More recent formulations of addiction tend to see these neuroadaptative processes as just part of the cluster of factors that make up the dependence syndrome.

The importance of the treatment and management of withdrawal should not be underestimated, however. The processes of neuroadaptation present problems both for the therapist and for the patient. Detoxification may act either as a barrier to recovery or as a springboard. Even though drug withdrawal is seldom medically serious and can be accomplished even with individuals dependent on high doses of heroin (Gossop 1989), many addicts are anxious about the prospect of detoxification, and their fears about withdrawal may deter some of them from seeking treatment. Further, the discomfort of withdrawal symptoms may interfere with treatment and may, in some circumstances, lead the patient to drop out of treatment. For these reasons, detoxification should be considered a critically important part of the total treatment plan and should be managed in a way that involves as little discomfort as possible.

The clinical features of the opiate withdrawal syndrome are well known and their underlying mechanisms relatively well understood. When heroin is discontinued, the agonist effects diminish for 6 to 8 hours. After about 8 hours, and certainly after 12 to 15 hours, addicts will start to feel uncomfortable. After about 18 hours, they will feel unwell, and withdrawal symptoms will increase in severity. After about 24 hours they are anxious and restless and find it difficult either to sleep or to rest comfortably. Glandular secretions increase: the eyes and nose run, and salivation and sweating are increased. Withdrawal symptoms are usually at their most intense between 24 and 72 hours. The bones, muscles, and joints ache, and the addict may also suffer from stomach cramps, vomiting, and diarrhea. Because of this cluster of symptoms, a commonly drawn analogy is that the opiate withdrawal syndrome is similar to a bad case of influenza (Kleber 1981). Thereafter, the symptoms will gradually lessen in intensity, though it may be more than a week or even 10 days before the dependent individual starts to feel well again.

Assessment of the opioid withdrawal syndrome can be accomplished by means of self-report instruments. One typical scale has patients rate the severity of ten commonly reported symptoms: feeling sick, stomach cramps, muscle spasms/twitching, feelings of coldness, heart pounding, muscular tension, aches and pains, yawning, runny eyes, and insomnia (Gossop 1990). Another similar scale is described by Wesson and Ling (2003), who also review the history of opioid withdrawal measurement in their paper. Such scales can provide valuable information, collected using standardized instruments, to the clinician about the effectiveness of detoxification procedures over time in individual patients. Use of standardized assessments is recommended because patients may differ initially in the severity of withdrawal and their response to treatment interventions.

The withdrawal syndrome is similar for all the opiates, though it tends to be less severe for less potent drugs such as codeine and propoxyphene (McKim 2000). One controversial topic is the widely held belief that withdrawal from methadone is more prolonged but less severe than withdrawal from heroin (Jaffe 1985). Little empirical evidence supports this view, however, which appears to be derived from early work by Isbell, Vogel, and others (Vogel et al. 1948). In general, withdrawal severity will depend on the dose and consistency of opiate use. Thus, sporadic use of heroin would be expected to result in less severe withdrawal than daily use, and persistent exposure to long-acting methadone might be expected to produce an even more severe withdrawal syndrome. One study investigated the withdrawal symptoms shown by opiate addicts who were using either heroin or methadone before detoxification treatment. During treatment, all received a 10-day methadone taper. Under these conditions, there were no differences in peak withdrawal severity or duration of withdrawal symptoms for the heroin and methadone users (Gossop and Strang 1991).

Drug withdrawal syndromes are powerfully influenced by neurophysiologic and neurochemical processes, as evidenced by the physiologic symptoms that are a prominent feature of the (opiate) withdrawal syndrome. In addition, detoxification often involves the administration of medication. For these reasons, detoxification is often seen primarily in physical terms, and the treatment of withdrawal is viewed primarily as a "medical" procedure. However, social and psychological factors have a considerable impact on the withdrawal syndrome. Anxiety-related factors, for example, increase the severity of the withdrawal response and can have a more powerful influence on withdrawal symptoms than the dose of heroin on which the addict was dependent before detoxification (Phillips et al. 1986). Physiologically based withdrawal symptoms also have psychological effects. For example, sleep disturbance is often found during withdrawal from many types of drugs. Lack of sleep is distressing for most people and, at times of particular stress such as during detoxification, it may sap the individual's motivation to change and commitment to treatment. Thus, the design of detoxification programs must take both physical and psychological factors into consideration.

The Goals of Detoxification

Reasons for the popularity of detoxification among both opiate users and some treatment providers are easy to understand. Detoxification attracts drug users who believe (generally incorrectly) that this is all they need to get off drugs and remain drug-free, as well as those who want only short-term relief from their habit. Treatment providers may view detoxification as an essential first step in a longer treatment process. Some residential rehabilitation programs, for example, require drug users to be drug free before they enter treatment, and some methadone maintenance programs require patients to have made at least one detoxification attempt before they are eligible to receive maintenance treatment. For other service providers, detoxification alone may offer the tempting prospect of a comparatively inexpensive treatment.

Detoxification alone, however, is seldom effective as a treatment for drug dependence. It has been shown repeatedly that there are high rates of relapse to addictive drug use after detoxification alone and that most patients achieve little long-term benefit. Thus, Simpson and Sells in the first large national drug abuse treatment outcome study (DARP) found that outcomes for patients in detoxification were consistently worse than for those who received methadone maintenance, therapeutic community, or outpatient drug-free treatment (Simpson and Sells 1990). In fact, outpatient detoxification offered no more therapeutic benefit than formal intake-only procedures without treatment (Simpson and Sells 1983). In the next large national treatment outcome study, TOPS, detoxification services were excluded from the possible treatment modalities because detoxification was regarded as "a short-term public health service that provides limited, if any, habilitation and rehabilitation services" (Hubbard et al. 1989, p. 14).

The purpose and role of detoxification in the larger picture of drug abuse treatment is often misunderstood. Detoxification should perhaps not be considered as a treatment modality in the same sense as methadone maintenance, Therapeutic Communities, chemical dependence, and psychosocial treatments because it does not produce, nor should it be expected to produce, the long-lasting psychological and behavioral changes that provide a secure foundation for sustained abstinence. Rather, the successful management of drug withdrawal during detoxification is a narrower and shorter-term goal than that of other treatments. Detoxification may be necessary but is not sufficient for recovery from an addiction disorder. Thus, the specific goals of detoxification are limited. This is a clearly delineated phase of treatment designed to eliminate or to reduce the severity of withdrawal symptoms when the physically dependent user stops taking drugs; it should be considered a precursor to other longer-term treatments that can tackle the problems of psychological dependence. Detoxification may also provide a period of respite from addictive drug use and its consequences, during which the individual may have an opportunity to reflect on the wisdom of further drug taking and possibly to engage with other types of treatment services (Mattick and Hall 1996).

Table 16.1   **Criteria for Judging the Effectiveness of Detoxification**

Criteria for Outcome	Specification of Outcome
Acceptability	Is the user willing to seek and undergo the intervention?
Availability	Is the treatment available and accessible, or can it be made available through existing treatment services?
Symptom severity	Is the treatment effective in the specific sense of reducing or eliminating the discomfort and distress of withdrawal?
Duration of withdrawal	Does the treatment reduce the overall duration of the withdrawal syndrome?
Side effects	The treatment should have no side effects, or only side effects that are less severe, and/or less medically serious than the untreated withdrawal symptoms.
Completion rate	Do a sufficient number of patients manage to complete the program and achieve a drug-free state at the end of the detoxification treatment?

The criteria by which the effectiveness of detoxification should be judged are shown in table 16.1.

When judged by the appropriate criteria, many current detoxification procedures can be considered effective, provided they are completed, in the sense that they permit a comfortable transition to abstinence with minimal symptoms of withdrawal.

Detoxification Methods

Although it is not the intent of this chapter to compare the effectiveness of methods of detoxification, it is necessary to say something about methods and procedures because of their implications for service delivery and because of the acceptability of different methods to the patient. Some heroin addicts attempt to manage their own detoxification without seeking formal treatment. Self-detoxification tends to be attempted more often during early stages of the individual's addiction career and may involve self-medication with benzodiazepines (Gossop et al. 1991).

Detoxification within the formal treatment system is not a uniform procedure. In fact, a large variety of procedures have been employed. Detoxification has been tried in both residential and outpatient settings with the use of various pharmacologic agents and nonpharmacologic interventions. It has been tried rapidly and slowly, and with and without counseling or other supportive services. A large assortment of medications has been used in heroin detoxification programs. Gowing and colleagues (2000) provide the following list of medications that have been used alone or in combination: tapered methadone, other opioid agonists (e.g., morphine), buprenorphine, adrenergic agonists, in particular, clonidine and lofexidine, opioid antagonists (e.g., naloxone, naltrexone, nalmefene) administered under anesthesia or sedation as a rapid detoxification or used as a follow-up to buprenorphine detoxification, antianxiety, antidepressant, or antipsychotic drugs used to modify receptor activity or treat concurrent psychiatric problems, and symptomatic medications (e.g., hypnotics to aid sleep).

One of the most widely used methods to manage withdrawal from opiates involves gradually reducing doses of an opiate agonist, usually oral methadone (Kreek 2000). Methadone is typically substituted for heroin before withdrawal, and detoxification is implemented by gradually reducing doses of methadone for periods of 10 to 28 days (Gossop et al. 1987, 1989b; Strang and Gossop 1990). One drawback of gradual methadone withdrawal, however, is that it leads to a protracted residual withdrawal response, with withdrawal symptoms persisting well beyond the last methadone dose (Bradley et al. 1989; Gossop et al. 1987, 1989b). Residual withdrawal symptoms may continue for as long as the original detoxification procedure. For example, when given for a 21-day period, patients are not fully recovered until 40 days after the beginning of withdrawal (Gossop et al. 1987, 1989b). The same residual withdrawal effect can be seen for 10-day reductions with symptoms persisting for about 20 days (Gossop and Strang 1991). In general, the period around the end of the methadone reduction schedule is associated with the greatest levels of discomfort. This can cause clinical management problems since many patients expect the last methadone dose to coincide with the last day of withdrawal discomfort, and the continued presence and relatively high severity of the residual withdrawal symptoms may be unsettling. Newer agents such as buprenorphine may provide a better profile of effects during detoxification (see chap. 11).

Although hospital or residential detoxification tends to be relatively brief (e.g., 2–21 days), outpatient detoxification is often implemented for prolonged periods. Methadone reduction treatment (MRT), for example, has been widely used in the United Kingdom for many years. Typically, MRT involves prescribing methadone for relatively long periods (6–12 months), with the expectation that the dose will gradually be reduced and that the patient will eventually be withdrawn from the drug and become abstinent from opiates. The policy of methadone reduction was formulated soon after the establishment of the British clinic system (Edwards

1969). Similar programs are implemented in other countries, and MRT is analogous to the gradual methadone detoxification programs described by Senay and colleagues (1977) and to the 90- and 180-day detoxification programs that have been implemented in the United States (Iguchi and Stitzer 1991; Reilly et al. 1995; Sees et al. 2000).

Studies of methadone reduction treatments, however, have raised questions about their ultimate effectiveness. Among patients receiving methadone maintenance, reductions in illicit heroin use are generally associated with higher methadone doses and longer retention in treatment (Gossop et al. 2001; Strain et al. 1999). In contrast, patients who receive MRT have poorer outcomes than those who receive stable dosing (Gossop et al. 2001; Sees et al. 2000; Senay et al. 1977). Faster dose reduction is associated with poorer outcomes than slower reduction (Gossop et al. 2001; Senay et al. 1977), and Capelhorn and colleagues (1994) also found worse outcomes for patients receiving abstinence-oriented rather than indefinite maintenance. MRT represents an uneasy compromise between maintenance and detoxification, with the danger that it may fail to achieve the full benefits of either form of treatment. For those patients receiving methadone who wish to detoxify and attempt to sustain their recovery without medication assistance, however, reasonably good outcomes can be achieved using slow, gradual detoxification schedules (Senay et al. 1977), even though success rates may not be as good as those achieved with continuing maintenance (e.g., only 53% of gradual withdrawal patients in the study by Senay et al. successfully completed their 30-week detoxification program).

In addition to studies showing that the speed of detoxification makes a difference in outcome, some attempts have been made to identify more effective methadone detoxification schedules. One attempt by Strang and Gossop, for example, involved modification of the slope of the reduction curve with proportionate (exponential) dose reductions rather than a fixed (linear) dose reduction schedule (Strang and Gossop 1990). It was hoped that a more rapid decrease in the earlier stages coupled with a more gradual reduction during the later stages would reduce withdrawal severity and/or reduce the duration of residual withdrawal symptoms. The study found that highly dependent addicts (those who needed to start their detoxification on methadone doses of 50 mg or higher) reported somewhat less withdrawal distress during the first 10 days of treatment under the linear as compared with the exponential schedule. Overall, however, the schedule showed no benefits on other measures of clinical outcome such as symptom severity during later phases of detoxification, time to symptom resolution, or treatment retention. Thus, detoxification rate may be a more fruitful parameter to manipulate than detoxification schedule is.

Psychological interventions can be used to support and improve the effectiveness of detoxification. The chances of successful detoxification are increased where both patient and clinician are in agreement about goals and procedures. Different people approach treatment services and enter treatment programs with differing expectations of what the therapeutic process will entail. To the extent that there are discrepancies between what the patient expects and what they receive, this may interfere with progress or reduce treatment adherence. It is useful to provide the patient with information about the procedures and requirements of treatment to reduce distress and improve treatment adherence rates (Katz et al. 2004; Meichenbaum and Turk 1987).

Providing addicts with accurate but reassuring information about withdrawal can alter the nature of the withdrawal response. Opiate addicts who had been informed of the nature and severity of their probable responses to detoxification experienced lower peak withdrawal scores and showed lower levels of residual withdrawal symptoms after a methadone reduction schedule than a noninformed group of heroin addicts (Green and Gossop 1988). In addition, the informed group was more likely to complete the detoxification program.

One factor that is sometimes believed to increase the successful completion of detoxification is the extent to which patients are involved in deciding their own rate of withdrawal from drugs. There has been considerable enthusiasm for adopting a more flexible and negotiable approach to clinical work with drug users including the management of detoxification (ACMD 1988), and it was hoped that the introduction of flexible detoxification schedules would be an improvement on existing "fixed" detoxification procedures. In a study addressing this question, Dawe and colleagues (1991) randomly allocated outpatient opiate addicts to either a fixed rate methadone reduction over a 6-week period, or a flexible, negotiable program that allowed patients to regulate the rate of their reduction within a 10-week period. Where patients negotiated a change in their detoxification regimen, this invariably resulted in a slower rate of reduction. Although the slower detoxification rate might be expected to produce better outcomes, in this study, no difference occurred between the fixed and negotiable groups in completion rates. It is possible that differences would be seen with longer periods available for the negotiated detoxification.

Treatment Setting: Residential versus Outpatient

Treatment consists of more than just clinical procedures and interventions. The total treatment package also includes program location, facilities, policies, services, and the aggregate characteristics of the patients and staff (Moos 1997). Detoxification can be provided in a variety of settings, including specialist inpatient drug dependence units, psychiatric hospital wards, residential rehabilitation programs, outpatient clinics, primary care clinics, and prisons. Different detoxification settings may be suitable for users with different circumstances and problems, or even for the same user at different stages of their addiction career.

The detoxification of opiate addicts on an outpatient basis, including detoxification in primary care settings, is widely used as part of national treatment responses in many countries. National policy in the United Kingdom is to encourage and expand the role of general practitioners (GPs) in the care and treatment of drug misusers; currently, British GPs have a substantial and increasing involvement with drug users (Gruer et al. 1997). In a U.K. survey, more than 40 percent of the methadone prescriptions given to addicts and filled by retail pharmacists were issued by GPs (Strang et al. 1996).

The U.S. Institute of Medicine reported in 1980 that detoxification may be undertaken successfully in most cases in a (nonhospital) residential, partial day care, or other community setting. This conclusion did not take completion rates into account, however. Whereas detoxification from opiates *can* be achieved in an outpatient setting, detoxification is less likely to be successful when attempted in this setting, where the key to successful completion of detoxification is compliance with the treatment protocol, and especially the avoidance of using illicit drugs during detoxification. In practice, success rates for outpatient detoxification programs are often poor, with many opiate addicts failing to complete their outpatient treatment program.

In an early review of the literature, Lipton and Maranda found completion rates of between 50 and 77 percent for inpatient detoxification and of about 20 percent for outpatient detoxification (Lipton and Maranda, 1983). This was borne out in later studies conducted in Great Britain, where it was found that the percentage of outpatients who achieve abstinence from opiates for even as little as 24 hours after treatment may be as low as 17 to 28 percent (Dawe et al. 1991; Gossop et al. 1986). This compares with initial abstinence rates for inpatient detoxification of 80 to 85 percent (Gossop et al. 1986; Gossop and Strang 1991). Thus, the reliance on outpatient or community-based detoxification occurs despite the consistently low completion rates that have been reported for such programs.

The most common reason for the failure of outpatient detoxification is the resumption of illicit drug use before program completion (Iguchi and Stitzer 1991). The poor completion rates for outpatient detoxification may be largely due to problems of drug availability and exposure to drug-related cues, including contact with other users and with neighborhoods where drug use is prevalent. Unnithan and colleagues (1992) found that more than three-quarters of the opiate addicts in an outpatient methadone reduction program had met other drug users during the previous week, and nearly one-quarter had met drug users every day; the majority had been offered drugs on at least one occasion during the previous week and some had been offered drugs every day. Such exposures clearly put outpatients at very high risk for lapse to drug taking, even when motivation to abstain is high. The study also pointed to other pressures toward relapse. Approximately one-half of the sample reported persistent feelings of depression, boredom, and anxiety, negative mood states that are themselves often associated with relapse (Bradley et al. 1989; Cummings et al. 1980). The many problems that are associated with the delivery of effective detoxification in outpatient settings raise questions about the continued reliance on this type of treatment service.

Inpatient treatments are an intensive form of treatment provided in a hospital or similar medical setting. In the United Kingdom, such services are mostly provided in psychiatric teaching hospitals and usually consist of a combination of detoxification and psychosocial rehabilitation. Inpatient treatments have several potential advantages over less intensive outpatient programs. A hospital setting permits a high level of medical observation, supervision, and safety for patients needing more intensive forms of care. In this respect, such services may be especially appropriate for the treatment of patients with complex dual-diagnosis disorders, because they permit a period of observation under drug-free conditions during which psychiatric symptoms may remit (Strain et al. 1991b). Residential treatment also may be useful for patients who do not respond to less intense interventions (Weiss 1999).

Detoxification in an inpatient setting may also be indicated where complicated detoxification treatment regimens are required for patients who are codependent on two or more drugs, a frequently encountered clinical problem (Strain et al. 1991a). The most common multiple dependencies requiring clinical management during withdrawal involve combinations of opiates, benzodiazepines, alcohol, and stimulants. Among heroin addicts treated at the Maudsley Hospital in London, for example, the percentage that were regular users of benzodiazepines doubled between 1988 and 1991. About one-third were found to be regular users of benzodiazepines, and about half of the regular users were physically dependent and required detoxification treatment for a benzodiazepine withdrawal syndrome (Davison and Gossop 1996). Similarly, in a national study of drug-dependent patients in U.K. services, about two-thirds were found to be current users of three or more substances during the period before admission to treatment, and more than one-third were using stimulants, especially crack cocaine (Gossop et al. 1998).

This issue of multiple dependencies and the need for detoxification from multiple substances is one that confronts clinicians every day. However, little in the literature provides guidance on specific protocols that should be used, such as guidelines as to whether detoxification treatments for multiple substances should be delivered simultaneously or consecutively. One thing that is advisable is that dual (or multiple) detoxification treatments should be administered in a hospital setting because of the risks of complex drug and withdrawal interactions and the possible need for reevaluation and adjustment of detoxification regimens (Weiss 1999). Inpatient detoxification is much more likely to ensure that abstinence is actually initiated from all drugs (including alcohol) on which the patient may be dependent (Gossop et al. 1986; Maddux et al. 1980). Inpatient detoxification can also provide a useful first phase of an integrated treatment program in which patients are returned to outpatient care in a drug-free state and ready for relapse prevention treatments (Chutuape et al. 1999).

Detoxification-only programs are easier to establish and cheaper to run than more comprehensive services. However, cost cutting may occur at the ultimate expense of individual patients, their families, and society. Gossop and Strang (2000) calculated that the unadjusted weekly cost of an inpatient detoxification was 24 times greater than that of an outpatient detoxification. However, discussion of treatment costs can be misleading if it is not informed by, and adjusted for, evidence of effectiveness. For example, Gossop and Strang (2000) found that the costs of a 10-day inpatient program, when adjusted for the different rates at which patients successfully completed the program, were almost identical with those of the outpatient program (indeed, they were marginally lower). Further, the patient's interests may be irreconcilable with crude calculations based solely on cost. It is unfortunate, therefore, that these are the calculations that so often appear to be made by purchasers and planners of treatment. For the individual patient, it is the prospect of improved clinical outcome that is paramount.

Overall, the choice between inpatient and outpatient settings should not be seen as a choice between better and worse alternatives. The issue is choosing a treatment setting appropriate to the circumstances, needs, and problems of individual patients at specific times, with psychiatric co-morbidities and multiple drug dependencies being among the criteria that would indicate the need for an inpatient detoxification (Finney et al. 1996). Further, the availability of psychological support, drug abuse counseling, and aftercare planning and services should also be considered when selecting a detoxification program.

Risks and Benefits of Detoxification

Although detoxification offers important benefits, the achievement of a drug-free state is not a risk-neutral event. Among patients who have been detoxified in inpatient or residential services, an initial lapse to opiate use often occurs very soon after leaving the program. The first few weeks after discharge represent a critical period in terms of the individual's chances of staying off drugs. Two studies have found that within one week of leaving an inpatient treatment program, nearly one-half of the sample had used opiates on at least one occasion, and within six weeks of discharge, almost three-quarters of them had used opiates (Chutuape et al. 2001a; Gossop et al. 1989a). Although this initial lapse to opiate use did not necessarily herald a full-blown relapse to addiction, the reduction or loss of tolerance that occurs during and after detoxification puts the individual at risk for a drug overdose if opiate use is resumed. Drug overdose continues to be one of the most frequent causes of death among opiate misusers, and increased rates of fatal overdose have been reported among recently detoxified opiate addicts (Strang et al. 2003). Detoxification programs need to be aware of the potential risks of overdose among patients who have partially or completely lost their tolerance to the effects of opiates after being successfully withdrawn from opiates. Note also that overdoses attributed to the use of opiates frequently involve the combined use of opiates and alcohol or other sedatives (Darke and Zador 1996; Gossop et al. 2002). Thus, special precautions may be needed when treating opiate users who also use alcohol or other sedatives, as these drug combinations are especially likely to increase the risk of death associated with respiratory depression.

Service Delivery Considerations: Integration of Care

Detoxification services could be improved by integration of care. Where drug misusers have multiple problems in different domains, this may require additional treatment input to meet their differing treatment needs (McLellan et al. 1993). This issue is especially relevant to patients who are dually dependent on drugs and alcohol, or who have concurrent mental health diagnoses, areas where services have traditionally been established and operated separately.

Treating dually diagnosed patients in separate mental health and addiction treatment services is often unsatisfactory, especially for those with severe psychiatric disorders. General psychiatrists and mental health clinicians may fail to obtain a thorough history of drug use, and drug problems are often overlooked and underdiagnosed in mental health treatment settings (Skipsey et al. 1997). Further, mental health staffs often lack the training, the expertise, and the confidence to respond appropriately to drug misuse among their patients. Conversely, addiction service staff may not respond effectively to mental health problems among their patients. The reliance on separate service systems can lead to a disconnect between mental health and addiction treatment services and to disagreement over treatment practices and treatment goals. In one study, improved outcomes were found among substance abusers with severe mental illnesses that were treated in integrated programs compared with those who received a traditional service intervention (Drake et al. 1993). The common problem of dual dependence on both drugs and alcohol, as well as the common comorbidity between drug addiction and mental health problems, raises challenging questions about the wisdom of continuing to maintain the traditional separation of services.

Summary and Future Directions

Despite the limited impact of detoxification programs on the long-term addiction career of patients, it seems likely that these services will continue to be extensively used. Detoxification has become an established part of the treatment system and provides an extremely useful source of palliative care in which opioid misusers can transition comfortably through the opioid withdrawal syndrome to a drug-free state. Detoxification services support high utilization rates because they are desirable to addicts, an important precursor to other longer-term treatments, and acceptable to treatment funders (e.g., insurance providers). For these reasons, it is necessary to consider how further supportive procedures or services can be used to improve program completion rates and patient outcomes. Of importance here would be better integration of services and especially closer ties between detoxification and aftercare services. When considering the topic of services integration, it is important to realize that drug-dependent patients may have difficulty in making desirable transitions from one service to another. Thus, special procedures may be needed to improve transition rates (Chutuape et al. 2001b). Although detoxification is often used as a stand-alone treatment or as a crisis management response, it is important that this service be viewed as one component within the broader context of long-term treatment and intervention strategies. This broader vision should help to lay the groundwork for better long-term treatment planning and cooperation across service providers as well as integration of service delivery.

References

ACMD (1988). AIDS and Drug Misuse: Part 1. Report by the U.K. Advisory Council on the Misuse of Drugs, London.

Bradley BP, Phillips G, Green L, Gossop M (1989). Circumstances surrounding the initial lapse to opiate use following detoxification. *Br J Psychiatry* 154: 354–9.

Caplehorn JR, Dalton MS, Cluff MC, Petrenas AM (1994). Retention in methadone maintenance and heroin addicts' risk of death. *Addiction* 89: 203–9.

Chutuape MA, Jasinski DR, Fingerhood MI, Stitzer ML (2001a). One-, three-, and six-month outcomes after brief inpatient opioid detoxification. *Am J Drug Alcohol Abuse* 27: 19–44.

Chutuape MA, Katz EC, Stitzer ML (2001b). Methods for enhancing transition of substance dependent patients from inpatient to outpatient treatment. *Drug Alcohol Depend* 61: 137–43.

Chutuape MA, Silverman K, Stitzer M (1999). Contingent reinforcement sustains post-detoxification abstinence from multiple drugs: a preliminary study with methadone patients. *Drug Alcohol Depend* 54: 69–81.

Cummings N, Gordon J, Marlatt G (1980). Relapse: strategies of prevention and prediction. In: Miller WR, ed. *The Addictive Behaviors*. Oxford: Pergamon.

Darke S, Zador D (1996). Fatal heroin 'overdose': a review. *Addiction* 91: 1765–72.

Davison S, Gossop M (1996). The problem of interviewing drug addicts in custody: a study of interrogative suggestibility and compliance. *Psychol Crime Law* 2: 185–95.

Dawe S, Griffiths P, Gossop M, Strang J (1991). Should opiate addicts be involved in controlling their own detoxification? A comparison of fixed versus negotiable schedules. *Br J Addict* 86: 977–82.

Drake RE, McHugo GJ, Noordsy DL (1993). Treatment of alcoholism among schizophrenic outpatients: 4-year outcomes. *Am J Psychiatry* 150: 328–9.

Edwards G (1969). The British approach to the treatment of heroin addiction. *Lancet* 1: 768–72.

Finney JW, Hahn AC, Moos RH (1996). The effectiveness of inpatient and outpatient treatment for alcohol abuse: the need to focus on mediators and moderators of setting effects. *Addiction* 91: 1773–96; discussion, 1803–20.

Gossop M (1989). The detoxification of high dose heroin addicts in Pakistan. *Drug Alcohol Depend* 24: 143–50.

Gossop M (1990). The development of a Short Opiate Withdrawal Scale (SOWS). *Addict Behav* 15: 487–90.

Gossop M, Battersby M, Strang J (1991). Self-detoxification by opiate addicts. A preliminary investigation. *Br J Psychiatry* 159: 208–12.

Gossop M, Bradley B, Phillips GT (1987). An investigation of withdrawal symptoms shown by opiate addicts during and subsequent to a 21-day in-patient methadone detoxification procedure. *Addict Behav* 12: 1–6.

Gossop M, Green L, Phillips G, Bradley B (1989a). Lapse, relapse and survival among opiate addicts after treatment. A prospective follow-up study. *Br J Psychiatry* 154: 348–53.

Gossop M, Griffiths P, Bradley B, Strang J (1989b). Opiate withdrawal symptoms in response to 10-day and 21-day methadone withdrawal programmes. *Br J Psychiatry* 154: 360–3.

Gossop M, Johns A, Green L (1986). Opiate withdrawal: inpatient versus outpatient programmes and preferred versus random assignment to treatment. *Br Med J (Clin Res Ed)* 293: 103–4.

Gossop M, Marsden J, Stewart D, Lehmann P, Edwards C, Wilson A, Segar G (1998). Substance use, health and social problems of service users at 54 drug treatment agencies. Intake data from the National Treatment Outcome Research Study. *Br J Psychiatry* 173: 166–71.

Gossop M, Marsden J, Stewart D, Treacy S (2001). Outcomes after methadone maintenance and methadone reduction treatments: two-year follow-up results from the National Treatment Outcome Research Study. *Drug Alcohol Depend* 62: 255–64.

Gossop M, Stewart D, Treacy S, Marsden J (2002). A prospective study of mortality among drug misusers during a 4-year period after seeking treatment. *Addiction* 97: 39–47

Gossop M, Strang J (1991). A comparison of the withdrawal responses of heroin and methadone addicts during detoxification. *Br J Psychiatry* 158: 697–9.

Gossop M, Strang J (2000). Price, cost and value of opiate detoxification treatments. Reanalysis of data from two randomised trials. *Br J Psychiatry* 177: 262–6.

Gowing L, Ali R, White J (2000). *The Management of Opioid Withdrawal: An Overview of the Research Literature.* Adelaide, South Australia: University of Adelaide.

Green L, Gossop M (1988). Effects of information on the opiate withdrawal syndrome. *Br J Addict* 83: 305–9.

Gruer L, Wilson P, Scott R, Elliott L, Macleod J, Harden K, Forrester E, Hinshelwood S, McNulty H, Silk P (1997). General practitioner centred scheme for treatment of opiate dependent drug injectors in Glasgow. *BMJ* 314: 1730–5.

Hubbard RL, Marsden ME, Rachal JV, Harwood HJ, Cavanaugh ER, Ginzburg HM (1989). *Drug Abuse Treatment: A National Study of Effectiveness.* Chapel Hill, NC: The University of North Carolina Press.

Iguchi MY, Stitzer ML (1991). Predictors of opiate drug abuse during a 90-day methadone detoxification. *Am J Drug Alcohol Abuse* 17: 279–94.

Jaffe J (1985). Drug addiction and drug abuse. In: Goodman A, Gilman L, Rall T, eds. *The Pharmacological Basis of Therapeutics.* New York: Macmillan.

Katz EC, Brown BS, Schwartz RP, Weintraub E, Barksdale W, Robinson R (2004). Role induction: a method for enhancing early retention in outpatient drug-free treatment. *J Consult Clin Psychol* 72: 227–34.

Kleber H (1981). Detoxification from Narcotics. In: Lowinson J, Ruiz P, eds. *Substance Abuse*. Baltimore, MD: Williams and Wilkins.

Kreek MJ (2000). Methadone-related opioid agonist pharmacotherapy for heroin addiction. History, recent molecular and neurochemical research and future in mainstream medicine. *Ann N Y Acad Sci* 909: 186–216.

Lipton D, Maranda M (1983). Detoxification from heroin dependency: an overview of method and effectiveness. In: Stimmel B, ed. *Evaluation of Drug Treatment Programs*, 31–55. New York: Haworth Press.

Maddux JF, Desmond DP, Esquivel M (1980). Outpatient methadone withdrawal for heroin dependence. *Am J Drug Alcohol Abuse* 7: 323–33.

Mattick RP, Hall W (1996). Are detoxification programmes effective? *Lancet* 347: 97–100.

McKim W (2000). *Drugs and Behaviour*. Upper Saddle River, NJ: Prentice Hall.

McLellan AT, Arndt IO, Metzger DS, Woody GE, O'Brien CP (1993). The effects of psychosocial services in substance abuse treatment. *JAMA* 269: 1953–9.

Meichenbaum D, Turk D (1987). *Facilitating Treatment Adherence*. New York: Plenum.

Moos RH (1997). *Evaluating Treatment Environments*. Somerset, NJ: Transaction Publishers.

Phillips GT, Gossop M, Bradley B (1986). The influence of psychological factors on the opiate withdrawal syndrome. *Br J Psychiatry* 149: 235–8.

Reilly PM, Sees KL, Shopshire MS, Hall SM, Delucchi KL, Tusel DJ, Banys P, Clark HW, Piotrowski NA (1995). Self-efficacy and illicit opioid use in a 180-day methadone detoxification treatment. *J Consult Clin Psychol* 63: 158–62.

SAMHSA (1999). Treatment Episode Data Set (TEDS) 1992–1997. Bethesda, MD: Substance Abuse and Mental Health Services Administration, Office of Applied Studies.

Sees KL, Delucchi KL, Masson C, Rosen A, Clark HW, Robillard H, Banys P, Hall SM (2000). Methadone maintenance vs 180-day psychosocially enriched detoxification for treatment of opioid dependence: a randomized controlled trial. *JAMA* 283: 1303–10.

Senay EC, Dorus W, Goldberg F, Thornton W (1977). Withdrawal from methadone maintenance. Rate of withdrawal and expectation. *Arch Gen Psychiatry* 34: 361–7.

Simpson D, Sells S (1983). Effectiveness for treatment of drug abuse: an overview of the DARP research programme. *Adv Alcohol Subst Abuse* 2: 7–29.

Simpson DD, Sells SB (1990). *Opioid addiction and treatment: a 12-year follow-up*. Malabar, FL: Robert E. Krieger Publishing Company.

Skipsey K, Burleson JA, Kranzler HR (1997). Utility of the AUDIT for identification of hazardous or harmful drinking in drug-dependent patients. *Drug Alcohol Depend* 45: 157–63.

Strain EC, Bigelow GE, Liebson IA, Stitzer ML (1999). Moderate- vs high-dose methadone in the treatment of opioid dependence: a randomized trial. *JAMA* 281: 1000–5.

Strain EC, Brooner RK, Bigelow GE (1991a). Clustering of multiple substance use and psychiatric diagnoses in opiate addicts. *Drug Alcohol Depend* 27: 127–34.

Strain EC, Stitzer ML, Bigelow GE (1991b). Early treatment time course of depressive symptoms in opiate addicts. *J Nerv Ment Dis* 179: 215–21.

Strang J, Gossop M (1990). Comparison of linear versus inverse exponential methadone reduction curves in the detoxification of opiate addicts. *Addict Behav* 15: 541–7.

Strang J, McCambridge J, Best D, Beswick T, Bearn J, Rees S, Gossop M (2003). Loss of tolerance and overdose mortality after inpatient opiate detoxification: follow up study. *BMJ* 326: 959–60.

Strang J, Sheridan J, Barber N (1996). Prescribing injectable and oral methadone to opiate addicts: results from the 1995 national postal survey of community pharmacies in England and Wales. *BMJ* 313: 270–2.

Unnithan S, Gossop M, Strang J (1992). Factors associated with relapse among opiate addicts in an out-patient detoxification programme. *Br J Psychiatry* 161: 654–7.

Vogel V, Isbell H, Chapman K (1948). Present status of narcotic addiction. *J Am Med Assoc* 138: 1019–26.

Weiss RD (1999). Inpatient treatment. In: Galanter M, Kleber HD, eds. *The American Psychiatric Press Textbook of Substance Abuse Treatment, 2nd ed.* Washington, DC: American Psychiatric Press.

Wesson DR, Ling W (2003). The Clinical Opiate Withdrawal Scale (COWS). *J Psychoactive Drugs* 35: 253–9.

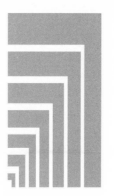

V

COMORBIDITIES IN
OPIOID DEPENDENCE

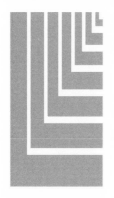

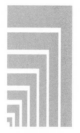

17

Other Substance Use Disorders: Prevalence, Consequences, Detection, and Management

Maxine L. Stitzer, Ph.D., and Stacey C. Sigmon, Ph.D.

Other drug use is common among patients in opioid treatment programs (OTPs). The substances abused by methadone patients during treatment include both those legally available (i.e., tobacco and alcohol) and drugs that can be obtained only on the illegal market (e.g., heroin and cocaine). The use of oral prescription medications is also seen in methadone patients, prominently including, but not limited to, benzodiazepines. Finally, new compounds surface periodically within the panoply of drugs favored by opioid-dependent patients, clonidine being an example, so clinicians must always be alert to new trends in drug use in their clinic. This chapter reviews the prevalence, consequences, and detection methods for drugs commonly used by patients during methadone treatment. It focuses on heroin, cocaine, benzodiazepines, alcohol, marijuana, and tobacco and makes recommendations for the clinical management of patients using various drug combinations.

PREVALENCE AND PATTERNS OF POLYDRUG USE

Table 17.1 shows representative data from a large-sample survey of patients enrolled in methadone maintenance at a community treatment program in Baltimore, Maryland (Brooner et al. 1997). Although regional and population differences in drug use may exist among methadone patients, this study makes the important point that most opioid-dependent

Table 17.1 Substance Abuse Disorders among Methadone Maintenance Patients

Abuse or Dependence	Lifetime Rates	Current Rates
Opioid	100.0	100.0
Cocaine	77.1	43.6
Alcohol	63.3	26.5
Cannabis	65.7	18.6
Sedative	57.6	18.4
Stimulant	30.7	0.3
Hallucinogen	27.3	0.7
Other*	20.4	3.2

Source: Data from Brooner et al. (1997). *Arch Gen Psychiatry,* 54: 71–80.
Note: Based on SCID interviews with 716 methadone patients in a Baltimore community clinic.
*Primarily inhalants, clonidine and promethazine

patients have a history of using multiple drugs. Each methadone patient may have as many as four to five substance abuse or dependence disorders, and for patients who have any comorbid psychiatric disorder (including antisocial personality disorder) this number is even greater. The Baltimore study also illustrates the relative prevalence of use across different types of drugs. In this study, cocaine was by far the more prevalent secondary drug of abuse among methadone patients, with a lifetime prevalence of 77 percent and current prevalence of 43 percent. Alcohol dependence is seen in about one-quarter of patients receiving methadone maintenance and poses another challenge for rehabilitation. The other two drugs with significant prevalence in the opioid-dependent population are marijuana and sedatives (usually benzodiazepines). About 20 percent of the treatment population was dependent on each of these two drugs in the Baltimore sample, although higher rates of marijuana use, including use that does not meet dependence criteria, have been reported in other samples (Epstein and Preston 2003; Nirenberg et al. 1996). The prevalence of tobacco dependence was not assessed in the Baltimore study, but another study conducted with methadone patients in Baltimore found that 92 percent of patients smoked cigarettes (Clemmey et al. 1997). This finding is consistent with the high rates of cigarette smoking reported for other groups of drug abusers.

As previously discussed, methadone blocks or attenuates the effects of heroin, and it is clear that heroin use declines substantially during methadone treatment as compared with pretreatment. Nevertheless, a substantial number of methadone patients continue to use heroin during treatment, with prevalence at specific sites influenced by factors including the maintenance dose of methadone (see chap. 6), time in treatment (rates tend to decrease over time), and the clinic's tolerance of this behavior. There may be several reasons why some methadone patients continue to use heroin during treatment despite withdrawal suppression and the opioid blockade provided by methadone. One study suggests that although a wide range of methadone doses are sufficient to suppress withdrawal, only doses of 120 mg or more can effectively block the effects of heroin during methadone maintenance (Donny et al. 2002). Thus, some patients may continue to use heroin to obtain euphoric effects, especially if they are maintained on an insufficient dose of methadone. One association consistently observed, however, is that between heroin and cocaine use. For example, it has been shown that methadone patients who used cocaine in the last three months were six times more likely to have used heroin than those patients who had not used cocaine (Hartel et al. 1995). It is possible that heroin continues to boost or otherwise modulate cocaine's effects even though patients are maintained on methadone.

Changes over Time in Treatment

It has been suggested that alcohol or other drug use may increase after entry into methadone maintenance treatment, but the validity of this belief is controversial. There are several reasons why an increase in use might occur, if this does happen. For example, patients who stop or greatly reduce heroin use after entering methadone treatment may now have more time and money to expend on other drugs such as cocaine and alcohol. Drugs such as benzodiazepines may become more readily available because of new associations formed at the methadone clinic. Finally, drug use could start or escalate because of the interaction between that drug and methadone. For example, methadone may increase the high obtained from using cocaine (Preston et al. 1996), and benzodiazepines can enhance the effects produced by methadone (Preston et al. 1984).

Studies examining this issue, however, have generally failed to document any increases in secondary drug use over time during methadone treatment; in fact, trends toward decreasing rates of drug use are more often reported. Decreases over time have been documented especially for opiate-positive urine samples, indicating that heroin use declines over time in treatment. For example, one study found that heroin use was reported by 40–50 percent of patients who had been in treatment for less than two years, but by only 12–20 percent of those in treatment more than two years (Hartel et al. 1995). Because such studies are generally cross-sectional rather than longitudinal, however, it is not entirely clear whether individual patients actually decrease their use over time or whether it is simply that those who stop using drugs early in treatment are more likely to remain in treatment. The main point is that most methadone patients come to treatment with an extensive history of multiple drug use and that, on the whole, drug use appears to decrease rather than increase during time in treatment.

Consequences of Polydrug Use during Methadone Treatment

There are medical, psychological, and behavioral risks inherent in using all drugs of abuse, and these risks continue when methadone patients use licit and illicit drugs of abuse during treatment. This section provides a brief overview of some of the risks and adverse consequences that methadone patients face when they continue to use drugs during treatment.

Heroin

Although heroin has no direct toxic effects unless a high, overdose amount is consumed, there may be several important adverse consequences of continued heroin use during treatment. One consequence, if use is by the intravenous route, is the potential for exposure to HIV infection. There is also a risk of infection with one of the viral hepatitides, abscesses, and other infections when drug preparations or injecting equipment are contaminated. A second potential risk that is currently based on speculation rather than research is that patients who continue to use heroin will tend to become even more physically dependent through exposure to the added short-acting opiate. This in turn could result in increasing levels of withdrawal discomfort and the need to continue use of short-acting opiates for withdrawal symptom relief. In this scenario, increasing the methadone dose could be a beneficial treatment strategy, because suppression of the excess withdrawal symptoms should result. Continued association with drug users and a drug-using lifestyle could be listed as a final adverse consequence of heroin use (as well as cocaine use) during treatment.

Cocaine

Cocaine has substantial medical risks (reviewed in Benowitz 1993). The most serious risks are related to intense central nervous system stimulation and vasoconstriction that can result in severe hypertension. This in turn can produce serious consequences, such as aortic rupture or restricted blood flow to organs, which can lead to heart attacks and damage to kidneys and intestines. Pregnant women who use cocaine can have spontaneous abortions and placental abruption. Most deaths that result from cocaine use are sudden and occur before medical help can be found. Despite these potentially serious complications, however, cocaine use may actually be associated more with traumatic deaths and injuries (including homicide, suicide, and accidents) than with medical complications. Cocaine intoxication can also produce mental confusion and other symptoms, including anxiety, panic attacks, agitated delirium, and paranoid psychosis. Symptoms produced by cocaine, including chest pains and mental confusion, are a common cause of visits to inner-city emergency departments.

Benzodiazepines

Problems associated with benzodiazepine use can include sedation, memory impairment, overdose, and physical dependence. Although tolerance develops to the sedative effects of these drugs, the use of benzodiazepines may be a factor in road accidents, in particular, when they are used in combination with other sedative drugs such as alcohol. Memory impairment is one of the most striking adverse effects of benzodiazepines (Curran 1991; 2000), and it is not clear how much tolerance develops to this effect. Clinically, memory impairment could be disruptive or dangerous to the extent that people forget important events or information, or engage in risky behaviors while under the influence of drugs. In general, an overdose with benzodiazepines alone is not lethal, but an overdose of a benzodiazepine combined with another sedating drug (including methadone) can be fatal (Gossop et al. 2002b). Thus, benzodiazepines are routinely found in toxicology screens of suicide victims or attempters, and suicide risk should be closely assessed and monitored in methadone patients who are taking benzodiazepines (Darke et al. 2004).

Perhaps the most prominent and relevant risk associated with benzodiazepine use in a drug-abusing population is that of physical dependence and withdrawal symptoms following discontinuation. When regular use of benzodiazepines is discontinued, patients can experience rebound anxiety and agitation, insomnia, tension, sweating, tremulousness, ringing in the ears, increased sensitivity to noises and to light, and sensory and perceptual distortions (Busto et al. 1986). In cases of severe dependence, withdrawal delirium and seizures (like those seen in severe alcohol withdrawal) may be observed. The extent and timing of symptoms will depend in part on the amount and duration of previous use and on the type of benzodiazepine being used. Because of the potentially dangerous symptoms that can appear, benzodiazepine detoxification should be conducted only under medical supervision (Dickinson et al. 2003).

Alcohol

Heavy alcohol use among opiate addicts has been associated with health problems, increased mortality, and disruptive behaviors at the OTP. Other common alcohol-related problems include blackouts, aggressive or violent behaviors, arrests, accidents, loss of employment, disruption of family life, and deterioration of mental and physical health. One study noted that heroin abusers codependent on alcohol tended to have poorer physical and psychological health and were more likely to have problems related to their injecting behavior, including abscesses, scarring, and overdoses (Gossop et al. 2002a). In another study that enrolled a sample of methadone-maintained problem drinkers for an alcoholism treatment project, half of the subjects had been hospitalized with an alcohol-related illness in the three months before participation (Ling et al. 1983). Liver disease is the best known and most common complication associated with excessive drinking. Alcohol is well known to produce toxic effects on other organs, however, and can result in both acute and chronic cognitive impairment and heart, kidney, and blood disorders. Alcohol use is a leading cause of death in methadone patients, estimated in different studies to account for 18–60 percent of all mortalities (Bickel et al. 1987). In a 12-year follow-up study of individuals previously enrolled in drug abuse treatment, heavy drinkers died at a rate seven times higher than an age-adjusted general population (Sells and Simpson 1987). Alcohol use is also a strong contributing factor to premature treatment discharges and has been estimated to account for about 25 percent of discharges from methadone programs, primarily because of its association with absenteeism and disruptive behavior at the clinic (Bickel and Amass 1993).

Marijuana

Marijuana use impairs a variety of cognitive and behavioral skills, including motor coordination, visual function, attention, and memory. These effects may interfere with the patient's ability to perform tasks and could contribute to accidents and intentional injuries (Macdonald et al. 2003). Marijuana can also have adverse psychological consequences, including anxiety and panic attacks, perceptual distortions, and, in extreme cases, toxic psychosis. The primary physiologic effects of marijuana are increased heart rate, increased appetite, and bloodshot eyes. Although increased heart rate can be a problem for people with cardiovascular disease, dangerous cardiovascular reactions to marijuana are rare. A well-confirmed danger of marijuana, however, is its effects on the lungs. Marijuana smoke contains the same carcinogens as tobacco smoke, usually in somewhat higher concentrations. Marijuana is inhaled deeply and held in the lungs longer than tobacco smoke, so there can be an increased risk of lung diseases, including bronchitis, emphysema, and lung cancer. These effects add to the potential damage caused by nearly universal cigarette smoking among patients in OTPs. Little evidence has emerged linking marijuana use during methadone treatment with use of other illicit drugs or with poor treatment response. In several studies, for example, marijuana abuse by methadone-maintained patients was not associated with use of other drugs or treatment outcome (Epstein and Preston 2003; Nirenberg et al. 1996; Saxon et al. 1993; Weizman et al. 2004; but see Wasserman et al. 1998). This is in contrast to the case with other secondary drugs of abuse, most notably cocaine and benzodiazepines, which are clearly associated with higher rates of heroin use, greater risk-taking behaviors, and poor treatment response. Although these conclusions are based on a growing number of studies, the role of marijuana smoking in patients receiving methadone maintenance needs to be further evaluated.

Tobacco

Tobacco use is associated with an elevated risk of morbidity and mortality in the general population, with more than 400,000 people in the United States dying annually of smoking-related causes, including heart attack, stroke, chronic lung diseases, and cancer. As in the general population, tobacco use among OTP patients is significantly associated with morbidity and mortality (Hser et al. 1994). Given the extremely high prevalence of tobacco use among opioid-dependent individuals (Clemmey et al. 1997; Stark and Campbell 1993), it seems likely that even if opioid abusers stopped using all illicit drugs and cut down on alcohol, they would still be at risk for premature death and disease due to cigarette smoking (Hser et al. 1994; Hurt et al. 1996). Moreover, tobacco use may be associated with treatment outcome among methadone-maintained patients. For example, one study found that heavy smokers, as compared with occasional smokers and nonsmokers, required a higher maintenance dose of methadone (Frosch et al. 2000). In that study, smoking status also was associated with use of other drugs, with illicit drug use increasing in a stepwise function from nonsmokers to occasional smokers and then heavy smokers.

DETECTION OF SECONDARY DRUGS

Given the high prevalence and associated risks of on-going substance use during methadone treatment, is clearly important to assess accurately the rates and patterns of secondary drug use among methadone patients to establish individual treatment plans and targets for intervention. Both self-report and objective assessment methods are available to accomplish this.

Self-report Assessments

Most clinics have their own questionnaires so that new patients can provide information about their history and rates of drug use and patterns and routes of current use. The Addiction Severity Index (ASI) (McLellan et al. 1980, 1992) is an interview-based instrument that has been widely adopted in the drug abuse treatment community for assessment of overall patient functioning. It contains detailed questions on drug and alcohol use, with a 30-day time-frame assessment. Thus, the instrument gathers systematic information about the number of days within the past 30 that a patient has used each of a variety of abused drugs, including heroin, methadone, alcohol, barbiturates, other sedatives and tranquilizers, cocaine, amphetamines, marijuana, hallucinogens, and inhalants. New patients are also asked how much money they spent in the past 30 days on drugs and on alcohol. Because the ASI is so widely used, OTPs should consider adopting it or at least incorporating the 30-day assessment time frame into their own questionnaires to gather data that can be compared with other treatment sites. Training in the administration of the instrument is available from the test developers (www.tresearch.org; 1-215-399-0980).

More in-depth and sophisticated information can be obtained by administration of the Structured Clinical Interview for DSM-IV (SCID) (First et al. 2001). This clinical interview provides information for making lifetime and current diagnoses of both mood (e.g., depression, anxiety) and personality (e.g., antisocial) disorders that are common among drug abusers as well as substance use diagnoses (abuse or dependence) for a range of drugs commonly used by methadone patients. The SCID is often used in research to characterize drug abusers, and is a lengthy interview that requires extensive training and the ability to make clinical judgments based on information derived from the interview. It is therefore infrequently used as a tool in clinical practice.

The Composite International Diagnostic Interview–Second Edition (CIDI-2) (Kessler et al. 1998) offers a briefer, clinically useful alternative to the SCID (Forman et al. 2004). This instrument includes a Substance Abuse Module that provides lifetime diagnoses (past and current) for substance use disorders according to DSM-IV and ICD-10 criteria. The CIDI-2 can be administered by trained lay interviewers who do not have a clinical background, it has demonstrated reliability and validity for substance use diagnoses (Robins et al. 1988), and typically requires only 20–30 minutes to administer.

Because of the high rates of documented alcohol dependence among methadone patients, careful clinical assessment should be included early in treatment to identify those patients with current and past alcohol problems. Two brief assessment instruments, the Michigan Alcoholism Screening Test (MAST) and Alcohol Use Disorders Identification Test (AUDIT), are the most commonly used and convenient instruments to administer; both have been shown to be useful for detecting current, excessive drinking in methadone maintenance populations (Bickel and Amass 1993; Maisto et al. 1995; Skipsey et al. 1997). The MAST is a 25-item instrument that assesses physical, behavioral, and psychosocial problems commonly associated with alcoholic drinking (table 17.2). The AUDIT is a shorter, 10-item instrument that includes an assessment of the amount of drinking and drinking-related problems (table 17.3). Both have norms and cutoffs that can be used to identify problem drinkers. The AUDIT has been specifically recommended for identification of hazardous or harmful drinking in drug-dependent populations (Skipsey et al. 1997). These screening instruments are not designed to assess histories of drinking and, thus, must be supplemented with an additional clinical interview to identify patients with alcoholism in remission. Also, none of these instruments can be used to obtain psychiatric diagnostic classification, which requires a more sophisticated clinical interview (e.g., the SCID).

Urine Testing: Types of Tests Available

Those working in drug abuse treatment are fortunate to have a method, urine testing, for obtaining objective evidence of recent use versus abstinence for a variety of drugs with which patients may be involved (see table 17.4). The two most common analytic methods available at commercial testing laboratories for urine testing are immunoassay tests (e.g., enzyme multiplied immunoassay test or EMIT) and thin-layer chromatography

Table 17.2 **Michigan Alcoholism Screening Test (MAST)**

Answer each question below with a YES or NO

1. Do you feel you are a normal drinker? (No-2)
2. Have you ever awakened the morning after some drinking the night before and found that you could not remember a part of the evening before? (Yes-2)
3. Does your wife (or do your parents) ever worry or complain about your drinking? (Yes-1)
4. Can you stop drinking without a struggle after one or two drinks? (No-2)
5. Do you ever feel bad about your drinking? (Yes-1)
6. Do friends or relatives think you are a normal drinker? (No-2)
7. Do you ever try to limit your drinking to certain times of the day or to certain places? (0)
8. Are you always able to stop drinking when you want to? (No-2)
9. Have you ever attended a meeting of Alcoholics Anonymous (AA)? (Yes-5)
10. Have you gotten into fights when drinking? (Yes-1)
11. Has drinking ever created problems with you and your wife? (Yes-2)
12. Has your wife (or other family member) ever gone to anyone for help about your drinking? (Yes-2)
13. Have you ever lost friends or girlfriends/boyfriends because of drinking? (Yes-2)
14. Have you ever gotten into trouble at work because of drinking? (Yes-2)
15. Have you ever lost a job because of drinking? (Yes-2)
16. Have you ever neglected your obligations, your family, or your work for two or more days in a row because you were drinking? (Yes-2)
17. Do you ever drink before noon? (Yes-1)
18. Have you ever been told you have liver trouble? Cirrhosis? (Yes-2)
19. Have you ever had delirium tremens (DTs), severe shaking, heard voices, or seen things that weren't there after heavy drinking? (Yes-2)
20. Have you ever gone to anyone for help about your drinking? (Yes-5)
21. Have you ever been in a hospital because of your drinking? (Yes-5)
22. Have you ever been a patient in a psychiatric hospital or on a psychiatric ward of a general hospital where drinking was part of the problem? (Yes-2)
23. Have you ever been seen at a psychiatric or mental health clinic, or gone to a doctor, social worker, or clergyman for help with an emotional problem in which drinking had played a part? (Yes-2)
24. Have you ever been arrested, even for a few hours, because of drunk behavior? (Yes-2)
25. Have you ever been arrested for drunk driving after drinking? (Yes-2)

Source: Selzer (1971). Reprinted with permission from the American Journal of Psychiatry. Copyright 1971. American Psychiatric Association.
Note: Responses shown in parentheses after each question indicate the direction for a significant answer, and the score for that answer. Question 7 is not scored and is dropped from some forms of the MAST. Total scores of 5 or greater are considered indicative of possible alcoholism.

(TLC). (A review of urine testing techniques can be found in Verebey 1992.) Immunoassay has become the most widespread technology in current use for urine testing. Specific methods include the FPIA (fluorescence polarization immunoassay) and EMIT. These methods are based on antigen-antibody reactions using the drug to form highly specific antigen-antibody complexes that are employed in the test. Immunoassay tests pro-

Table 17.3 Alcohol Use Disorders Identification Test (AUDIT)

1. How often do you have a drink containing alcohol? (0) Never. (1) Monthly or less.
   (2) 2 to 4 times a month. (3) 2 to 3 times a week. (4) 4 or more times a week.

2. How many drinks containing alcohol do you have on a typical day when you are drinking? (0) 1 or 2. (1) 3 or 4. (2) 5 or 6. (3) 7 to 9. (4) 10 or more standard drinks.*

3. How often do you have six or more drinks on one occasion? (0) Never. (1) Less than
   monthly. (2) Monthly. (3) Weekly. (4) Daily or almost daily.

4. How often during the past year have you found that you were not able to stop drinking
   once you had started? (0) Never. (1) Less than monthly. (2) Montly. (3) Weekly. (4) Daily
   or almost daily.

5. How often during the past year have you failed to do what was normally expected from
   you because of drinking? (0) Never. (1) Less than monthly. (2) Monthly. (3) Weekly.
   (4) Daily or almost daily.

6. How often during the past year have you needed a first drink in the morning to get your-
   self going after a heavy drinking session? (0) Never. (1) Less than monthly. (2) Monthly.
   (3) Weekly. (4) Daily or almost daily.

7. How often during the past year have you had a feeling of guilt or remorse after drinking?
   (0) Never. (1) Less than monthly. (2) Monthly. (3) Weekly. (4) Daily or almost daily.

8. How often during the past year have you been unable to remember what happened
   the night before because you had been drinking? (0) Never. (1) Less than monthly.
   (2) Monthly. (3) Weekly. (4) Daily or almost daily.

9. Have you or someone else been injured as a result of your drinking? (0) No. (2) Yes, but
   not in the past year. (4) Yes, during the past year.

10. Has a relative or friend or a doctor or other health worker been concerned about your
    drinking or suggested you cut down? (0) Never. (2) Yes, but not in the past year. (4) Yes,
    during the past year.

Source: Saunders et al. (1993). Development of the Alcohol Use Disorders Identification Test (AUDIT):
WHO Collaborative Project on Early Detection of Persons with Harmful Alcohol Consumption. Addiction
88: 791–804.
Note: Numbers in parentheses are scoring weights. AUDIT Core total score is the sum of the scoring weights.
The AUDIT manual contains scoring procedures and interpretation (Babor TF, De La Fuente JR, Saunders
J, Grant M [1989]. The Alcohol Use Disorders Identification Test: Guidelines for Use in the Primary Health
Care. WHO Publ. No. 89.4. Geneva: World Health Organization).
*One "standard drink" contains 10 g of alcohol.

vide a specific and sensitive assay for most common drugs of abuse based
on their metabolites. Thus, for example, all drugs with morphine as a
metabolite will be detected by the opiate test, whereas only cocaine will
be detected by the cocaine test based on the benzoylecgonine metabolite.

TLC, one of the oldest technologies to be developed for drug testing,
is based on the observation that molecules with differing sizes and properties will reliably migrate to a certain spot on a wet plate when appropriate solvents are applied. Thus, the presence of a particular drug mole-
cule in urine can be reliably detected by comparing its migration with that
of a known standard. TLC allows for detection of a wide range of com-

pounds, including some for which immunoassay reagents are not available. The primary advantage of TLC is its high specificity for detecting use of specific drugs within a given category. For example, because the immunoassay opiate test is based on morphine, it detects only drugs metabolized to morphine and does not distinguish among them. In contrast, TLC can differentiate meperidine (Demerol) and codeine as well as morphine. Testing for new drugs of abuse can sometimes be developed by using TLC. Recent examples are oxycodone (OxyContin), tramadol (Ultram), and clonazepam (Klonopin). Thus, TLC is a relatively inexpensive method of obtaining a broad range of urine-testing information.

Other convenient technologies have been developed for on-site drug testing (for a recent review, see George and Braithwaite 2002). These on-site testing methods consist of compact devices containing the reagents needed for drug detection in a lightweight plastic cup, dipstick, or panel, with visual changes in color or density indicating the presence versus absence of the specified drug. On-site testing products are available for all major drugs of abuse, including cocaine, opiates, amphetamine, benzodiazepines, and marijuana. These new technologies have sensitivity and specificity similar to immunoassay tests and can be used to obtain immediate (typically within 5 minutes) test results when clinically desired. On-site products are also reasonably cost-effective, with the approximate cost per drug tested averaging about $2.00 (although this can vary across manufacturers and depends on the number of products purchased). These products are offered by several manufacturers (see table 17.4), and each company typically offers multiple products that can test for a single drug or for multiple drugs simultaneously, allowing the user to choose a combination of drug tests that best fits clinic needs. More information can be obtained by contacting the National On-site Testing Association, 203 N. Main Street, Flemington, NJ (www.checkfordrugs.com; 888-387-9378) or by consulting a book that reviews numerous issues and products related to on-site drug testing (Jenkins and Goldberger 2002).

Hair testing is another technology for assessing drug exposure (for a review on hair testing, see Karacic and Skender 2003). This method requires chemical testing expertise to perform, however, and it is primarily useful for determining in a gross manner whether a person used drugs during the past several months. It does not appear to have immediate utility in an opioid treatment program. Of more relevance to clinical practice is quantitative urine testing, which is now offered by some laboratories. By determining the actual concentration of drug in the urine and tracking this over successive days, it is possible to determine whether the patient has had a new use of drug or whether instead a "positive" urine (whose concentration exceeds the cutoff value used in qualitative testing) may simply represent carryover from an episode of use that occurred previously (Preston et al. 1997). Although potentially useful to the clinician, quantitative testing is currently rather expensive (about $10 or more per sample), and frequent collection of samples is required; these cost factors make quantitative testing unreasonable for most clinics at the present time.

Urine Testing for Opiates and Cocaine

Immunoassay tests such as EMIT provide a highly sensitive and specific assay for both morphine, the metabolite of heroin, and for benzoylecgonine, the metabolite of cocaine; a cutoff of 300 ng/ml is used to determine positive versus negative samples for each. In general, both morphine and benzoylecgonine can be detected with the EMIT assay for one to three days after use of either heroin or cocaine. The duration of time during which a drug can be detected, however, will depend significantly on the amount, recency, and duration of last use and on individual differences in drug metabolism and elimination. Thus, individual patients may have positive urine samples for a longer time after cessation of use. Note that EMIT will not reliably detect a variety of synthetic opioid compounds, including meperidine (Demerol), oxycodone (Percodan, OxyContin), dextromethorphan (used in cough syrup), propoxyphene (Darvocet), and fentanyl (an important drug to test for among impaired health care workers). TLC can detect some of these synthetic opioids but only in relatively high concentrations. Clinicians should check with individual laboratories to determine which opioid drugs are assayed and reported.

Urine Testing for Benzodiazepines

The EMIT method provides a specific assay for benzodiazepines using lormetazepam as the reference calibrator; most commonly used benzodiazepines can be detected by EMIT. This test is somewhat less sensitive to clonazepam (Klonopin) and lorazepam (Ativan) than to other benzodiazepines, however. Furthermore, the test may fail to detect potent, short-acting benzodiazepines, such as triazolam (Halcion), which may not be present in sufficient concentrations at commonly used doses. EMIT reagents are available for both 300 ng/ml and 200 ng/ml cutoffs; the lower cutoff provides greater sensitivity and is recommended for clinical use with drug abusers. The duration of detection will depend on the length of time that the benzodiazepine drug stays in the body. Drugs such as diazepam that are long acting, or have long-acting metabolites to which tests are sensitive, may be detected for up to two weeks after use stops. Shorter-acting benzodiazepines (e.g., alprazolam or Xanax) can generally be detected for only two to three days. Because of the large number of benzodiazepine drugs available and the limitations of EMIT, it may be necessary to conduct more extensive urinalysis testing to obtain a comprehensive picture of benzodiazepine use by methadone patients. TLC testing can provide additional information about the specific benzodiazepines that patients may be abusing. Triage (see table 17.4) is an on-site test system that has been specifically developed to detect benzodiazepine glucuronide metabolites, which are the most prevalent metabolites. This method could provide a more sensitive assay for use of benzodiazepines by methadone patients, if desired.

Objective Monitoring for Alcohol

Recent drinking can be detected by analyzing blood, breath, urine, or saliva samples, all of which will provide roughly the same information about current concentration of alcohol in the body. Breath alcohol levels can be conveniently monitored at the OTP using a hand-held commercially available sensor (table 17.4), and saliva tests have been developed as well. Most immunoassay and on-site urine tests also have specific reagents for alcohol testing. Because alcohol is metabolized at a steady rate, the duration over which it can be detected in body fluids depends significantly on the amount and recency of consumption. In general, however, alcohol levels will drop below those that can be detected within a few hours after consumption stops. Thus, these tests are useful only for detection of recent drinking. On-site alcohol testing is primarily useful as a means to verify recent drinking, particularly in patients that appear intoxicated when they come to the clinic.

Urine Testing for Other Drugs

Certification standards for urine-testing laboratories differ from state to state in the United States, and available testing services differ from one laboratory to another both in the range and sophistication of testing available. For example, some offer an immunoassay for initial screening with TLC for confirmation and additional specificity information about substances used. Some laboratories offer gas chromatography-mass spectrometry, a highly sensitive and specific but expensive technique that is needed to detect drugs such as 3,4-methylenedioxymethamphetamie

Table 17.4 **Objective Methods for Detecting Abused Substances**

Method	Features
Urine testing	
Thin-layer chromatography	Broad-spectrum testing with high specificity for particular drugs within a pharmacologic class; available at specialty laboratories
Immunoassay techniques	High specificity and sensitivity for most common
EMIT*	drugs of abuse; testing can be conducted at an
FPIA†	outside laboratory or equipment and reagents can be purchased for on-site use
On-site testing‡	Convenient, immediate results; no special training
Syva Rapid Test§	needed; sensitive and specific for most common
OnTrak Testcard 9¶	drugs of abuse
Triage Drugs of Abuse Panel‖	
Breath alcohol testing	Accurate index of current blood alcohol levels
Alco-sensor#	

*Enzyme multiplied immunoassay test (Dade Behring, Deerfield, IL)
†Florescence polarization immunoassay (Abbot Diagnostics, Abbot Park, IL)
‡Listed are the three largest commercial manufacturers currently supporting these types of products.
§Dade Behring, Deerfield, IL
¶Roche, Indianapolis, IN
‖Biosite, San Diego, CA
#Intoximeter, Inc., St. Louis, MO

(MDMA, Ecstasy) and methylphenidate (Ritalin). Because of this variability, it is essential that clinicians obtain detailed information about the capabilities and limitations of the laboratory they use for urine testing. Clinicians should understand which drugs are included and not included in routine screens and the relative sensitivities of the testing methods used. In laboratories using TLC technology, for example, routine screens will generally provide information on opiates (heroin and some synthetic opioids such as Darvon and Demerol), cocaine, amphetamine, benzodiazepines, antidepressants, barbiturates and other nonbarbiturate sedatives (e.g., phenothiazines), as well as quinine, which is used as a cutting agent for heroin and cocaine sold on the street. Tests for alcohol and marijuana, although available, may not be routinely included in urine screens and may need to be specially requested. If cannabinoid testing is desired for marijuana screening, the clinician must remember that this drug is stored in body lipids and excreted slowly; therefore, it may be detected for a week or longer after just a single use, and for up to six weeks after cessation of chronic use. Certain drugs may not be detected by either immunoassay or TLC, for example, clonidine, fentanyl, MDMA, and other designer drugs. If it becomes important to test for particular drugs owing to use patterns that develop in specific locales, other sophisticated testing methodologies can be used, but these are generally costly to implement. Overall, it is important to recognize the variability that can exist across laboratories and to learn about the capabilities and limitations of the laboratory selected to conduct urine testing for a given clinic.

Information Obtained from Urine Testing

A negative urine test provides extremely useful evidence of recent abstinence. In contrast, a positive urine test in fact gives little useful information about amount or frequency of recent use. Thus, urine test results for a patient who uses heroin twice a week might appear identical with those for a patient who uses heroin several times a day. This insensitivity suggests that urine testing needs to be supplemented with self-report or quantitative testing if more detailed information is desired. The minimal information provided by a positive result also suggests that urine testing might be most useful in cases in which patients deny drug use or are involved in therapeutic procedures that require confirmation of abstinence. This strategy conserves scarce urine-testing resources for their most useful application.

Treatment and Clinical Recommendations

Heroin

Treatment

Increasing the methadone dose is the primary therapeutic strategy available to deal with continued opiate use (usually heroin) during treatment. In a study of heroin outcomes among methadone-maintained patients, for example, higher maintenance doses were predictive of reduced heroin use, with each milligram of prescribed methadone producing a 2 percent reduction in the likelihood of regular heroin use (Gossop et al. 2001). Although a clear inverse relationship exists between dose and overall rates of opiate use (as discussed in chap. 6), additional systematic research is needed about the reliability or time course of individual subject response to an increase in methadone dose. Beneficial effects of methadone dose increases may require several weeks to appear. Furthermore, some patients will clearly continue to use opiates even on methadone doses of 80–100 mg per day. Because higher-dose methadone is safe to administer to individuals who are already methadone-tolerant, more research is warranted to determine whether the greater opioid blockade provided by doses higher than 100 mg per day might be clinically beneficial. Finally, heroin use can be indirectly affected by interventions designed to reduce use of cocaine, a principle that has been supported in several studies using contingency management interventions to reduce cocaine use (see chap. 8). This effect of reduced heroin use by targeting cocaine use is probably due to the common practice of combining heroin and cocaine (a so-called "speedball").

Clinical Recommendations

Methadone doses should be raised for patients who have evidence of continued heroin use (e.g., opioid-positive urine samples). Dose increases should continue until heroin use stops or the clinic's maximum dose is reached. Monitoring with urine testing should continue, to evaluate whether this strategy has been effective. If methadone dose raises are insufficient, the next step should be behavior therapy interventions designed to place consequences on drug use (chap. 8). If the patient is also using cocaine, clinical intervention targeting both heroin and cocaine simultaneously is indicated.

Cocaine

Treatment

Cocaine has become the most prevalent supplemental drug of abuse among patients in OTPs and is therefore a dominant concern in the management of continued illicit drug use. Methadone as a medication does not directly address the problem of cocaine use, but the process of methadone treatment does bring cocaine abusers into daily contact with a therapeutic environment where cocaine use can be addressed. It would be quite feasible to include a specific anticocaine pharmacotherapy in the treatment of methadone patients, for example, if such a medication existed. Unfortunately, although a vigorous search is being conducted to identify useful pharmacologic treatments for cocaine addiction, there are no known effective treatments at the present time.

Increased counseling and surveillance is usually considered the first step in treating concurrent cocaine abuse, although these strategies may have little impact unless they are combined with motivational interventions specifically designed to promote cessation of cocaine use. One commonly used, though controversial, strategy is to gradually lower methadone doses and eventually discharge patients from treatment after they have had a succession of positive urine tests for cocaine. Because patients usually value methadone maintenance and want to continue in treatment, the possibility of being withdrawn from methadone because of continued cocaine (or other drug) use may motivate some patients to discontinue such use. Research suggests that this aversive control strategy may be effective with approximately one-half the patients who receive it (e.g., Dolan et al. 1985). Even when the threat of methadone withdrawal does not successfully motivate a particular patient, adherence to this policy may have beneficial effects on the program overall by discouraging other patients from beginning or continuing to use cocaine. It may also have a delayed impact on the patient who is discharged from the methadone program after submitting cocaine-positive urine samples; on subsequent readmission, the patient may be less likely to begin or to continue cocaine use for fear of being withdrawn from methadone.

Proponents of this approach believe failure to respond to a patient's continued cocaine use with a series of progressively stringent consequences allows patients to ignore the negative impact of their on-going drug use. Opponents of this view argue that because of the increasing HIV infection rates among injecting drug users, there are strong public health reasons for retaining injecting drug users in treatment under any circumstances; indeed, the consequences of treatment discharge can be significant, including increased risk of death. Programs remain divided on both this policy in general and its application to specific patients. A new approach for motivating behavior change that incorporates treatment discharge as a final negative event (called motivated stepped care) has proven effective for increasing patient compliance in stopping drug use and is described in chapter 7. In this program, a rapid readmission policy allows noncompliant patients to be readmitted within 24 hours after discharge provided they agree to immediately pursue predischarge treatment goals, including cessation of cocaine use. In addition to the motivated stepped care approach, behavioral interventions that employ positive reinforcers to reward cocaine abstinence have also been developed that also appear quite promising. These are described in chapter 8.

Clinical Recommendations

Cocaine use is a serious problem among methadone patients because of its high prevalence and the harmful consequences associated with its use. Identifying those who use cocaine during treatment is an important priority, with urine testing being the preferred method for obtaining objective data. Cocaine use should be addressed as part of the treatment plan. Intensified counseling and urine surveillance may be a good first step in treating cocaine-using patients, with more potent motivational interventions utilizing either positive or negative incentives for those patients who continue to use cocaine. Programs should remember that individuals injecting cocaine while on methadone remain at risk for HIV and should carefully consider whether discharging such patients is in the best interests of either the patient or the program. For many patients, engaging in methadone treatment can result in decreased injecting drug use and other risky behavior, even though complete abstinence may not be initially achieved.

Benzodiazepines and Other Sedative-Hypnotics

Treatment

Benzodiazepines are unique from the other drugs discussed in this chapter because they have legitimate uses for treatment of both physical and psychological complaints, especially anxiety. They are also among the most widely prescribed psychotropic medications in the world. There are disproportionately high rates of benzodiazepine use in methadone patients as compared with rates in the general population, however, and it appears that this use is usually a form of drug abuse rather than self-medication of an underlying psychiatric disorder (Barnas et al. 1992; Iguchi et al. 1993). Research has also shown that patients who continue to use benzodiazepines while in treatment are more likely to engage in high-risk behaviors (i.e., injection of heroin, use of more amphetamines and cocaine, and sharing of needles) (Darke et al. 1993). Therefore, it is important to detect and address benzodiazepine use in methadone patients because of the increased potential of abuse in this population, dangerous patterns of use, and adverse consequences associated with chronic use of these drugs.

When a methadone patient has been taking one or more benzodiazepine drugs for a period and the use is no longer medically indicated, or when there are signs of abuse and dependence, detoxification may be indicated. The detoxification of someone who is dependent on sedative, hypnotic, or antianxiety substances requires careful supervision because of the serious and, at times, life-threatening withdrawal symptoms that may appear after abrupt cessation of these medications. An inpatient rather than outpatient detoxification setting is recommended to facilitate medical monitoring and enhance compliance with abstinence expectations. Detoxification is generally accomplished with either a gradual step-by-step reduction of the medication itself or by the substitution of a cross-tolerant, longer-acting medication such as phenobarbital that is then gradually withdrawn over time (Dickinson et al. 2003).

Clinical Recommendations

Benzodiazepines may be medically appropriate for the treatment of anxiety or sleeplessness, symptoms that are often present among patients in OTPs. Given the relatively high abuse potential of benzodiazepines among opiate abusers, however, their prescription can be problematic and alternative medications should be used if possible. For those who are currently using benzodiazepines on a regular basis, discontinuation of use should be incorporated into the treatment plan. If possible, an inpatient detoxification should be arranged followed by an intensive aftercare plan designed to prevent relapse back to drug use. A comprehensive reevaluation of psychiatric status is warranted once the patient is benzodiazepine-free to detect and address any concurrent anxiety or depression that may have been masked by drug use. Because benzodiazepine abusers generally use other drugs as well and have a poor prognosis in treatment, they should be engaged in whatever forms of intensive treatment services are available at the OTP, including abstinence incentive programs.

Alcohol

The high rates of alcohol dependence observed in methadone patients, combined with the substantial risk of death and disease associated with heavy alcohol use, suggest it would be beneficial to vigorously treat alcoholism in this patient group. Clinicians should place a priority on treating alcoholic patients because heavy drinking poses a threat to recovery from other drug use and because drinking-related problems have an impact on the operation of the OTP. Heavy drinkers can be disruptive at an OTP when they arrive intoxicated, and staff must deal with decisions about whether the daily methadone dose can be safely administered to an alcohol-intoxicated patient.

Psychosocial and Behavioral Treatment for Alcoholism

Daily contact with patients at the OTP makes it convenient to deliver a variety of specific alcohol treatment interventions. One approach is to offer psychosocial treatment (individual or group) specifically targeted at the use of alcohol. However, one study that tried this approach found poor patient compliance with the treatment offered and high rates of dropouts among active alcoholics in methadone treatment (Stimmel et al. 1983). Thus, the utility of psychosocial interventions for addressing alcohol use among methadone patients has not been documented to date. It has been suggested that regular monitoring of breath alcohol readings, combined with contingencies based on these readings, could be the basis for a useful intervention with alcoholic methadone patients (Bickel et al. 1987), although this strategy has not been evaluated for efficacy and would potentially affect only the excessive drinking of those patients who routinely come to an OTP intoxicated. Other interventions may be needed for those patients judged to have serious alcohol problems that interfere with recovery and lifestyle.

Medications for Alcoholism Treatment

Three medications are currently used to maintain abstinence in patients with alcoholism: naltrexone (ReVia), acamprosate (Campral), and disulfiram (Antabuse). *Naltrexone cannot be used for methadone patients* because it is an opiate antagonist and thus would precipitate severe withdrawal symptoms in a methadone-dependent individual. There are no known studies testing the efficacy and safety of acamprosate in methadone-maintained patients, although the same contraindications do not exist with acamprosate as with naltrexone. Disulfiram has been used successfully in methadone patients and is the recommended pharmacologic approach to treating alcoholism in this population. The following sections give more details on the pharmacology of disulfiram and clinical considerations in its use and then briefly address the use of acamprosate.

Disulfiram Pharmacology

Disulfiram is a medication that blocks the normal metabolism of alcohol. The result of this metabolic blockade is that a toxic by-product of alcohol, acetaldehyde, builds up in the body if the patient drinks after having taken disulfiram. Thus, disulfiram has an effect only if the patient drinks, in which case a very unpleasant acetaldehyde reaction occurs, consisting of sweating, flushing, palpitations, nausea, and blurred vision. Disulfiram can be a very useful tool in the treatment of severe alcoholism, because patients will generally discontinue drinking during periods in which the medication is used regularly to avoid the unpleasant acetaldehyde reaction. There are no methadone-disulfiram interactions that would preclude concurrent administration of the two medications.

Research on Disulfiram Efficacy

Results from clinical trials of disulfiram's efficacy have varied depending on the conditions under which the medication was prescribed. At least two clinical trials (Fuller et al. 1986; Ling et al. 1983) found no difference in treatment outcome between patients assigned to active versus placebo disulfiram under double-blind conditions (i.e., patients did not know whether they were assigned to active or placebo medication). One possible reason for these no-difference outcomes is that all patients in a study of disulfiram must be warned about the potential adverse consequences of drinking alcohol, and unless these patients are willing to take a chance and "test" their medication by drinking, those on placebo will be equally likely to avoid drinking because they believe that they may be on disulfiram. Another possible reason for no difference outcomes is that some patients may not be taking their prescribed medication.

Disulfiram Compliance

Several studies have concluded that the benefits of disulfiram are directly related to compliance with medication ingestion. One large study conducted with alcoholic veterans concluded that when alcoholic patients are simply given a disulfiram prescription only about 20 percent can be expected to comply and actually take the medication (Fuller et al. 1986). Thus, it appears that many alcoholics will not take disulfiram voluntarily if given a choice, but among those who do, drinking usually stops immediately. This understanding about the importance of compliance has led to the development of monitored disulfiram strategies that can increase compliance.

It should be clear that the OTP is an ideal place to dispense disulfiram under monitored conditions, because it can be given daily along with the methadone dose. A study by Liebson and colleagues (1978) illustrates this point. The study showed that alcoholic methadone patients who were required to drink disulfiram (250 mg) mixed in with their methadone dose each day had substantially better outcomes than patients who were given disulfiram supplies weekly and urged to take their daily dose each morning at home. Figure 17.1 shows results for a measure of reported drinking days, but the difference between the two groups is actually understated because drinking in the control groups was substantial, both by clinical observation (intoxication, ataxia, belligerence) and by breath alcohol readings, whereas drinking in the treatment condition generally involved the patients' "cautious experimentation with the alcohol-disulfi-

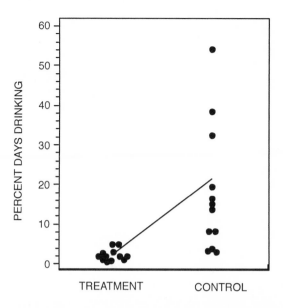

Figure 17.1. Each point represents a patient enrolled in the study and shows the percentage of days that person drank alcohol while in the treatment condition (on the left) or the control condition (on the right). All patients were maintained on methadone. When in the treatment group, they took disulfiram under supervision; when in the control condition, they took disulfiram on their own. Liebson et al. 1978.

ram reaction." Improved outcomes were also reflected in arrest rates, which were substantially lower for disulfiram-treated versus control patients. Compliance was achieved in this study by offering disulfiram as an alternative to treatment termination.

Disulfiram Treatment: Practical Issues

The most certain method for ensuring immediate and sustained remission of alcohol problems is to place patients on disulfiram, mixing it with the daily methadone dose as part of their required treatment. Once patients stop drinking alcohol, alcohol-related disruptive behaviors usually end abruptly. In addition, psychological problems such as depression frequently resolve. Several practical issues surround the use of disulfiram, however.

1. *Motivating participation.* Motivating acceptance of disulfiram remains a clinical challenge. Either positive or negative incentive procedures can be useful in this regard. For example, because alcohol drinking is often closely tied to use of other illicit drugs, some patients may be per-

suaded to stop drinking with the use of disulfiram if they are simultaneously offered the chance to earn incentives for stopping their other illicit drug use.

2. *Detoxification.* Because patients must stop alcohol use for at least 12 hours before beginning disulfiram treatment, there may be cases in which brief, medically supervised inpatient detoxification is needed to ensure sobriety for the start of disulfiram treatment. Medically supervised inpatient detoxification is recommended whenever there are medical complications or when a patient has a history of difficult alcohol withdrawal with delirium tremens and/or seizures. From a behavioral viewpoint, however, brief hospitalization may be needed simply to ensure there is sufficient alcohol-free time to begin disulfiram. Long-acting benzodiazepine drugs (e.g., chlordiazepoxide, diazepam, oxazepam) are frequently administered during an alcohol detoxification (Sellers et al. 1983). These medications can effectively suppress withdrawal discomfort and symptoms and do not interfere with starting disulfiram.

3. *Dosing regimens.* The usual daily dose of disulfiram is 250 mg, but patients are often started on a higher "loading" dose of 500 mg per day for the first few days. It may take several days before a full alcohol-disulfiram reaction is elicited with ingestion of alcohol, and sensitivity increases gradually over time during chronic ingestion. Once chronic administration has begun, single missed doses should not be a problem since disulfiram accumulates in the body. In fact, the medication can be effectively used on a three-day-per-week dosing schedule (250 mg on Monday and Wednesday, 500 mg on Friday). Disulfiram administration can be continued indefinitely and should be discontinued only when clinical judgment suggests that adequate social stability has been established to support continued abstinence. However, this is a difficult judgment, and relapse is always a possibility, with the resultant need to reintroduce more intensive treatment. Once disulfiram is discontinued, the patient should be advised that there is still at least a one-week period after the last dose during which a disulfiram reaction can occur, because it takes this long for the medication to be eliminated from the body.

4. *Safety and side effects.* Patients who have had previous toxic reactions with disulfiram or who have conditions that could be medically compromised by the disulfiram-alcohol interaction should not be placed on this therapy. Such conditions include ischemic heart disease, cardiomyopathy, cardiac arrhythmia, hepatic or pulmonary insufficiency, or renal failure (Wright and Moore 1990). Whether patients with impaired liver function due to chronic alcohol use can receive disulfiram is controversial. There is obviously a catch 22 here, because these may be the patients

who could most benefit from the medication. If the patient can be hospitalized and observed during the start of therapy, the risk of liver problems would be reduced. Otherwise, frequent liver function testing is advised. Because disulfiram-related liver problems usually occur early in treatment, testing should be done every two weeks for the first two months, followed by testing at three- to six-month intervals thereafter (Wright et al. 1988). In most cases, liver function should improve once drinking stops.

Side effects associated with disulfiram can include skin eruptions, drowsiness, headache, impotence, and a metallic taste in the mouth. These are most often reported during the first two weeks and typically disappear with longer-term treatment. Potentially more serious side effects include liver damage and neurotoxicity. Liver damage and hepatitis are relatively rare but potentially fatal reactions to disulfiram. Disulfiram has also been associated with serious neurotoxicity. Symptoms include fatigue, forgetfulness, and confusion and can progress to affective changes, ataxia, stupor, and frank psychosis. Because of daily interaction with staff, the methadone clinic is an ideal place to monitor patients for altered psychological status. If problems with liver function or psychiatric status are noted during disulfiram therapy, the medication should be discontinued immediately. Note, however, that if a placebo can be substituted for an active drug without informing the patient, it is possible that the patient will continue to abstain indefinitely to avoid a potential disulfiram reaction.

5. *Drinking alcohol while taking disulfiram.* Patients must be informed about the dangers of contact with any alcohol while taking disulfiram. Contact can occur through medications with an alcohol base or even through externally applied alcohol, as in shaving lotions. Sensitization to the alcohol-disulfiram reaction increases over time and, therefore, these warnings should be repeated periodically. Despite such warnings, there are reports, both anecdotal and published, of alcoholic or drug abuse patients who can drink while maintained on disulfiram. Presumably, this is accomplished by ingesting alcohol at a sufficiently slow rate as to make the acetaldehyde reaction tolerable. The first clinical response to such a report would be to make sure that compliance-monitoring procedures are operating as expected and that the patient is actually taking the disulfiram. The next step would be to raise the disulfiram dose to 500 mg per day or more. If drinking still continues, questioning the patient about extent and frequency of alcohol use would provide helpful clinical insight and might reveal that alcohol intake is very much reduced from predisulfiram amounts and that it is occurring at clinically acceptable levels.

Clinical Recommendations

Because substantial rates of alcohol use and alcohol dependence occur in the OTP patient population, early identification of problem patients is essential. This can be done using self-report questionnaires, clinical interviews, and breath alcohol testing, as discussed previously. It is common in clinical practice to withhold a portion of the daily methadone dose and any scheduled take-home bottles for patients who come into the clinic with positive breath alcohol readings. This strategy is consistent with safety considerations, although its effectiveness as a behavior change strategy is uncertain. In contrast, the use of monitored disulfiram treatment in which the medication is administered at the clinic along with the daily methadone dose can be a highly effective method to counteract the medical complications and behavioral problems associated with ongoing alcohol dependence among patients receiving methadone and should be utilized whenever possible. Administration at the clinic addresses compliance problems typically associated with disulfiram and ensures that doses are taken. More research is needed, however, on which patients should be selected for disulfiram treatment (e.g., how much drinking is too much?) and on the most effective methods for convincing patients to participate in a disulfiram program (e.g., mandated versus voluntary versus incentive-motivated).

Acamprosate

Acamprosate is a synthetic compound used to treat alcohol dependence that is structurally related to the amino acid homotaurine and the neurotransmitter gamma-aminobutyric acid (GABA). It has been available and used in Europe for several years and was approved for use in the United States in 2004. Although the mechanism of acamprosate's effects is not entirely clear, it appears to exert its primary effects by inhibiting excitatory amino acids in the central nervous system and may also exert effects on calcium channels and other neurotransmitter systems (Littleton and Zieglgansberger 2003; Wilde and Wagstaff 1997).

 Clinical trials have shown that acamprosate can be more effective than placebo in maintaining abstinence from alcohol for persons with alcohol dependence who have undergone detoxification (Baltieri and De Andrade 2004; Kiefer et al. 2003; Mann et al. 2004; Poldrugo 1997; Sass et al. 1996; Soyka and Chick 2003), and it appears that persons who relapse while on acamprosate have less alcohol use when compared with persons who relapse while treated with placebo (Chick et al. 2003). Although acamprosate is effective, the strength of this effect is modest and not all persons respond to it. It appears that combining acamprosate with naltrexone may produce greater efficacy than either medication alone (Kiefer et al. 2003).

One relative disadvantage to acamprosate's use is that dosing is usually thrice daily (e.g., 666 mg is given orally three times per day for a total daily dose of 1,998 mg). It is generally well tolerated; the primary side effect is gastrointestinal (diarrhea). As noted earlier, there are no known studies in which acamprosate has been used with methadone (or buprenorphine). However, in contrast to naltrexone, there are no known pharmacologic contraindications to its use with either of these medications. It will be important for studies to determine the optimal use and safety of acamprosate for patients with both opioid and alcohol dependence. In the meantime, it is probably best to recommend caution if a clinician wishes to use acamprosate in a patient maintained on methadone.

Marijuana

The prevailing ideology in substance abuse treatment programs, including methadone programs, usually emphasizes abstinence from all drugs of abuse. This philosophy stems from clinical beliefs that use of any drug can have a domino effect leading to relapse to other drugs, that use of any drug can interfere with social functioning, and that medical and psychological complications associated with drug use are harmful to patients. Despite this prevailing philosophy, marijuana use is often ignored or given only lip service, and testing for cannabinoids is frequently not included in routine urine-screening assays at OTPs. This may actually be a sensible approach. As previously noted, there does not, in fact, appear to be a clear relationship between use of marijuana and use of other drugs (heroin, cocaine, benzodiazepines) during treatment, nor is there evidence to support a relationship between marijuana use and poor treatment response in methadone programs. Clinics may not want to ignore marijuana completely, but these findings suggest that clinics should consider ranking marijuana use relatively low in their priorities for clinical attention and resources. This is a choice that each clinic must make, however, because there may nevertheless be excellent reasons related to health and well being for patients to stop their use of marijuana, and programs may choose to address marijuana use and to include this in their ongoing treatment protocols.

Tobacco

Treatment

The observation that cigarette smoking is nearly universal among patients receiving methadone, combined with associated risks of disease and premature death, suggests that treatment for tobacco dependence would be quite beneficial to the future health of the OTP population. Nevertheless, substance abuse treatment programs have historically not targeted tobacco smoking, because conventional wisdom argued against addressing tobacco dependence in the context of treating other drug dependencies (Hughes 1993). Both clinicians and researchers alike have begun to challenge this philosophy, however. Several survey studies have suggested that drug and alcohol abusers are interested in smoking cessation (Clemmey et al. 1997; Richter et al. 2001), and a growing number of substance abuse programs have begun offering some form of smoking cessation treatment. Few controlled evaluations of smoking cessation interventions among patients receiving methadone have been performed. In two studies, a behavioral intervention significantly reduced cigarette smoking by offering patients receiving methadone rewards contingent on smoking abstinence (Shoptaw et al. 1996, 2002). Both of these studies also demonstrated decreases in other drug use, such as illicit opiates and cocaine, when cigarette smoking was reduced. These studies support the feasibility of introducing smoking cessation programs to reduce cigarette smoking among patients receiving methadone. Future research should examine the types of treatments that are best suited to this clinical subpopulation, as well as the success rates that can be achieved compared with those in the general population.

Clinical Recommendations

Opioid treatment programs should offer smoking cessation programs to their patients. Based on a review of the scientific literature, clinical guidelines have been published that outline elements of effective smoking cessation treatment (DHHS 2000; Hughes et al. 1996). Cessation rates in the general population can be doubled with the use of nicotine replacement therapy, including products currently available over the counter (e.g., nicotine patches and gum) and by prescription (e.g., nicotine spray and inhaler). Furthermore, rates of cessation have been directly related to the amount of face-to-face therapy delivered as part of the smoking cessation program. Specifically, programs that involve four to seven hours of therapy spread over the first eight postcessation weeks have achieved the best results (DHHS 2000). Active elements of smoking cessation therapy include social support from the counselor and relapse prevention problem solving. Although these methods have not been specifically tested in patients receiving methadone, there is every reason to believe that they will be effective. Furthermore, the OTP provides a convenient setting in which to provide smoking cessation treatment. Patients can be frequently monitored for smoking status by using breath carbon monoxide, which can be measured using a handheld device. Nicotine replacement products (patches or gum) can be dispensed along with opioid treatment medication, and face-to-face counseling can be included as part of drug abuse treatment or provided as a special service. Outlines of behavioral treatment programs for smoking cessation are readily available from the American Lung Association (www.lunguse.org) and the U.S. National Cancer Institute (www.nci.nih.gov). Offering smoking cessation treatment in methadone clinics could be an important step toward limiting smoking-related death and disease among these patients (Hser et al. 1994; Hurt et al. 1996).

SUMMARY

When all drug classes are considered, other drug use can be quite common among OTP patients, with tobacco being the most prevalent drug used (80–90% prevalence) followed by cocaine and heroin (40–60%). Alcohol and sedative dependence (particularly benzodiazepines) are also of concern and occur in a significant portion of this population (approximately 20–25%). Use of more than one drug is a common finding, with an average of four to five lifetime drug dependencies found in patients receiving methadone maintenance. Other drug use in patients receiving methadone is a concern, in part, because of adverse medical and psychological consequences associated with other drug use, including continued risk of exposure to HIV infection.

Identifying secondary drug use in patients is the first step in treatment. Identification can be accomplished by using a combination of interviews and self-reports, with urine testing being an essential tool to verify recent use. Once the type and pattern of other drug use is identified, targeted clinical interventions for each abused substance should be developed. These interventions can include initial detoxification (for alcohol and sedative-tranquilizers), medications (e.g., disulfiram for alcohol, the nicotine patch or gum for tobacco), intensive counseling services, and behavioral treatments. A more detailed discussion of appropriate behavioral treatment interventions, such as contingency management therapies, is provided in chapters 7 and 8.

References

Baltieri DA, De Andrade AG (2004). Acamprosate in alcohol dependence: a randomized controlled efficacy study in a standard clinical setting. *J Stud Alcohol* 65: 136–9

Barnas C, Rossmann M, Roessler H, Riemer Y, Fleischhacker WW (1992). Benzodiazepines and other psychotropic drugs abused by patients in a methadone maintenance program: familiarity and preference. *J Clin Psychopharmacol* 12: 397–402.

Benowitz NL (1993). Clinical pharmacology and toxicology of cocaine. *Pharmacol Toxicol* 72: 3–12.

Bickel WK, Amass L (1993). The relationship of mean daily blood alcohol levels to admission MAST, clinic absenteeism and depression in alcoholic methadone patients. *Drug Alcohol Depend* 32: 113–8.

Bickel WK, Marion I, Lowinson JH (1987). The treatment of alcoholic methadone patients: a review. *J Subst Abuse Treat* 4: 15–9.

Brooner RK, King VL, Kidorf M, Schmidt CW, Jr., Bigelow GE (1997). Psychiatric and substance use comorbidity among treatment-seeking opioid abusers. *Arch Gen Psychiatry* 54: 71–80.

Busto U, Sellers EM, Naranjo CA, Cappell H, Sanchez-Craig M, Sykora K (1986). Withdrawal reaction after long-term therapeutic use of benzodiazepines. *N Engl J Med* 315: 854–9.

Chick J, Lehert P, Landron F (2003). Does acamprosate improve reduction of drinking as well as aiding abstinence? *J Psychopharmacol* 17: 397–402.

Clemmey P, Brooner R, Chutuape MA, Kidorf M, Stitzer M (1997). Smoking habits and attitudes in a methadone maintenance treatment population. *Drug Alcohol Depend* 44: 123–32.

Curran HV (1991). Benzodiazepines, memory and mood: a review. *Psychopharmacology (Berl)* 105: 1–8.

Curran HV (2000). Psychopharmacological approaches to human memory. In: Gazzaniga MS, ed. *The New Cognitive Neurosciences,* 797–804. Boston, MA: MIT Press.

Darke S, Ross J, Lynskey M, Teesson M (2004). Attempted suicide among entrants to three treatment modalities for heroin dependence in the Australian Treatment Outcome Study (ATOS): prevalence and risk factors. *Drug Alcohol Depend* 73: 1–10.

Darke S, Swift W, Hall W, Ross M (1993). Drug use, HIV risk-taking and psychosocial correlates of benzodiazepine use among methadone maintenance clients. *Drug Alcohol Depend* 34: 67–70.

DHHS (2000). Treating Tobacco Use and Dependence: A Clinical Practice Guideline. Bethesda, MD: U.S. Department of Health and Human Services.

Dickinson WE, Mayo-Smith MF, Eickelberg SJ (2003). Management of sedative-hypnotic intoxication and withdrawal. In: Graham AW, Schultz TK, Mayo-Smith MF, Ries RK, Wilford BB, eds. *Principles of Addiction Medicine, 3rd ed.,* 633–49. Chevy Chase, MD: American Society of Addiction Medicine.

Dolan MP, Black JL, Penk WE, Robinowitz R, DeFord HA (1985). Contracting for treatment termination to reduce illicit drug use among methadone maintenance treatment failures. *J Consult Clin Psychol* 53: 549–51.

Donny EC, Walsh SL, Bigelow GE, Eissenberg T, Stitzer ML (2002). High-dose methadone produces superior opioid blockade and comparable withdrawal suppression to lower doses in opioid-dependent humans. *Psychopharmacology (Berl)* 161: 202–12.

Epstein DH, Preston KL (2003). Does cannabis use predict poor outcome for heroin-dependent patients on maintenance treatment? Past findings and more evidence against. *Addiction* 98: 269–79.

First MB, Spitzer RL, Gibbon M, Williams JBW (2001). Structured Clinical Interview for DSM-IV-TR Axis I Disorders (SCID-I/P). New York: Biometrics Research, New York State Psychiatric Institute.

Forman RF, Svikis D, Montoya ID, Blaine J (2004). Selection of a substance use disorder diagnostic instrument by the National Drug Abuse Treatment Clinical Trials Network. *J Subst Abuse Treat* 27: 1–8.

Frosch DL, Shoptaw S, Nahom D, Jarvik ME (2000). Associations between tobacco smoking and illicit drug use among methadone-maintained opiate-dependent individuals. *Exp Clin Psychopharmacol* 8: 97–103.

Fuller RK, Branchey L, Brightwell DR, Derman RM, Emrick CD, Iber FL, James KE, Lacoursiere RB, Lee KK, Lowenstam I, et al. (1986). Disulfiram treatment of alcoholism. A Veterans Administration cooperative study. *JAMA* 256: 1449–55.

George S, Braithwaite RA (2002). Use of on-site testing for drugs of abuse. *Clin Chem* 48: 1639–46.

Gossop M, Marsden J, Stewart D (2002a). Dual dependence: assessment of dependence upon alcohol and illicit drugs, and the relationship of alcohol dependence among drug misusers to patterns of drinking, illicit drug use and health problems. *Addiction* 97: 169–78.

Gossop M, Marsden J, Stewart D, Treacy S (2001). Outcomes after methadone maintenance and methadone reduction treatments: two-year follow-up results from the National Treatment Outcome Research Study. *Drug Alcohol Depend* 62: 255–64.

Gossop M, Stewart D, Treacy S, Marsden J (2002b). A prospective study of mortality among drug misusers during a 4-year period after seeking treatment. *Addiction* 97: 39–47.

Hartel DM, Schoenbaum EE, Selwyn PA, Kline J, Davenny K, Klein RS, Friedland GH (1995). Heroin use during methadone maintenance treatment: the importance of methadone dose and cocaine use. *Am J Public Health* 85: 83–8.

Hser YI, McCarthy WJ, Anglin MD (1994). Tobacco use as a distal predictor of mortality among long-term narcotics addicts. *Prev Med* 23: 61–69.

Hughes JR (1993). Treatment of smoking cessation in smokers with past alcohol/drug problems. *J Subst Abuse Treat* 10: 181–7.

Hughes JR, Fiester S, Goldstein M, Resnick M, Rock N, Ziedonis D (1996). Practice guideline for the treatment of patients with nicotine dependence. *Am J Psychiatry* 153: 1–31.

Hurt RD, Offord KP, Croghan IT, Gomez-Dahl L, Kottke TE, Morse RM, Melton LJ, III (1996). Mortality following inpatient addictions treatment. Role of tobacco use in a community-based cohort. *JAMA* 275: 1097–1103.

Iguchi MY, Handelsman L, Bickel WK, Griffiths RR (1993). Benzodiazepine and sedative use/abuse by methadone maintenance clients. *Drug Alcohol Depend* 32: 257–66.

Jenkins AJ, Goldberger BA (2002). *On-site Drug Testing*. Totowa, NJ: Humana Press

Karacic V, Skender L (2003). Hair testing for drugs of abuse. *Coll Antropol* 27: 263–9.

Kessler RC, Wittchen H-U, Abelson JM, McGonagle KA, Schwarz N, Kendler KS, Knäuper B, Zhao S (1998). Methodological studies of the Composite International Diagnostic

Interview (CID) in the U.S. National Comorbidity Survey. *Int J Methods Psychiatric Res* 7: 33–55.

Kiefer F, Jahn H, Tarnaske T, Helwig H, Briken P, Holzbach R, Kampf P, Stracke R, Baehr M, Naber D, Wiedemann K (2003). Comparing and combining naltrexone and acamprosate in relapse prevention of alcoholism: a double-blind, placebo-controlled study. *Arch Gen Psychiatry* 60: 92–99.

Liebson IA, Tommasello A, Bigelow GE (1978). A behavioral treatment of alcoholic methadone patients. *Ann Intern Med* 89: 342–4.

Ling W, Weiss DG, Charuvastra VC, O'Brien CP (1983). Use of disulfiram for alcoholics in methadone maintenance programs. A Veterans Administration Cooperative Study. *Arch Gen Psychiatry* 40: 851–4.

Littleton J, Zieglgansberger W (2003). Pharmacological mechanisms of naltrexone and acamprosate in the prevention of relapse in alcohol dependence. *Am J Addict* 12 Suppl 1: S3–S11

Macdonald S, Anglin-Bodrug K, Mann RE, Erickson P, Hathaway A, Chipman M, Rylett M (2003). Injury risk associated with cannabis and cocaine use. *Drug Alcohol Depend* 72: 99–115.

Maisto SA, Connors GJ, Allen JP (1995). Contrasting self-report screens for alcohol problems: a review. *Alcohol Clin Exp Res* 19: 1510–6.

Mann K, Lehert P, Morgan MY (2004). The efficacy of acamprosate in the maintenance of abstinence in alcohol-dependent individuals: results of a meta-analysis. *Alcohol Clin Exp Res* 28: 51–63.

McLellan AT, Kushner H, Metzger D, Peters R, Smith I, Grissom G, Pettinati H, Argeriou M (1992). The Fifth Edition of the Addiction Severity Index. *J Subst Abuse Treat* 9: 199–213.

McLellan AT, Luborsky L, Woody GE, O'Brien CP (1980). An improved diagnostic evaluation instrument for substance abuse patients. The Addiction Severity Index. *J Nerv Ment Dis* 168: 26–33.

Nirenberg TD, Cellucci T, Liepman MR, Swift RM, Sirota AD (1996). Cannabis versus other illicit drug use among methadone maintenance patients. *Psychol Addict Behav* 10: 222–7.

Poldrugo F (1997). Acamprosate treatment in a long-term community-based alcohol rehabilitation programme. *Addiction* 92: 1537–46.

Preston KL, Griffiths RR, Stitzer ML, Bigelow GE, Liebson IA (1984). Diazepam and methadone interactions in methadone maintenance. *Clin Pharmacol Ther* 36: 534–41.

Preston KL, Silverman K, Schuster CR, Cone EJ (1997). Assessment of cocaine use with quantitative urinalysis and estimation of new uses. *Addiction* 92: 717–27.

Preston KL, Sullivan JT, Strain EC, Bigelow GE (1996). Enhancement of cocaine's abuse liability in methadone maintenance patients. *Psychopharmacology (Berl)* 123: 15–25.

Richter KP, Gibson CA, Ahluwalia JS, Schmelzle KH (2001). Tobacco use and quit attempts among methadone maintenance clients. *Am J Public Health* 91: 296–9.

Robins LN, Wing J, Wittchen HU, Helzer JE, Babor TF, Burke J, Farmer A, Jablenski A, Pickens R, Regier DA. (1988). The Composite International Diagnostic Interview. An epidemiologic instrument suitable for use in conjunction with different diagnostic systems and in different cultures. *Arch Gen Psychiatry* 45: 1069–77.

Sass H, Soyka M, Mann K, Zieglgänsberger W (1996). Relapse prevention by acamprosate: results from a placebo-controlled study of alcohol dependence. *Arch Gen Psychiatry* 53: 673–80.

Saxon AJ, Calsyn DA, Greenberg D, Blaes P, Haver VM, Stanton V (1993). Urine screening for marijuana among methadone-maintained patients. *Am J Addict* 2: 207–11.

Sellers EM, Naranjo CA, Harrison M, Devenyi P, Roach C, Sykora K (1983). Diazepam loading: simplified treatment of alcohol withdrawal. *Clin Pharmacol Ther* 34: 822–6.

Sells SB, Simpson DD (1987). Role of alcohol use by narcotic addicts as revealed in the DARP research on evaluation of treatment for drug abuse. *Alcohol Clin Exp Res* 11: 437–9.

Shoptaw S, Jarvik ME, Ling W, Rawson RA (1996). Contingency management for tobacco smoking in methadone-maintained opiate addicts. *Addict Behav* 21: 409–12.

Shoptaw S, Rotheram-Fuller E, Yang X, Frosch D, Nahom D, Jarvik ME, Rawson RA, Ling W (2002). Smoking cessation in methadone maintenance. *Addiction* 97: 1317–28; discussion 1325.

Skipsey K, Burleson JA, Kranzler HR (1997). Utility of the AUDIT for identification of hazardous or harmful drinking in drug-dependent patients. *Drug Alcohol Depend* 45: 157–63.

Soyka M, Chick J (2003). Use of acamprosate and opioid antagonists in the treatment of alcohol dependence: a European perspective. *Am J Addict* 12 Suppl 1: S69–S80.

Stark MJ, Campbell BK (1993). Cigarette smoking and methadone dose levels. *Am J Drug Alcohol Abuse* 19: 209–17.

Stimmel B, Cohen M, Sturiano V, Hanbury R, Korts D, Jackson G (1983). Is treatment for alcoholism effective in persons on methadone maintenance? *Am J Psychiatry* 140: 862–6.

Verebey K (1992). Diagnostic laboratory: screening for drug abuse. In: Lowinson JH, Ruiz P, Millman RB, Langrod JG, eds. *Substance Abuse: A Comprehensive Textbook*. Baltimore, MD: Williams and Wilkins.

Wasserman DA, Weinstein MG, Havassy BE, Hall SM (1998). Factors associated with lapses to heroin use during methadone maintenance. *Drug Alcohol Depend* 52: 183–92.

Weizman T, Gelkopf M, Melamed Y, Adelson M, Bleich A (2004). Cannabis abuse is not a risk factor for treatment outcome in methadone maintenance treatment: a 1-year prospective study in an Israeli clinic. *Aust N Z J Psychiatry* 38: 42–46.

Wilde MI, Wagstaff AJ (1997). Acamprosate: a review of its pharmacology and clinical potential in the management of alcohol dependence after detoxification. *Drugs* 53: 1038–53.

Wright C, Moore RD (1990). Disulfiram treatment of alcoholism. *Am J Med* 88: 647–55.

Wright C, Vafier JA, Lake CR (1988). Disulfiram-induced fulminating hepatitis: guidelines for liver-panel monitoring. *J Clin Psychiatry* 49: 430–4.

18

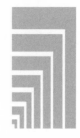

Comorbid Medical Disorders

Michael I. Fingerhood, M.D.

The provision of medical care to patients in opioid treatment programs (OTPs) depends on a trusting, caring relationship between care providers and patients. Especially because of the AIDS epidemic, medically ill addicts need lifetime medical care and associated support services. Historically, medical care for substance-abusing patients has been, at best, episodic and mostly lacking. Medical providers may avoid caring for patients with substance abuse, including those receiving an opioid agonist medication such as methadone. Patients, in turn, sense this often unspoken displeasure and appear demanding or manipulative. A better understanding of the approach to patients taking methadone and knowledge of the comorbid medical conditions will benefit the doctor-patient relationship and ultimately lead to a change in attitude of both the physician and the patient. In a comfortable setting, care can be provided to patients treated with opioid agonists with a high rate of visit compliance, similar to that of any other type of patient.

Medical illness occurs frequently in patients with substance abuse. Although opioid agonist treatment such as methadone maintenance is associated with reduced risk for many medical complications, including acquisition of viruses spread by needle sharing (e.g., HIV, hepatitis B and C), endocarditis, and soft tissue infections, many patients on opioid agonists still present with the same complications seen in injecting-drug users. Often these complications are related to cocaine use, which is frequently injected by patients in OTPs. Additionally, by the time patients enter methadone treatment they often have already developed complications from their pretreatment injecting-drug use. This chapter focuses on the provision of medical care to individuals receiving opioid agonist medications such as methadone, including issues related to the management of health maintenance and the myriad of health complications that can occur in this population.

Basic Primary Care

Patients dependent on opioids report high rates of physical problems at the time of entry to methadone treatment (Ryan and White 1996), and providing on-site primary medical care at the OTP can result in better compliance when treating medical problems (Herman and Gourevitch 1997; Umbricht-Schneiter et al. 1994). On-site primary medical care is often unavailable at OTPs, however, and patients needing medical services are referred to outside medical providers. Under these circumstances, close coordination between the OTP and off-site medical providers is essential.

The provision of primary care to patients in an OTP focuses on screening and prevention. The medical history should include questions, discussion, and counseling related to HIV risk factors, including needle sharing (and, if available, the use of needle-exchange programs) and sexual practices (including the use of condoms). In a nonjudgmental fashion, histories of sexually transmitted diseases (STDs), domestic violence, and tuberculosis exposure should be explored. Focused questions should be asked regarding any history of medical complications of injecting-drug use outlined in this chapter, including endocarditis, HIV, skin infections, and liver disease (especially hepatitis C).

The physical examination should always include a thorough examination of the skin (for signs of abscesses or cellulitis), heart (for presence of a murmur), liver (for size), pelvis (for signs of herpes, genital warts, or discharge), and nose (for septal perforation). The laboratory evaluation should be based on the patient's history. All individuals with a history of needle sharing or high-risk sexual activity should be encouraged to be tested for HIV. For similar reasons, they should undergo screening for hepatitis B (surface antigen and antibody) and hepatitis C (antibody). Individuals with a history of hepatitis should undergo liver function tests (aspartate aminotransferase [AST], alanine aminotransferase [ALT], gamma-glutamyltransferase [GGT], alkaline phosphatase, and bilirubin). Syphilis screening (RPR), which is inexpensive, is also recommended. Screening for tuberculosis with a purified protein derivative (PPD) should be done annually. Individuals with a newly positive PPD (10 mm if HIV-negative and 5 mm if HIV-positive) should be referred for a chest x-ray. If coordinated, treatment with isoniazid (INH) for a positive PPD can be directly observed with dosing of medication (e.g., methadone). All women should undergo screening annually for cervical cancer with a Papanicolaou (Pap) smear.

Routine immunization guidelines should be followed for all patients. Usually, this means a tetanus booster every ten years; and, if individuals test negative for hepatitis B, they should be immunized with a series of three injections. Patients with chronic liver disease should be immunized for hepatitis A.

For patients treated with methadone, side effects can occur even in individuals undergoing long-term treatment. These effects include increased sweating, constipation, and menstrual abnormalities. Laboratory changes include lymphocytosis and increased prolactin levels. Constipation is by far the most commonly occurring side effect, and individuals on methadone maintenance should be encouraged to be on a high-fiber diet. Chronic use of laxatives should be discouraged, but if constipation is severe, occasional doses of magnesium citrate, sorbitol, or lactulose can be prescribed.

General Guidelines for Prescribing

Individuals attending an OTP are at high risk for abusing prescription drugs with abuse liability. Prescription drug abuse can be best avoided by careful and thoughtful prescribing of medications. Practitioners must not be "duped"—that is, acquiesce to demanding patients by prescribing medications inappropriately. To avoid possible abuse, medications should always be prescribed on a fixed schedule. Such scheduling improves symptom control, minimizes the development of symptoms (rather than reacting to symptoms after they occur), and keeps patients from focusing on immediate relief. Medications should be prescribed for short periods during treatment of acute symptoms. Individuals should be frequently seen for reassessment, and the practitioner should avoid refilling medications by telephone.

Unfortunately, there is a risk that some patients will steal prescription blanks or alter their prescription. All prescription pads should be safeguarded and, ideally, marked "not for scheduled drugs." Prescriptions should be written clearly, and the number of pills to be dispensed and the number of refills should be written out (not just a number). If no refills are to be given, "no refill" should be noted. All prescribing of scheduled drugs should be documented clearly in the chart. Practitioners should beware of patients who lose prescriptions or medications, obtain prescriptions from multiple physicians, or repeatedly run out of medications earlier than expected.

In general, two classes of medications with abuse liability, barbiturates and benzodiazepines, should be avoided in patients taking methadone. Barbiturates are prescribed infrequently, and, in addition to abuse potential, another reason that the use of barbiturates should be avoided in patients receiving methadone is that they can induce methadone metabolism. Benzodiazepines also can interact with methadone, and they enhance methadone's effects (Preston et al. 1984). This interaction may account for the observation of substantial rates of illicit benzodiazepine use in some patients receiving methadone. Thus, the physician working in an OTP should be sensitive to the risk of inappropriate use of a prescribed benzodiazepine or diversion of the prescription to the illicit market. It is common practice to recommend avoiding any use of prescription benzodiazepines for patients treated in an OTP.

Note, however, that given these cautions, some practitioners report successful use of prescribed benzodiazepines for selected methadone-maintained patients, such as those with a clear anxiety disorder. In such cases, benzodiazepines with high abuse potential, for example, diazepam (most commonly marketed as Valium), lorazepam (Ativan), and alprazolam (Xanax) are typically avoided and instead low-abuse-potential benzodiazepines such as oxazepam (Serax) are prescribed. (For a review of the relative abuse potential of benzodiazepines, see Griffiths and Wolf 1990.)

Other potentially abusive medications that generally should be avoided in an OTP population include muscle relaxants, methylphenidate (Ritalin), amphetamines, and clonidine. Clonidine use is not detected in routine urine screening, and abuse of clonidine has been reported to be quite high in some areas and populations (Beuger et al. 1998). Because of this potential for clonidine abuse or the diversion of a prescription to the illicit market (resulting in subsequent poor blood pressure control for the patient), clonidine should not be used in the management of hypertension for patients maintained on an opioid agonist. Other medications that need to be used cautiously in OTP patients include antiemetics (promethazine and compazine), amitriptyline, and cough syrups. Oxaprozin (Daypro), a nonsteroidal anti-inflammatory drug, should be avoided because it can give a false-positive result for benzodiazepines in a drug screen. Efavirenz (Sustiva), a commonly used medication for HIV infection, can give a false-positive screen for marijuana.

Pain Management

Pain management can be extremely challenging in OTP patients. Furthermore, patients with drug abuse have a high rate of pain complaints (Rosenblum et al. 2003). Several general rules can help physicians in their approach to the management of acute pain in this population (Payte and Khuri 1993). First and most important, for patients experiencing acute pain, the physician should not discontinue the patient's daily dose of opioid agonist (e.g., methadone). If the patient is unable to take methadone orally, doses can be divided and delivered by intramuscular injection. No decrease in the daily maintenance dose should be made if the dose is given by injection. Maintenance on methadone does not mean the patient is in a chronic state of analgesia; experimental evidence indicates that pain perception adapts to a normal range for patients maintained on methadone (Schall et al. 1996).

Second, alternatives to pharmacologic therapy, such as relaxation techniques, exercise, acupuncture, biofeedback, and massage, should be initially attempted when possible. Third, if pharmacologic therapy is indicated, nonopioids such as nonsteroidal anti-inflammatory drugs (NSAIDs) should be used first. Even these medications, however, can cause adverse effects, such as hepatotoxicity and gastrointestinal effects (e.g., bleeding, ulceration) with chronic or high doses, so they should be used with caution.

Fourth, if an opioid is to be used for pain control, mixed agonist-antagonists, such as pentazocine, butorphanol, nalbuphine, and buprenorphine, in general, should be avoided. Use of these compounds in a patient maintained on an opioid agonist such as methadone could result in a precipitated withdrawal syndrome, further complicating the patient's management.

Fifth, when opioids are indicated, weaker opioids (codeine and propoxyphene) should be tried first, with a progression to stronger opioids (oxycodone and hydrocodone) and finally morphine. If morphine is to be used, a long-acting formulation of morphine may have lower abuse liability. Finally, it is important to stress the need to communicate clearly to patients plans for controlling their pain and to treat aggressively patients' pain (Scimeca et al. 2000).

Methadone can be used as an effective analgesic, but it is not recommended for the treatment of pain in methadone-maintained patients (i.e., as supplemental doses of methadone added to the daily dose). Acute doses of methadone in non-opioid-dependent patients provide analgesia for about six to eight hours. Thus, if methadone is used in pain management, three to four doses per day will be necessary.

DRUG INTERACTIONS WITH METHADONE

Although no drugs are absolutely contraindicated with methadone, some medications should be avoided (table 18.1). For example, administration of an opiate antagonist would cause opiate withdrawal, so under routine clinical circumstances opiate antagonists such as naloxone, nalmefene, and naltrexone should be avoided.

A variety of drugs have an impact on the metabolic clearance of methadone and may cause opiate withdrawal and opiate craving. For example, rifampin has been shown to have a clinically significant impact on methadone clearance, requiring an adjustment in the dosing of methadone (Kreek et al. 1976; Raistrick et al. 1996). Individuals treated for tuberculosis with rifampin need an upward adjustment of their methadone dose or split methadone dosing. Rifabutin, structurally similar to rifampin and

Table 18.1 **Medications That May Alter Methadone Blood Levels or Alter Methadone's Effects**

Drugs decreasing methadone blood levels
    Barbiturates (for example, phenobarbital)
    Carbamezepine
    Efavirenz
    Estrogens*
    Nevaripine
    Phenytoin
    Protease inhibitors*
    Rifampin
    Spironolactone*
    Verapamil*
Drugs increasing methadone blood levels
    Amitriptyline*
    Cimetidine
    Fluvoxamine
    Sertraline
Drug acutely producing opioid withdrawal symptoms
    Metyrapone
Drug acutely increasing methadone's effects
    Ethanol

*May influence methadone blood levels, although there is limited evidence for this effect.

used in HIV-positive patients for prevention of mycobacterium avium-intracellular, does not appear to cause a similar effect on methadone blood levels (Brown et al. 1996).

Several anticonvulsants that induce liver enzymes can increase methadone metabolism, and patients have reported withdrawal symptoms later in the day after having received their dose of methadone (Bell et al. 1988; Tong et al. 1981). Anticonvulsants that can produce such effects include phenytoin, carbamazepine, and barbiturates (e.g., phenobarbital).

Several other medications may decrease methadone blood levels (table 18.1) (Plummer et al. 1988). Two commonly prescribed HIV medications, efavirenz and nevaripine, can have profound effects by increasing methadone clearance, thus requiring a significant increase in the dose of methadone (Faragon and Piliero 2003). Another class of HIV medication, protease inhibitors, may also increase metabolism of methadone, but clinical symptoms requiring change in methadone dosing is not common (Faragon and Piliero 2003). In addition, some medications can increase methadone blood levels or acutely potentiate the effects of methadone. Most notably, cimetidine and fluvoxamine can increase methadone blood levels, and alcohol can potentiate the effects of methadone (Bertschy et al. 1994; Donnelly et al. 1983).

In addition to drugs affecting methadone levels, methadone can alter the blood levels and effects of other medications. For example, pharmacokinetic studies have found the concentration of zidovudine (AZT) to be elevated in some patients treated with methadone (Jatlow et al. 1997; Schwartz et al. 1992). It is unclear if this increase is clinically significant, but increased risk of zidovudine toxicity (lethargy, nausea, headache, and anemia) is possible, and therefore individuals on methadone should be followed closely. Similarly, methadone appears to increase blood levels of tricyclic antidepressants (Maany et al. 1989). Finally, methadone can delay alcohol elimination.

HIV Infection

Much data, direct and indirect, support the use of opioid agonist treatment as a deterrent to the spread of HIV (De Castro and Sabate 2003). Nevertheless, many patients receiving methadone are HIV positive, which is partially related to previous needle use but, especially for women, also to the heterosexual spread of HIV. In the United States, 50 percent of HIV-positive women are positive as a result of injecting-drug use and another 25 percent as a result of heterosexual activity with an injecting-drug user (Squires 2003).

The care of the HIV-positive patient taking methadone requires sensitivity to specific issues related to substance abuse as well as to those related to methadone. In studies of HIV-positive patients, comparing those who acquired HIV through injecting-drug use with those who acquired HIV through homosexual activity, there is little difference in disease progression or opportunistic infections (Des Jarlais 1999; Selwyn et al. 1992). The major difference is in morbidity related to injecting-drug use—endocarditis, abscesses, and viral hepatitis (Cohen 2002). In addition, those who inject drugs have a higher rate of bacterial pneumonia and tuberculosis.

More than ever, the aim of HIV care is to attack the virus aggressively with triple-medication therapy (HAART) to decrease the amount of circulating virus (viral load) to an undetectable level. Such medical regimens can be complicated and are expensive. There is also the risk of viral resistance if the medications are not taken reliably (Lucas et al. 2002; Stein et al. 2000). Therefore, complicated regimens consisting of multiple drugs should not be initiated until an HIV-positive patient has demonstrated compliance with medical visits (Lucas et al. 2001). Linkage between the OTP and HIV primary care can have a synergistic effect, benefiting patients in both areas and enhancing compliance (O'Connor et al. 1992). Many HIV regimens are now taken only once daily and can potentially be linked with opioid agonist dosing to improve adherence and outcome.

The medical approach to providing care to HIV-infected individuals is shown in table 18.2. The initiation of therapy is based on viral load and

Table 18.2 **HIV Standards of Care**

A. Baseline
1. Documentation of HIV serology
2. Blood work: CBC (complete blood count), HIV viral load, CD4, chemistry panel, RPR, hepatitis serology
3. Screening: PPD, Pap smear (women)
4. Immunizations: pneumococcal vaccine if CD4 >200, flu vaccine if season, tetanus if needed, hepatitis B if negative serology

B. Monitoring
1. Viral load: every 3 to 4 months, or more often if indicated, to evaluate changes in therapy
2. CD4: every 3 to 4 months
3. CBC: every 3 to 4 months (if taking AZT will need closer follow-up initially)
4. Pap smear: repeat in 6 months and then annually
5. RPR: annually
6. PPD: annually

CD4. The number of approved medications directed against the HIV virus has increased and, therefore, only providers who are well versed in providing HIV care and up to date regarding current therapies should initiate treatment.

SKIN AND SOFT TISSUE INFECTIONS

Skin and soft tissue infections are the most common complications of injecting-drug use (CDC 2001; Harris and Young 2002). These infections result from abusers using nonsterile techniques when injecting and from their inability to inject properly into a vein. Although cultured samples of heroin have grown a wide range of organisms including staphylococcus, clostridium, and aspergillus, most likely the addict's skin is the primary source of the infection. Organisms isolated from abusers' works or paraphernalia are rarely found in the bloodstreams of infected users (Tuazon and Elin 1981).

The injection of cocaine causes blood vessels to spasm, which can result in the injection of drug and diluents (cutting agents) into soft tissue. Cocaine injection may also cause thrombus distant to the injection site. When veins in the arms are no longer available, drug users often turn to injecting in their legs, neck, and groin. In addition, "skin popping" into subcutaneous tissue is common. Complications from these various forms of injecting drugs can include cellulitis, abscess, septic thrombophlebitis, pyomyositis, and pseudoaneurysms (Ebright and Pieper 2002). Furthermore, osteomyelitis or septic arthritis may occur, owing to bacterial spread from contiguous soft tissue or from bacteremia (Kak and Chandrasekar 2002). Other problems associated with the process of injecting drugs can include lymphatic obstruction and edema, which can result from chronic skin popping, and foreign-body reactions to needle fragments that become lodged subcutaneously (which also can migrate centrally) (Galdun et al. 1987).

Staphylococcus aureus is the most likely microorganism to cause tissue infection, followed by streptococci, and Gram-negative rods. The initial management of tissue infections often requires incision and drainage. Infection may or may not be accompanied by fever and an elevated white blood cell count. Minor abscesses and infections can often be managed with an oral antibiotic (cephalexin or dicloxacillin) after incision and drainage. More severe infections require hospitalization for administration of intravenous antibiotics. Resistant organisms, including methicillin-resistant staphylococcus, have been increasingly isolated in injecting-drug users who have attempted to treat their own infections by using antibiotics bought from the street market.

CARDIAC COMPLICATIONS

The most common cardiac complication of injection-drug use is endocarditis. Chronic injecting-drug use likely results in chronic low-grade bacteremia and creates endothelial valvular damage and platelet fibrin deposition. Some injecting-drug users are particularly prone to repeated bouts of endocarditis. The diagnosis of endocarditis is based on the presence of a murmur on examination, positive blood cultures, and echocardiographic evidence. At least four sets of blood cultures should be drawn from different sites and at different times to maximize the detection of the infectious agent. Although bacteremia is often indicative of endocarditis, 35–60 percent of bacteremias are unrelated to endocarditis and are most often related to soft tissue infections. If transthoracic echocardiogram is unable to detect valvular vegetation and clinical suspicion for endocarditis is high, a transesophageal echocardiogram should be performed.

The incidence of bacterial endocarditis in injecting-drug users is estimated at 2 to 5 percent per year (Miro et al. 2002; Sande et al. 1992). Unlike endocarditis in individuals without a history of injecting-drug use, individuals with a history of injecting-drug use develop predominantly right-sided endocarditis, most often affecting the tricuspid valve. *Staphylococcus aureus* is the most frequently isolated organism. It is easily treatable, but large vegetations, greater than 1 cm, increase treatment failure. Methicillin-resistant organisms are increasingly being seen.

Streptococcus typically causes left-sided, aortic or mitral valve endocarditis. Left-sided infections have a higher medical failure rate and more commonly have subsequent morbidity and mortality. Complications include sequelae of emboli (e.g., stroke), conduction disturbance, and valve damage resulting in regurgitant flow and heart failure.

Less common causes of endocarditis include *Pseudomonas aeruginosa, Serratia, Haemophilus, Neisseria, Enterobacteriaceae,* and *Candida. Pseudomonas* infection may cause coexisting right- and left-sided endocarditis, with a poor prognosis. Candidal endocarditis is related to the presence of candida in the diluents or cutting agents mixed with heroin (Leen and Brettle 1991). With rare exceptions, when treating endocarditis, intravenous antibiotics should be administered on an inpatient basis for the duration of therapy.

Most noninfection cardiac complications of drug abuse are attributed to cocaine. Cocaine has been reported to cause myocardial infarction, coronary artery spasm with angina, and cardiomyopathy (Lange and Hillis 2001).

Sexually Transmitted Diseases (STDs)

All STDs are commonly seen in drug abusers, even those treated with opioid agonist medications such as methadone. Especially among women, sexual intercourse is often exchanged for drugs. Additionally, unprotected sexual intercourse is common in crack houses, placing non-injecting-drug users at risk for sexually transmitted diseases and HIV. Guidelines for the treatment of STDs are shown in table 18.3.

Chlamydia is a common sexually transmitted disease; it is often asymptomatic, which makes transmission easy. Gonorrhea is also easily transmitted and can be seen as a cause of septic arthritis in drug users. The presence of genital herpes infection appears to increase the likelihood of sexual transmission of HIV infection. Additionally, HIV-infected individuals often shed herpes virus even when they do not have active disease.

The diagnosis of syphilis in a person with a history of injecting-drug use is confounded by an approximately 25 percent biologic false-positive rate for the standard serologic test for syphilis (STS or RPR). False-positive titers are rarely at greater than a 1:4 titer. All positive STS or RPR titers should be sent for the more specific assay of free treponemal antibody (FTA). Syphilis screening should be performed yearly on all sexually active individuals, and all new positive results should be treated. Presentation of advanced syphilis can be seen among injecting-drug users. A person who presents with an erythematous rash affecting the palms and soles should be diagnosed as having secondary syphilis until proven otherwise.

Individuals who test positive for syphilis with unknown previous testing and no history of symptomatic disease (a primary chancre) should be treated as if they have latent disease with three consecutive weekly injections of 2.4 million units of benzathene penicillin. Because penicillin is the most effective treatment, individuals who claim penicillin allergy, but who do not have a history of anaphylaxis, should be tested for penicillin allergy. The treatment of syphilis in HIV-infected individuals is identical, but there are reports of increased treatment failures in such individuals (Hall et al. 2004).

Evidence has shown that human papilloma virus (HPV), another sexually transmitted disease, is the causative agent in most cases of cervical cancer. Sexual intercourse at an early age and higher numbers of sexual partners correlate as risk factors for cervical cancer. Women with a his-

Table 18.3   **Treatment of Sexually Transmitted Diseases**

Type of Disease	Drug of Choice	Dosage	Alternatives
Chlamydia trachomatis Urethritis, cervicitis	Azithromycin	1 g oral once	Ofloxacin 300 mg oral bid for 7 days Levofloxacin 500 mg oral qD for 7 days
	Doxycycline	100 mg oral bid for 7 days	Erythromycin 500 mg oral qid for 7 days
Gonorrhea Urethral, cervical, rectal, or pharyngeal	Ceftriaxone	125 mg IM once	Ciprofloxacin 500 mg oral once Ofloxacin 400 mg oral once
Syphilis Early (primary or latent less than one year)	Penicillin G benzathine	2.4 million units IM once	Doxycycline 100 mg oral bid for 14 days
Late (more than one year's duration, late-latent)	Penicillin G benzathine	2.4 million units IM weekly for 3 weeks	Doxycycline 100 mg oral bid for 4 weeks
Chancroid	Ceftriaxone Azithromycin Ciprofloxacin	250 mg IM once 1 g oral once 500 mg oral once	
Herpes simplex First episode genital	Acyclovir	400 mg oral tid for 7–10 days	Acyclovir 200 mg oral 5 times per day for 7–10 days
First episode proctitis	Acyclovir	800 mg oral tid for 7–10 days	Acyclovir 400 mg oral 5 times per day for 7–10 days

Abbreviations: bid, two times a day; qD, every day; qid, four times a day; tid, three times a day; IM, intramuscular.

tory of injecting-drug use, including those on methadone, have a high rate of abnormalities on Pap smears and all should undergo yearly testing. If a significant abnormality is found, referral should be made for colposcopy. Mild abnormalities should be followed up with a repeat smear in six months. HIV-positive women tend to have particularly aggressive forms of cervical cancer linked to HPV, and invasive cervical cancer is an AIDS-defining illness. Hence, HIV-positive women should have screening Pap smears every six months until they have two consecutive normal test results. Thereafter, only yearly screening is necessary.

Hepatitis

Despite the onslaught of AIDS, liver disease is the most prevalent medical problem among individuals with addiction, including those receiving opioid agonist treatments. Liver damage ranges from alcohol-induced liver damage to viral hepatitis in injecting-drug users. It now appears that hepatitis C poses the greatest risk. In Baltimore, Maryland, a study of individuals with a history of injecting-drug use presenting for detoxification found that 86 percent had hepatitis C (Fingerhood et al. 1993). These patients had elevated aminotransferase enzymes indicative of active hepatitis. It is estimated that 50 percent of individuals testing positive for hepatitis C develop chronic hepatitis, with 20 percent of those with chronic hepatitis later developing cirrhosis (Liang et al. 2000). Alcohol use increases the likelihood of disease progression. Hepatitis C tends to have an asymptomatic acute phase, with a slow progression of disease over many years. Presently, it is difficult to predict why certain individuals have a more fulminant course. Coinfection with HIV and hepatitis has been shown to hasten the progression to cirrhosis (Romeo et al. 2000; Sulkowski and Thomas 2003; Tedaldi et al. 2003). Transmission of the hepatitis C virus is through needle use, and the risk of sexual transmission is low, but possible. In addition, it is not understood why 25 percent of alcoholics without a history of injecting-drug use test positive for hepatitis C. Any injecting-drug user with elevated aminotransferases should be evaluated for hepatitis C. All individuals who test positive for hepatitis C should be considered for treatment. Treatment consists of ribavirin pills taken twice daily and injections of pegylated interferon weekly. Duration of therapy is 24 or 48 weeks depending on the hepatitis C genotype. The likelihood of cure also depends on the genotype, with cure rates ranging from 40 to 65 percent (Davis et al. 2003). Side effects of therapy (fever, arthralgias, fatigue, and depression) often cause patients to abandon treatment.

Chronic hepatitis B (carriers of HBSAg) is less common, affecting an estimated 5 percent of injecting-drug users (Fingerhood et al. 1993). Such individuals can transmit hepatitis B via needle sharing and sexual contact. Most individuals exposed to hepatitis B will develop immunity, as expressed by the development of hepatitis B surface antibody. During the acute phase of hepatitis B, all individuals are contagious but not all individuals are symptomatic. Hepatitis B carriers may all be coinfected with delta virus (hepatitis D), increasing the risk of development of fulminant hepatitis (Bean 2002). A biphasic pattern of illness with relapse a few weeks after an initial episode of hepatitis B suggests delta infection. Several treatments for chronic hepatitis B are now available (lamivudine, adefovir, and interferon) that can potentially limit the progression of hepatitis B.

Maintenance on an opioid agonist such as methadone, or halting injecting-drug use, does not halt or limit the progression of chronic viral hepatitis. Cessation of alcohol use and avoidance of drugs that are hepatotoxic is essential, however. In individuals who have chronic hepatitis or cirrhosis, isoniazid (INH) should not be used to treat tuberculosis. Additionally, disulfiram should be used with caution in these individuals. Alcoholic hepatitis typically improves with the cessation of drinking. Diagnosis and prognosis for alcohol-related liver disease is based on the pathology present from a liver biopsy, because individuals may present with severe jaundice and ascites that is reversible with abstinence, or they may already have cirrhosis. Rapid improvement with abstinence makes hepatitis the more likely diagnosis rather than cirrhosis.

When chronic acute hepatitis of any etiology progresses to liver failure, treatment becomes supportive. Unfortunately, many liver transplant programs will not consider individuals for transplant if they are taking an opioid agonist treatment such as methadone, although some transplant surgeons educated about methadone treatment will now consider patients receiving methadone for liver transplantation. A decision as to whether the individual is sufficiently stable to wean off methadone, however, must be made before consideration for transplantation.

PULMONARY COMPLICATIONS

Most pulmonary complications seen in injecting drug users are directly related to HIV–pneumocystis pneumonia and frequent bacterial pneumonias. Studies imply that HIV-negative drug users are also at a greater risk for bacterial pneumonia. The fact that more than 90 percent of drug users smoke cigarettes may account for this higher risk. Additionally, aspiration pneumonia commonly occurs as a result of alcohol abuse or overdosing.

Secondary lung infections can occur in injecting-drug users as a result of septic emboli from endocarditis or thrombophlebitis. Chest x-rays in these patients will show wedge-shaped lesions. Septic emboli may cause an abscess, an empyema, or a pulmonary infarction. Antibiotics are targeted at the cause of infection and, in the case of empyema, a chest tube is indicated.

Tuberculosis must always be considered in an injecting-drug user with pulmonary symptoms, fever, and weight loss. A history of incarceration and HIV infection each add to the risk for tuberculosis. Chest x-ray may not show the typical upper-lobe infiltrate. Any patient who is highly suspected of having tuberculosis should be hospitalized with respiratory isolation. If the diagnosis is confirmed, the use of direct observed therapy, the standard of care in many cities, adds dramatically to the success of completed treatment. All patients in an OTP should be screened for tuberculosis yearly, using the standard PPD; anergy testing is not necessary. In non-HIV-infected individuals, 10 mm of induration indicates a positive response, whereas in HIV-infected individuals, 5 mm of induration indicates a positive response. Newly positive responses should be strongly considered for treatment with INH for nine months. Pyridoxine generally should be coadministered. Compliance with INH therapy is greatly enhanced when it is administered daily at the OTP.

In addition, drug users are at high risk for noninfectious pulmonary disease (Gotway et al. 2002). For example, heroin overdose may present with pulmonary edema, a complication that may be delayed for hours after the overdose (Sporer and Dorn 2001). The occurrence of heroin-induced pulmonary edema is correlated with the purity or grade of heroin used. The chest x-ray of a patient with heroin-related pulmonary edema will show a widespread interstitial and alveolar pattern with a normal-sized heart, and heart function is normal in these patients. Treatment is supportive, and although patients are usually treated with intravenous naloxone, no good evidence shows that this has an impact on survival. Hypoventilation, although present, is not the cause of the pulmonary edema, and the mechanism of heroin-related pulmonary edema is likely related to capillary leak. Although the exact mechanism of this capillary leakage is not known, it has been postulated that opiate-induced histamine release is the cause.

Chronic lung disease can occur directly as a result of injecting drugs. Most likely it results from the injection of contaminants that are not fully dissolved and that cause emboli. Cotton and starch are often injected and cause granulomas. Pills that are ground and then injected (e.g., methylphenidate) may contain talc. Talc lung disease is progressive and causes reduced single-breath-diffusing capacity (Dlco) and expiratory obstruction (reduced forced expiratory volume in 1 second [FEV_1]). Chest x-ray in these patients will show increased interstitial markings, often with micronodules, bullae, and flattened diaphragms (Goldstein et al. 1986). Cigarette smoking can add to the progression of this disease, and pulmonary hypertension can develop as a result of hypoxia. Treatment for chronic lung disease includes steroids and bronchodilators, which provide symptomatic relief, and progression of the disease leads to the need for supplemental oxygen.

Bronchospasm is commonly seen in drug users after the smoking of heroin or cocaine. Local inflammation occurs and treatment with bronchodilators and steroids ameliorates symptoms. The smoking of freebase cocaine has also been reported to cause atelectasis, alveolar hemorrhage, pulmonary infarction, and bronchiolitis obliterans (Haim et al. 1995).

Pneumothorax is an acute complication of injecting-drug use that can occur when attempting to inject drugs into a neck vein. Hemothorax or a large hematoma in the neck may also be present. Symptoms of pneumothorax include sudden shortness of breath and pleuritic chest pain on the side of the attempted injection. Individuals with these symptoms require immediate medical attention and a chest x-ray. A pneumothorax is a medical emergency, most often requiring placement of a chest tube. Pneumothorax may also occur as a complication of *Pneumocystis carini* pneumonia, but in this setting, individuals have a history of cough, fever, and progressive shortness of breath.

RENAL COMPLICATIONS

Kidney failure in injecting-drug users has been termed "heroin nephropathy" despite the lack of evidence to support heroin as the etiologic factor (Cunningham et al. 1980, 1983; Rao et al. 1974). Many reported cases are likely related to hepatitis C infection (do Sameiro Faria et al. 2003). Renal biopsy usually shows focal segmental to diffuse sclerosing glomerulonephritis. Seen almost exclusively in men, often without a history of hypertension, the kidney failure begins with nephrotic syndrome and rapidly progresses to a stage that requires dialysis.

Renal amyloidosis can occur in injecting-drug users who skin-pop or have severe chronic abscesses from injecting-drug use and can lead to chronic renal failure requiring dialysis (Neugarten et al. 1986). Renal biopsy reveals AA-protein amyloid, which can also be found in the skin, pleura, and liver. Progression to chronic renal failure is more gradual than for heroin nephropathy, often taking years.

The costs of maintaining drug users on dialysis for a lifetime are tremendous and complications are more likely if injecting-drug abuse continues. Dialysis access sites are likely to become infected and often require repeated surgery. The controlled setting of an OTP is particularly important for injecting-drug users on dialysis because it may prevent further severe complications related to ongoing injecting-drug use.

Acute renal diseases that affect injecting-drug users include myoglobinuria and glomerulonephritis related to endocarditis or infection with hepatitis B or C (do Sameiro Faria et al. 2003). Myoglobinuria related to injection of heroin and cocaine may occur without immobilization or limb compression (Rice et al. 2000). Focal muscle tenderness may not be present, but blood tests reveal elevated levels of serum myoglobin and creatine phosphokinase associated with elevations in blood urea nitrogen and creatine; in general, treatment with intravenous saline reverses the disorder. Methadone can be safely used in patients on dialysis; in such patients, methadone is not removed by dialysis, nor does the absence of renal function lead to methadone accumulation (Furlan et al. 1999; Kreek et al. 1980).

Acute and chronic hepatitis B infection and chronic hepatitis C infection are associated with a variety of pathologic renal diseases (Meyers et al. 2003). Individuals may often have asymptomatic hepatitis, and chronic hepatitis may be present for years before the onset of renal dysfunction. Pathologic changes associated with hepatitis B and C include membranous, membranoproliferative, and minimal change diseases. The prognosis for glomerulonephritis associated with acute hepatitis is better than that with chronic hepatitis.

NEUROLOGICAL COMPLICATIONS

Neurological complications seen in drug-abusing patients may be infectious or noninfectious (Brust 2002). Changes in mental status suggest a wide range of possible diagnoses, especially in HIV-infected individuals, resulting in an often-extensive workup that may include imaging (computed tomography [CT] or magnetic resonance imaging [MRI]) and cerebrospinal fluid analysis (lumbar puncture). Delirium and hallucinations are most commonly related to alcohol but may also be related to the use of contaminated batches of heroin or cocaine from the street market. In 1996 scopolamine was sold as heroin on the Baltimore, Maryland, street market, and its use resulted in anticholinergic poisoning that presented as delirium. Individuals on opioid agonist treatment also commonly abuse benzodiazepines, which in large amounts can cause delirium.

Seizures are the most common noninfectious neurological complication of drug abuse. Overdose-related seizures are usually related to hypoxia from respiratory depression and are usually of the grand mal type. Seizures may also occur as a result of cocaine-induced vasospasm, abscess, HIV-related infection, embolic or thrombotic stroke, meningitis, subdural hematoma, and alcohol withdrawal.

Traumatic mononeuropathies may occur directly at injection sites from hitting a nerve, or they may occur from persistent, direct pressure on a nerve after a change in mental status. Atraumatic mononeuropathies have been reported at a distance from the injection site, perhaps related to vasospasm. Additionally, Bell's palsy, a facial nerve palsy, is commonly seen in injecting-drug users who are HIV positive. Most mononeuropathies improve over time and do not require surgical intervention.

Infectious neurological complications of intravenous drug use are most commonly related to bacteremia. Meningitis, brain abscess, subdural and epidural abscesses, and mycotic aneurysms have all been reported. Simple complaints of back pain or headache may deserve particular attention in the injecting-drug user. Fever or an elevated sedimentation rate accompanied by subacute back pain that has not resolved with conservative measures warrants imaging with a CT scan or MRI to pursue a diagnosis of epidural abscess or vertebral osteomyelitis (Sapico and Montgomerie 1980).

IMMUNOLOGY

Immunologic abnormalities are common in injecting-drug users, independent of HIV infection. Many of the abnormalities have unclear clinical consequences. Most long-time addicts have hypergammaglobulinemia (attributed to chronic antigenic stimulation) with elevated total protein levels and normal or low albumin levels. Chronic liver disease may potentiate the abnormality. Serum protein electrophoresis will reveal a polyclonal gammopathy in such patients. These excess globulins contribute to the high rate of false-positive syphilis tests in injecting-drug users. Other false-positive tests found in addicts include Coombs, smooth muscle antibodies, monospot (heterophile antibody) and rheumatoid factor.

The most clinically relevant immunologic disorder in injecting-drug users is thrombocytopenic purpura (Ryan 1979). This disorder results from circulating immune complexes reacting with platelets. Quinine used as a cutting agent is the most commonly implicated causative agent. Despite very low platelet counts, severe bleeding is unusual. Platelets that are present are functional. Treatment with steroids (prednisone, 15 mg every six hours) is indicated if the platelet count is very low (less than 10,000 without bleeding or less than 30,000 with bleeding). Individuals who continue to inject drugs are at high risk for recurrence.

WOMEN AND DOMESTIC VIOLENCE

Women with a history of substance abuse, including those in an OTP and on methadone maintenance, have a high rate of domestic violence. Screening for domestic violence should be incorporated into the medical interview for all women on opioid agonist maintenance treatment. It is important to deal with the issue sensitively as the individual may be reluctant to disclose information because of shame, humiliation, and low self-esteem. Some women believe they deserve the abuse and therefore do not deserve help, or they may feel the need to protect a partner who is a source of support. Occasionally, the victim believes that medical providers will not find her claim of abuse to be plausible.

Complaints from victims of domestic violence may range from those related to obvious evidence of physical trauma to nonspecific complaints of fatigue, insomnia, or difficulty concentrating. Once a diagnosis of domestic violence is made, the medical provider must validate the seriousness of the situation to the patient. The immediate safety of the woman should be assessed. If safety is in question, the woman should be advised to stay with family or friends or in a shelter that provides special care for abused women. The National Domestic Violence Hotline (1-800-799-SAFE) is a 24-hour service that will help women find a safe place to stay in their community. However, women with ongoing substance abuse are often refused shelter at such places.

SUMMARY

Comorbid medical conditions are commonly found among patients maintained on opioid agonist therapy. However, this is a population whose medical needs are often inadequately addressed. Treatment with an opioid agonist provides a unique opportunity to intervene and provide the necessary medical care for patients dependent on opioids, and this care can decrease morbidity, mortality, and long-term health care costs. Some aspects of the provision of medical care to opioid-agonist-maintained patients can be unique (e.g., the selection of appropriate medications that won't interact with methadone), and many of the conditions seen in this patient population can be related to their drug use (e.g., diseases transmitted through drug injecting). However, central to the treatment of this patient population, including in the context of an OTP, is a staff familiar with substance abuse and willing to provide care that is responsive to patients' needs in a trusting and caring setting. In this respect the treatment of this patient population is no different from the treatment that should be provided to all patients with medical needs.

References

Bean P (2002). Latest discoveries on the infection and coinfection with hepatitis D virus. *Am Clin Lab* 21: 25–27.

Bell J, Seres V, Bowron P, Lewis J, Batey R (1988). The use of serum methadone levels in patients receiving methadone maintenance. *Clin Pharmacol Ther* 43: 623–9.

Bertschy G, Baumann P, Eap CB, Baettig D (1994). Probable metabolic interaction between methadone and fluvoxamine in addict patients. *Ther Drug Monit* 16: 42–45.

Beuger M, Tommasello A, Schwartz R, Clinton M (1998). Clonidine use and abuse among methadone program applicants and patients. *J Subst Abuse Treat* 15: 589–93.

Brown LS, Sawyer RC, Li R, Cobb MN, Colborn DC, Narang PK (1996). Lack of a pharmacologic interaction between rifabutin and methadone in HIV-infected former injecting drug users. *Drug Alcohol Depend* 43: 71–77.

Brust JC (2002). Neurologic complications of substance abuse. *J Acquir Immune Defic Syndr* 31 Suppl 2: S29–S34.

CDC (2001). Soft tissue infections among injection drug users-San Francisco, California. *MMWR Morb Mortal Wkly Rep* 50: 381–4.

Cohen JA (2002). HIV-1 infection in injection drug users. *Infect Dis Clin North Am* 16: 745–70.

Cunningham EE, Brentjens JR, Zielezny MA, Andres GA, Venuto RC (1980). Heroin nephropathy. A clinicopathologic and epidemiologic study. *Am J Med* 68: 47–53.

Cunningham EE, Zielezny MA, Venuto RC (1983). Heroin-associated nephropathy. A nationwide problem. *JAMA* 250: 2935–6.

Davis GL, Wong JB, McHutchison JG, Manns MP, Harvey J, Albrecht J (2003). Early virologic response to treatment with peginterferon alfa-2b plus ribavirin in patients with chronic hepatitis C. *Hepatology* 38: 645–52.

De Castro S, Sabate E (2003). Adherence to heroin dependence therapies and human immunodeficiency virus/acquired immunodeficiency syndrome infection rates among drug abusers. *Clin Infect Dis* 37 Suppl 5: S464–S467.

Des Jarlais DC (1999). Psychoactive drug use and progression of HIV infection. *J Acquir Immune Defic Syndr Hum Retrovirol* 20: 272–4.

do Sameiro Faria M, Sampaio S, Faria V, Carvalho E (2003). Nephropathy associated with heroin abuse in Caucasian patients. *Nephrol Dial Transplant* 18: 2308–13.

Donnelly B, Balkon J, Lasher C, Lynch V, Bidanset JH, Bianco J (1983). Evaluation of the methadone-alcohol interaction. I. Alterations of plasma concentration kinetics. *J Anal Toxicol* 7: 246–8.

Ebright JR, Pieper B (2002). Skin and soft tissue infections in injection drug users. *Infect Dis Clin North Am* 16: 697–712.

Faragon JJ, Piliero PJ (2003). Drug interactions associated with HAART: focus on treatments for addiction and recreational drugs. *AIDS Read* 13: 433–4, 437–41, 446–50.

Fingerhood MI, Jasinski DR, Sullivan JT (1993). Prevalence of hepatitis C in a chemically dependent population. *Arch Intern Med* 153: 2025–30.

Furlan V, Hafi A, Dessalles MC, Bouchez J, Charpentier B, Taburet AM (1999). Methadone is poorly removed by haemodialysis. *Nephrol Dial Transplant* 14: 254–5.

Galdun JP, Paris PM, Weiss LD, Heller MB (1987). Central embolization of needle fragments: a complication of intravenous drug abuse. *Am J Emerg Med* 5: 379–82.

Goldstein DS, Karpel JP, Appel D, Williams MH, Jr. (1986). Bullous pulmonary damage in users of intravenous drugs. *Chest* 89: 266–9.

Gotway MB, Marder SR, Hanks DK, Leung JW, Dawn SK, Gean AD, Reddy GP, Araoz PA, Webb WR (2002). Thoracic complications of illicit drug use: an organ system approach. *Radiographics* 22 Spec No: S119–S135.

Griffiths RR, Wolf B (1990). Relative abuse liability of different benzodiazepines in drug abusers. *J Clin Psychopharmacol* 10: 237–43.

Haim DY, Lippmann ML, Goldberg SK, Walkenstein MD (1995). The pulmonary complications of crack cocaine. A comprehensive review. *Chest* 107: 233–40.

Hall CS, Klausner JD, Bolan GA (2004). Managing syphilis in the HIV-infected patient. *Curr Infect Dis Rep* 6: 72–81.

Harris HW, Young DM (2002). Care of injection drug users with soft tissue infections in San Francisco, California. *Arch Surg* 137: 1217–22.

Herman M, Gourevitch MN (1997). Integrating primary care and methadone maintenance treatment: implementation issues. *J Addict Dis* 16: 91–102.

Jatlow P, McCance EF, Rainey PM, Kosten T, Friedland G (1997). Methadone increases zidovudine exposure in HIV-infected injection drug users. In: Harris LS, ed. Problems of Drug Dependence 1996: Proceedings of the 58th Annual Scientific Meeting, College on Problems of Drug Dependence, pp 136. Rockville, MD: National Institute on Drug Abuse.

Kak V, Chandrasekar PH (2002). Bone and joint infections in injection drug users. *Infect Dis Clin North Am* 16: 681–95.

Kreek MJ, Garfield JW, Gutjahr CL, Giusti LM (1976). Rifampin-induced methadone withdrawal. *N Engl J Med* 294: 1104–6.

Kreek MJ, Schecter AJ, Gutjahr CL, Hecht M (1980). Methadone use in patients with chronic renal disease. *Drug Alcohol Depend* 5: 197–205.

Lange RA, Hillis LD (2001). Cardiovascular complications of cocaine use. *N Engl J Med* 345: 351–8.

Leen CL, Brettle RP (1991). Fungal infections in drug users. *J Antimicrob Chemother* 28 Suppl A: 83–96.

Liang TJ, Rehermann B, Seeff LB, Hoofnagle JH (2000). Pathogenesis, natural history, treatment, and prevention of hepatitis C. *Ann Intern Med* 132: 296–305.

Lucas GM, Cheever LW, Chaisson RE, Moore RD (2001). Detrimental effects of continued illicit drug use on the treatment of HIV-1 infection. *J Acquir Immune Defic Syndr* 27: 251–9.

Lucas GM, Gebo KA, Chaisson RE, Moore RD (2002). Longitudinal assessment of the effects of drug and alcohol abuse on HIV-1 treatment outcomes in an urban clinic. *AIDS* 16: 767–74.

Maany I, Dhopesh V, Arndt IO, Burke W, Woody G, O'Brien CP (1989). Increase in desipramine serum levels associated with methadone treatment. *Am J Psychiatry* 146: 1611–3.

Meyers CM, Seeff LB, Stehman-Breen CO, Hoofnagle JH (2003). Hepatitis C and renal disease: an update. *Am J Kidney Dis* 42: 631–57.

Miro JM, del Rio A, Mestres CA (2002). Infective endocarditis in intravenous drug abusers and HIV-1 infected patients. *Infect Dis Clin North Am* 16: 273–95, vii–viii.

Neugarten J, Gallo GR, Buxbaum J, Katz LA, Rubenstein J, Baldwin DS (1986). Amyloidosis in subcutaneous heroin abusers ("skin poppers' amyloidosis"). *Am J Med* 81: 635–40.

O'Connor PG, Molde S, Henry S, Shockcor WT, Schottenfeld RS (1992). Human immunodeficiency virus infection in intravenous drug users: a model for primary care. *Am J Med* 93: 382–6.

Payte JT, Khuri ET (1993). Principles of methadone dose determination. In: Parrino MW, ed. *State Methadone Treatment Guidelines (Treatment Improvement Protocol (TIP)).* Rockville, MD: U.S. Department of Health and Human Services, 47–58.

Plummer JL, Gourlay GK, Cherry DA, Cousins MJ (1988). Estimation of methadone clearance: application in the management of cancer pain. *Pain* 33: 313–22.

Preston KL, Griffiths RR, Stitzer ML, Bigelow GE, Liebson IA (1984). Diazepam and methadone interactions in methadone maintenance. *Clin Pharmacol Ther* 36: 534–41.

Raistrick D, Hay A, Wolff K (1996). Methadone maintenance and tuberculosis treatment. *BMJ* 313: 925–6.

Rao TK, Nicastri AD, Friedman EA (1974). Natural history of heroin-associated nephropathy. *N Engl J Med* 290: 19–23.

Rice EK, Isbel NM, Becker GJ, Atkins RC, McMahon LP (2000). Heroin overdose and myoglobinuric acute renal failure. *Clin Nephrol* 54: 449–54.

Romeo R, Rumi MG, Donato MF, Cargnel MA, Vigano P, Mondelli M, Cesana B, Colombo M (2000). Hepatitis C is more severe in drug users with human immunodeficiency virus infection. *J Viral Hepat* 7: 297–301.

Rosenblum A, Joseph H, Fong C, Kipnis S, Cleland C, Portenoy RK (2003). Prevalence and characteristics of chronic pain among chemically dependent patients in methadone maintenance and residential treatment facilities. *JAMA* 289: 2370–8.

Ryan CF, White JM (1996). Health status at entry to methadone maintenance treatment using the SF-36 health survey questionnaire. *Addiction* 91: 39–45.

Ryan DH (1979). Heroin and thrombocytopenia. *Ann Intern Med* 90: 852–3.

Sande MA, Lee BL, Mills J, Chambers HF (1992). Endocarditis in intravenous drug users. In: Kaye D, ed. *Infective Endocarditis.* New York: Raven Press.

Sapico FL, Montgomerie JZ (1980). Vertebral osteomyelitis in intravenous drug abusers: report of three cases and review of the literature. *Rev Infect Dis* 2: 196–206.

Schall U, Katta T, Pries E, Kloppel A, Gastpar M (1996). Pain perception of intravenous heroin users on maintenance therapy with levomethadone. *Pharmacopsychiatry* 29: 176–9.

Schwartz EL, Brechbuhl AB, Kahl P, Miller MA, Selwyn PA, Friedland GH (1992). Pharmacokinetic interactions of zidovudine and methadone in intravenous drug-using patients with HIV infection. *J Acquir Immune Defic Syndr* 5: 619–26.

Scimeca MM, Savage SR, Portenoy R, Lowinson J (2000). Treatment of pain in methadone-maintained patients. *Mt Sinai J Med* 67: 412–22.

Selwyn PA, Alcabes P, Hartel D, Buono D, Schoenbaum EE, Klein RS, Davenny K, Friedland GH (1992). Clinical manifestations and predictors of disease progression in drug users with human immunodeficiency virus infection. *N Engl J Med* 327: 1697–703.

Sporer KA, Dorn E (2001). Heroin-related noncardiogenic pulmonary edema: a case series. *Chest* 120: 1628–32.

Squires KE (2003). Treating HIV infection and AIDS in women. *AIDS Read* 13: 228–34, 239–40.

Stein MD, Rich JD, Maksad J, Chen MH, Hu P, Sobota M, Clarke J (2000). Adherence to antiretroviral therapy among HIV-infected methadone patients: effect of ongoing illicit drug use. *Am J Drug Alcohol Abuse* 26: 195–205.

Sulkowski MS, Thomas DL (2003). Hepatitis C in the HIV-Infected Person. *Ann Intern Med* 138: 197–207.

Tedaldi EM, Baker RK, Moorman AC, Alzola CF, Furhrer J, McCabe RE, Wood KC, Holmberg SD (2003). Influence of coinfection with hepatitis C virus on morbidity and mortality due to human immunodeficiency virus infection in the era of highly active antiretroviral therapy. *Clin Infect Dis* 36: 363–7.

Tong TG, Pond SM, Kreek MJ, Jaffery NF, Benowitz NL (1981). Phenytoin-induced methadone withdrawal. *Ann Intern Med* 94: 349–51.

Tuazon CU, Elin RJ (1981). Endotoxin content of street heroin. *Arch Intern Med* 141: 1385–6

Umbricht-Schneiter A, Ginn DH, Pabst KM, Bigelow GE (1994). Providing medical care to methadone clinic patients: referral vs on-site care. *Am J Public Health* 84: 207–10.

19

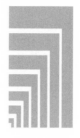

Comorbid Psychiatric Disorders

Van L. King, M.D., Jessica Peirce, Ph.D.,
and Robert K. Brooner, Ph.D.

Substantial psychiatric comorbidity exists among opioid abusers in the form of both other substance use disorders and other psychiatric disorders. This chapter focuses on nonsubstance use psychiatric disorders in patients maintained on opioid-agonist medications (methadone or buprenorphine). A review of comorbid substance abuse disorders in these patients can be found in chapter 17.

This chapter has three sections. The first section reviews the prevalence of comorbid psychiatric disorders in opioid abusers, and the second discusses mechanisms for screening, assessing, and diagnosing comorbid conditions in these patients. The third section reviews treatment for these disorders. This chapter does not comprehensively review all aspects and treatments for psychiatric disorders, such as the relative strengths and weaknesses of different medications for the treatment of major depression. The interested reader can find a more detailed discussion of such topics in one of several excellent general psychiatric textbooks (for example, Sadock and Sadock 2005, or Tasman et al. 2003). Rather, the purpose of this chapter is to provide information about those aspects of treating comorbid psychiatric disorders in patients receiving opioid-agonist medication that are unique to this population.

Prevalence of Psychiatric Comorbidity in Patients Dependent on Opioids

Several studies have examined the rate of other psychiatric disorders in patients with opioid dependence (table 19.1). Comparisons across studies can be difficult, because investigators use different interviews and criteria to make diagnoses and because the population (drug-dependent persons in the community versus patients receiving opioid-agonist treatment) and the length of time patients have been in treatment vary. This last point is illustrated in a study that examined self-reported depressive symptoms in patients on the day they started methadone treatment and then at weekly intervals (Strain et al. 1991b). Results showed that average scores on the Beck Depression Inventory (BDI) declined significantly from the day of admission to the first week in treatment and that scores plateaued rapidly thereafter (fig. 19.1). These results suggest that rates of depression can appear elevated in patients evaluated at the time of treatment entry versus those who have been enrolled in methadone treatment for just a few days. Similarly, rates of major depression and depressive symptoms in opioid abusers entering treatment decrease after six months of methadone maintenance even though no specific intervention is used (Rounsaville et al. 1982a).

Although rates of particular disorders vary across studies, essentially all studies find high rates of comorbid conditions in this population, with particularly high rates of mood, anxiety, and personality disorders. The prevalence of these conditions and other less common but equally problematic disorders is reviewed in this section.

Mood Disorders

Studies of mood disorders in patients dependent on opioids typically focus on diagnoses of major depression, bipolar disorder, and dysthymic disorder. Major depression is the most common serious psychiatric condition in the general population, and across studies rates of major depression in opioid abusers clearly appear to be higher than rates found in the general population. For example, in a study conducted by Brooner and colleagues (1997) (table 19.1) the rate of major depression was three times higher than the Baltimore sample of the Epidemiological Catchment Area (ECA) survey, a study that evaluated psychiatric disorder in the general population (Robins et al. 1984). There is considerable variability across studies in reported rates of both lifetime and current major depression in patients dependent on opioids, with the prevalence of a lifetime diagno-

Table 19.1 Studies of Prevalence of Comorbid Psychiatric Disorders in Opioid-Dependent Patients

Study	Sample Size	Assessment	Lifetime Psychiatric Disorder	Current Major Depression	Lifetime Major Depression	Current Anxiety Disorder	Lifetime Anxiety Disorder	Personality Disorder	APD
					Percent of Patients with Diagnosis of				
Abbott et al. 1994	144	SCID	84.7	7.6	25.0	16.7	27.1	45.8	31.3
Brooner et al. 1997	716	SCID	47.5	3.2	15.8	5.0	8.2	34.8	25.1
Khantzian and Treece 1985	133	Clinical	93.2	26.3	34.6		11.3	65	34.6
Kosten et al. 1982	384	SADS							54.7
Rounsaville et al. 1982	533	SADS-L	86.9	23.8	53.9		16.1	68	26.5
Strain et al. 1991	66	ARC	47.0	0.0	19.7				30.3
Woody et al. 1983	110	SADS-L			42.7				14.5

Abbreviations: APD, antisocial personality disorder; ARC, Alcohol Research Center Intake Interview (results are diagnoses using DSM-III-R criteria); Clinical, patients were assessed with a semistructured clinical interview and diagnosed by using DSM-III criteria; SADS, Schedule for Affective Disorders and Schizophrenia (results are diagnoses using DSM-III); SADS-L, Schedule for Affective Disorders and Schizophrenia–Lifetime version (results are diagnoses using the Research Diagnostic Criteria [RDC]; SCID, Structured Clinical Interview for DSM-III-R.

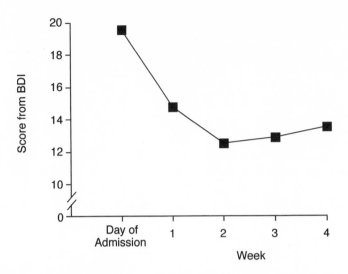

Figure 19.1. Self-reported depressive symptoms in 58 opioid-dependent patients entering methadone treatment (day of admission) and at each subsequent week of treatment. BDI, Beck Depression Inventory. Adapted from Strain et al. 1991b.

sis of major depression as low as 15.8 percent and as high as 53.9 percent (table 19.1). Similarly, the prevalence of current major depression can be as low as 0 percent and as high as 26.3 percent. The lower rates of depression found in some studies may result, in part, from a longer stabilization period in treatment before diagnostic evaluation (Brooner et al. 1997; Strain et al. 1991b) and from the evaluation of patients both in and out of methadone treatment in some studies. The absence of a standard time frame for evaluation may also account for differences between studies (Khantzian and Treece 1985; Rounsaville et al. 1982a).

Most studies reporting on the prevalence of bipolar disorder in patients dependent on opioids have found low rates (both lifetime and current rates of about 1%), which are consistent with rates found in the general population (APA 2000). On the other hand, the prevalence of dysthymic disorder in patients dependent on opioids is somewhat higher—at least 3 to 4 percent (Brooner et al. 1997)—and some studies have found rates around 15 percent (Abbott et al. 1994; Khantzian and Treece 1985).

Anxiety Disorders

Studies examining the rates of anxiety disorders in patients dependent on opioids have typically reported on five conditions: posttraumatic stress disorder (PTSD), panic disorder, generalized anxiety disorder (GAD), obsessive-compulsive disorder (OCD), and the phobias. Arguably, the most common anxiety disorder found in opioid-dependent patients is PTSD. Though PTSD has not been routinely assessed in patients dependent on opioids, it has been found to occur at rates of up to 50 percent in non-opioid-drug-dependent patients (Dansky et al. 1997). On the other hand, Cottler and colleagues reported a lifetime rate of 8.3 percent for PTSD among cocaine or opiate abusers and a rate of 6.5 percent in a study of inner-city drug users (Cottler et al. 2001). These rates are similar to those found in a general survey of young adults living in the Detroit area (8%) (Breslau et al. 1991). Likewise, in the few studies specifically targeting treatment-seeking opioid abusers, investigators have documented lifetime rates of PTSD in patients entering methadone maintenance treatment as high as 29 percent (Clark et al. 2001) and as low as 4 percent (Peirce et al. 2002). Rates of current PTSD in methadone maintenance patients are similarly variable, ranging from 20 percent (Hien et al. 2000) to 1 percent (Peirce et al. 2002). One of the likely reasons for the widely divergent rates of PTSD in these studies is the absence of standardized procedures and measures for assessing the disorder in a drug-using population. Reports that use standard psychiatric assessment interviews and document the assessment methodology tend to find lower rates of PTSD (Cottler et al. 2001; Peirce et al. 2002), but more work is needed to further develop reliable and valid methods for detection of PTSD. Untreated PTSD is associated with greater psychiatric distress and greater drug use severity in methadone maintenance patients (Clark et al. 2001; Hien et al. 2000), findings that emphasize the need to identify and treat this disorder.

In the general population, the most commonly found anxiety disorders are the phobias. Lifetime rates of phobias range between 2.3 (Khantzian and Treece 1985) and 9.6 percent (Rounsaville et al. 1982b) in opioid abusers. Rates for a current diagnosis of a phobia are probably lower, although at least one study found rates as high as 9.2 percent (Rounsaville et al. 1982b).

The next most common anxiety disorder is GAD, with lifetime rates ranging as high as 5.4 percent (Rounsaville et al. 1982b). However, current rates of GAD appear to be closer to 1 percent. Similarly, lifetime rates of panic disorder can be as high as 2 percent (Brooner et al. 1997), but current rates are less than 1 percent. Finally, OCD also is relatively rare, with most studies finding lifetime rates of less than 2 percent and current rates of 1 percent or less (Brooner et al. 1997; Rounsaville et al. 1982b; Woody et al. 1983).

Personality Disorders

Personality disorders are highly prevalent comorbid conditions found in patients dependent on opioids, and overall rates of personality disorder across studies range from 34.8 to 68 percent. Antisocial personality disorder (APD) (either with or without another personality disorder diagnosis) is the most common personality disorder (table 19.1). Although rates of APD vary across studies, from 14.5 percent (Woody et al. 1983) to as high as 54.7 percent (Kosten et al. 1982), in general, it appears that about one-quarter to one-third of patients can be diagnosed with APD. For example, Brooner and colleagues documented a 25.1 percent rate of APD in their study of treatment-seeking opioid abusers (Brooner et al. 1997), which is eight times the rate of APD in the general population, as measured in the ECA study (Robins et al. 1984). The lower rates of APD in some studies reflect the higher proportion of females in those studies (Brooner et al. 1997; Strain et al. 1991a). The most common other personality disorders in the Brooner et al. (1997) study were borderline (5%), avoidant (5%), passive-aggressive (4%), and paranoid (3%). The other studies listed in table 19.1 reported rates of borderline personality disorder between 3.7 and 12.1 percent (Kosten et al. 1982), and rates for other personality disorders are less than 5 percent.

Other Psychiatric Disorders

Although relatively uncommon, patients dependent on opioids in opioid-agonist treatment can have evidence of other comorbid psychiatric disorders. Some of these, such as schizophrenia, are relatively rare (i.e., a current prevalence of 1–2%). Others, such as eating disorders, can have a higher lifetime prevalence (i.e., greater than 1% in women) but are rarely found as a current diagnosis (Abbott et al. 1994; Brooner et al. 1997).

The diagnosis of attention-deficit hyperactivity disorder (ADHD) has historically received little attention in patients dependent on opioids, although it may be a relatively common disorder in this population (Eyre et al. 1982). For example, a study of 125 new admissions to a methadone clinic found that one-fifth had a retrospective childhood history of ADHD, although only 12 percent had three or more significant current symptoms warranting specific treatment for ADHD. These patients were also more likely to have a history of comorbid anxiety and mood disorders and APD (King et al. 1999). The detection of this condition can be important because impulsivity and poor attention may affect a patient's ability to engage in treatment.

Detection and Assessment of Comorbid Psychiatric Disorders

Assessment and diagnosis of comorbid psychiatric disorder in opioid abusers can be a complex undertaking. It is clear, looking across studies, that there is no widely accepted strategy. This section describes several instruments that can be useful in the process of evaluation and our own clinical approach to psychiatric evaluation and diagnosis. It is important to emphasize, however, that the best methods for obtaining reliable and valid diagnoses are unresolved and that this remains an important area for further research.

Several standardized instruments can be used to screen and diagnose psychiatric disorders in patients receiving opioid-agonist treatment. In general, these instruments fall into two categories: self-rating questionnaires (i.e., the patient completes a form) and interviewer-based instruments (i.e., the patient answers questions presented by a trained interviewer). The former require less work on the part of staff, who simply need to review a form and score it. However, self-rating questionnaires do not provide diagnoses; rather, they provide assessments of symptoms. On the other hand, interviews can provide diagnoses and the patient's responses can be checked, thereby increasing the probability that the interview results are valid. However, interviews take time and effort on the part of staff, and therefore can be expensive and time consuming. Examples of commonly used questionnaires and interviews are summarized in this section.

Questionnaires

Beck Depression Inventory (BDI)

The BDI is a rapidly administered questionnaire that rates significant depressive features over the previous week (Beck et al. 1961). It is a useful screening tool for identifying patients with possible depression, but it does not provide a diagnosis of depression. The BDI contains 21 items and a patient can typically complete the form in less than 10 minutes.

Symptom Checklist-90-R (SCL-90-R)

The SCL-90-R is a standardized self-report that measures psychological distress along nine primary symptom dimensions and three summary indices (Derogatis 1983). Like other self-report measures, it does not produce a diagnosis, but it does provide valuable information about self-reported psychological distress (and the particular areas of such distress, such as depression, anxiety, etc.).

Interviews

Addiction Severity Index (ASI)

The ASI is a structured interview assessing seven life domains relevant to patients with substance use disorder (alcohol use, drug use, family/social, psychiatric, legal, medical, employment) (McLellan et al. 1980). Although the ASI does not diagnose psychiatric disorders, it does provide quantitative responses in areas of interest to drug abuse treatment programs. Patients are assessed by using a 30-day interval, and sequential administrations of the ASI (e.g., at 1-month intervals) can be used to track changes over time on measures of drug use, health, and quality of life. The ASI takes approximately 45 minutes to administer and can be very helpful in identifying problem areas to address in treatment and to monitor progress in treatment.

Structured Clinical Interview for DSM-IV (SCID)

The Structured Clinical Interview for DSM-IV-TR Axis I Disorders (SCID I) and the Structured Clinical Interview for DSM-IV Axis II Personality Disorders (SCID II) are semistructured interviews that yield diagnoses for Axis I and Axis II disorders based on DSM criteria (First et al. 1996, 2001). They cover a broad range of diagnoses, including substance abuse and dependence, mood, psychotic, anxiety, eating, and personality disorders. The SCID requires extensive training and is best administered by clinicians with experience in evaluating patients in the diagnostic categories covered, because its use requires the ability to make clinical judgments.

Diagnostic Interview Schedule (DIS)

The DIS is a structured interview that provides diagnoses of psychiatric disorders based on DSM criteria (Robins et al. 1995). However, unlike the SCID, the DIS requires less training and may be helpful in case identification for referral to professional staff for further diagnostic evaluation. Staff without clinical training can learn to use the DIS. Whereas the SCID is a semistructured interview (interviewers must ask questions in the interview, but then can reword and ask their own questions if needed to clarify the diagnosis), the DIS is a structured interview (specific instructions are given for questions and how they are to be asked).

Clinical Evaluation

Although standard assessments for screening and evaluating patients are useful, many clinicians evaluate patients without using these tools. Such an approach can be used efficiently and provide a comprehensive review of psychiatric conditions commonly found in patients with opioid dependence. However, when using such an approach, the clinician should still depend on standardized diagnostic criteria such as those found in DSM-IV-TR (APA 2000) for determining diagnoses. In addition, it is important that the clinician probe for those conditions most commonly found in patients dependent on opioids (e.g., major depression, dysthymic disorder, APD and other personality disorders, anxiety disorders, ADHD, as well as other substance use disorders). Furthermore, it is also recommended that patients be briefly assessed for conditions with high morbidity such as psychotic disorders and bipolar disorder, although such disorders are uncommon in opioid abusers entering opioid-agonist treatment.

Rarely, if ever, does treatment of a comorbid condition obviate the need for extensive substance abuse and rehabilitative treatment in patients who require opioid-agonist treatment. Once patients abstain from drug use, dysphoria often subsides, and they feel more encouraged and less in need of additional support. Thus, it is important for staff to emphasize to the dysphoric patient the need to become abstinent since depressive symptoms improve with abstinence. The support of a drug counselor is often sufficient to help the patient through the early stages of drug treatment and the achievement of abstinence. However, if a patient continues to have significant psychiatric complaints after two or more weeks of abstinence, referral for psychiatric evaluation is certainly indicated.

When initially evaluating the patient with complaints of psychiatric symptomatology, the most relevant factor in the initial history is whether the patient is abstinent from abused drugs. A systematic review and meta-analysis included studies that examined the treatment of combined depression and substance use disorder between the years 1970 and 2003 (Nunes and Levin 2004). The results from this analysis concluded that the diagnosis of depression in substance abusers was best determined after at least a one-week period of abstinence, because patients who abuse substances frequently experience transient mood changes related to substance use. Unfortunately, patients typically have scant drug-free history as adults and, consequently, have never had an adequate psychiatric evaluation. A thorough history with reference to recent physical examination and laboratory work will determine whether a patient is able to receive outpatient treatment for his or her psychiatric complaints or whether a drug abuse treatment residential unit or inpatient psychiatric unit is needed. If a patient is intoxicated in the clinic on a daily basis or is using large amounts of substances daily, the probability of outpatient treatment producing a drug-free state quickly enough to evaluate serious psychiatric complaints (e.g., suicidal tendencies, prominent neurovegetative complaints, paranoia) will be small. Similarly, if the patient is continually positive for abused drugs on urine toxicology screens but does not claim to use large amounts of substances, the patient's feelings of hopelessness about his or her situation may necessitate an inpatient stay. The judicious use of a residential unit for several days to two weeks can greatly aid the process of sorting out substance-induced symptoms from independent depression or bipolar disorder.

If a patient is to be managed as an outpatient, a minimal period of abstinence (one to two consecutive weeks of negative urine toxicology screens) is required. Often, however, a patient is not able to accomplish this goal without being substantially pressured by the staff of the treatment program. It is often a mistake to prescribe psychotropic medications unless the patient is abstinent for at least one to two weeks. Exceptions to this rule would be patients who have a definite independent psychotic disorder that requires antipsychotic medication, or patients who have been previously diagnosed with a mood or anxiety disorder when abstinent, who had subsequently stopped taking medication. Requiring intensive work on drug rehabilitation allows time for a thorough evaluation, and the anticipation of pharmacotherapy (e.g., antidepressant medication) can act as a significant positive reinforcement for drug abstinence. The dysphoria associated with continued drug use is associated not only with the chemical effects of the drug or its withdrawal, but also with the discouragement and guilt a patient feels in connection with continued drug use. Mood may often improve markedly within days of successful drug abstinence, even if a patient's use was less frequent than daily and the patient had no appreciable physical withdrawal state. More frequent supportive psychotherapy or counseling contact is often needed to encourage patients during the first few days of abstinence. Short, weekly visits to a psychiatrist can serve as a powerful motivator for drug abstinence in some patients.

The alternative to abstinence before medication treatment for a psychiatric disorder is problematic at best. If the patient is still abusing drugs, the clinician must rely heavily on a previous history of specific symptoms and on the patient's response to specific medication or treatments. Sometimes, a reliable (preferably drug-free) friend or family member can provide valuable information about the patient's previous psychiatric and family history. Records from psychiatric hospitalizations or from significant episodes of outpatient treatment can be helpful, although patients are usually not observed long enough in an abstinent state to determine independent psychiatric symptoms reliably. In addition, physicians who are inexperienced in treating severely drug-dependent patients may have started patients on medication regimens during previous treatment episodes without good rationale. It is not uncommon for patients to be put on antidepressants or mood stabilizers on the day of admission to a psychiatric hospital or rehabilitation unit even though they were still using drugs heavily and on a daily basis. Rapidly treating these patients with such medications is more likely to confuse them and their future care. It can be argued that starting a medication treatment for mood or anxiety symptoms without several days of abstinence may help the patient become abstinent if a mood or anxiety disorder is complicating their drug or alcohol use problems. Rapid changes in mood are common during early abstinence, however, and the patient may take medication unnecessarily. An even greater risk is that patients will view medication as the easy route to alleviating their distress and believe they do not need to engage in the more difficult work of substance abuse rehabilitation. In certain instances, patients come to believe that the "depression" or "anxiety" needs to be treated first, before they can become abstinent, because they are "only self-medicating" this distressing condition. The results from the meta-analysis noted earlier (Nunes and Levin 2004) reinforce this perspective. They emphasize the need for concurrent substance abuse and depression treatment because treatment of depression alone rarely results in abstinence from abused drugs. A clear message regarding the separate nature of the patients' substance use disorder and the comorbid psychiatric condition is vital from the outset of treatment.

Substance-Induced versus Independent Comorbid Disorders

Determining whether the initiation or continuation of comorbid psychiatric disorder is in some way related to concurrent substance use disorder can be challenging (Brooner et al. 1997; Miller 1993). Some authors describe the disorders as *primary* or *secondary* to elucidate this relationship. These terms often refer to the condition that was first apparent (primary), which in some way determines either the initiation or course of the secondary diagnosis. For example, if alcohol abuse temporally precedes a depressive disorder, then the alcohol use disorder would be primary. Because of the early onset of substance use in opioid-agonist patients, however, virtually all other psychiatric conditions will occur after the onset of the substance use disorder. Although it is especially apparent in opioid-agonist maintenance patients, this oversimplified approach generally has limited heuristic value. In addition, these designations have not been consistently used in the literature, thus further limiting their clinical and teaching value.

Other authors use the designations *major* and *minor*. Again, few conditions would be more impairing than chronic opioid dependence, and one could imagine various situations in which the "minor" condition (e.g., dysthymic disorder) might be the "major" focus of treatment for a patient who was abstinent yet still on opioid-agonist maintenance treatment. These designations suffer from many of the same problems as the primary and secondary designations.

Another, more satisfactory, approach is use of the designations *substance-induced* versus *independent* psychiatric disorder. With this classification, emphasis is placed on the temporal relationship between changes in drug use (either increases or decreases) and the symptoms being evaluated. It is also important to know whether the patient had similar symptoms during times of significant drug abstinence (preferably of several weeks or months of duration). Substance-induced disorders are self-limiting if the appropriate steps are taken to abstain from abused drugs and the appropriate drug abuse treatment is undertaken. By using this classification, the naturalistic history of the onset of the psychiatric disorder (e.g., major depression) can be determined in relation to the pattern of substance use to best determine whether the condition's initiation, continuation, or offset was connected to the substance use. For example, using this approach, Brooner et al. (1997) reported that 77 percent of treatment-seeking opioid abusers who met criteria for lifetime major depression had a substance-induced rather than independent disorder.

The presence of untreated or poorly controlled medical disorders (e.g., HIV disease, hepatitis, diabetes mellitus, chronic obstructive pulmonary disease [COPD], thyroid disease) or treatment for medical conditions (e.g., interferon treatment for chronic active hepatitis; steroid treatment for asthma, COPD, or rheumatologic disease) are other important factors to consider. These conditions and treatments can substantially affect mood and neurovegetative symptoms and can be confused with an independent psychiatric disorder. It is vital to rule out medical or substance-induced mood changes and to treat any independent psychiatric disorder to improve the patient's ability to engage in drug abuse treatment via counseling, medication treatments, and medical management.

TREATMENT OF COMORBID PSYCHIATRIC CONDITIONS

Comorbid disorders are associated with increased risk of drug use while patients are in treatment. For example, depression was associated with continued drug use in a six-month treatment follow-up of opioid-dependent subjects (Rounsaville et al. 1986). In addition, depression was found to be associated with continued drug use in a 2.5-year follow-up of opiate abusers (Kosten et al. 1986b). Methadone maintenance patients who have a comorbid psychiatric disorder have higher lifetime rates of other substance abuse disorders (in addition to their opioid dependence) when compared with patients receiving methadone who do not have a comorbid psychiatric disorder (Brooner et al. 1997; Rutherford et al. 1994; Strain et al. 1991a). Personality disorder is associated with higher rates of substance abuse (Brooner et al. 1997; King et al. 2001; Rutherford et al. 1994) and poorer treatment outcome (Reich and Green 1991; Woody et al. 1985). APD may convey more risk than other personality disorders (Brooner et al. 1997), although not all studies find this relationship (Rutherford et al. 1994). Thus, the identification of comorbid psychiatric conditions can serve as a useful indicator for patients who may be at increased risk for poor treatment performance. These patients may need further treatment resources targeting these vulnerabilities. In addition, they may need treatment for their comorbid psychiatric conditions, both to improve compliance with treatment goals and to decrease morbidity associated with these conditions.

Coordination of Treatment Services

Coordinated substance abuse and other psychiatric treatments are essential for best treatment outcomes. Because more than 50 percent of patients entering opioid-agonist treatment will have additional psychiatric diagnoses, many will require treatment for their comorbid conditions. Nevertheless, low adherence to scheduled counseling sessions and other clinic appointments often undermines the treatment of comorbid disorders in substance abuse treatment clinics. A few studies have examined how to improve adherence in opioid-agonist treatment settings (Kidorf and Stitzer 1999), though it is clear that low rates of treatment adherence are a major factor leading to poor treatment outcome in a variety of treatment settings (Stein et al. 2000; Thompson et al. 2000; Umbricht-Schneiter et al. 1994).

A model of integrated care that reinforces attendance to scheduled appointments has been developed and operationalized (Brooner and Kidorf 2002). In this model, the OTP plays a key role in the coordination of various treatment services, including psychiatric services, both in the clinic and in other settings. To this end, the structure of the OTP can be of great benefit in and of itself in helping patients in the process of rehabilitation. Regular daily attendance, with clear contingencies and expectancies, can provide a stabilizing environment. Personality characteristics of avoidance, argumentativeness, manipulation, poor organization, and untimeliness can be addressed in a straightforward, therapeutic manner. Psychiatric medications can be given at the medication window to ensure that patients are receiving treatment for their psychotic or mood disorders. Patients can be required to make appropriate appointments for psychiatric or medical evaluation if clinic staff believe (or the patient would have the staff believe) that a condition is interfering with their substance abuse treatment. Intensive and continuing efforts to integrate the care of patients in the program can mean the difference between treatment retention or dropout.

Many patients in methadone maintenance treatment have health care providers outside the clinic, psychiatric and otherwise. These patients can be required to submit prescriptions, written by outside health care providers, to the medical director of the OTP for approval, to avoid problems with drug interactions and abuse. The OTP should consider having a policy that reserves the right to require an independent evaluation in the clinic if staff are concerned about a patient's outside care or are concerned that the patient is not telling his or her complete history to an outside provider (e.g., being in an OTP or actively abusing drugs; it is common for a patient to not tell his or her private physician about being in an OTP). If a patient is doing poorly in treatment and abusing drugs, the clinic should consider requiring that the patient allow clinic staff to speak with outside providers to discuss and coordinate the patient's substance abuse and other treatments.

Adequate medical care is an essential part of the rehabilitation process and, when relevant, can be incorporated as a required element of the treatment plan. Our clinic uses a general philosophical approach that allows patients the maximum latitude in their treatment involvement as long as they are doing well in their substance abuse treatment. Thus, the clinic requires gradually increasing the amounts of accountability and coordination of services both inside and outside the clinic if the patient is doing poorly in substance abuse treatment. However, some patients have an adversarial relationship with the treatment program because of contingencies on drug use and may not be entirely honest with program staff. For these patients off-site psychological counseling or psychiatric care can be helpful; this approach, however, prevents patients from receiving the most comprehensive care because of constraints on coordination with outside providers.

Because of the decreased treatment structure in most physician offices compared with OTPs, coordination of care may be more challenging for patients who receive opioid-agonist medication in this setting. For treatment in this setting, most physicians will want to choose patients with fewer and less severe comorbid psychiatric and other substance use disorders (see chap. 12). Once the physician decides that a patient can be managed with opioid-agonist treatment in the office setting, he or she should explain explicitly to the patient the treatment criteria and expectations for continued office-based management as well as criteria for transfer to a more structured and intensive level of care if the office-based setting is not adequate to meet the needs of the patient.

Integrating psychiatric services with substance abuse treatment services for patients receiving opioid-agonist treatment is the ideal, but few studies have been conducted that can guide practice in this area (Ley et al. 2000). This is true not only for OTPs, but also especially for office-based opioid-agonist treatment. Future psychiatric services research is needed to identify models of care relevant to the spectrum of opioid-agonist treatment that can address these clinical challenges in a scientifically rigorous fashion.

Counseling and Psychotherapy

Once a diagnosis is made, an appropriate treatment plan must be formulated. Unfortunately, many patients who require opioid-agonist treatment have scant financial means or psychological-mindedness to access and benefit from sophisticated psychotherapy. If medication for comorbid conditions is not warranted, counseling from a clinic counselor with support from a supervisor or doctoral staff member may be adequate. At times, referral to the local community mental health center may be necessary for more expert regular psychotherapy. Several studies have shown the efficacy of psychotherapy for improving general psychiatric symptoms and drug abuse treatment outcome (see chap. 7), but unfortunately, in the

OTP, patient needs often exceed the availability of funds to pay for such resources as psychotherapy. These concerns may also apply to physician office-based opioid treatment.

The relationship between the patient and the treatment staff is vitally important. Patients will not rehabilitate well without sound support; the treatment staff must constantly encourage patients to attain abstinence. In our treatment program, patients who continue to use drugs after they are stabilized on opioid-agonist medication are required to attend cognitive-behavioral group therapy sessions in addition to individual counseling sessions. These group therapy sessions are conducted by the most experienced senior staff members. Individual counselors can then receive valuable input from more experienced therapists who assess their patients in the group setting, and the patients benefit from therapy with the more highly trained senior staff members. The group therapists also act as important supports for patients who have not connected well with their individual counselor or for patients whose individual counselor has left and before a new counselor can be assigned. Strong interpersonal bonds to multiple treatment providers can help to retain patients who are struggling to meet their treatment plan goals. Patients must believe that the treatment program can help them attain abstinence and that staff members care about them and have their best interests in mind during the difficult process of rehabilitation.

An important aspect of treatment for many psychiatric conditions is work activity, either paid or volunteer. Work activity builds confidence and enhances self-attitude and can substantially improve psychiatric symptoms in chronically unproductive patients. In addition, it can provide structure and prosocial behavior, which can greatly benefit the process of drug abuse rehabilitation. If a patient with a comorbid psychiatric disability is not able to participate in work, a psychiatric psychosocial rehabilitation program may be appropriate. Participation in such a program can make evident any incompletely treated disorders and promote further psychosocial rehabilitation (e.g., an undetected social phobia or extensive negative symptoms of schizophrenia in an otherwise minimally symptomatic person). Clinic staff members need to monitor compliance with this aspect of treatment, however, because it can be a difficult commitment for many patients.

Treatment of Depression

Substance-Induced Depressive Disorder

A substantial proportion of depressive disorders in methadone maintenance patients are substance induced. For example, one study found that

77 percent of treatment-seeking opioid abusers who met criteria for lifetime major depression had a substance-induced rather than independent disorder (Brooner et al. 1997). It is worthwhile to review the propensity for various abused drugs to cause depression, concentrating on those other drugs most commonly abused by opioid dependent patients: alcohol, cocaine, and benzodiazepines.

Alcohol. Alcohol use is often associated with dysphoria and complaints of both depression and anxiety (Schuckit and Monteiro 1988). Numerous studies have shown high rates of alcohol dependence in methadone maintenance patients (see chap. 17), and some evidence suggests that alcohol use may increase over time among patients receiving methadone maintenance (Kosten et al. 1986a). Patients often fail to appreciate that chronic alcohol use can have a dramatic impact on mood.

Unfortunately, covert alcohol use is difficult to detect with routine urine toxicology screens and breathalyzers if a patient drinks in the afternoons and evenings, after attending the clinic. Obtaining serum liver function tests (aspartate aminotransferase [AST], alanine aminotransferase [ALT], and gamma-glutamyltransferase [GTT]) can be quite helpful in this regard, because these test results are often elevated if the patient is using alcohol regularly. The use of disulfiram administered daily with the methadone dose is an effective deterrent and is well tolerated in most patients (see chap. 17). Disulfiram can be effective in certain patients if given three times per week, and this dosing interval may be especially useful in an office setting (e.g., where buprenorphine is used as the treatment medication). To maintain disulfiram compliance, ingestion should be supervised to ensure the patient receives the medication's benefit. Depressive symptoms are not uncommon in alcoholics, but abstinence improves these complaints in most patients within two to four weeks (Brown and Schuckit 1988). Nevertheless, alcohol-induced mood symptoms can linger for weeks after initial abstinence; therefore, it can be difficult to determine whether they are symptomatic of an independent mood disorder.

Benzodiazepines and other sedative/hypnotics. Patients with chronic benzodiazepine abuse can present with a lethargic, unmotivated, anhedonic, and tearful depression. Alternately, patients can present with delirium, or in agitated, disinhibited states of intoxication or withdrawal that can mimic manic states. Popular benzodiazepines currently abused by patients dependent on opioids include alprazolam (Xanax) and clonazepam (Klonopin). Clonazepam is favored most, primarily because of prominent sedative effects. It is also difficult to detect on standard benzodiazepine urine screens, except at very high levels (at times, over 5 mg per day, which is a very high dose), but this threshold for detection varies among individuals. Some laboratories have specific urine tests available for the detection of clonazepam; however, these tests may not detect the drug in patients taking as little as 1 mg per day. A clonazepam serum level is a more sensitive method of detecting covert, daily clonazepam use. This test is quite expensive, so it should be used judiciously.

Concern about low-dose benzodiazepine abuse may seem misguided to clinicians who are simply glad to reduce injecting-drug abuse in these patients. The effects of these "low" doses of benzodiazepines are clinically obvious, however, and can make an individual lethargic and mentally dull and impair the rehabilitation process. Along with undetected alcoholics, patients using low doses of benzodiazepines may present to a psychiatrist with treatment refractory mood symptoms. The therapeutic process is undermined both psychologically and psychopharmacologically if clinicians do not address continuing drug use, even if the drug use is "low dose" or difficult to detect. Many patients have little appreciation for a healthy mental state and will be satisfied with a new, less impaired baseline if staff are willing to collaborate with them. In addition, it is important not to ignore low-dose benzodiazepine use because rarely does a patient on opioid agonist treatment abuse any drug at "low" doses for more than a short period.

Other sedating drugs commonly abused include clonidine, promethazine (Phenergan), and antihistamines in over-the-counter sleeping and cold remedy preparations. Besides the obvious problems of toxicity, tolerance, and hemodynamic instability associated with abuse of these medications at high doses, the incidence of substance-induced depressive symptoms with chronic use does not seem as great as with the benzodiazepines. Patients typically will be sedated, so abuse of these substances is reasonably easy to monitor on a clinical basis. One must remember that some opioid agonist patients have a high toleration of (and often preference for) sedation, and even frank mental impairment, if they do not need to work or be around others. This condition has profound ramifications for the rehabilitation process. Patients are not able to reliably meet treatment or other important responsibilities, and family members and friends begin to view the problems as caused by the opioid-agonist (patients will sometimes blame methadone for sedating effects rather than admit to sedative abuse). This makes it difficult for family and friends to support opioid agonist treatment if they believe it is impairing the patient. This issue also emphasizes the importance of involving the patient's family in the treatment process; patients will not do well in treatment if their families do not understand the treatment process and instead undermine the treatment plan.

Cocaine and other stimulants. Cocaine use can also present as a mood disorder. For example, a patient may describe a severe depressive syndrome after binging on cocaine for several days. This condition can take several days to remit. Cocaine intoxication can present with agitation, hallucinations, paranoia, repetitive behavior patterns, and formication. Again, these symptoms typically remit rapidly after cessation of drug use. The mood effects of other stimulants such as amphetamines can be similar to the effects of cocaine.

Marijuana. Marijuana use is commonly found among persons in OTPs, and studies show that depressive symptoms and cognitive impairment related to memory and learning difficulties can be secondary to marijuana use. Studies of methadone maintenance patients who use marijuana have not shown that marijuana use is correlated with increased use of other illicit drugs compared with patients receiving methadone who do not use marijuana (Nirenberg et al. 1996; Saxon et al. 1993). Some important measures of treatment outcome in methadone maintenance patients, such as retention, employment, or cognitive function, have been found to be unaffected by marijuana use (Budney et al. 1998; Saxon et al. 1993). On the other hand, there is some evidence of elevated schizoid and schizotypal traits in methadone maintenance patients who are regular marijuana users (Saxon et al. 1993), and similar findings have been noted in non-opioid-dependent marijuana abusers (Nunn et al. 2001). Regular marijuana users also report a higher incidence of depression in studies not limited to opioid abusers (Bovasso 2001; Degenhardt et al. 2003). Using extensive neuropsychological testing batteries, other researchers found significant impairments in cognitive performance in long-term, heavy users of marijuana (Solowij et al. 2002); heavy users demonstrate impairment in memory and attention compared with short-term users or nonusing controls. Though occasional marijuana use may not cause serious problems, results from these studies suggest that long-term and/or chronic use, especially in persons with comorbid psychiatric problems, could interfere with substance abuse rehabilitation. These problems are not likely to be detected in small studies of opioid-agonist patients.

In the authors' experience, patients with comorbid anxiety and depressive disorders frequently experience exacerbation of their psychiatric symptoms with marijuana use, and their symptoms improve when they stop marijuana use. Other patients without Axis I disorder may use marijuana as a way to decrease daily stress, but then experience impaired motivation to meet new people, to expand their drug-free support networks, and to work on the social and recreational aspects of substance abuse rehabilitation. Marijuana dependence is clearly present in a significant proportion of long-term marijuana users in opioid-agonist treatment and so can act as a significant deterrent to important rehabilitation activities. In our treatment program we treat marijuana use like any other drug use: it is not healthy, it is clearly detrimental to rehabilitation for many patients, and it continues links to illegal behavior and must be acquired from individuals who often sell other drugs that are more harmful. Marijuana use is best stopped in the interest of the patient's rehabilitation.

Other drugs and medications. Psychiatric symptoms in patients receiving opioid agonist therapy may be related to their opioid-agonist dose. For example, complaints of sleeplessness, irritability, poor appetite, and general dysphoria are common if patients are not maintained on an adequate opioid-agonist dose, or if they are rapidly metabolizing a medication such as methadone (e.g., concurrent use of certain medications can alter the metabolism of methadone; see chap.18). If such symptoms are caused by inadequate dosing, they can be rapidly alleviated with an increase in the opioid-agonist dose. There are limitations in this regard for buprenorphine, however, and sometimes a patient is not able to obtain an adequate agonist effect despite buprenorphine dose increases. In this case, a switch to methadone may be required to stabilize the patient. This is also an important consideration for patients who are tapering their opioid-agonist dose; for example, significant increases in depressive symptoms occur in patients as their methadone dose is tapered (Kanof et al. 1993). Patients tapering off buprenorphine can also experience these symptoms, though they are often milder due to the long half-life of buprenorphine. In stable patients who are tapering their dose, reassurance and time-limited prescription of adjunctive, nonopioid medications can help manage mild withdrawal symptoms at the end of the taper. Occasionally, these patients must slow down, stop, or even reverse the opioid-agonist taper for a time to adjust to the lower dose before continuing the taper. Paradoxically, some patients complain of sleeplessness if they are dosed with methadone too late in the day. In this case, switching to a morning methadone-dosing schedule can help with this complaint.

Ongoing complaints of sleeplessness and lethargy, but only mild or inconsistently present mood disturbance, can sometimes be attributed to caffeinism or excessive smoking at night. Often patients do not view these substances as drugs and are sincerely surprised to learn of their potent effects. Caffeine and nicotine can also interfere with the management of depressive or manic symptoms. At times patients need to taper off over-the-counter sleep remedies that they believe to be "nonaddicting" yet have grown habituated to taking.

Antidepressant Medication Treatment

Studies of the use of antidepressants for the treatment of depression in methadone maintenance patients show outcomes for patients receiving methadone that are no different than those found in the general population. Tricyclic antidepressants (TCAs) are the best-studied antidepressant medications in methadone-maintained patients, and methadone-maintained patients who have major depression respond well to TCAs (Nunes et al. 1991, 1998; Woody et al. 1975). Adverse effects of the TCAs can be problematic, however, especially in conjunction with the effects of methadone. For example, both methadone and TCAs can cause constipation, and adequate bowel hygiene including a high-fiber diet and sometimes a stool softener are important. Dry mouth can be a common side effect with TCAs, and patients need to be counseled to brush their teeth regularly and to avoid sugary snacks and soft drinks to prevent dental caries. Dental problems are quite common in many patients dependent on opioids, and, curiously, some patients believe that methadone causes dental problems (rather than years of personal neglect). It is possible that the analgesic effects of chronic methadone administration may impair early detection of dental problems by patients, so this may partially explain the association of methadone with dental problems.

Increased serum levels of the TCA desipramine when methadone was added to a stable dosing regimen have been reported (Maany et al. 1989). These increases are probably related to methadone's ability to impair the metabolism of TCAs (Kosten et al. 1990). Thus, somewhat lower doses of TCAs may be needed in methadone-maintained patients. A patient who is being stabilized on a TCA should undergo regular testing for TCA blood levels.

In general, most of the selective serotonin reuptake inhibitors (SSRIs: fluoxetine, sertraline, paroxetine, citalopram, escitalopram) and other newer antidepressants (bupropion, mirtazapine, venlafaxine, nefazadone) are as well tolerated in patients receiving methadone as in the general population. Fuvoxamine can increase methadone blood levels, however, and is probably best avoided for this reason (table 18.1). Certain SSRIs (sertraline, citalopram, escitalopram, fluvoxamine) can cross-react with the benzodiazepine enzyme-multiplied immunoassay test (EMIT) typically used in urinalysis screens. To avoid the confusion that may result from false-positive urinalysis results, paroxetine or fluoxetine may be better SSRI antidepressant choices. The efficacy of SSRIs to treat depression in methadone-maintained patients has been quite low in some studies (Dean et al. 2002; Petrakis et al. 1998), although this class of medications may be more effective in methadone-treated patients when used with persons who live in a more positive environment with respect to employment, living situation, and support networks (Carpenter et al. 2004).

Buprenorphine is metabolized by the cytochrome P450 3A4 isozyme, so medications that may inhibit (e.g., some SSRIs) or induce (e.g., protease inhibitors) this system should be carefully monitored if combined with buprenorphine treatment. Monoamine oxidase inhibitors (MAOIs) are not recommended for use in opioid-agonist treatment patients, and severe and even fatal adverse interactions can occur with the combination of an MAOI and certain opioids. Furthermore, MAOIs are contraindicated in patients with cocaine and alcohol use disorders.

Methadone itself has mood-altering effects (Dyer et al. 2001). Many patients feel a mild euphoria one to two hours after methadone dosing and may feel sedated during that time. Patients tapering off methadone maintenance often describe feeling more "alive" and "feeling emotions more intensely" once their methadone dose is in the range of 10–20 mg per day. Conversely, some patients experience a mild dysthymia with chronic low-dose opioids (methadone or other opioids), although higher doses produce the expected euphoric effect. Though less pronounced, patients maintained on buprenorphine may experience similar effects.

On the other hand, methadone and buprenorphine appear to blunt the emotional pain of depression and may have antidepressant effects in some patients. Opioids have been used for the treatment of refractory depressive disorders. For example, in a study of ten patients with chronic refractory major depression who were treated with low-dose buprenorphine, four had marked benefits that lasted at least through the end of a six-week trial (Bodkin et al. 1995).

Treatment of Anxiety Disorders

Like depression, complaints of anxiety are common in substance-dependent patients. This complaint is especially common in alcoholics and benzodiazepine-dependent patients and is also heard in cocaine/stimulant users and users of psychedelics and marijuana. Complaints are usually general, but panic anxiety is sometimes described. Symptoms reminiscent of OCD can be seen with cocaine or stimulant intoxication, though specific anxiety disorders are not frequently substance-induced. The same general approach applies to the evaluation of substance-induced anxiety as to the evaluation of substance-induced depression. A period of abstinence is essential; because of the long half-life of many benzodiazepines, detoxification and then observation on a residential unit for one to two weeks is invaluable for proper assessment. Anxiety symptoms from alcohol use can also have a protracted course, so some time in a protected setting can be beneficial for diagnostic purposes.

Once substance-induced symptoms are ruled out, the evaluation and treatment of anxiety should be approached similarly to that of any non-drug-dependent patient. Using an approach that parallels the one described for depression is reasonable. Medical causes and medication adverse effects should be ruled out. The patient's history should be thoroughly examined to determine psychosocial problems that are contributing to anxiety, and cognitive-behavioral strategies should be utilized. If the anxiety is accompanied by a depressive syndrome that is responsive to medication, the depression should be treated aggressively. PTSD, GAD, panic, or other anxiety disorders are better treated with specific cognitive-behavioral therapy combined with antidepressant or buspirone treatment. Even if good-quality cognitive-behavioral therapy is not available, most patients will do well with medication and supportive counseling. Opioid agonists can have mild, nonspecific anxiolytic effects, but are not effective for specific anxiety disorders.

In general, benzodiazepines should be avoided in the treatment of anxious patients maintained on an opioid agonist. The high risk for abuse outweighs the potential benefit for patients treated with methadone, and this class of medications is relatively contraindicated for persons treated with buprenorphine (see chap. 11). Buspirone may be relatively ineffective for treating anxiety in these patients (McRae et al. 2004), and a TCA or SSRI medication treatment is probably a better choice than use of a benzodiazepine or buspirone. If the clinician wishes to try a trial of a benzodiazepine in an opioid agonist-maintained patient with a clear anxiety disorder who has no concurrent drug or alcohol abuse, then low doses of a long half-life compound for a short treatment period is the preferred strategy, and supervised dose administration by a responsible family member should be considered. Use of benzodiazepines in opioid agonist-maintained patients should be considered only under special circumstances.

Treatment of Personality Disorders

Personality disorder (primarily antisocial personality) is the most frequent comorbid disorder in patients dependent on opioids. Various studies have shown that patients with personality disorder respond more poorly to treatment of Axis I disorders, including substance use disorders (King et al. 2001; Reich and Green 1991; Rounsaville et al. 1987). Woody and colleagues compared methadone maintenance patients with and without APD under two conditions: standard drug counseling and professional psychotherapy (Woody et al. 1985). As expected, APD patients did not respond as well to treatment as non-APD patients. APD patients with an additional comorbid Axis I disorder improved as much as non-APD patients, however. This finding suggests that patients with APD may be more likely to benefit from treatment under certain circumstances (e.g., when distressed) than at other times.

Other authors (Vaillant 1975) have recommended highly structured behavioral programs to improve the effectiveness of treatment for APD patients. Evidence from a behavioral study that targets patients with APD gives some encouragement in this regard (Brooner et al. 1998). The experimental and control groups were treated using two different, highly structured, behaviorally contingent approaches. Patients improved significantly in both conditions, though there was no significant difference between groups. Management and treatment of patients with severe personality disorder is challenging, but cautious optimism may be warranted in certain subgroups of APD patients or with certain highly structured behavioral interventions.

Treatment of Schizophrenia and Bipolar Disorder

As mentioned, few schizophrenic patients apply for opioid-agonist treatment, and rates of schizophrenia in the clinic are similar to rates in the community at large. Several factors may account for these low observed rates, including the need to be timely and to behave properly in the clinic, which can be difficult for many patients with schizophrenia. In addition, patients with schizophrenia may not be physically dependent on illicit opioids because the lifestyle of a person dependent on opioids is beyond their capability, given their psychotic symptoms. If they do use illicit opioids, this use may only be sporadic.

Diagnosing psychotic disorder is often more straightforward than diagnosing mood or anxiety disorder in an opioid-dependent person. The mean age of patients in methadone treatment is midthirties, whereas schizophrenia typically has a younger age of onset. Thus, patients with schizophrenia who apply for opioid-agonist treatment have typically had a long history of psychiatric treatment to support the diagnosis of schizophrenia. Also, patients with schizophrenia frequently request antipsychotic medication treatment or find that antipsychotic medications quickly improve their symptoms. Patients with substance-induced symptoms, on the other hand, are often unwilling to endure routine antipsychotic medication treatment. Close psychiatric follow-up is needed when a patient with schizophrenia is symptomatic and, therefore, treatment by an on-site psychiatrist or closely involved mental health center is essential.

Although there may be additive sedative effects from concurrent opioid-agonist and antipsychotic medication treatment, in practice, antipsychotic medications are effective and tolerated at doses similar to those prescribed for patients who are not taking an opioid agonist. Clinically, opioid agonists do not appear to decrease the incidence of extrapyramidal adverse effects or akathisia from antipsychotic medication treatment. The general calming effect of chronic opioid-agonist treatment may help to stabilize the affective state of the chronically psychotic patient, however. There are case reports that both buprenorphine and methadone can have antipsychotic effects for patients with schizophrenia (Brizer et al. 1985; Groves and Nutt 1991; Miotto et al. 2001; Schmauss et al. 1987), so some individuals may benefit from a possible antipsychotic effect associated with these medications. In addition, the regular clinic attendance and routine contact can be stabilizing for these patients. Antipsychotic medications can also be given at the medication window with methadone if the patient is nonadherent, thereby further integrating care. Not surprisingly, psychotic patients may have additional substance abuse problems, including alcohol dependence. Disulfiram can be used in conjunction with antipsychotic medication treatment for alcohol-dependent patients with schizophrenia if they are judged to comprehend the aversive nature of the disulfiram treatment. Patients need to be monitored for sedation and possible exacerbation of psychosis when initiating disulfiram and, consequently, the risk-to-benefit ratio needs to be carefully weighed (Banys 1988).

Severe bipolar disorder is not common in patients receiving opioid-agonist treatment, for reasons similar to those for schizophrenia. However, bipolar II disorder (hypomania and major depression) is more common. Typically, bipolar II patients will come to clinical attention with either a depressive, or a mixed depressive/anxious, presentation. Hypomania can result from treatment with antidepressant medications. Frequently, they have limited or no appreciation of the hypomanic condition, and substance use often escalates during this time. If a patient is abusing cocaine or another stimulant, hypomania may be undetected if the patient is not seen by an experienced clinician who will consider a primary psychiatric illness in the differential diagnosis.

Appropriate medication treatment for bipolar disorder begins with mood stabilizers, in particular, lithium carbonate and divalproex sodium

(Depakote). Lamotrigine (Lamictal) is also useful and is gaining wider popularity as a treatment for bipolar disorder. Carbamazepine (Tegretol) is best avoided because of hepatic induction. If carbamazepine is used in a methadone-maintained patient, the patient's methadone dose may need to be raised almost twofold, or the patient may need dosing on a more frequent basis (i.e., twice per day). Antipsychotic medications are needed at times on an adjunctive basis for the treatment of bipolar disorder. Methadone or buprenorphine may be of some help in the manic patient, through a general calming effect. Benzodiazepines are contraindicated, including clonazepam (which has not shown specific antimanic activity in any case).

Attention-Deficit Hyperactivity Disorder

Although some reports suggest that rates of ADHD in substance-abusing patients may be high, the information about rates of ADHD among patients dependent on opioids is limited. Not infrequently, patients may self-diagnose ADHD either as a way of explaining their erratic behaviors to themselves or in a clear attempt to seek drugs. When establishing the diagnosis of ADHD in a patient receiving opioid-agonist treatment, it is important to determine the necessary childhood behaviors, using corroborating informants (such as the patient's parents or old school or medical records). Because most adult patients with childhood histories of ADHD do not require specific, ongoing psychiatric care (particularly the use of medications), it is important to observe the patient free of abused drugs for some time to assess any impairment before considering the use of medications.

For significant, impairing symptoms of ADHD (prominent distractibility or hyperactivity), the first pharmacologic interventions should be medications without significant abuse liability. A new selective norepinephrine reuptake inhibitor, atomoxetine (Strattera), has shown excellent benefit for ADHD symptoms, so this medication may be a good choice for patients dependent on opioids who are otherwise stable in substance abuse treatment. Other medications that have demonstrated utility in the treatment of ADHD are TCAs with significant norepinephrine reuptake inhibition (e.g., desipramine), bupropion (Wellbutrin), or venlafaxine (Effexor). Because many patients dependent on opioids have chronic viral hepatitis, pemoline (Cylert) should probably not be used because of its potential to cause hepatic dysfunction. If trials of nonabusable medications fail, then a final option is to attempt a course of either methylphenidate (e.g., Ritalin) or amphetamine (e.g., Adderall). Amphetamine abuse is experiencing a resurgence, so use of a stimulant to treat ADHD in a patient treated with an opioid agonist should be reserved for the most symptomatic patients who are resistant to nonabusable medications and who are otherwise doing well in treatment.

Summary

Psychiatric diagnosis and treatment of patients with severe substance use disorder is extremely challenging. Studies indicate high rates of comorbid psychiatric disorder in these patients, in particular, personality disorders. In addition, high rates of HIV risk behavior and poor outcome are more common in patients with comorbid disorders. Because of the intensive needs of these patients, a structured, consistent treatment setting is invaluable. Psychiatric, substance abuse, and medical treatment must be integrated for optimal outcome. Careful assessment of psychiatric symptoms when in a drug-free state is important so that appropriate additional therapy can be offered to maximize the opportunity for rehabilitation. Patients with independent comorbid psychiatric disorders need access to psychiatric services combined with appropriate, individualized treatment planning for optimal response to substance abuse treatment.

References

Abbott PJ, Weller SB, Walker SR (1994). Psychiatric disorders of opioid addicts entering treatment: preliminary data. *J Addict Dis* 13: 1–11.

APA (2000). *Diagnostic and Statistical Manual of Mental Disorders, 4th ed. Text Revision.* Washington, DC: American Psychiatric Association.

Banys P (1988). The clinical use of disulfiram (Antabuse): a review. *J Psychoactive Drugs* 20: 243–61.

Beck AT, Ward CH, Mendelson M (1961). An inventory for measuring depression. *Arch Gen Psychiatry* 4: 53–63.

Bodkin JA, Zornberg GL, Lukas SE, Cole JO (1995). Buprenorphine treatment of refractory depression. *J Clin Psychopharmacol* 15: 49–57.

Bovasso GB (2001). Cannabis abuse as a risk factor for depressive symptoms. *Am J Psychiatry* 158: 2033–7.

Breslau N, Davis GC, Andreski P, Peterson E (1991). Traumatic events and posttraumatic stress disorder in an urban population of young adults. *Arch Gen Psychiatry* 48: 216–22.

Brizer DA, Hartman N, Sweeney J, Millman RB (1985). Effect of methadone plus neuroleptics on treatment-resistant chronic paranoid schizophrenia. *Am J Psychiatry* 142: 1106–7

Brooner RK, Kidorf M (2002). Using behavioral reinforcement to improve methadone treatment participation. *Science Practice Perspectives* 1: 38–48.

Brooner RK, Kidorf M, King VL, Stoller K (1998). Preliminary evidence of good treatment response in antisocial drug abusers. *Drug Alcohol Depend* 49: 249–60.

Brooner RK, King VL, Kidorf M, Schmidt CW, Jr., Bigelow GE (1997). Psychiatric and substance use comorbidity among treatment-seeking opioid abusers. *Arch Gen Psychiatry* 54: 71–80.

Brown SA, Schuckit MA (1988). Changes in depression among abstinent alcoholics. *J Stud Alcohol* 49: 412–7.

Budney AJ, Bickel WK, Amass L (1998). Marijuana use and treatment outcome among opioid-dependent patients. *Addiction* 93: 493–503.

Carpenter KM, Brooks AC, Vosburg SK, Nunes EV (2004). The effect of sertraline and environmental context on treating depression and illicit substance use among methadone maintained opiate dependent patients: a controlled clinical trial. *Drug Alcohol Depend* 74: 123–34.

Clark HW, Masson CL, Delucchi KL, Hall SM, Sees KL (2001). Violent traumatic events and drug abuse severity. *J Subst Abuse Treat* 20: 121–7.

Cottler LB, Nishith P, Compton WM, 3rd (2001). Gender differences in risk factors for trauma exposure and post- traumatic stress disorder among inner-city drug abusers in and out of treatment. *Compr Psychiatry* 42: 111–7.

Dansky BS, Saladin ME, Coffey SF, Brady KT (1997). Use of self-report measures of crime-related posttraumatic stress disorder with substance use disordered patients. *J Subst Abuse Treat* 14: 431–7.

Dean AJ, Bell J, Mascord DJ, Parker G, Christie MJ (2002). A randomised, controlled trial of fluoxetine in methadone maintenance patients with depressive symptoms. *J Affect Disord* 72: 85–90.

Degenhardt L, Hall W, Lynskey M (2003). Exploring the association between cannabis use and depression. *Addiction* 98: 1493–1504.

Derogatis LR (1983). SCL-90R; Administration, Scoring and Procedures Manual II, 2nd ed. Baltimore: Clinical Psychometric Research.

Dyer KR, White JM, Foster DJ, Bochner F, Menelaou A, Somogyi AA (2001). The relationship between mood state and plasma methadone concentration in maintenance patients. *J Clin Psychopharmacol* 21: 78–84.

Eyre SL, Rounsaville BJ, Kleber HD (1982). History of childhood hyperactivity in a clinic population of opiate addicts. *J Nerv Ment Dis* 170: 522–9.

First MB, Spitzer RL, Gibbon M, Williams JBW (1996). *Structured Clinical Interview for DSM-IV Axis II Personality Disorders (SCID II)*. Washington, DC: American Psychiatric Press.

First MB, Spitzer RL, Gibbon M, Williams JBW (2001). *Structured Clinical Interview for DSM-IV-TR Axis I Disorders (SCID-I/P)*. New York: Biometrics Research, New York State Psychiatric Institute.

Groves S, Nutt D (1991). Buprenorphine and schizophrenia. *Hum Psychopharmacol* 6: 71–73.

Hien DA, Nunes E, Levin FR, Fraser D (2000). Posttraumatic stress disorder and short-term outcome in early methadone treatment. *J Subst Abuse Treat* 19: 31–7.

Kanof PD, Aronson MJ, Ness R (1993). Organic mood syndrome associated with detoxification from methadone maintenance. *Am J Psychiatry* 150: 423–8.

Khantzian EJ, Treece C (1985). DSM-III psychiatric diagnosis of narcotic addicts. Recent findings. *Arch Gen Psychiatry* 42: 1067–71.

Kidorf MS, Stitzer ML (1999). Contingent access to clinic privileges reduced drug abuse in methadone maintenance patients. In: Higgins S, Silverman K, eds. *Motivating behav-*

ior change among illicit-drug abusers: contemporary research on contingency management interventions. Washington, DC: American Psychological Association Books.

King VL, Brooner RK, Kidorf MS, Stoller KB, Mirsky AF (1999). Attention deficit hyperactivity disorder and treatment outcome in opioid abusers entering treatment. *J Nerv Ment Dis* 187: 487–95.

King VL, Kidorf MS, Stoller KB, Carter JA, Brooner RK (2001). Influence of antisocial personality subtypes on drug abuse treatment response. *J Nerv Ment Dis* 189: 593–601.

Kosten TR, Gawin FH, Morgan C, Nelson JC, Jatlow P (1990). Evidence for altered desipramine disposition in methadone-maintained patients treated for cocaine abuse. *Am J Drug Alcohol Abuse* 16: 329–36.

Kosten TR, Rounsaville BJ, Kleber HD (1982). DSM-III personality disorders in opiate addicts. *Compr Psychiatry* 23: 572–81.

Kosten TR, Rounsaville BJ, Kleber HD (1986a). A 2.5 year follow-up of treatment retention and reentry among opioid addicts. *J Subst Abuse Treat* 3: 181–9.

Kosten TR, Rounsaville BJ, Kleber HD (1986b). A 2.5-year follow-up of depression, life crises, and treatment effects on abstinence among opioid addicts. *Arch Gen Psychiatry* 43: 733–8.

Ley A, Jeffery DP, McLaren S, Siegfried N (2000). Treatment programmes for people with both severe mental illness and substance misuse. *Cochrane Database Syst Rev* CD001088.

Maany I, Dhopesh V, Arndt IO, Burke W, Woody G, O'Brien CP (1989). Increase in desipramine serum levels associated with methadone treatment. *Am J Psychiatry* 146: 1611–3.

McLellan AT, Luborsky L, Woody GE, O'Brien CP (1980). An improved diagnostic evaluation instrument for substance abuse patients. The Addiction Severity Index. *J Nerv Ment Dis* 168: 26–33.

McRae AL, Sonne SC, Brady KT, Durkalski V, Palesch Y (2004). A randomized, placebo-controlled trial of buspirone for the treatment of anxiety in opioid-dependent individuals. *Am J Addict* 13: 53–63.

Miller NS (1993). Comorbidity of psychiatric and alcohol/drug disorders: interactions and independent status. *J Addict Dis* 12: 5–16.

Miotto P, Preti A, Frezza M (2001). Heroin and schizophrenia: subjective responses to abused drugs in dually diagnosed patients. *J Clin Psychopharmacol* 21: 111–3.

Nirenberg TD, Cellucci T, Liepman MR, Swift RM, Sirota AD (1996). Cannabis versus other illicit drug use among methadone maintenance patients. *Psychol Addict Behav* 10: 222–7.

Nunes EV, Levin FR (2004). Treatment of depression in patients with alcohol or other drug dependence: a meta-analysis. *JAMA* 291: 1887–96.

Nunes EV, Quitkin FM, Brady R, Stewart JW (1991). Imipramine treatment of methadone maintenance patients with affective disorder and illicit drug use. *Am J Psychiatry* 148: 667–9.

Nunes EV, Quitkin FM, Donovan SJ, Deliyannides D, Ocepek-Welikson K, Koenig T, Brady R, McGrath PJ, Woody G (1998). Imipramine treatment of opiate-dependent patients with depressive disorders. A placebo-controlled trial. *Arch Gen Psychiatry* 55: 153–60.

Nunn JA, Rizza F, Peters ER (2001). The incidence of schizotypy among cannabis and alcohol users. *J Nerv Ment Dis* 189: 741–8.

Peirce JM, Waesche MC, Kendrick A, Kindbom K, Brooner RK (2002). Association between PTSD and drug use and psychosocial problems in drug abusers. The Annual Scientific Conference of The College on Problems of Drug Dependence, Quebec City, Canada

Petrakis I, Carroll KM, Nich C, Gordon L, Kosten T, Rounsaville B (1998). Fluoxetine treatment of depressive disorders in methadone-maintained opioid addicts. *Drug Alcohol Depend* 50: 221–6.

Reich JH, Green AI (1991). Effect of personality disorders on outcome of treatment. *J Nerv Ment Dis* 179: 74–82.

Robins LN, Cottler LB, Bucholz K, Compton WM (1995). Diagnostic Interview Schedule (DIS) for DSM-IV, St. Louis, MO: Washington University.

Robins LN, Helzer JE, Weissman MM, Orvaschel H, Gruenberg E, Burke JD, Jr., Regier DA (1984). Lifetime prevalence of specific psychiatric disorders in three sites. *Arch Gen Psychiatry* 41: 949–58.

Rounsaville BJ, Dolinsky ZS, Babor TF, Meyer RE (1987). Psychopathology as a predictor of treatment outcome in alcoholics. *Arch Gen Psychiatry* 44: 505–13.

Rounsaville BJ, Kosten TR, Weissman MM, Kleber HD (1986). Prognostic significance of psychopathology in treated opiate addicts. A 2.5-year follow-up study. *Arch Gen Psychiatry* 43: 739–45.

Rounsaville BJ, Weissman MM, Crits-Christoph K, Wilber C, Kleber H (1982a). Diagnosis and symptoms of depression in opiate addicts. Course and relationship to treatment outcome. *Arch Gen Psychiatry* 39: 151–6.

Rounsaville BJ, Weissman MM, Kleber H, Wilber C (1982b). Heterogeneity of psychiatric diagnosis in treated opiate addicts. *Arch Gen Psychiatry* 39: 161–8.

Rutherford MJ, Cacciola JS, Alterman AI (1994). Relationships of personality disorders with problem severity in methadone patients. *Drug Alcohol Depend* 35: 69–76

Sadock BJ, Sadock VA (2005). *Kaplan and Sadock's Comprehensive Textbook of Psychiatry, 8th ed.* Philadelphia: Lippincott Williams and Wilkins.

Saxon AJ, Calsyn DA, Greenberg D, Blaes P, Haver VM, Stanton V (1993). Urine screening for marijuana among methadone-maintained patients. *Am J Addict* 2: 207–11.

Schmauss C, Yassouridis A, Emrich HM (1987). Antipsychotic effect of buprenorphine in schizophrenia. *Am J Psychiatry* 144: 1340–2.

Schuckit MA, Monteiro MG (1988). Alcoholism, anxiety and depression. *Br J Addict* 83: 1373–80.

Solowij N, Stephens RS, Roffman RA, Babor T, Kadden R, Miller M, Christiansen K, McRee B, Vendetti J (2002). Cognitive functioning of long-term heavy cannabis users seeking treatment. *JAMA* 287: 1123–31.

Stein MD, Rich JD, Maksad J, Chen MH, Hu P, Sobota M, Clarke J (2000). Adherence to antiretroviral therapy among HIV-infected methadone patients: effect of ongoing illicit drug use. *Am J Drug Alcohol Abuse* 26: 195–205.

Strain EC, Brooner RK, Bigelow GE (1991a). Clustering of multiple substance use and psychiatric diagnoses in opiate addicts. *Drug Alcohol Depend* 27: 127–34.

Strain EC, Stitzer ML, Bigelow GE (1991b). Early treatment time course of depressive symptoms in opiate addicts. *J Nerv Ment Dis* 179: 215–21.

Tasman A, Kay J, Lieberman JA (2003). *Psychiatry.* West Sussex, England: John Wiley and Sons.

Thompson C, Peveler RC, Stephenson D, McKendrick J (2000). Compliance with antidepressant medication in the treatment of major depressive disorder in primary care: a randomized comparison of fluoxetine and a tricyclic antidepressant. *Am J Psychiatry* 157: 338–43.

Umbricht-Schneiter A, Ginn DH, Pabst KM, Bigelow GE (1994). Providing medical care to methadone clinic patients: referral vs on-site care. *Am J Public Health* 84: 207–10.

Vaillant GE (1975). Sociopathy as a human process. A viewpoint. *Arch Gen Psychiatry* 32: 178–83.

Woody GE, Luborsky L, McLellan AT, O'Brien CP, Beck AT, Blaine J, Herman I, Hole A (1983). Psychotherapy for opiate addicts. Does it help? *Arch Gen Psychiatry* 40: 639–45.

Woody GE, McLellan AT, Luborsky L, O'Brien CP (1985). Sociopathy and psychotherapy outcome. *Arch Gen Psychiatry* 42: 1081–6.

Woody GE, O'Brien CP, Rickels K (1975). Depression and anxiety in heroin addicts: a placebo-controlled study of doxepin in combination with methadone. *Am J Psychiatry* 132: 447–50.

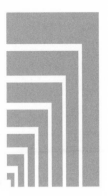

VI

SPECIAL TREATMENT ISSUES

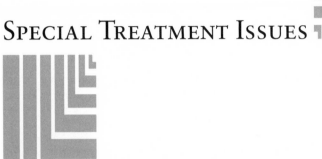

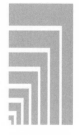

20

Specialty Treatment for Women

Hendrée E. Jones, Ph.D., Michelle Tuten, M.S.W.,
Lori Keyser-Marcus, M.A., and Dace S. Svikis, Ph.D.

This chapter covers two related topics. The first section deals with gender differences in drug abuse prevalence, in drug abuse-related comorbidities, and in treatment outcomes. These topics are important because they provide guidance for the type of treatment services from which women can derive the most benefit. The second section deals with the critically important topic of treatment for pregnant women dependent on drugs. Pregnancy is an event that may bring women dependent on drugs into the treatment system, and it is important to have services available that are tailored to their particular needs. The use of methadone and other pharmacotherapies in pregnant women is a controversial topic that will be considered in this section.

GENDER DIFFERENCES IN THE PREVALENCE OF OPIOID USE

Clear gender differences exist in the prevalence of illicit opioid use within the adult population of the United States. After adjusting for persons incarcerated or in drug treatment, data on heroin use in the U.S. adult population indicate that 2.9 million people reported lifetime use and 663,000 reported use in the past year of opioids, with reported use in the past year being three times more common in men (0.3%) than in women (0.1%) (Epstein and Gfroerer 1997). Males were also more likely than females (14.3% versus 11.0%, respectively) to have used prescription pain relievers for nonmedical purposes in their lifetime (http://oad.samhsa.gov/

2k4/pain/pain.pdf). Although more men than women report heroin and other opioid use overall, women are somewhat more likely to report heroin/opioid use at treatment entry than men (19% of women versus 16% of men entering treatment report opioid use). The gender differences in lifetime use and treatment entries observed with opioids are similar to other illegal drugs, including cocaine. More men than women report lifetime cocaine use (17.9% versus 11.2%, respectively) (http://oas.samhsa .gov/nhsda/2k2nsduh/sect1peTabs36to40.pdf), but the percentage of women entering treatment who report cocaine use (22%) is higher than the percentage of men entering treatment who report cocaine use (14%) (SAMHSA 2001).

Similar to heroin and cocaine, more men than women report use of alcohol and marijuana in their lifetime. For alcohol, 57.3 percent of males aged 12 years or older were current drinkers compared with 43.2 percent of females (SAMHSA 2004). In contrast to heroin and cocaine, percentages of men and women reporting alcohol use at treatment entry are similar to their respective prevalence of lifetime use (53% of men versus 40% of women report alcohol use at treatment entry) (SAMHSA 2001). For marijuana, 45.1 percent of males aged 12 years and older used marijuana in their lifetime compared with 36.0 percent of females (http://oas.samhsa .gov/MJ.htm#Tables), and a higher percentage of men than women reported marijuana use at treatment entry (10% versus 7%, respectively) (SAMHSA 2001).

Thus, epidemiology data show that gender differences exist in rates of both licit and illicit drug use, in particular, with regard to the prevalence of lifetime drug use. It seems that women who use opiates and cocaine are more likely than their male counterparts to enter treatment, however. This contrasts with the situation for alcohol and marijuana, where men and women enter treatment roughly in proportion to the relative rates of their use of these substances.

Special Issues Associated with Opiate and Other Drug Use among Women

Women have different risk factors and reasons for initiation of drug use relative to men (Stein and Cyr 1997). Women usually initiate substance use at a later age than men and seek treatment after fewer years of drug use (Brady and Randall 1999). Compared with males, female drug abusers have a poorer functioning in many aspects of life, including physical health, psychological well-being, and economic stability (Jones et al. 2004), as well as relationships, social functioning, and HIV/AIDS risk behaviors. Females are also more likely to report exposure to violence than males (Wechsberg et al. 1998). In contrast, females appear to have less legal involvement, criminal activity, and severe alcohol problems than their male counterparts (Kosten et al. 1985; Rowan-Szal et al. 2000; Wechsberg et al. 1998). Although women appear to have a more complicated picture of addiction, they tend to have treatment outcomes similar to men (Brady and Randall 1999). The next section will characterize the special needs of addicted women with special emphasis placed on opioid abuse.

Medical Issues

Drug-abusing women have more severe medical problems relative to their male counterparts (Kosten et al. 1985). Many of these medical problems are related to gynecological problems and sexually transmitted diseases (STDs) (Schoenbaum et al. 1989; Solomon et al. 1993). Compared with women in the general population, women who use drugs are at increased risk for reproductive complications, including amenorrhea, anovulation, ovarian atrophy, luteal phase dysfunction, spontaneous abortion, and premature menopause (Lex 1991). Drug use is the largest risk factor for contraction of HIV infection among women. The number of HIV incident and prevalent cases is rising for women (CDCP 2001; Zablotsky and Kennedy 2003), with the latest estimates indicating that 20 percent of new cases are female. Approximately 50 percent of AIDS cases in women result from intravenous drug use by the woman herself, and an additional 20 percent are from intravenous drug use by her sexual partner(s) (CDC 1994). Compared with men, drug-abusing women are at greater risk for HIV infection because the virus is more easily transmitted by sexual intercourse from men to women. Women are likely to have unprotected sex to finance their addiction, and women's sexual partners are more often individuals who engage in high-risk behaviors. Men and women appear equally likely to benefit from HAART regimens for the treatment of HIV infection (Moore et al. 2003).

Most other medical complications associated with opiate abuse are the consequences of needle use (Stein 1990), with hepatitis C being the most common infectious disease among injection-drug users regardless of gender. Other medical complications common to both genders are the dental consequences of opioid use, which are often overlooked. Although dental problems are commonly found among drug users and are often due to inattention to overall health and the lack of financial resources to attend to dental hygiene, illicit opioid use can complicate dental problems. For example, opioids are known to decrease saliva production, and this along with other medical complications (e.g., infections) can lead to exacerbation of already compromised dental health (Carter 1978; Titsas and Ferguson 2002).

Psychological Issues

Women with substance abuse disorders are at increased risk for several psychological problems, including affective disorders (Helzer and Pryzbeck 1988) and suicide attempts (Gomberg 1989), relative to the general population of women. Compared with substance-abusing males, substance-abusing females have higher rates of psychopathology (Brooner et al. 1997; Jones et al. 2004; Marsh and Simpson 1986), more often report suicidal thoughts and attempts (Rowan-Szal et al. 2000), have lower self-esteem, greater anxiety, depression, and simple phobias (Bartholomew et al. 1994; Brooner et al. 1997; Colten 1979; Cuskey et al. 1977; Jones et al. 2004; Rowan-Szal et al. 2000), show lower levels of coping skills for everyday life events (Luthar et al. 1993), and higher levels of overall psychological distress (Kosten et al. 1985; Luthar et al. 1996).

Family and Social Issues

In addition to the greater risk of psychological problems drug-abusing women face, they also have more difficulty in their relationships and social functioning. Drug-abusing women, compared with their male counterparts, tend to lack confidence in their communication skills (Colten 1979), be more passive in their relationships with partners, are more likely to be divorced or separated, and are more likely to report feelings of loneliness (Tucker 1979). They also have smaller networks of social support and a higher frequency of unresolved sexual issues (Bartholomew et al. 1994; Colten 1979; Cuskey et al. 1977). In general, female substance abusers are more socially isolated, with fewer friends and romantic relationships, and have more difficulty socializing than male substance abusers (Wallen 1992). One study found that among patients hospitalized for cocaine treatment, women had more severe family and social problems than men at intake, although these differences were not evident at a six-month follow-up when women were more likely than men to be cocaine abstinent (Weiss et al. 1997).

Substance-abusing women report higher rates of alcohol and drug dependence in their family of origin than substance-abusing men (Beckwith et al. 1994; Haller et al. 1993; Wallen 1992; Zilberman et al. 2003). Among patients enrolled in methadone maintenance treatment, 70 percent of women reported a history of illicit drug use by at least one sibling (Pivnick et al. 1994).

Physical, Sexual, and Emotional Abuse

High rates of reported childhood sexual abuse are present in the female drug-abusing population. In one study of alcoholic women, 66 percent reported childhood sexual abuse, compared with 35 percent of the general population of women (Miller et al. 1989). For many women, these patterns of childhood exposure to substance-abusing family members and physical/mental/sexual abuse continue into adulthood. One-third to one-half of substance-abusing women live with a substance-abusing man (Griffin et al. 1989; Kosten et al. 1985). In fact, women who experienced severe violence were twice as likely to report that their partners had been intoxicated and six times as likely to report that their partners had been high on drugs at some point in the past year (Kantor and Straus 1989).

Women who abuse substances report a history of high rates of emotional, physical, and sexual abuse. Among pregnant women asked shortly after admission to treatment about previous violence exposure, 66 percent reported a history of emotional, physical and/or sexual abuse (Moylan et al. 2001; Tuten et al. 2004). These rates increase to more than 90 percent when questions were repeated later in treatment, once a solid therapeutic rapport had been established. Studies have shown that men who use alcohol and illicit drugs are more likely than nonusers to perpetrate sexual violence against women (Abbott et al. 1995). Substance use by the woman herself places her at increased risk of becoming a victim of physical and sexual violence (Amaro et al. 1990; El-Bassel et al. 2000). Several studies have shown that women place themselves at elevated risk for assault when they and/or their sexual partner are intoxicated (Downs et al. 1993). Women are three times as likely to experience violence while drunk and six times as likely if they have used drugs in the past year (Kantor and Straus 1989). A recent study found more severe alcohol, family, and psychiatric problems at treatment entry among women reporting versus not reporting a history of abuse victimization (Tuten et al. 2004). Furthermore, the sexual partners of the abused women had higher rates of alcohol and drug use than the partners of nonabused women.

Parenting Issues

Drug-exposed children respond positively to stable and nurturing environments, but drug-abusing women may have inadequate parenting skills. In a review of the mother–child interaction literature, more than 60 percent of the studies observed that maternal substance abuse had a negative impact on the interaction between mother and child. The degree of detrimental impact was related to the extent of maternal substance abuse and its continuation postpartum (Johnson 2001). Mother–infant interaction styles have been compared between drug-dependent and non-drug-dependent mothers (Fitzgerald et al. 1988). At birth, drug-dependent mothers and their newborns had a lower quality of dyadic interaction, less social engagement, more negative affect, and greater detachment, whereas infants exhibited fewer social promotion behaviors relative to comparison children. At four months of age, the drug-dependent mother–infant dyads were more similar to their comparisons although drug-dependent mothers reported greater levels of stress and their infants were hypertonic and less coordinated. These findings suggest that the initial mother–child relationship is difficult for drug-involved women, but it improves over time. Nevertheless, parenting is a life area that may be of special concern and challenge to drug-involved women. Recently, several interventions have been developed for improving the parenting of drug-abusing women. Few of these have received rigorous testing, however, and those that have undergone experimental scrutiny had modest effects (Barnard and McKeganey 2004; Black et al. 1994; Catalano et al. 1999). More research is clearly needed to develop effective parenting interventions for this population. These interventions can be challenging given the need to develop therapeutic relationships with mothers while also focusing on the safety and development of the child.

In addition to parenting, several programs have focused on preventing the development of substance abuse in children of substance-abusing parents. These programs appear most effective when they incorporate elements that target the whole family rather than just parenting interventions. These elements include increasing parenting ability skills, enhancing family cohesion and communication, and improving the child's prosocial and school behavior. One successful example of this type of program is the Strengthening Families Program (SFP). The positive results of this program have been replicated in different cultural groups and children of varying ages (Aktan et al. 1996; Kumpfer et al. 2003).

Economic and Legal Issues

Drug-abusing women tend to be at an economic disadvantage to men in that they have poorer occupational functioning (Ellinwood et al. 1966) and can be dependent on men for economic support, often via prostitution or exchanging sex for drugs or daily needs. They tend to report low levels of vocational training and job skills and high rates of unemployment (Allen 1995). Drug-abusing women display a large incongruity between the types of jobs they rate as most interesting and their current skills levels (Silverman et al. 1995).

Although these women have many problems, they are less likely than men to display socially deviant behaviors that result in involvement with the legal system (Kosten et al. 1985; Luthar et al. 1993, 1996; Rowan-Szal et al. 2000). Most women dependent on drugs have had at least one legal conviction, however (Stevens and Arbiter 1995). Evidence shows that legal involvement can improve enrollment and retention in substance abuse services (Haller et al. 2003; Knisley et al. 1993). Although fewer women than men are involved in illegal activities such as drug sales and theft, a common legal problem women face is involvement with Child Protective Services (CPS). In fact, the fear of being reported to CPS can be a deterrent to treatment entry. Alternately, once a child is removed from the woman's custody the desire to reunite with the child can be a motivating factor in treatment compliance.

Overall, women as compared with men have special problems in a variety of life areas. This array of problems suggests that women could benefit from tailored treatment approaches.

Drug Treatment for Women

Barriers to Care for Women Entering Drug Treatment

It has been estimated that the ratio of men to women enrolled in drug treatment is 2.3 to 1 (SAMHSA 2001). This discrepancy in treatment entry may simply reflect gender differences in the prevalence of drug abuse, but there are likely to be other influences as well. The difference could be due in part to the differing ways the two sexes are referred to treatment. More men than women enter treatment via the criminal justice system, whereas women are most often self-referred or referred by a social relation (SAMHSA 2001). The lower enrollment rates of women may also be due to social and practical barriers. Women may be hindered from entering treatment by insufficient outreach focused on women not highly motivated to enter treatment, gender and cultural insensitivity in program composition, fear of legal consequences such as loss of children, lack of child care, lack of transportation, lack of health insurance coverage, inability to find another person to care for dependent family members, ineligibility of women for treatment medications if pregnant or not using reliable birth control, the social stigmatization of being a female drug user, and the lack of support (sometimes even sabotage of treatment efforts) by family and friends (Chasnoff 1991; Ehrmin 2001).

Addressing Barriers through Specialty Programs for Women

Because women appear to have unique treatment needs, researchers have recommended comprehensive drug treatment services for women (Finnegan 1988; Finnegan et al. 1993; Grella 1997). Table 20.1 shows typical areas that a woman's drug abuse treatment program should address. Outreach to increase women's access to care should include utilizing workers from the community, developing liaisons with community-based organizations, and providing transportation. Furthermore, women-only groups are an effective way for treatment programs to deal with sensitive issues such as self-esteem, anxiety, depression, sexuality, communication skills, and personal health (Blume 1990). This specialized women's programming appears to increase knowledge and self-esteem and to provide social support, which may lead to decreased anxiety (Bartholomew et al. 1994). Screening for partner violence can be more readily accomplished in a specialty program and is necessary because women who return to violent relations tend to relapse to drug use (Miller et al. 1989). Interventions should also address HIV, hepatitis, and sexually transmitted diseases and work on vocational training and skills needed to acquire and maintain a job. As long as women remain economically dependent on men via prostitution or exchanging sex for drugs or daily needs, they will continue to be at high risk for relapse.

A special topic of importance to women is treatment for drug abuse disorders during pregnancy. Here, there are special considerations as the health of the fetus as well as the mother must be taken into account in the treatment process, and options for specialized services are more limited than those treatment services available for nonpregnant women. These issues are discussed in more detail in the next section.

METHADONE TREATMENT OF PREGNANT WOMAN

History

The occurrence of neonatal drug withdrawal associated with maternal opiate use was recognized as early as the late 1800s; however, the increased use of heroin in the 1950s and 1960s among women of childbearing age sparked renewed interest and concern about the in utero effects of opiates on the developing child. In 1956, the first review of reported cases of prenatal heroin use was documented (Goodfriend et al.

Table 20.1 Specific Treatment Needs of Drug-Abusing Women

Medical	Psychological
General health care	Depression and anxiety
Obstetric-gynecological care	Sexual abuse
HIV prevention	Sexuality
Nutritional counseling	Issues of loss
Family planning	Self-esteem
Relationships and social functioning	Economic
Parenting skills	Interview and job skills training
Communication skills	Employment
Conflict resolution	Maintaining a job
Developing a support network	Money management
Special considerations	
Child care during treatment	
Transportation	
Housing	
Literacy	

1956). In 1973, the U.S. Food and Drug Administration declared that all women with confirmed pregnancies would undergo detoxification within 21 days after acceptance into a methadone program. This ruling was then reversed after two, single patient case reports of adverse consequences, including death of the fetus related to neonatal opioid withdrawal (Rementeria and Nunag 1973; Zuspan et al. 1975). This led to the practice of methadone maintenance treatment rather than withdrawal for pregnant women dependent on opiates starting in the early 1970s and also prompted researchers to begin examining the effects of this pharmacotherapy on pre- and postnatal development.

As a result of studies conducted in the late 1960s and 1970s (Parrino 1993), methadone became the standard of care for pregnant opioid addicts and is the only medication currently recommended (Category B, low risk within the FDA classification system of medications for risk during pregnancy) for their treatment. Methadone has been one of the most scrutinized drugs ever prescribed for pregnant women, with almost four decades of research on its effects during and after pregnancy. The weight of this evidence supports the contention that methadone is a safe and efficacious medication for mother and child.

Benefits of Methadone Treatment in Pregnant Women Dependent on Drugs

Compared with heroin abuse, methadone maintenance treatment during pregnancy has been associated with better prenatal care, increased fetal growth, reduced fetal mortality, decreased risk of HIV infection, decreased rates of preeclampsia and neonatal withdrawal, and, importantly, an increased likelihood of the infant being discharged to his/her parents (Finnegan 1991; Kandall et al. 1977). Furthermore, under conditions where drug-free and methadone treatment are both available, treatment retention has been shown to be considerably better for methadone treatment (Jones et al. 2001; Laken and Ager 1996; Svikis et al. 1997).

A caveat to the preceding is that most of the research on methadone treatment of pregnant women has been performed in comprehensive care settings where women had access to obstetrical/medical services, psychiatric care, social workers, and counseling services. Thus, conclusions about the benefits of methadone *itself* in producing improved birth outcomes are limited. One study addressing this issue showed that 70 percent of infants whose mothers received both regular prenatal care and methadone had problems at birth, as compared with rates of 75 and 82 percent in infants whose mothers received methadone with little or no prenatal care, respectively (Connaughton et al. 1977).

Controversies in Use of Methadone: The Neonatal Abstinence Syndrome

Despite evidence of positive benefits associated with methadone treatment during pregnancy, the use of methadone in the treatment of pregnant drug abusers is not without controversy. Concerns surrounding methadone are a result, in part, of contradictory or unclear findings from human studies about the problems associated with maternal methadone treatment during pregnancy. Furthermore, this problem can be exacerbated by dissemination and amplification of inaccurate information regarding the problems of children born to methadone-treated mothers. One of the most misunderstood issues surrounding prenatal exposure to methadone is the neonatal abstinence syndrome (NAS), which will be discussed in more detail below.

In utero exposure to all commonly used opioids, including heroin and methadone, can result in a neonatal abstinence syndrome. It has been estimated that between 55 and 94 percent of infants prenatally exposed to methadone will have withdrawal symptoms (Finnegan 1988; Johnson et al. 2003). The neonatal abstinence syndrome is characterized by a constellation of signs and symptoms, including central nervous system hyperirritability, gastrointestinal dysfunction, respiratory distress, and autonomic symptoms that include yawning, sneezing, skin discoloration, and fever (table 20.2). Neonates experiencing abstinence often attempt to suck frantically on their fists or thumbs, yet their sucking reflex may be uncoordinated and ineffectual. Infants undergoing abstinence frequently develop mild tremors that occur only when the infant is disturbed; however, tremors can progress to a point at which they occur spontaneously without stimulation. High-pitched crying, increased muscle tone, tremors, greater irritability (Finnegan and Kaltenbach 1992), decreases in cuddliness, and decrements in responsiveness to visual stimulation also may develop (Chasnoff et al. 1984; Jeremy and Hans 1985; Kaplan et al. 1976; Strauss et al. 1976, 1979). Methadone-exposed infants also have been observed to be deficient in their ability to interact with the environment, with a reduced capacity for attention and less social responsiveness immediately after birth (Kaltenbach and Finnegan 1988). These deficits in interaction were present until infants were symptom free and completely withdrawn from the drug.

Although the onset of withdrawal symptoms can vary from minutes to hours after birth, most symptoms are present within 72 hours of delivery. Many factors influence the onset of withdrawal in infants, including the timing of the last dose of methadone relative to parturition, character of the labor, the type and amount of anesthesia or analgesic administered during labor, and the gestational age, nutrition, and health of the infant (Finnegan 1991). Premature, methadone-exposed infants have

Table 20.2 **Withdrawal Symptoms in Infants Prenatally Exposed to Opioids**

Autonomic	CNS	Respiratory	Gastrointestinal
Yawning	Coarse tremors	Rhinorrhea	Salivation
Wakefulness	Seizures (myoclonic jerks)	Stuffy nose	Hiccups
Lacrimation	Twitching	Sneezing	Disorganized suck
Fever	Hyperactivity	Respiratory distress	Vomiting
Rub or scratch marks	Hypertonicity	Respiratory alkalosis	Diarrhea
Diaphoresis	High-pitched cry		Weight loss or
Skin mottling	Hyperreflexia		failure to gain
Voracious sucking	Hyperacusis		weight
Unpatterned sucking	Photophobia		
Hypothermia	Apneic spells		
Poor sleep pattern	Irritability		
Sneezing	Tremulous		

a less severe abstinence syndrome relative to full-term infants. This may be due to the immaturity of the infant, which may either mitigate the expression of abstinence or delay methadone metabolism, thus delaying or preventing manifestations of abstinence (Doberczak et al. 1991). Alternatively, the reduction in total methadone exposure during a shorter parturition may result in a less severe expression of withdrawal.

The relationship between maternal methadone dose and the presence or severity of infant withdrawal has been difficult to establish. Studies that do versus those that do not show dose-response relationships are represented about equally in the scientific literature, with 13 studies suggesting there is a relationship between methadone dose and NAS, and 16 studies suggesting no such relationship occurs (references available on request). Note that papers showing a relationship between maternal methadone dose and NAS often examined very low methadone doses and also often included women who were not receiving methadone at the time of delivery (Dashe et al. 2002). The inability to establish a clear dose-response relationship between methadone dose and NAS severity also may be due to other mitigating factors, such as tobacco exposure, which can contribute to the severity of NAS. Support for this is found in the results of a study that categorized methadone-treated pregnant women into light (10 or fewer cigarettes per day) or heavy (more than 10 cigarettes per day) smokers, and examined the effect of prenatal tobacco exposure on NAS. Heavy as compared with lighter smokers had significantly higher NAS peak scores (9.8 versus 4.8) and a shorter time to peak symptom onset (37.8 hr versus 113.0 hr) (Choo et al. 2004).

Other possible reasons for the discrepancy between studies on maternal methadone dosing and NAS include that the assessment of clinical severity of neonatal narcotic withdrawal has been based on individual hospital guidelines in some reports and that the NAS assessment has been conducted under open conditions (which can be subject to rater biases) in other studies. Although standardized withdrawal assessment tools such as the Neonatal Abstinence Score Chart by Finnegan have been developed to solve this problem, many hospitals adopt their own version of the scale, thus reducing the ability to compare outcome scores between settings. In summary, the data are conflicting, and although the NAS has been described and clearly associated with methadone administration during pregnancy, a clear relationship between maternal methadone dose and withdrawal severity has not been established.

Treatment of the Neonatal Abstinence Syndrome

NAS is readily treated and seldom life threatening to the infant. Several pharmacologic treatments for NAS have been explored, but the recommended treatment is diluted opium tincture because it contains opioid medication without the undesirable constituents contained in paregoric (e.g., camphor, benzoic acid). As yet, neither the dosage nor the therapeutic level necessary to control withdrawal symptoms have been systematically investigated, although a starting dose schedule of 0.2–0.4 mg/ml every three hours has been recommended (Levy and Spino 1993). Although morphine could theoretically be used, to the best of our knowledge, there are no published reports examining the use of morphine in the treatment of NAS. The use of methadone appears controversial. Some researchers state it should not be used because it has a prolonged half-life (26 hours), which makes dosage adjustment difficult (Rosen and Pippenger 1975); however, others believe it is "an excellent agent" for alleviating opioid withdrawal in newborns and suggest an initial dose of 1 to 2 mg of methadone twice a day (Hoegerman and Schnoll 1991). In addition to pharmacotherapy, a supportive environment can help alleviate symptoms of NAS. For instance, the environment should be calm, quiet, and warm. Gentle handling, swaddling to decrease sensory stimulation and help the infant regulate body temperature, a pacifier to relieve irritability and increased sucking urge, and frequent small feedings also help the infant maintain homeostasis.

It is possible that a methadone-exposed infant would receive sufficient methadone via breast-feeding to alleviate symptoms of the NAS. Data on breast-feeding have been reviewed (Jansson et al. 2004), and it appears that infants receive less than 1 mg of methadone via breast milk. This small quantity is unlikely to either produce significant direct effects in the infant or to be adequate to prevent neonatal abstinence symptoms (Begg et al. 2001). There is one report of two patients whose infants developed NAS signs and symptoms after the abrupt cessation of breast-feeding (the daily maternal methadone doses were 70 and 130 mg). These authors suggest that methadone-maintained women should wean breast-feeding infants gradually (Malpas and Darlow 1999). Provided women do not have HIV and are abstinent from illicit drugs and alcohol, they should be encouraged to breast feed to gain the nutritional and immunologic benefits associated with this feeding method (Jansson et al. 2004).

In summary, NAS can occur as a result of maintenance on an opioid substitution medication such as methadone. Although potentially disturbing to observers, this syndrome can be readily treated and does not appear to be associated with long-term developmental consequences (see below). In fact, methadone maintenance during pregnancy serves a number of valuable functions. It reduces or eliminates the illicit opiate-seeking behavior of the pregnant women and prevents the marked fluctuation in the maternal heroin level that often occurs with use of short-acting opiates. Furthermore, maintaining a woman on a steady-state dose of methadone that is sufficient to prevent withdrawal and reduce craving enables her to focus on other areas of her life, such as birthing preparations and other issues including nutrition, housing, education, employment, and relationships.

Methadone Treatment for Pregnant Women: Entry Criteria

As noted previously, methadone maintenance has become the standard treatment for pregnant women. In the United States, federal guidelines dictating methadone treatment state that methadone should only be prescribed to patients fulfilling the criteria for a current opioid dependence with signs of withdrawal and that this dependence should be present for more than one year. Exceptions to these guidelines may be made when a patient is pregnant or recently released from jail, however (Parrino 1993). In general, however, the diagnosis of opioid dependence in the pregnant woman is akin to that of a nonpregnant opioid addict and should be based on a comprehensive and detailed medical and drug abuse history as well as physical examination (see chap. 9), and urine toxicology is needed to document opioid and possibly other drug abuse.

Assessment of Pregnant Drug-Abusing Women

Most drug-abusing women who are pregnant do not seek prenatal care and are therefore vulnerable to medical and obstetrical complications. A program enrolling pregnant women dependent on drugs will want to obtain a detailed medical history, including previous compliance with prenatal care and laboratory work. Other important information can also be gathered during this interview that is related to the special needs of female drug abusers. This includes information about family use of alcohol and drugs and presence of drug-associated diseases (e.g., hepatitis or bacterial endocarditis). A history of arrests, incarcerations, or legal problems and intentional periods of abstinence can also aid in the assessment of drug abuse (Finnegan 1991; Hoegerman and Schnoll 1991). It is recommended that substance abuse questions be postponed until later in the examination because time is needed to establish rapport, and the medical history and physical examination can provide needed information with which to then probe about substance abuse.

When asking sensitive questions about abuse, it is important to use the same tone of voice as the other questions were asked and not apologize for asking these questions, as it would imply that the responder should apologize for the events happening to them. The limits of confidentiality should also be given to the women before she answers any questions. In some states, the health provider will be required to report child abuse if they are given the perpetrator's name, even if that person is dead or the event happened many years ago. The order of the questions is also important. Begin by asking about emotional abuse and define what is meant by this term (e.g., "By emotional abuse I mean has anyone ever said things to make you feel particularly bad?"). This can then be followed with questions about physical abuse, again defining the terms used (e.g., "Have you ever been hit, slapped, or held down against your will?"). At times women will have experienced such events but not characterize them as physical abuse. Finally, the interviewer should ask about sexual abuse (e.g., "Have you ever been forced to have sex against your will?"). Asking the patient to provide a list of individuals who may have conducted any of these types of abuse can help to take the "spotlight" off any one person.

Regardless of the drug used, all pregnant substance abusers are at high risk for pregnancy complications. These medical complications may vary because of the drug or combination of drugs used, the time during pregnancy when the drug was used, the route of drug administration, possible withdrawal or cycling between intoxication and withdrawal during pregnancy, lack of prenatal care, and the failure to identify and treat the medical problems in a timely manner. (See also chap. 18 for a review of the medical problems found in patients dependent on opioids.) An electrocardiogram should be performed because of the cardiac toxicity associated with the abuse of stimulant drugs. Infections comprise a high percentage of medical complications and can cause harm to mother and child if not properly treated. The treatment and management of HIV is sometimes required not only for the mother but also for the infant (Finnegan 1991). Drug-abusing women should also undergo liver function testing because they may have active or postviral hepatitis. Frequent urine cultures should be conducted to rule out urinary tract infections. A tuberculin skin test should be done, because this population is at higher risk for tuberculosis. Inspection of the skin and venous access sites for infection and cellulitis should be made; note that pregnancy can result in expanded injection sites such as the breast. In addition to medical complications, there are also possible obstetrical complications in women dependent on drugs. These include gestational diabetes, spontaneous abortion, intrauterine death, postpartum hemorrhage, preeclampsia, abruptio placentae, eclampsia, chorioamnionitis, thrombophlebitis, stillbirth, placental insufficiency, intrauterine growth retardation, premature rupture of membranes, and premature labor. A sonogram should be done because intrauterine growth retardation is seen in this population. In summary, the woman's health status should be carefully and thoroughly evaluated.

In addition to the physical consequences of drug use, depression and personality disorders commonly occur in pregnant addicts. The latter can frequently interfere with treatment and can lead to conflicts with health care staff (Hoegerman and Schnoll 1991). A mental status assessment is an important part of the initial evaluation, and follow-through should occur with referral or in-house psychiatric care.

Comprehensive Care Guidelines

Guidelines for comprehensive prenatal care of pregnant drug-abusing women have been established (Finnegan 1988; Jansson et al. 1996) and are shown in figure 20.1. Recommended program components include intensive perinatal management for high-risk pregnancy, psychosocial counseling, prenatal/parenting education classes, psychiatric therapy, and methadone maintenance when needed. A residential component is also advisable for assisting pregnant women in abstaining from drugs (both initially at entry to the program and later should relapses occur) and optimizing a healthy birth for the developing fetus. Getting women involved in these types of comprehensive care settings is often challenging, however. Primary barriers to care for drug-abusing women include a fear of criminal prosecution and removal of their children by the penal system, a lack of transportation services, an absence of child care resources for existing children, poor access to obstetrical care, social stigmatization by the medical community, and a lack of treatment services addressing women's issues (Jansson et al. 1996).

The most effective treatment for pregnant addicts is delivered in the context of well-organized comprehensive services. In addition to the methadone and psychological services for the treatment of addiction, general medical care and obstetrical care is needed. Many of these women have been disenfranchised by their community and society and need education about nutrition, parenting, and money management. Many pregnant addicts have unstable living situations, are unemployed, and have

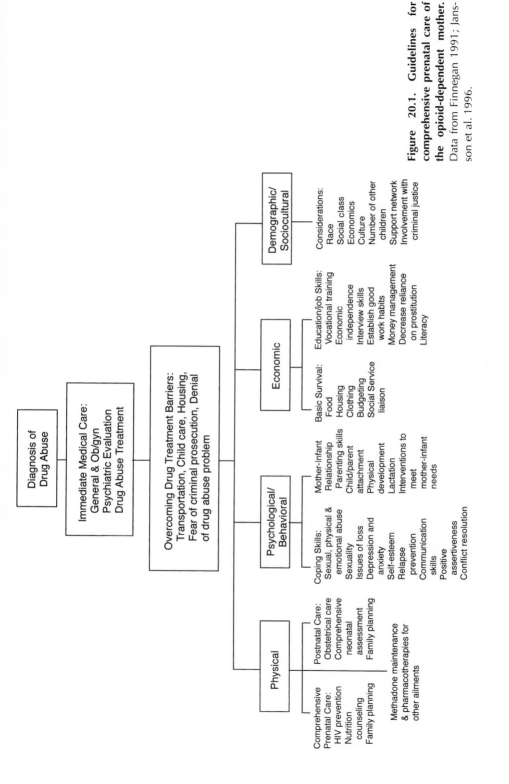

Figure 20.1. Guidelines for comprehensive prenatal care of the opioid-dependent mother. Data from Finnegan 1991; Jansson et al. 1996.

poor or nonexistent literacy skills; thus, social services advocates are critical.

Methadone Dosing

As previously reviewed, methadone is the recommended medication for opioid-dependent pregnant women. Those who are already in methadone maintenance before pregnancy can be maintained on the pre-pregnancy dose. Many women do not seek treatment, however, until they are already pregnant. Ideally, they should be admitted to a hospital or treatment program for medical and psychological evaluation as well as the determination of an adequate methadone dose. The opioid-dependent patient should initially be evaluated for signs and symptoms of withdrawal including those specific to pregnancy: abdominal cramping, uterine irritability, and increased fetal activity. If evidence of withdrawal is present, several different suggestions for methadone dosing are available. For inpatients, one option is to give an initial dose of 10 mg of methadone, with additional 5-mg doses given every four to six hours if withdrawal symptoms are present during the first 24 hours. On the second day, the previous day's total dose is administered as the maintenance dose. The patient is then evaluated for withdrawal over the next 24 hours, and additional doses given as needed (Finnegan and Wapner 1987). The current protocol used at the Center for Addiction and Pregnancy (CAP) located on the Johns Hopkins Bayview Medical Campus provides an example of dose induction. An initial 30- to 45- mg dose of methadone is given on the first day and increases of 5 mg per day follow until a comfortable dose is achieved (with an average methadone dose of 70 mg at CAP).

For women starting in outpatient treatment without a residential component, an initial dose of 15 mg should be given on the morning of the first day followed by close observation for intoxication or withdrawal and possible administration of additional medication (10–25 mg) in the afternoon. The dose should be increased 10 mg per day until withdrawal complaints subside (Smith et al. 1989). In general, methadone is administered once daily. However, methadone-maintained women frequently complain of increasing withdrawal symptoms as pregnancy progresses and may need increases of their dose to maintain the same plasma level and remain free from withdrawal. Kreek and others have demonstrated that, for a given dose of methadone, the plasma levels are significantly lower and withdrawal symptoms are increased during the third trimester of pregnancy (Gazaway et al. 1993; Kreek 1979; 1986; Kreek et al. 1974). The reduced methadone plasma levels coincide with increased methadone metabolism and faster clearance during the third trimester (Pond et al. 1985). Thus, when determining an appropriate maintenance dose of methadone, it is advisable to consider the serum trough level of methadone rather than the milligrams of methadone provided in each daily dose. A trough serum level of 0.3 mg/L of methadone should be adequate to prevent withdrawal symptoms in pregnancy. Daily methadone doses given to achieve this serum level are typically between 50 and 150 mg; however, a great deal of individual variability can occur in dosing, especially in the third trimester (Drozdick et al. 2002).

One of the factors to consider when dosing with methadone is whether to use a single daily dose or to split the dose. It has been found that a single dose significantly affects the behavior of the fetus, whereas a more stable pattern of fetal behavior is noted with the split dosing (Wittmann and Segal 1991). Split dosing may be especially relevant during the third trimester of pregnancy, when metabolism and clearance rates increase and steady-state methadone levels decline, but there are drawbacks to split dosing. Multiple daily doses require more frequent treatment attendance and may necessitate more staff time. If take-home doses are provided, there is a risk of diversion of medication and underdosing for the woman. For these reasons, the risks and benefits of split dosing should be carefully considered.

Detoxification during Pregnancy

Most treatment practitioners in perinatal addiction believe that methadone should be maintained during pregnancy to reduce the possibility of illicit drug use and to reduce the risk of HIV infection. The necessity of daily, supervised methadone administration also gives the treatment provider an opportunity to maintain close contact with the woman that might not occur if she was not maintained on methadone. Although the prevailing opinion of treatment providers supports continuation of methadone throughout pregnancy, there may be occasions when this is not possible. Jarvis and Schnoll (1995) have written about four circumstances under which the pregnant woman may need to be withdrawn from, or not treated with, methadone. First, the patient may refuse to be placed on methadone maintenance treatment; second, the woman may live in an area where methadone treatment is not available; third, the woman may request a methadone detoxification before delivery; or fourth, the patient may be too disruptive in the treatment environment and must be removed from the setting. If the pregnant addict meets any one of these criteria, then the risks of withdrawal should be clearly explained before it is initiated. It is important to explain to the patient that if she is to be withdrawn, and relapses or requests to be placed back on methadone with her goal being methadone withdrawal again while pregnant, then she should know that this cycling on and off the medication places her fetus at greater risk than maintaining a constant level of methadone. If she chooses to be withdrawn, it is recommended that intensive psychosocial support be provided throughout and after the withdrawal period.

When implementing opiate withdrawal for pregnant women, methadone tapers as short as seven days have been examined (Jones et al. 2001). Withdrawal from methadone or any drug should be done with the patient naive to the dose and speed of the detoxification. The medication should be placed in a fixed volume of liquid, preferably with a flavor mask, so that the patient receives the same volume of fluid, which tastes the same throughout the withdrawal period. The dose should decrease at a rate of no greater than 10 mg per week (Jarvis and Schnoll 1995), and 5 mg every two weeks has been recommended (Finnegan 1991). No matter how slowly the dose is decreased, intensive physiologic monitoring of the mother and fetus should be conducted. If detoxification must be done, it is not advised to begin withdrawal before the fourteenth week of pregnancy because of the potential risk of inducing abortion (Finnegan 1991). Detoxification during the last trimester of pregnancy has been shown to be associated with increased fetal adrenal response and increased levels of epinephrine and norepinephrine in the amniotic fluid; these physiologic responses are reduced when methadone dose is increased. Because of these changes associated with methadone withdrawal in the final trimester, it has been concluded that withdrawal late in pregnancy is not recommended unless the fetus can be monitored for stress (Rementeria and Nunag 1973; Zuspan et al. 1975).

Overall, the weight of the evidence suggests that it is possible to withdraw pregnant women during any trimester; however, the maternal and infant outcomes are likely to be less optimal than on methadone maintenance. Only one study has systematically examined withdrawal compared with methadone maintenance (Jones et al. 2001). In this retrospective records review, pregnant opioid-dependent women enrolled in a comprehensive treatment program and received either a 3-day MS Contin (morphine sulfate) taper ($N = 85$), a 3-day methadone taper ($N = 58$), a 7-day methadone taper ($N = 82$), or methadone maintenance ($N = 82$). Despite similar demographic and drug use characteristics, patients from all three medication taper groups were more likely than methadone-maintained patients to prematurely leave treatment and to deliver an infant with a drug-positive urine toxicology. Detoxification was not associated with adverse fetal outcomes in those who remained in treatment to complete the detoxification program, however. Thus, although detoxification may have less desirable outcomes than methadone maintenance, it can be used if necessary or wanted by the patient.

Is Maternal Methadone Treatment during Pregnancy Safe?

In addition to the neonatal abstinence syndrome discussed previously, it is theoretically possible that infants exposed to methadone in utero could have developmental abnormalities, and it is important to consider this possibility when assessing the risk–benefit ratio of methadone treatment for pregnant women. Several studies have reported *higher* birth weights in infants born to methadone-maintained women relative to neonates of heroin-dependent women not maintained on methadone (Kandall et al. 1976, 1977; Stimmel et al. 1982; Zelson 1973). This is a good finding, as low birth weight can be a predictor of slow infant development. Furthermore, a significant dose–effect relationship has been reported between methadone dose and birth weight, with higher methadone doses being associated with higher birth weights (Hagopian et al. 1996; Kandall et al. 1976). When birth weights of methadone-exposed neonates are compared with birth weights of neonates from non-drug-dependent women, however, babies exposed to methadone, though within normal limits for gestational age, generally weigh less than unexposed babies (Kaltenbach and Finnegan 1987; Chasnoff et al. 1982; Lifschitz et al. 1983; Hans 1989).

Children who are prenatally exposed to methadone have small head circumference at birth, suggesting the possibility that methadone has a potential structural effect on the brain (Chasnoff et al. 1982; Hans 1989; Kaltenbach and Finnegan 1987; Lifschitz et al. 1983; Rosen and Johnson 1982). This smaller head size at birth can often be accounted for by birth weight, however (Kaltenbach and Finnegan 1987). In follow-up studies, head circumference was smaller in methadone-exposed children at two (Hans 1989) and three (Rosen and Johnson 1985) years of age compared with nonexposed children. By preschool, however, this difference between groups disappears (Lifschitz et al. 1985). Furthermore, a study examining growth rates found catch-up growth was evident between one and six months of age, with neurological development as assessed by the Bayley Scales of Infant Development in the normal range for methadone-exposed infants (Patso et al. 1989).

Few studies using adequate methodology have monitored children prenatally exposed to methadone beyond the first weeks of life. In general, the studies that have been done show that methadone-exposed infants function within the normal range for the first two years of life and beyond. For example, when methadone-exposed children were compared to non-drug-exposed children at 3, 6, and 12 months of age (Kaltenbach and Finnegan 1987; Strauss et al. 1976), no differences were found using the Bayley Mental Development Index (BMDI). Similarly, no differences were observed between methadone-exposed and comparison children in several studies that have administered the McCarthy Scales of Children's Abilities (MSCA) (McCarthy 1972) at the ages of 3 and 6 (Lifschitz et al. 1985), 4½ years (Kaltenbach and Finnegan 1989), and 5 years (Strauss et al. 1979). Finally, when children prenatally exposed to methadone are compared with nonexposed children, no differences have been found on academic performance and externalizing problems when methadone-exposed children reach school age and adolescence (Hans 1996).

Although methadone-exposed children appear normal when standardized tests such as the BMDI and MSCA are administered, researchers often describe poorer performance of methadone-exposed children in areas such as fine and gross motor coordination, attention, and language when compared with control groups (Chasnoff et al. 1984; Rosen and Johnson 1985; Strauss et al. 1976; Wilson et al. 1981). Furthermore, methadone-exposed children are more likely to meet criteria for attention deficit hyperactivity disorder and to display deficits in basic attention processes, impulsivity, and disruptive behaviors when compared with a nonexposed control group (Hans 1996). Thus, more research is needed to explore basic functions in methadone-exposed children, such as information-processing performance and use of language in early childhood, and cognitive development and performance in later childhood to fully understand the possible sequelae of prenatal methadone exposure.

Risk–Benefit of Methadone Treatment during Pregnancy

In weighing the risk–benefit ratio for methadone maintenance treatment during pregnancy, it is important to consider both maternal and child outcomes. The most important benefit to both is the reduction or elimination of injection-drug use. Methadone suppresses opiate craving and provides a stable blood level of opioid maintenance that eliminates exposure of the neonate to the repeated cycling between opiate high and opiate withdrawal. Furthermore, it reduces the likelihood of exposure to other diseases including HIV and hepatitis C virus (HCV) that can pose a danger to both mother and infant. Risks to the neonate are primarily those associated with NAS and possibly developmental delays in cognitive functioning. The NAS is generally short-lived, readily treated, and relatively benign. Methadone-exposed children appear to fall within the normal range of developmental processes and to catch up in growth to non-drug-exposed children by two to three years of age. Thus, methadone maintenance, although not without some drawbacks, currently continues to be the recommended treatment for pregnant women dependent on opioids.

Prenatal Buprenorphine Exposure

As discussed elsewhere in this book (chap. 11), buprenorphine has an excellent safety profile. It has been reported to produce mild autonomic signs and symptoms of opioid withdrawal after abrupt discontinuation in nonpregnant adults. Because of buprenorphine's unusual pharmacologic profile, there has been interest in its possible use for the treatment of the pregnant, opioid-dependent woman. This interest has been driven by several lines of reasoning. First, the minimal withdrawal profile with discontinuation of buprenorphine seen in adults could mean that buprenorphine will produce a mild NAS in a newborn. Second, the poor oral bioavailability of buprenorphine suggests that breast-feeding by a buprenorphine-maintained mother should not result in appreciable buprenorphine blood levels in the breast-fed infant. And finally, in the United States and elsewhere, the availability of buprenorphine through office-based treatment rather than opioid treatment programs may make it easier for women dependent on opioids to receive medication treatment. However, in the United States the FDA has not approved buprenorphine for the treatment of pregnant patients, although its use during pregnancy is currently being investigated.

Through March 2004, 23 reports were published, representing approximately 16 samples of infants prenatally exposed to buprenorphine (references available on request from the author). Of approximately 338 infants exposed, the number of patients in each sample ranged between 1 and 153, with a median of 6 per report. A NAS has been reported in 205 (61%) of infants with 161 (48%) requiring treatment. Though data are quite limited in many of the reports, more than 40 percent report concomitant drug use by buprenorphine-exposed mothers, and a diversity of procedures was used to determine and treat the NAS. The NAS associated with buprenorphine generally appears within 12–48 hours, peaks at approximately 72–96 hours, and lasts for 120–168 hours (Johnson et al. 2003). Studies are currently ongoing to determine whether the patterns of NAS signs are different between buprenorphine and methadone. From a review of the literature, buprenorphine appears to be as safe and effective as methadone in both mother and infant. Under controlled conditions where concomitant drug use is quite low, the NAS following buprenorphine exposure may be qualitatively and quantitatively different from methadone. The long-term outcomes following buprenorphine exposure are not known, but this is a topic that deserves study, especially in comparison with the current standard treatment, methadone.

Conclusions

Important medical, psychological, and social differences exist between male and female drug abusers. These differences have implications for the content and delivery of therapeutic services to drug-abusing women. The importance of recognizing the illness of drug addiction as a complex health issue best treated with comprehensive and coordinated services is highlighted with the pregnant woman. Methadone maintenance is currently the recommended treatment for pregnant opioid-dependent women. It should be provided in a comprehensive care setting that meets the pregnant woman's unique requirements and addresses not only the substance abuse disorder itself, but also the concurrent problem areas such as personal health and psychological stressors, including violence, relationships, and daily life requirements. The dose of methadone should be carefully monitored throughout the gestation and adjustments made in the dose and/or the dosing regimen as needed with particular attention given to the third trimester, because this is a time during which methadone metabolism is increased. Detoxification is not recommended during pregnancy, although it may be necessary under certain circumstances. The NAS that is associated with prenatal methadone exposure is treatable and, in combination with methadone exposure itself, does not appear to produce long-term effects on development. Buprenorphine is the latest medication to be investigated for treating pregnant patients dependent on opioids. Preliminary data suggest it is beneficial to the mother and may be optimal for reducing the risk of the NAS. Overall, it appears that when the physical, psychological, and economic issues of the pregnant opioid abuser are addressed concurrently with methadone treatment, the benefits far outweigh the risks for the mother, the fetus, and the infant.

References

Abbott J, Johnson R, Koziol-McLain J, Lowenstein SR (1995). Domestic violence against women. Incidence and prevalence in an emergency department population. *JAMA* 273: 1763–7.

Aktan GB, Kumpfer KL, Turner CW (1996). Effectiveness of a family skills training program for substance use prevention with inner city African-American families. *Subst Use Misuse* 31: 157–75.

Allen K (1995). Barriers to treatment for addicted African-American women. *J Natl Med Assoc* 87: 751–6.

Amaro H, Fried LE, Cabral H, Zuckerman B (1990). Violence during pregnancy and substance use. *Am J Public Health* 80: 575–9.

Barnard M, McKeganey N (2004). The impact of parental problem drug use on children: what is the problem and what can be done to help? *Addiction* 99: 552–9.

Bartholomew NG, Rowan-Szal GA, Chatham LR, Simpson DD (1994). Effectiveness of a specialized intervention for women in a methadone program. *J Psychoactive Drugs* 26: 249–55.

Beckwith L, Espinosa M, Howard J (1994). Psychological profile of pregnant women who abuse cocaine, alcohol, and other drugs, In Harris LS, ed. Problems of Drug Dependence, 1993: Proceedings of the 55th Annual Scientific Meeting The College on Problems of Drug Dependence, pp. 116. Bethesda, MD: National Institute on Drug Abuse, U.S. Department of Health and Human Services.

Begg EJ, Malpas TJ, Hackett LP, Ilett KF (2001). Distribution of R- and S-methadone into human milk during multiple, medium to high oral dosing. *Br J Clin Pharmacol* 52: 681–5.

Black MM, Nair P, Kight C, Wachtel R, Roby P, Schuler M (1994). Parenting and early development among children of drug-abusing women: effects of home intervention. *Pediatrics* 94: 440–8.

Blume SB (1990). Chemical dependency in women: important issues. *Am J Drug Alcohol Abuse* 16: 297–307.

Brady KT, Randall CL (1999). Gender differences in substance use disorders. *Psychiatr Clin North Am* 22: 241–52.

Brooner RK, King VL, Kidorf M, Schmidt CW, Jr., Bigelow GE (1997). Psychiatric and substance use comorbidity among treatment-seeking opioid abusers. *Arch Gen Psychiatry* 54: 71–80.

Carter EF (1978). Dental implications of narcotic addiction. *Aust Dent J* 23: 308–10.

Catalano RF, Gainey RR, Fleming CB, Haggerty KP, Johnson NO (1999). An experimental intervention with families of substance abusers: one-year follow-up of the focus on families project. *Addiction* 94: 241–54.

CDC (1994). HIV/AIDS Surveillance Report 6. Atlanta, GA: Centers for Disease Control.

CDCP (2001). HIV/AIDS Surveillance Report, Midyear 2000, 12–14. Atlanta, GA: Centers for Disease Control and Prevention.

Chasnoff IJ (1991). Drugs, alcohol, pregnancy, and the neonate. Pay now or pay later. *JAMA* 266: 1567–8.

Chasnoff IJ, Hatcher R, Burns WJ (1982). Polydrug- and methadone-addicted newborns: a continuum of impairment? *Pediatrics* 70: 210–3.

Chasnoff IJ, Schnoll SH, Burns WJ, Burns K (1984). Maternal nonnarcotic substance abuse during pregnancy: effects on infant development. *Neurobehav Toxicol Teratol* 6: 277–80.

Choo RE, Huestis MA, Schroeder JR, Shin AS, Jones HE (2004). Neonatal abstinence syndrome in methadone-exposed infants is altered by level of prenatal tobacco exposure. *Drug Alcohol Depend* 75: 253–60.

Colten ME (1979). A descriptive and comparative analysis of self perceptions and attitudes of heroin-addicted women. Addicted Women: Family Dynamics, Self-perceptions and Support Systems. Washington, DC: U.S. Government Printing Office.

Connaughton JF, Jr., Reeser D, Finnegan LP (1977). Pregnancy complicated by drug addiction. In: Bolognese R, Schwartz R, eds. *Perinatal Medicine,* 265–76. Baltimore, MD: Williams and Wilkins.

Cuskey WR, Berger LH, Densen-Gerber J (1977). Issues in the treatment of female addiction: a review and critique of the literature. *Contemp Drug Probl* 7: 307–71.

Dashe JS, Sheffield JS, Olscher DA, Todd SJ, Jackson GL, Wendel GD (2002). Relationship between maternal methadone dosage and neonatal withdrawal. *Obstet Gynecol* 100: 1244–9.

Doberczak TM, Kandall SR, Wilets I (1991). Neonatal opiate abstinence syndrome in term and preterm infants. *J Pediatr* 118: 933–7.

Downs WR, Miller BA, Panek DD (1993). Differential patterns of partner-to-woman violence: a comparison of samples of community, alcohol abusing and battered women. *J Fam Violence* 8: 113–35.

Drozdick J, III, Berghella V, Hill M, Kaltenbach K (2002). Methadone trough levels in pregnancy. *Am J Obstet Gynecol* 187: 1184–8.

Ehrmin JT (2001). Unresolved feelings of guilt and shame in the maternal role with substance-dependent African American women. *J Nurs Scholarsh* 33: 47–52.

El-Bassel N, Gilbert L, Schilling R, Wada T (2000). Drug abuse and partner violence among women in methadone treatment. *J Fam Violence* 15: 209–28.

Ellinwood EH, Smith WG, Vaillant GE (1966). Narcotic addiction in males and females: a comparison. *Int J Addict* 12: 541–51.

Epstein JF, Gfroerer JC (1997). Heroin Abuse in the United States. OAS Working Paper. Rockville, MD: Substance Abuse and Mental Health Services Administration, 1–8.

Finnegan LP (1988). Influence of maternal drug dependence on the newborn. In: Kacew S, Lock S, eds. *Toxicology and Pharmacologic Principles in Pediatrics.* New York: Hemisphere Publishing Corporation.

Finnegan LP (1991). Treatment issues for opioid-dependent women during the perinatal period. *J Psychoactive Drugs* 23: 191–201.

Finnegan LP, Davenny K, Hartel D (1993). Drug use in HIV-infected women. In: Johnson MA, Johnstone FD, eds. *HIV Infection in Women,* 133–55. Edinburgh: Churchill Livingstone.

Finnegan LP, Kaltenbach K (1992). Neonatal abstinence syndrome. In: Hoekelman RA, Friedman SB, Nelson NM, Seidel HM, eds. *Primary Pediatric Care.* St. Louis, MO: Mosby Year Book.

Finnegan LP, Wapner RJ (1987). Drug use in pregnancy. In: Neibyl JR, ed. *Narcotic Addiction in Pregnancy.* Philadelphia: Lea and Febiger.

Fitzgerald E, Kaltenbach K, Finnegan LP (1988). Patterns of interaction among drug dependent women and their infants. *Pediatr Res* 24: 44.

Gazaway PM, Bigelow GE, Brooner RK (1993). The influence of pregnancy upon trough plasma levels of methadone and its' opioid effects. In: Harris L, ed. Problems of Drug Dependence, 1992: Proceedings of the 54th Annual Scientific Meeting The College on Problems of Drug Dependence, Inc. Rockville, MD; U.S. Department of Health and Human Services.

Gomberg ES (1989). Suicide risk among women with alcohol problems. *Am J Public Health* 79: 1363–5.

Goodfriend MJ, Shey IA, Klein MD (1956). The effects of maternal narcotic addiction on the newborn. *Am J Obstet Gynecol* 71: 29–36

Grella CE (1997). Services for perinatal women with substance abuse and mental health disorders: the unmet need. *J Psychoactive Drugs* 29: 67–78.

Griffin ML, Weiss RD, Mirin SM, Lange U (1989). A comparison of male and female cocaine abusers. *Arch Gen Psychiatry* 46: 122–6.

Hagopian GS, Wolfe HM, Sokol RJ, Ager JW, Wardell JN, Cepeda EE (1996). Neonatal outcome following methadone exposure in utero. *J Matern Fetal Med* 5: 348–54.

Haller DL, Knisely JS, Dawson KS, Schnoll SH (1993). Perinatal substance abusers. Psychological and social characteristics. *J Nerv Ment Dis* 181: 509–13.

Haller DL, Miles DR, Dawson KS (2003). Factors influencing treatment enrollment by pregnant substance abusers. *Am J Drug Alcohol Abuse* 29: 117–31.

Hans SL (1989). Developmental consequences of prenatal exposure to methadone. *Ann N Y Acad Sci* 562: 195–207.

Hans SL (1996). Prenatal drug exposure: behavioral functioning in late childhood and adolescence. *NIDA Res Monogr* 164: 261–76.

Helzer JE, Pryzbeck TR (1988). The co-occurrence of alcoholism with other psychiatric disorders in the general population and its impact on treatment. *J Stud Alcohol* 49: 219–24.

Hoegerman G, Schnoll S (1991). Narcotic use in pregnancy. *Clin Perinatol* 18: 51–76.

Jansson LM, Svikis D, Lee J, Paluzzi P, Rutigliano P, Hackerman F (1996). Pregnancy and addiction. A comprehensive care model. *J Subst Abuse Treat* 13: 321–9.

Jansson LM, Velez M, Harrow C (2004). Methadone maintenance and lactation: a review of the literature and current management guidelines. *J Hum Lact* 20: 62–71.

Jarvis MA, Schnoll SH (1995). Methadone use during pregnancy. *NIDA Res Monogr* 149: 58–77.

Jeremy RJ, Hans SL (1985). Behavior of neonates exposed in utero to methadone as assessed on the Brazelton Scale. *Infant Behav Dev* 8: 323–36.

Johnson MO (2001). Mother-infant interaction and maternal substance use/abuse: an integrative review of research literature in the 1990s. *Online J Knowl Synth Nurs* 8: 2.

Johnson RE, Jones HE, Fischer G (2003). Use of buprenorphine in pregnancy: patient management and effects on the neonate. *Drug Alcohol Depend* 70: S87-S101.

Jones HE, Johnson RE, Bigelow GE, Strain EC (2004). Differences at treatment entry between opioid-dependent and cocaine-dependent males and females. *Addict Disord Their Treatment* 3: 110–21.

Jones HE, Johnson RE, Tuten M (2001). Detoxification of Pregnant Opiate Dependent Addicted Women using Methadone: Safety and Efficacy. St. Louis, MO: American Methadone Treatment Association.

Kaltenbach K, Finnegan LP (1987). Perinatal and developmental outcome of infants exposed to methadone in-utero. *Neurotoxicol Teratol* 9: 311–3.

Kaltenbach K, Finnegan LP (1988). The influence of neonatal abstinence syndrome and mother infant interactions. In: Anthony EJ, Chiland C, eds. *Perilous Development: Child Raising and Identity Formation Under Stress*. New York: John Wiley and Sons.

Kaltenbach K, Finnegan LP (1989). Children exposed to methadone in-utero: assessment of developmental and cognitive ability. *Ann N Y Acad Sci* 562: 360–62.

Kandall SR, Albin S, Gartner LM, Lee KS, Eidelman A, Lowinson J (1977). The narcotic-dependent mother: fetal and neonatal consequences. *Early Hum Dev* 1: 159–69.

Kandall SR, Albin S, Lowinson J, Berle B, Eidelman AI, Gartner LM (1976). Differential effects of maternal heroin and methadone use on birthweight. *Pediatrics* 58: 681–5.

Kantor GK, Straus MA (1989). Substance abuse as a precipitant of wife abuse victimizations. *Am J Drug Alcohol Abuse* 15: 173–89.

Kaplan SL, Kron RE, Phoenix MD, Finnegan LP (1976). Brazelton neonatal assessment at three and twenty-eight days of age: a study of passively addicted infants, high risk infants and normal infants. In: Alksne H, Kaufman E, Schecter A, eds. *Critical Concerns in the Field of Drug Abuse. Proceedings of the Third National Drug Abuse Conference.* New York: Marcel Dekker.

Knisley JS, Christmas JT, Dinsmoore M, Spear E, Schnoll SH (1993). The impact of intensive prenatal and substance abuse care on pregnancy outcome. In: Harris L, ed. Problems of Drug Dependence, 1992: Proceeding of the 54th Annual Scientific Meeting, The College on Problems of Drug Dependence, Inc. Rockville, MD: U.S. Department of Health and Human Services.

Kosten TR, Rounsaville BJ, Kleber HD (1985). Ethnic and gender differences among opiate addicts. *Int J Addict* 20: 1143–62.

Kreek MJ (1979). Methadone disposition during the perinatal period in humans. *Pharmacol Biochem Behav* 11: 7–13.

Kreek MJ (1986). Drug interactions with methadone in humans. *NIDA Res Monogr* 68: 193–225.

Kreek MJ, Schecter A, Gutjahr CL, Bowen D, Field F, Queenan J, Merkatz I (1974). Analyses of methadone and other drugs in maternal and neonatal body fluids: use in evaluation of symptoms in a neonate of mother maintained on methadone. *Am J Drug Alcohol Abuse* 1: 409–19.

Kumpfer KL, Alvarado R, Whiteside HO (2003). Family-based interventions for substance use and misuse prevention. *Subst Use Misuse* 38: 1759–8.

Laken MP, Ager JW (1996). Effects of case management on retention in prenatal substance abuse treatment. *Am J Drug Alcohol Abuse* 22: 439–48.

Levy M, Spino M (1993). Neonatal withdrawal syndrome: associated drugs and pharmacologic management. *Pharmacotherapy* 13: 202–11.

Lex BW (1991). Some gender differences in alcohol and polysubstance users. *Health Psychol* 10: 121–32.

Lifschitz MH, Wilson GS, Smith EO, Desmond MM (1983). Fetal and postnatal growth of children born to narcotic-dependent women. *J Pediatr* 102: 686–91.

Lifschitz MH, Wilson GS, Smith EO, Desmond MM (1985). Factors affecting head growth and intellectual function in children of drug addicts. *Pediatrics* 75: 269–74.

Luthar SS, Cushing G, Rounsaville BJ (1996). Gender differences among opioid abusers: pathways to disorder and profiles of psychopathology. *Drug Alcohol Depend* 43: 179–89.

Luthar SS, Glick M, Zigler E, Rounsaville BJ (1993). Social competence among cocaine abusers: moderating effects of comorbid diagnoses and gender. *Am J Drug Alcohol Abuse* 19: 283–98.

Malpas TJ, Darlow BA (1999). Neonatal abstinence syndrome following abrupt cessation of breastfeeding. *N Z Med J* 112: 12–3.

Marsh KL, Simpson DD (1986). Sex differences in opioid addiction careers. *Am J Drug Alcohol Abuse* 12: 309–29.

McCarthy DA (1972). Manual for the McCarthy Scales of Children's Abilities. Marrickville NSW 2204 Australia: The Psychological Corporation

Miller BA, Downs WR, Gondoli DM (1989). Spousal violence among alcoholic women as compared to a random household sample of women. *J Stud Alcohol* 50: 533–40.

Moore AL, Kirk O, Johnson AM, Katlama C, Blaxhult A, Dietrich M, Colebunders R, Chiesi A, Lungren JD, Phillips AN (2003). Virologic, immunologic, and clinical response to highly active antiretroviral therapy: the gender issue revisited. *J Acquir Immune Defic Syndr* 32: 452–61.

Moylan PL, Jones HE, Haug NA, Kissin WB, Svikis DS (2001). Clinical and psychosocial characteristics of substance-dependent pregnant women with and without PTSD. *Addict Behav* 26: 469–74.

Parrino MW (1993). State Methadone Treatment Guidelines. Rockville, MD: Substance Abuse and Mental Health Services Administration, U.S. Department of Health and Human Services.

Patso ME, Ehrlich S, Kaltenbach K, Graziani L, Kurtz A, Goldberg B, Finnegan LP (1989). Cerebral sonographic characterizations and maternal and neonatal risk factors in infants of opiate-dependent mothers. *Ann N Y Acad Sci* 562: 355–7.

Pivnick A, Jacobson A, Eric K, Doll L, Drucker E (1994). AIDS, HIV infection, and illicit drug use within inner-city families and social networks. *Am J Public Health* 84: 271–4.

Pond SM, Kreek MJ, Tong TG, Raghunath J, Benowitz NL (1985). Altered methadone pharmacokinetics in methadone-maintained pregnant women. *J Pharmacol Exp Ther* 233: 1–6.

Rementeria JL, Nunag NN (1973). Narcotic withdrawal in pregnancy: stillbirth incidence with a case report. *Am J Obstet Gynecol* 116: 1152–6.

Rosen TS, Johnson HL (1982). Children of methadone-maintained mothers: follow-up to 18 months of age. *J Pediatr* 101: 192–6.

Rosen TS, Johnson HL (1985). Long-term effects of prenatal methadone maintenance. *NIDA Res Monogr* 59: 73–83.

Rosen TS, Pippenger CE (1975). Disposition of methadone and its relationship to severity of withdrawal in the newborn. *Addict Dis* 2: 169–78.

Rowan-Szal GA, Chatham LR, Joe GW, Simpson DD (2000). Services provided during methadone treatment. A gender comparison. *J Subst Abuse Treat* 19: 7–14.

SAMHSA (2001). Drug and Alcohol Services Information Report: How Men and Women Enter Substance Abuse Treatment. Rockville, MD: Substance Abuse and Mental Health Services Administration, Office of Applied Studies.

SAMHSA (2004). Results from the 2003 National Survey on Drug Use and Health: National Findings. DHHS Pub. No. SMA 04-3964. Rockville, MD: Substance Abuse and Mental Health Services Administration, Office of Applied Studies.

Schoenbaum EE, Hartel D, Selwyn PA, Klein RS, Davenny K, Rogers M, Feiner C, Friedland G (1989). Risk factors for human immunodeficiency virus infection in intravenous drug users. *N Engl J Med* 321: 874–9.

Silverman K, Chutuape MA, Svikis DS, Bigelow GE, Stitzer ML (1995). Incongruity between occupational interests and academic skills in drug abusing women. *Drug Alcohol Depend* 40: 115–23.

Smith DE, Wesson DR, Tusel DJ (1989). *Treating Opiate Dependency.* Center City, MN: Hazelden Foundation.

Solomon L, Astemborski J, Warren D, Munoz A, Cohn S, Vlahov D, Nelson KE (1993). Differences in risk factors for human immunodeficiency virus type 1 seroconversion among male and female intravenous drug users. *Am J Epidemiol* 137: 892–8.

Stein MD (1990). Medical complications of intravenous drug use. *J Gen Intern Med* 5: 249–57.

Stein MD, Cyr MG (1997). Women and substance abuse. *Med Clin North Am* 81: 979–98.

Stevens SJ, Arbiter N (1995). A therapeutic community for substance-abusing pregnant women and women with children: process and outcome. *J Psychoactive Drugs* 27: 49–56.

Stimmel B, Goldberg J, Reisman A, Murphy RJ, Teets K (1982). Fetal outcome in narcotic-dependent women: the importance of the type of maternal narcotic used. *Am J Drug Alcohol Abuse* 9: 383–95.

Strauss ME, Lessen-Firestone JK, Chavez CJ, Stryker JC (1979). Children of methadone-treated women at five years of age. *Pharmacol Biochem Behav* 11 Suppl: 3–6.

Strauss ME, Starr RH, Ostrea EM, Chavez CJ, Stryker JC (1976). Behavioural concomitants of prenatal addiction to narcotics. *J Pediatr* 89: 842–6.

Svikis DS, Lee JH, Haug NA, Stitzer ML (1997). Attendance incentives for outpatient treatment: effects in methadone- and nonmethadone-maintained pregnant drug dependent women. *Drug Alcohol Depend* 48: 33–41.

Titsas A, Ferguson MM (2002). Impact of opioid use on dentistry. *Aust Dent J* 47: 94–98.

Tucker MB (1979). A descriptive and comparative analysis of the social support structure of heroin addicted women. Addicted Women: Family Dynamics, Self-perceptions and Support Systems. DHEW Pub. No. 80-762. Rockville, MD: U.S. Department of Health, Education and Welfare, pp. 130.

Tuten M, Jones HE, Tran G, Svikis DS (2004). Partner violence impacts the psychosocial and psychiatric status of pregnant, drug-dependent women. *Addict Behav* 29: 1029–34.

Wallen J (1992). A comparison of male and female clients in substance abuse treatment. *J Subst Abuse Treat* 9: 243–8.

Wechsberg WM, Craddock SG, Hubbard RL (1998). How are women who enter substance abuse treatment different than men? A gender comparison from the Drug Abuse Treatment Outcome Study (DATOS). *Drugs Soc* 13: 97–115.

Weiss RD, Martinez-Raga J, Griffin ML, Greenfield SF, Hufford C (1997). Gender differences in cocaine dependent patients: a 6 month follow-up study. *Drug Alcohol Depend* 44: 35–40.

Wilson GS, Desmond MM, Wait RB (1981). Follow-up of methadone-treated and untreated narcotic-dependent women and their infants: health, developmental, and social implications. *J Pediatr* 98: 716–22.

Wittmann BK, Segal S (1991). A comparison of the effects of single- and split-dose methadone administration on the fetus: ultrasound evaluation. *Int J Addict* 26: 213–8.

Zablotsky D, Kennedy M (2003). Risk factors and HIV transmission to midlife and older women: knowledge, options, and the initiation of safer sexual practices. *J Acquir Immune Defic Syndr* 33 Suppl 2: S122–S130.

Zelson C (1973). Infant of the addicted mother. *N Engl J Med* 288: 1393–5.

Zilberman ML, Hochgraf PB, Andrade AG (2003). Gender differences in treatment-seeking Brazilian drug-dependent individuals. *Subst Abus* 24: 17–25.

Zuspan FP, Gumpel JA, Mejia-Zelaya A, Madden J, Davis R (1975). Fetal stress from methadone withdrawal. *Am J Obstet Gynecol* 122: 43–6.

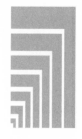

21

Treatment of Persons under Legal Restrictions

Carl G. Leukefeld, D.S.W., Michele Staton, Ph.D.,
J. Matthew Webster, Ph.D., and Hope Smiley McDonald, M.A.

The relationship between drug use, particularly heroin use, and crime has been well documented in the literature (Leukefeld et al. 2002). As a result, numerous drug abusers are receiving community-based treatment that are on probation or parole or who have been referred to treatment from other criminal justice programs, such as drug courts. The drug–crime connection is costly to society, with more than a third ($31.8 billion) of the estimated costs associated with drug abuse being related to crime (French 1995; French and Martin 1996). Further, cost-effectiveness and cost-offset studies have consistently reported that drug abuse treatment is cost-effective because the reductions in crime costs are greater than the cost of delivering treatment (French 1995; French and Martin 1996). For example, one well-publicized study from California (CALDATA) concluded that for every $1 spent on treatment there was a $7 cost savings, with the largest savings coming from reductions in crime (Gerstein et al. 1994). Thus, crime cost reductions associated with drug abuse treatment provide the economic foundation for approaches that meld criminal sanctions with community drug abuse treatment.

This chapter first examines the association between drugs and crime in more detail and then focuses on new models of drug abuse treatment delivered within criminal justice settings, including jails and prisons. Next, the characteristics of programs that meld treatment and sanctions by diverting drug abusers into community treatment through the criminal justice system are described. A major theme is that patients in treatment under legal restrictions or because of legal pressure, though treatment providers may view them as a special population, do not in fact differ substantively from non-criminal-justice-involved patients in major demographic or psychosocial characteristics or in their response to treatment. Note also that the criminal justice system has traditionally operated under referral practices that give preference to drug-free psychosocial treatment settings, including therapeutic communities, and that preclude referral to opioid substitution therapy modalities. The rationale for this referral pattern is discussed along with current trends in criminal justice referral mechanisms and practices.

THE DRUG–CRIME ASSOCIATION

Although drug use is not the only path leading to crime, early drug use can foster a criminal behavior pattern that continues into adulthood (Leukefeld and Tims 1988). Since the 1970s, the National Institute on Drug Abuse has supported studies on the drug–crime connection and, as a result, the association of chronic drug abuse and crime is well documented (Leukefeld et al. 2002; Leukefeld 1985). Research has shown that heroin addiction is specifically associated with high rates of criminal behavior (Ball et al. 1982; Inciardi 1979; Nurco et al. 1985) and that heavy drug users are more likely to engage in a more diverse array of criminal activities (Farabee et al. 2001). In an early study, for example, Inciardi reported that a cohort of 239 male heroin addicts from Miami committed 80,644 criminal acts during the 12 months before being interviewed (Inciardi 1979). Similarly, Ball and colleagues (1982) found that during an 11-year period a Baltimore, Maryland, cohort of 243 heroin addicts committed crimes on 248 days per year while addicted, with theft followed by drug sales being the most frequent types of crime. When not addicted, the same cohort had only 41 days of criminal activity per year. This relationship suggests that drug treatment engendering abstinence could be highly beneficial for reducing criminal activity of drug-involved individuals.

One consequence of the drug–crime connection is that many drug abusers enter the criminal justice system, a trend that has been exacerbated by changing policy in the United States during the early 1980s. Specifically, policy during that time began to strongly emphasize controlling the supply of drugs and invoking determinate sentencing for drug offenders and long prison terms as a strategy to decrease drug abuse. As expected, these efforts were followed by rapid increases in incarcerated drug abusers. The number of drug-involved offenders is evident from a survey of inmates in state and federal institutions which found that 83 percent of state prisoners reported past drug/alcohol use and 52 percent reported using drugs/alcohol in the month before their offense (Mumola 1999). This is consistent with an earlier report that 50 percent of federal inmates and 80 percent of state inmates had been drug-involved before incarceration (Innes 1988). In addition, data from the Arrestee Drug Abuse Monitoring (ADAM) system indicates that 64 percent of male arrestees and 67 percent of female arrestees in major U.S. cities tested positive for drugs (National Institute of Justice [NIJ] 2000), a finding that has been consistent over the years.

The increase in criminal justice involvement of drug abusers is further substantiated by a special report from the Bureau of Justice Statistics (Scalia 2001), which indicates that the number of defendants charged with drug offenses in federal courts increased 147 percent from 1984 to 1999. Sixty-two percent of convicted drug defendants were subject to minimum prison terms, and two-thirds of defendants with drug offenses in U.S. District Courts had prior arrests. Of this group, 44 percent had been arrested more than five times. By 1999 more than 100,000 drug offenders were under federal correctional supervision. In addition, probationers under community supervision now represent over one-half of the U.S. correctional population with 47 percent reporting they were high at the time of their offense and 70 percent having a history of drug use (Scalia 2001).

In-custody Drug Abuse Treatment

Given the large number of drug abusers involved in the criminal justice system, it seems logical to provide drug treatment services within a system where the target population is readily available and where treatment compliance may be less of an issue than it is in outpatient treatment settings. There are currently a limited but growing number of drug abuse treatment programs for individuals in the U.S. criminal justice system, and a growing body of research has highlighted the virtues of prison-based drug abuse treatment (Leukefeld et al. 2002). Similarly, programs in Australia, Canada, and Europe have been instituted (Darke et al. 1998; Dolan and Wodak 1996; Dolan et al. 2003; Howells et al. 2002; Sibbald 2002). Research has also shown that rehabilitation-focused programming can reduce criminality and drug use after incarceration. Furthermore, the cost of treatment within prison is generally less than community-based treatment (McCollister and French 2002).

Therapeutic Community Treatment Models

In the United States, long-term residential treatment programs modeled after therapeutic communities have been the most popular models of prison-based treatment. Programs implemented and described have included the Stay'n Out Program in New York (Wexler and Williams 1986), the Cornerstone Program in Oregon (Field 1985), and the Amity Program in California (Wexler and Graham 1994). Therapeutic community (TC) treatment focuses on drug use and related behavior using confrontation groups, program structure, job requirements, and behaviorally based restrictions and privileges within the treatment community (Hartman et al. 1997). A specific goal of TC prison treatment is drug abstinence and a lifestyle free from antisocial behaviors and attitudes. Evaluations of these programs have shown their ability to enhance postrelease outcomes, in particular, for males (Martin et al. 1999; Wexler et al. 1990). Specifically, several large-scale evaluations of in-prison therapeutic communities have found that this modality of treatment is associated with reduced rearrest and reconviction rates and with better parole outcomes (Knight et al. 1999; Martin et al. 1999; Wexler et al. 1990; Wexler and Williams 1986). Although TC programs are effective in reducing recidivism among those who participate (Wexler et al. 1999), however, there is also typically a high dropout rate, even for in-prison programs, which reduces the overall impact of this treatment approach within the criminally involved drug-abusing population.

Methadone Treatment for Incarcerated Opioid Abusers

In general, methadone treatment has been underutilized by the criminal justice system, especially in the United States, because of antimethadone attitudes that view methadone treatment as substituting one addiction for another. One exception to this general rule is Project KEEP (Key Extended Entry Program), one of the few criminal justice-based methadone treatment programs that have been implemented in the United States. Project KEEP provides methadone treatment to heroin users in the New York Rikers Island central jail with follow-up community methadone treatment (Magura et al. 1993). An evaluation of the project found high retention rates following jail release with no differences in gender. In addition, KEEP participants were 27 times more likely to apply for treatment and seven times more likely to be in treatment at the six-month follow-up, compared with the non-KEEP control group participants (Magura et al. 1993). Although these encouraging findings have not been sufficient to alter policy with regard to in-prison treatment programs in the United States, which continues to favor a therapeutic community model, there is interest in and research on the use of opioid-agonist treatment for prisoners (Kinlock et al. 2002).

However, prison-based methadone treatment has been instituted in other countries (for a review on this topic, see Dolan and Wodak 1996). Although some of these are reports on the use of methadone for relatively brief withdrawal periods at the initiation of incarceration (Howells et al. 2002; Jeanmonod et al. 1991), of more interest is use of maintenance methadone while persons are incarcerated. Institution of prison-based methadone maintenance treatment has been motivated, in part, by the observation of continued injecting-drug use (Clarke et al. 2001; Dye and Isaacs 1991; Gore et al. 1995a, 1995b; Malliori et al. 1998; van Haastrecht et al. 1998) and even HIV seroconversion (Dolan and Wodak 1999; Mutter et al. 1994) by persons in jail. Clinical experience on the use of methadone maintenance treatment while in prison has been reported most extensively from Australia, where it has been available in some locations since 1987 (Byrne and Dolan 1998; Hall et al. 1994). Prison-based methadone treatment is associated with markedly low rates of in-prison drug use and drug injecting (Darke et al. 1998; Dolan et al. 2003), especially when adequate methadone doses are utilized (Dolan et al. 1996).

COMMUNITY TREATMENT OF DRUG ABUSERS WITH LEGAL RESTRICTIONS

In addition to the growing number of in-prison drug treatment programs, the criminal justice system has actively embraced a strategy of coerced drug abuse treatment referral as a way to address the drug–crime connection. For example, U.S. drug abuse treatment admission data indicate that more than one-third (36%) of client admissions are directly referred from the criminal justice system (SAMHSA 2002). This strategy has taken diverse forms that meld monitoring, community treatment, and sanctions.

Coerced Treatment Models

In community-based corrections programs, drug testing and treatment referral combined with incarceration and other court sanctions can be used to foster entry of drug abusers into community treatment and to sustain treatment participation. Early studies generally supported the importance of involuntary community treatment of opioid addicts with court coercion as a key factor in controlling narcotic addiction (Brill and Lieberman

1969). Prison and jail treatment programs often incorporate case management to link offenders with drug treatment and other community services on release. Referral is usually to intensive outpatient programs that employ psychoeducational and 12-step approaches. The effectiveness of in-custody programs is greatly enhanced when followed by transitional services as prisoners return to the community (Martin et al. 1995), and those programs found to be more likely to reduce recidivism were at least several months in duration, targeted criminal thinking, and incorporated social skills training (Gendreau 1996).

In addition, several models of coerced treatment have been developed and evaluated over the years. For example, civil commitment programs have utilized close supervision of parolees and probationers via urine testing with jail sanctions for detected relapse to drug use (McGlothlin et al. 1977). A similar strategy is used in community-based corrections programs called Criminal Justice Authority, which includes treatment as part of probation, parole, or drug court. Treatment Accountability for Safer Communities (TASC) (Leukefeld et al. 2002) also uses court authority to "divert" drug abusers from prison to community treatment combined with drug testing and intermediate judicial sanctions for noncompliance.

Interest in community drug abuse treatment and criminal justice sanctions has also intensified with the proliferation of drug courts, which has increased the number of criminal justice referrals receiving community treatment (Belenko 2001). Drug courts, which began in Dade County, Florida, combine judicial criminal justice supervision with long-term drug abuse treatment (Harrell 2003). Drug courts currently operate in each of the states in the United States and in other parts of the world, such as Australia (Shanahan et al. 2004); as of December 2003, there are more than 1,098 courts and another 550 being planned in the United States. The increase in the number of drug courts is associated with reported positive outcomes in reduced recidivism, criminality, and drug use (Belenko 2001).

Evaluation of Coerced Residential and Outpatient Treatment

Because many drug-involved offenders enter treatment via criminal justice sanctions, it is important to understand how they fare once in treatment. Evaluation of treatment outcomes for those who enter under legal restrictions or criminal justice coercion has shown mixed results (Leukefeld et al. 2002). For example, Farabee, Prendergast, and Anglin (1998) reviewed eleven coercion-based treatment outcome studies, some of which dated from the 1970s. Of the eleven, five reported a positive relationship between the criminal justice referral and community treatment outcomes, four showed no difference, and two reported negative outcomes. These findings are challenging to interpret because of many factors, including lack of consistent terminology, neglect of internal motivation assessment, lack of program consistency, and lack of fidelity to protocols. Nevertheless, the overall strategy appeared promising.

More recent studies have indicated that criminal justice referrals look similar to substance abusers who are voluntarily referred or, in some cases, have more positive rearrest rates (Hiller et al. 1998). It has been consistently reported that criminal-justice-involved offenders remain in community treatment at least as long as others in treatment who are not criminal justice involved, and the perceived level of coercion can be a predictor of both treatment retention and treatment engagement (Rempel and Destefano 2001). In addition, Gregoire and Burke (2004) found that those who were legally coerced into treatment demonstrated increased motivation for treatment compared with nonlegally involved clients. Thus, although the literature is mixed, it seems that entry into treatment under court authority or other compulsory pathways, a condition that is becoming increasingly prevalent, should not be viewed by treatment programs and staff as a deterrent to good treatment outcome.

Treatment Referral Patterns

Criminal justice referrals to community treatment have tended to show a preference for certain modalities over others. The long-term nature of methadone treatment, for example, runs contrary to the treatment philosophy of many criminal justice administrators, who believe that methadone is merely substituting one drug for another, effectively negating the "drug-free" goal. The dilemma was highlighted in early work by Hubbard and colleagues who reported in a three-year follow-up study that less than 3 percent of patients in outpatient methadone treatment were referred to treatment by the criminal justice system as compared with about 30 percent of residential and outpatient drug-free clients (Hubbard et al. 1988). A striking example of this situation occurred recently in California, where legislation known as Proposition 36 allowed adults convicted of nonviolent drug possession offenses and/or parole or probation violations to choose community drug treatment rather than incarceration. In a preliminary study examining how this policy worked, Hser and colleagues (2003) found that although overall treatment admissions increased after the passage of the law, methadone treatment admissions actually dropped considerably in a sample of five California counties, and some of the sampled counties did not make methadone treatment referrals at all.

Thus, methadone treatment, which is in fact a highly effective drug abuse treatment modality for opioid users, is the treatment used the least by the criminal justice system. This dilemma has been sustained over time even though studies consistently indicate that methadone treatment is effective and that methadone treatment combined with criminal justice authority is a powerful combination for decreasing drug abuse and enhancing positive behaviors. Further, one small-scale study has specifically substantiated the benefits of methadone treatment for criminally involved patients (Brecht et al. 1993). In that study, methadone treatment clients were divided into high, medium, and low levels of legal coercion to determine whether any differences existed between these three groups in background characteristics and in treatment outcomes. Few differences were found on pretreatment characteristics, and all three groups showed substantial decreases in narcotics use, criminal activities, and other negative behaviors after methadone treatment. The authors concluded that their results supported legal coercion as a motivation for treatment entry and that coerced patients responded to methadone treatment in ways similar to voluntary patients, regardless of gender or ethnicity.

SUMMARY: MELDING DRUG ABUSE TREATMENT AND CRIMINAL JUSTICE SANCTIONS

With the well-established relationship between drug abuse and crime, persons dependent on opioids, in particular, are frequently involved in the criminal justice system as part of their drug abuse career and their criminal lifestyle. The goals of community treatment and criminal justice sanctions are in fact quite compatible. An artificial distinction is sometimes made between treatment and legal control, however, with treatment perceived as a helping hand and control from the criminal justice system as a coercive force (Leukefeld et al. 1992). In the extreme case, community treatment providers may point to criminal justice authority as disruptive to the therapeutic relationship. There are other ways of conceptualizing treatment and control, however, if the assumption is that all interventions incorporate a mixture of both treatment and control. For example, a therapeutic community or residential treatment facility typically provides a high and intensive level of both treatment and control, whereas outpatient treatment generally provides a comparably lower level of both treatment exposure and control (depending on the particular programs involved).

Thus, treatment and control can be viewed as complementary aspects of the therapeutic process that vary along a continuum as a function of different settings.

Diverse and creative attempts have been made over the years to meld the two approaches, including in-prison treatment, community aftercare programs operated by the criminal justice system, and referral to community treatment programs through case management, probation, and parole or drug courts. Although legal authority derived from the criminal justice system, in particular, probation and parole, can clearly be used to enhance community treatment participation, differential referral patterns have been apparent by the reluctance of criminal justice practitioners to utilize methadone programs as a referral option. Methadone treatment providers clearly have not taken a lead in working with criminal justice agencies to achieve the parallel goals of decreasing drug use as well as changing behavior and lifestyles. It is hoped that these attitudes will change in the future as new models of opioid substitution treatment and of criminal justice referral practices develop. In the meantime, research in additional services can make an important contribution to identifying the most beneficial methods for combining the powerful and complimentary forces of drug abuse treatment with criminal justice monitoring and sanctions.

References

Ball JC, Lawrence R, Flueck JA, Nurco DN (1982). Lifetime criminality of heroin addicts in the United States. *J Drug Issues* Summer: 225–39.

Belenko S (2001). *Research on Drug Courts: A Critical Review: 2000 Update.* New York: National Center on Addiction and Substance Abuse at Columbia University.

Brecht ML, Anglin MD, Wang JC (1993). Treatment effectiveness for legally coerced versus voluntary methadone maintenance clients. *Am J Drug Alcohol Abuse* 19: 89–106.

Brill L, Lieberman L (1969). *Authority and Addiction.* Boston, MA: Little, Brown.

Byrne A, Dolan K (1998). Methadone treatment is widely accepted in prisons in New South Wales. *BMJ* 316: 1744–5.

Clarke JG, Stein MD, Hanna L, Sobota M, Rich JD (2001). Active and Former Injection Drug Users Report of HIV Risk Behaviors During Periods of Incarceration. *Subst Abus* 22: 209–16.

Darke S, Kaye S, Finlay-Jones R (1998). Drug use and injection risk-taking among prison methadone maintenance patients. *Addiction* 93: 1169–75.

Dolan K, Hall W, Wodak A (1996). Methadone maintenance reduces injecting in prison. *BMJ* 312: 1162.

Dolan K, Wodak A (1996). An international review of methadone provision in prisons. *Addict Res* 4: 85–97.

Dolan KA, Shearer J, MacDonald M, Mattick RP, Hall W, Wodak AD (2003). A randomised controlled trial of methadone maintenance treatment versus wait list control in an Australian prison system. *Drug Alcohol Depend* 72: 59–65.

Dolan KA, Wodak A (1999). HIV transmission in a prison system in an Australian State. *Med J Aust* 171: 14–17.

Dye S, Isaacs C (1991). Intravenous drug misuse among prison inmates: implications for spread of HIV. *BMJ* 302: 1506.

Farabee D, Joshi V, Anglin M (2001). Addiction careers and criminal specialization. *Crime Delinq* 47: 196–220.

Farabee D, Prendergast M, Anglin MD (1998). The effectiveness of coerced treatment for drug-abusing offenders. *Fed Probat* 62: 3–11.

Field G (1985). The Cornerstone Program: a client outcome study. *Fed Probat* 49: 50–55

French MT (1995). Economic evaluation of drug abuse treatment programs: methodology and findings. *Am J Drug Alcohol Abuse* 21: 111–35.

French MT, Martin RF (1996). The costs of drug abuse consequences: a summary of research findings. *J Subst Abuse Treat* 13: 453–66.

Gendreau P (1996). Offender rehabilitation: what we know and what needs to be done. *Crim Justice Behav* 23: 144–61.

Gerstein DR, Johnson RA, Harwood HJ, Fountain D, Suter N, Mallow K (1994). Evaluating Recovery Services: The California Drug and Alcohol Treatment Assessment (CALDATA) General Report. Sacramento, CA: California Department of Alcohol and Drug Programs.

Gore SM, Bird AG, Burns SM, Goldberg DJ, Ross AJ, Macgregor J (1995a). Drug injection and HIV prevalence in inmates of Glenochil prison. *BMJ* 310: 293–6.

Gore SM, Bird AG, Ross AJ (1995b). Prison rites: starting to inject inside. *BMJ* 311: 1135–6.

Gregoire TK, Burke AC (2004). The relationship of legal coercion to readiness to change among adults with alcohol and other drug problems. *J Subst Abuse Treat* 26: 337–43.

Hall W, Ward J, Mattick R (1994). Methadone maintenance treatment in prisons: the New South Wales experience. *Psychiatry Psychol Law* 1: 33–44.

Harrell A (2003). Judging drug courts: balancing the evidence. *Crim Public Policy* 2: 207–12.

Hartman DJ, Wolk JL, Johnston JS, Colyer CJ (1997). Recidivism and substance abuse outcomes in a prison-based therapeutic community. *Fed Probat* 61: 18–25.

Hiller ML, Knight K, Broome KM, Simpson DD (1998). Legal pressure and treatment retention in a national sample of long-term residential programs. *Crim Justice Behav* 25: 463–81.

Howells C, Allen S, Gupta J, Stillwell G, Marsden J, Farrell M (2002). Prison based detoxification for opioid dependence: a randomised double blind controlled trial of lofexidine and methadone. *Drug Alcohol Depend* 67: 169–76.

Hser YI, Teruya C, Evans EA, Longshore D, Grella C, Farabee D (2003). Treating drug-abusing offenders. Initial findings from a five-county study on the impact of California's Proposition 36 on the treatment system and patient outcomes. *Eval Rev* 27: 479–505.

Hubbard RL, Collins JJ, Rachal JV, Cavanaugh ER (1988). The criminal justice client in drug abuse treatment. *NIDA Res Monogr* 86: 57–80.

Inciardi JA (1979). Heroin use and street crime. *Crime Delinq* 25: 335–46.

Innes CA (1988). Profile of state prison inmates, 1986. Washington, DC: U.S. Department of Justice.

Jeanmonod R, Harding T, Staub C (1991). Treatment of opiate withdrawal on entry to prison. *Br J Addict* 86: 457–63.

Kinlock TW, Battjes RJ, Schwartz RP (2002). A novel opioid maintenance program for prisoners: preliminary findings. *J Subst Abuse Treat* 22: 141–7.

Knight K, Simpson DD, Hiller ML (1999). Three-year reincarceration outcomes for in-prison therapeutic community treatment in Texas. *Prison J* 79: 337–51.

Leukefeld C, Matthews T, Clayton R (1992). Treating the drug-abusing offender. *J Ment Health Adm* 19: 76–82

Leukefeld C, Tims F, Farabee D (2002). *Treatment of Drug Offenders*. New York: Springer.

Leukefeld CG (1985). The clinical connection: drugs and crime. *Int J Addict* 20: 1049–64.

Leukefeld CG, Tims FM (1988). Compulsory treatment: a review of findings. *NIDA Res Monogr* 86: 236–51.

Magura S, Rosenblum A, Lewis C, Joseph H (1993). The effectiveness of in-jail methadone maintenance. *J Drug Issues* 23: 75–99.

Malliori M, Sypsa V, Psichogiou M, Touloumi G, Skoutelis A, Tassopoulos N, Hatzakis A, Stefanis C (1998). A survey of bloodborne viruses and associated risk behaviours in Greek prisons. *Addiction* 93: 243–51.

Martin SS, Butzin CA, Inciardi JA (1995). Assessment of a multistage therapeutic community for drug-involved offenders. *J Psychoactive Drugs* 27: 109–16.

Martin SS, Butzin CA, Saum CA, Inciardi JA (1999). Three-year outcomes of therapeutic community treatment for drug-involved offenders in Delaware: from prison to work release to aftercare. *Prison J* 79: 294–320.

McCollister K, French MT (2002). The economic cost of substance abuse treatment in criminal justice settings. In: Leukefeld CG, Tims F, Farabee D, eds. *Treatment of Drug Offenders: Policies and Issues*, 22–37. New York: Springer Publishing Company.

McGlothlin WH, Anglin MD, Wilson BD (1977). *An Evaluation of the California Addict Program*. Rockville, MD; National Institute on Drug Abuse.

Mumola C (1999). Substance Abuse and Treatment, State and Federal Prisoners, 1997. National Criminal Justice (NCJ) Pub. No. 172871. Washington, DC: Department of Justice.

Mutter RC, Grimes RM, Labarthe D (1994). Evidence of intraprison spread of HIV infection. *Arch Intern Med* 154: 793–5.

National Institute of Justice (NIJ) (2000). 1999 Annual Report on Drug Use among Adult and Juvenile Arrestees. NCJ Pub. No. 181426. Washington, DC: U.S. Department of Justice.

Nurco DN, Ball JC, Shaffer JW, Hanlon TE (1985). The criminality of narcotic addicts. *J Nerv Ment Dis* 173: 94–102

Rempel M, Destefano CD (2001). Predictors of engagement in court-mandated treatment: findings at the Brooklyn Treatment Court, 1996–2000. *J Offender Rehab* 33: 87–124

SAMHSA (2002). Treatment Episode Data Set (TEDS): 1992–2000. National Admissions to Substance Abuse Treatment Services. DHHS Pub. No. (SMA) 02-3727. Rockville, MD: Substance Abuse and Mental Health Services Administration, Office of Applied Studies.

Scalia J (2001). Federal Drug Offenders, 1999. Washington, DC: U.S. Department of Justice.

Shanahan M, Lancsar E, Haas M, Lind B, Weatherburn D, Chen S (2004). Cost-effectiveness analysis of the New South Wales adult drug court program. *Eval Rev* 28: 3–27.

Sibbald B (2002). Methadone maintenance expands inside federal prisons. *CMAJ* 167: 1154.

van Haastrecht HJ, Bax JS, van den Hoek AA (1998). High rates of drug use, but low rates of HIV risk behaviours among injecting drug users during incarceration in Dutch prisons. *Addiction* 93: 1417–25.

Wexler H, Falkin G, Lipton D (1990). Outcome evaluation of a prison therapeutic community for substance abuse treatment. *Crim Justice Behav* 17: 71–92.

Wexler H, Graham W (1994). Prison based therapeutic community for substance abusers: retention, rearrest, and reincarceration, presented at Annual Meeting of the American Psychological Association, Los Angeles, California, August 13, 1994.

Wexler HK, Melnick G, Lowe L, Peters J (1999). Three-year incarceration outcomes for Amity in-prison therapeutic community and aftercare in California. *Prison J* 79: 320–36.

Wexler HK, Williams R (1986). The stay 'n out therapeutic community: prison treatment for substance abusers. *J Psychoactive Drugs* 18: 221–30.

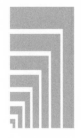

22

Treatment of Adolescents

Lisa A. Marsch, Ph.D.

In the United States, abuse of and dependence on heroin and other opioids is increasing among adolescents, and levels of use for this population are similar to those last observed in the 1960s. Data from the U.S. Drug Abuse Warning Network (DAWN) survey indicate that the absolute number of annual emergency department visits related to heroin among 12–17 year olds, while low, did increase more than twofold from 1995 to 2002 (from 396 to 813 visits) (accessed at http://DAWNinfo.samhsa.gov/pubs_94_02 on September 13, 2004). During the same period, the number of emergency department visits with a heroin mention among 18–19 year olds increased more than threefold (from 981 in 1995 to 3046 in 2002). Additionally, 27 percent (or 40,000) of those individuals who reported trying heroin for the first time in 2000 were less than 18 years of age (SAMHSA 2002a). Moreover, although the prevalence of past-year use of marijuana, club drugs, and tobacco products among youth has decreased in recent years, the prevalence of past-year heroin use among eighth, tenth, and twelfth graders has increased from 0.4–0.7 percent in the early 1990s to 1.0–1.5 percent in recent years (Johnston et al. 2003) (fig. 22.1). These trends are not specific to heroin use; youth are reporting high rates of use for other opiates as well. Specifically, 1.7 percent of eighth graders, 3.6 percent of tenth graders, and 4.5 percent of twelfth graders reported past-year use of OxyContin in 2003, and 2.8 percent of eighth graders, 7.2 percent of tenth graders, and 10.5 percent of twelfth graders reported past-year use of Vicodin in 2003 (accessed at www.mon-

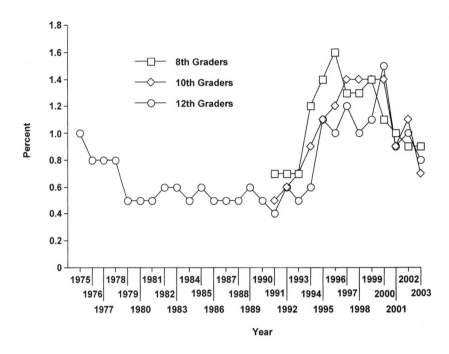

Figure 22.1. Annual use of heroin among eighth (squares), tenth (diamonds), and twelfth graders (circles) in the United States, 1975–2003. Note that this study did not begin tracking eighth and tenth graders' use of heroin until 1991. Data from Johnston et al. 2003.

itoringthefuture.org/data/03data/pro3t2.pdf on September 14, 2004) (fig. 22.2).

This marked increase in the number of young heroin users in the United States has been largely attributed to the dramatically decreased price and increased purity of heroin that occurred in the 1990s (Harling 1998; Hartnoll 1994; Hopfer et al. 2002; Schwartz 1998). Indeed, a report by the U.S. Drug Enforcement Administration (DEA) indicates that the average purity of heroin available in the United States in 2000 was 36.8 percent, a substantial increase from the 3.6 percent purity of heroin reported in 1980 (accessed at www.usdoj.gov:80/dea/pubs/intel/02025/02025.html#table1 on September 14, 2004). As a result of the increased availability of high-potency, low-cost heroin, many adolescents initiate heroin use by snorting it (accessed at www.monitoringthefuture.org/data/03data/pro3t1.pdf on September 14, 2004); however, it is not uncommon for some to progress to injection of heroin (Neaigus et al. 1998).

Studies of illicit opioid use in other countries also suggest that a small

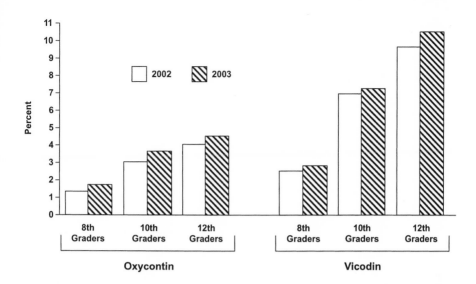

Figure 22.2. **Annual use of OxyContin (left) and Vicodin (right) among eighth, tenth, and twelfth graders in the United States.** Note that this study did not begin tracking annual use of these drugs until 2002. Data from Johnston et al. 2003.

but substantial number of youth at least experiment with illicit opioids such as heroin. For example, the European School Survey Project on Alcohol and Other Drug Use (ESPAD), an assessment of drug and alcohol use among 16-year-old students that is conducted in 30 European countries, found that in 1999 an average of 1 percent of students had a lifetime history of smoking heroin (Hibell et al. 2000). Rates of lifetime heroin use varied greatly between countries and by sex. For girls, the highest rates of lifetime heroin smoking were in Romania (9%), Latvia (6%), and Croatia (5%), whereas the highest rates for boys were in Romania (8%), Poland (7%), Latvia (6%), and Italy and Lithuania (5% each). Experimentation with heroin by youth was found throughout Europe, however, and was not limited to a few countries. These findings suggest that just as in adults, heroin experimentation and use should not be viewed as a unique phenomenon of a particular local geographical area. And, as in the United States, these rates suggest a potential growing problem with heroin use among youth.

The extent of illicit opioid use, the trends in its use, and the potential consequences of these trends emphasize the importance of understanding the characteristics of a science-based treatment for adolescent heroin and opioid users. In this chapter, we provide an overview of scientific knowledge to date regarding adolescent opiate use. First, we provide an overview of the characteristics of adolescent heroin and opiate users. Second, we describe treatments for opioid-abusing and opiate-dependent youth. Finally, we propose several clinically important areas where further study is needed to identify strategies to optimize treatment interventions for this population.

Characteristics of Adolescent Opioid Users

Data from Clinical Reports

Several studies were conducted in the 1960s and 1970s to examine the clinical profile of adolescent heroin users (Khuri et al. 1984; Kreek et al. 1986; Millman et al. 1978). These studies generally reported that heroin use among youth was strongly associated with delinquency, family dysfunction, deprived social and economic conditions, polydrug use, and psychiatric comorbidity (Chien et al. 1964; Noble and Barnes 1971; Wiener and Egan 1973). Studies of adolescent heroin users were then largely absent from the scientific literature for about 25 years, and only recently have a few studies systematically characterized the rapidly emerging cohort of adolescent heroin and opioid abusers (Crome et al. 1998; Gordon 2002; Hopfer et al. 2000, 2002; Marsch et al. 2003). These few reports have shown that, in general, adolescents who use heroin typically initiate drug use (including nicotine and alcohol) as early as 10 years of age, and many continue to abuse or become dependent on other drugs, including marijuana, cocaine, amphetamine, and other opiates, along with heroin. In addition, according to these reports, most adolescents using heroin appear to be male (about 53–68%) and white (about 80–97%) and report daily use of heroin (about 60%). About half of adolescent heroin users report use via an injection route of administration (approximately 45–57%). Moreover, many heroin-using adolescents have a number of legal problems and comorbid psychiatric problems, with the latter appearing to be particularly evident among female adolescent heroin users. Heroin-using adolescents have the highest rate of injection-drug use when compared with youth using other substances (Hopfer et al. 2000). Undoubtedly, injection-drug use by adolescent heroin users increases their risk of contracting and spreading hepatitis, the human immunodeficiency virus (HIV), and other serious diseases (Curran et al. 1988; Deas-Nesmith et al. 1999; Neaigus et al. 1998).

National Treatment Admission Data from the United States

Data from the U.S. Treatment Episode Data Set (TEDS), which characterizes admissions to the majority of substance abuse treatment facilities in the United States, reflect trends similar to those observed in the clinical reports described above (SAMHSA 2002b). Specifically, TEDS data indicate that male youth (aged 12–17 years) who use heroin and/or other opiates enter treatment with greater frequency than their female counterparts. Indeed, 51.4 and 63.1 percent of annual treatment admissions for youth using heroin and other opiates, respectively, are male, whereas 48.6 and 36.9 percent of admissions for youth using these substances, respectively, were female. Additionally, most treatment admissions for youth using heroin or other opiates are white (70.2 and 87.1%, respectively) and are typically referred to treatment either via the criminal justice system (approximately 30%) or via self-referral (approximately 26–33%).

National School Survey Data from the United States

Demographic data from the U.S., school-based Monitoring the Future study are also consistent with clinical reports and national treatment admissions data and indicate that the prevalence of heroin use among youth in eighth, tenth, and twelfth grades is slightly higher in males (0.8–1.3%) than females (0.8–1.0%) and among whites (1.0%) and Hispanics (0.8–1.2%) than blacks (0.3–0.6%). Additionally, 2.3 to 2.9 percent of youth in these grades who report they either do not plan to attend or graduate from college also report heroin use, whereas only about 0.7 percent of youth who report that they plan to complete college report use of heroin. Parental level of education is inversely related to heroin use among youth, with youth whose parents completed grade school or less having the highest rates of use (1.2–2.1%). Finally, heroin use among youth does not appear to be concentrated in a specific geographic location in the United States, but it is generally reported at comparable levels by youth in the Northeast, North Central, Southern, and Western areas of that country. Trends in the characteristics of youth who report sporadic use of narcotics other than heroin are similar to those reported for heroin-using youth, although level of parental education is not as strongly correlated with sporadic narcotic use among youth (Johnston et al. 2003).

Treatment of Adolescent Opioid Use

Although the scientific literature on the treatment of opioid dependence in adults is voluminous, only a small (but growing) body of research has examined effective treatments for adolescent opioid users. A few small-scale treatment studies were conducted in the 1960s and 1970s with adolescents who were abusing and dependent on opioids (see Hopfer et al. 2002 for a review of this literature). Unfortunately, these studies typically did not include control groups or random assignment to treatments. Additionally, many of these studies did not specifically focus on youth less than 18 years of age. Nonetheless, as reviewed in this section, several treatment options for adolescent opioid users exist, and rigorous scientific research to identify effective treatments for the emerging cohort of adolescent opioid users has recently been launched by our group and others.

Much of the current treatment offered to adolescent opioid users is medication free and is often offered in residential treatment settings, such as Therapeutic Communities (Sells and Simpson 1979). Although medication-free treatment may be useful with some opiate-abusing adolescents (Hopfer et al. 2002), the effectiveness of such treatment has not been systematically studied. Furthermore, medication-free treatment is unlikely to be effective with adolescents who meet criteria for opioid dependence (Hopfer et al. 2002). Although offering pharmacotherapy as part of a multicomponent intervention for youth dependent on opioids remains controversial in some settings (Crome 1999; Gilvarry 2000), providing a medication to this population to assist with discontinuation of illicit opiate use is likely critical to the success of the intervention. Specifically, because of the nature and pharmacology of opiate drugs, individuals who are physically dependent on opioids will experience a painful physical withdrawal syndrome if they abruptly discontinue their opiate use. The scientific literature examining effective treatments for adults dependent on opioids clearly indicates that pharmacotherapy is typically a necessary and acceptable component of effective opioid-withdrawal regimens. In addition, pharmacotherapy can be used in maintenance regimens to stabilize the brain neurochemistry of individuals dependent on opioids and prevent them from experiencing opiate withdrawal symptoms (Leshner 1997). Adolescents dependent on opioids would undoubtedly have a similar need for medication to aid them in successfully discontinuing illicit opiates. Moreover, offering pharmacotherapy to youth dependent on opioids is not markedly different from offering other medications to adolescents to treat psychiatric disorders and may be viewed simply as a subset to pediatric psychopharmacology.

Several opioid-agonist medications shown to be effective in the treatment of adults dependent on opioids may be similarly useful in medication-assisted detoxification or maintenance treatment with adolescents dependent on opioids. One such medication, the full mu opioid agonist methadone, has repeatedly been shown to produce marked reductions in illicit opioid use, criminal activity, and behavior that may place one at risk for infection with HIV, hepatitis, or other infectious diseases among adults dependent on opioids (Marsch 1998) (see chap. 6). Methadone may be similarly useful in the treatment of adolescents dependent on opioids. Indeed, some uncontrolled trials conducted in the early 1970s suggested that methadone treatment is associated with decreased heroin use and high treatment retention rates among heroin-using adolescents (DeAngelis and Lehmann 1973; Lloyd et al. 1974; Rosenberg and Patch 1972; see Hopfer et al. 2002 for a review). Additionally, clinical experience with methadone treatment for adolescents dependent on opioids further suggests its ability to promote high rates of treatment retention and improvements in employment and educational status (Hopfer et al. 2003).

In the United States, the Department of Health and Human Services (DHHS) has approved the limited use of methadone as a withdrawal agent for patients dependent on opioids who are less than 18 years of age. DHHS requirements indicate that withdrawal must be the first choice of treatment for individuals under the age of 18 who are addicted to narcotics. Individuals under 18 years of age may only be placed in maintenance treatment after they have at least two unsuccessful attempts at short-term detoxification or drug-free treatment. Moreover, adolescents may be admitted to maintenance treatment only if a "parent, legal guardian or responsible adult designated by the relevant State authority consents in writing to such treatment" (21 CFR Part 291). Note that this same DHHS regulation applies to the use of the full mu opioid agonist, LAAM, in the treatment of youth dependent on opioids. The effectiveness of LAAM, however, has not been systematically studied with adolescents dependent on opioids, nor is this medication currently being marketed for use in drug abuse treatment (see chap. 13).

The partial mu agonist buprenorphine may be a particularly useful medication in the treatment of adolescents dependent on opioids. Because of its pharmacologic profile, buprenorphine has a ceiling effect on its agonist activity, a lower abuse liability, and a better safety profile relative to full mu opioid agonists (see chap. 10). Buprenorphine's safety and efficacy as a pain medication has been clearly established in individuals as young as 9 months of age (Girotra et al. 1993; Harcus et al. 1980; Kamal and Khan 1995; Maunuksela et al. 1988), and it has been approved by the

Food and Drug Administration (FDA) in the United States for use in children, adolescents, and adults for this purpose. Buprenorphine has generally been shown to be as efficacious as methadone in adults dependent on opioids when equieffective doses of these medications are provided (see chap. 11). Buprenorphine may be similarly useful in the treatment of adolescents dependent on opioids who may have a shorter history of opioid use and/or lower levels of opioid dependence relative to their adult counterparts. In the United States, buprenorphine can be prescribed via a qualified physician in an office-based setting and via an opioid treatment program (see chap. 12). Thus, youth may have expanded treatment options with buprenorphine relative to methadone or LAAM.

To our knowledge, our group has conducted the only controlled trial evaluating the efficacy of buprenorphine in the treatment of adolescents dependent on opioids (Marsch et al. 2003). In this double-blind, double-dummy trial, we compared the relative efficacy of buprenorphine and the centrally active alpha$_2$-adrenergic agonist, clonidine, in a 28-day outpatient detoxification with adolescents dependent on opioids. Both medications were provided along with intensive and demonstrably efficacious behavioral interventions, including the Community Reinforcement Approach designed to increase nondrug sources of reinforcement for youth (Budney and Higgins 1998), thrice weekly urinalysis testing, monetary voucher incentives contingent on opiate abstinence and attendance, and thrice weekly individual counseling. Family counseling with an adolescent and his/her parent(s) was also provided and strongly encouraged. All participants were then offered the opportunity to transition to naltrexone treatment after the 28-day detoxification. During this aftercare phase, they received the opiate antagonist (blocker), naltrexone, for two months along with continued behavioral counseling and urinalysis testing.

Results indicated that a significantly greater percentage of participants who received buprenorphine (72%) were retained for the entire duration of the detoxification compared with participants receiving clonidine (39%). Additionally, participants in the buprenorphine group achieved greater opiate abstinence than members of the clonidine group (means of 64% and 32% opiate negative urine samples, respectively). Adolescents' self-reported risky drug-injection practices that may place them at risk for infection with HIV and hepatitis was markedly reduced from baseline levels to levels observed during treatment for both groups; however, the magnitude of this effect was greater among participants in the buprenorphine condition. In addition, the numerous measures we obtained to assess the safety of medication administration indicated that both medications were highly safe and did not produce adverse effects in participants. Importantly, 61 percent of participants in the buprenorphine group but only 5 percent of those in the clonidine group participated in the naltrexone aftercare phase of the study. This research demonstrates that combining buprenorphine with behavioral interventions is an effective treatment for youth dependent on opioids. In the United States, the FDA approval of buprenorphine for the treatment of opioid dependence allows for its use in patients dependent on opioids who are as young as 16 years of age (FDA 2002).

SUMMARY AND FUTURE DIRECTIONS

As reviewed in this chapter, a new cohort of adolescents abusing and dependent on opioids has emerged in recent years. Clearly, this trend and its associated potential consequences underscore the importance of expanded prevention and treatment interventions targeting this population. Recent research activities have provided important information regarding the clinical profile of this population. In addition, although several promising treatment interventions for adolescent opioid users are currently available to clinicians, additional research is needed to evaluate ways to optimize outcomes from both behavioral and pharmacologic treatments for adolescent opioid users. For example, our group plans to examine varying durations of pharmacotherapeutic interventions, including both detoxification and maintenance dosing regimens, to determine whether improved treatment outcomes can be achieved if the duration of the pharmacotherapy is lengthened. This research will help identify treatment durations that best minimize opiate withdrawal symptomatology and promote treatment retention and opiate abstinence. Another important research endeavor is the identification of optimal behavioral interventions that best help adolescent opiate users learn new skills and behaviors addressing how they might best discontinue their opiate use, prevent relapse to opiate use, and achieve their treatment goals. Moreover, understanding effective relapse prevention strategies for this population is critical. Such efforts may include the provision of the opioid antagonist naltrexone to youth. Naltrexone can be safely administered to both children (Campbell et al. 1993) and adolescents (Lifrak et al. 1997) for disorders other than opioid dependence. It may also be useful to provide naltrexone to youth who withdraw from illicit opiates to further increase the efficacy of opiate detoxification interventions, because, due to its pharmacology, naltrexone functions to prevent relapse to opioid use. These research activities will provide important empirical information regarding enhancing effective interventions for adolescent opioid use.

Acknowledgment

Preparation of this chapter was supported in part by National Institute on Drug Abuse Grant R03 DA 14570.

References

Budney AJ, Higgins ST (1998). A Community Reinforcement Plus Vouchers Approach: Treating Cocaine Addiction. DHHS Pub. No. 98-4309. Rockville, MD: U.S. Department of Health and Human Services.

Campbell M, Anderson LT, Small AM, Adams P, Gonzalez NM, Ernst M (1993). Naltrexone in autistic children: behavioral symptoms and attentional learning. *J Am Acad Child Adolesc Psychiatry* 32: 1283–91.

Chien I, Gerald DL, Lee RS, Rosenfeld E, Wilner DM (1964). *The Road to H: Narcotics, Delinquency, and Social Policy.* New York: Basic Books.

Crome IB (1999). Treatment interventions-looking towards the millennium. *Drug Alcohol Depend* 55: 247–63.

Crome IB, Christian J, Green C (1998). Tip of the national iceberg? Profile of adolescent patients prescribed methadone in an innovative community drug service. *Drug/Educ Prev Policy* 5: 195–7.

Curran JW, Jaffe HW, Hardy AM, Morgan WM, Selik RM, Dondero TJ (1988). Epidemiology of HIV infection and AIDS in the United States. *Science* 239: 610–6.

DeAngelis GG, Lehmann WX (1973). Adolescents and short term, low dose methadone maintenance. *Int J Addict* 8: 853–63.

Deas-Nesmith D, Brady KT, White R, Campbell S (1999). HIV-risk behaviors in adolescent substance abusers. *J Subst Abuse Treat* 16: 169–72.

FDA (2002). Suboxone (buprenorphine hydrochloride and naloxone hydrochloride)/Subutex (buprenorphine hydrochloride). Drug Label. Rockville, MD: U.S. Food and Drug Administration (www.fda.gov/cder/foi/label/2002/20732lbl.pdf)

Gilvarry E (2000). Substance abuse in young people. *J Child Psychol Psychiatry* 41: 55–80.

Girotra S, Kumar S, Rajendran KM (1993). Caudal buprenorphine for postoperative analgesia in children: a comparison with intramuscular buprenorphine. *Acta Anaesthesiol Scand* 37: 361–4.

Gordon SM (2002). Surprising data on young heroin users. *Brown Univ Child Adolesc Behav Lett* 18: 1, 3.

Harcus AW, Ward AE, Smith DW (1980). The monitored release of buprenorphine: results in the young. *J Int Med Res* 8: 153–5.

Harling R (1998). Heroin use among young people is increasing in England and Wales. *BMJ* 317: 431.

Hartnoll RL (1994). Opiates: prevalence and demographic factors. *Addiction* 89: 1377–83.

Hibell B, Andersson B, Ahlström S, Balakireva O, Bjarnason T, Kokkevi A, Morgan M (2000). *The 1999 ESPAD Report.* Stockholm: The Swedish Council for Information on Alcohol and Other Drugs, CAN Council of Europe.

Hopfer CJ, Khuri E, Crowley TJ (2003). Treating adolescent heroin use. *J Am Acad Child Adolesc Psychiatry* 42: 609–11.

Hopfer CJ, Khuri E, Crowley TJ, Hooks S (2002). Adolescent heroin use: a review of the descriptive and treatment literature. *J Subst Abuse Treat* 23: 231–37.

Hopfer CJ, Mikulich SK, Crowley TJ (2000). Heroin use among adolescents in treatment for substance use disorders. *J Am Acad Child Adolesc Psychiatry* 39: 1316–23.

Johnston LD, O'Malley PM, Bachman JG (2003). Monitoring the Future National Survey

Results on Drug Use, 1975–2002. Vol. I: Secondary School Students. NIH Pub. No. 03-5375. Bethesda, MD: National Institute on Drug Abuse.

Kamal RS, Khan FA (1995). Caudal analgesia with buprenorphine for postoperative pain relief in children. *Paediatr Anaesth* 5: 101–6.

Khuri ET, Millman RB, Hartman N, Kreek MJ (1984). Clinical issues concerning alcoholic youthful narcotic abusers. *Adv Alcohol Subst Abuse* 3: 69–86.

Kreek MJ, Khuri E, Fahey L, Miescher A, Arns P, Spagnoli D, Craig J, Millman R, Harte EH (1986). Long-term followup studies of the medical status of adolescent former heroin addicts in chronic methadone maintenance treatment: liver disease and immune status. *NIDA Res Monogr* 67: 307–9.

Leshner AI (1997). Addiction is a brain disease, and it matters. *Science* 278: 45–47.

Lifrak PD, Alterman AI, O'Brien CP, Volpicelli JR (1997). Naltrexone for alcoholic adolescents. *Am J Psychiatry* 154: 439–41.

Lloyd RA, Katon RN, DuPont RL (1974). Evolution of a treatment approach for young heroin addicts. Comparison of three treatment modalities. *Int J Addict* 9: 229–39.

Marsch LA (1998). The efficacy of methadone maintenance interventions in reducing illicit opiate use, HIV risk behavior and criminality: a meta-analysis. *Addiction* 93: 515–32.

Marsch LA, Bickel WK, Badger GJ, Stothart ME, Quesnel KJ, Stanger C (2003). Pharmacological and behavioral interventions for opioid-dependent adolescents: a randomized, controlled trial. Proceedings of the 65th Annual Scientific Meeting of the College on Problems of Drug Dependence. Bethesda, MD: National Institute on Drug Abuse, U.S. Department of Health and Human Services.

Maunuksela EL, Korpela R, Olkkola KT (1988). Comparison of buprenorphine with morphine in the treatment of postoperative pain in children. *Anesth Analg* 67: 233–9.

Millman RB, Khuri ET, Nyswander ME (1978). Therapeutic detoxification of adolescent heroin addicts. *Ann N Y Acad Sci* 311: 153–64.

Neaigus A, Atillasoy A, Friedman SR, Andrade X, Miller M, Ildefonso G, des Jarlais D (1998). Trends in the noninjecting use of heroin and factors associated with the transition to injecting. In: Inciardi JA, Harrison LD, eds. *Heroin in the Age of Crack Cocaine,* 131–59. Thousand Oaks, CA; Sage.

Noble P, Barnes GG (1971). Drug taking in adolescent girls: factors associated with the progression to narcotic use. *Br Med J* 2: 620–3.

Rosenberg CM, Patch VD (1972). Methadone use in adolescent heroin addicts. *JAMA* 220: 991–3.

SAMHSA (2002a). Results from the 2001 National Household Survey on Drug Abuse. Vol. II. Technical Appendixes and Selected Data Tables. DHHS Pub. No. SMA 02-3759. Rockville, MD: Substance Abuse and Mental Health Services Administration, Office of Applied Studies.

SAMHSA (2002b). Treatment Episode Data Set (TEDS): 1992–2000. National Admissions to Substance Abuse Treatment Services. DHHS Pub. No. (SMA) 02-3727. Rockville, MD: Substance Abuse and Mental Health Services Administration, Office of Applied Studies.

Schwartz RH (1998). Adolescent heroin use: a review. *Pediatrics* 102: 1461–6.

Sells SB, Simpson DD (1979). Evaluation of treatment outcome for youths in the Drug Abuse Reporting Program (DARP): a follow-up study. In: Beschner GM, Friedman AS, eds. *Youth Drug Abuse: Problems, Issues and Treatment.* Lanham, MD: Lexington Books.

Wiener JM, Egan JH (1973). Heroin addiction in an adolescent population. *J Am Acad Child Psychiatry* 12: 48–58.

23

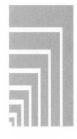

Prescription Opioid Nonmedical Use and Abuse

James P. Zacny, Ph.D.

Prescription opioid nonmedical use and abuse is not a new problem. It is a problem of growing concern, however, with survey data indicating that nonmedical use and abuse of prescription opioids is on the rise. This chapter reviews issues related to prescription opioid use and abuse in the United States, but misuse of prescription opioids is certainly not limited to the United States. The growing problem with prescription opioid use and abuse in the United States, data available about this misuse, and the response by both U.S. governmental agencies and professional organizations provide a particularly interesting example that may be instructive and useful for clinicians in the United States and in other parts of the world.

The rise of this misuse in the United States is impressive. For example, according to the 2000 report from the National Household Survey on Drug Abuse (NHSDA) (SAMHSA 2001), approximately 1.5 million persons used prescription opioids nonmedically for the first time in 1999. This number was quadruple the number of users in the mid-1980s, when the figure was less than 400,000 new users per year (see chap. 3).

Table 23.1 lists examples of prescription opioids available in the United States. Opioids can vary by being immediate-release (IR) versus controlled-release (CR) products. CR formulations are absorbed over a longer period than their IR counterparts. They can also vary with respect to being single-entity products and combination products (i.e., the latter

Table 23.1 **Some Prescription Opioids Currently Available**

Generic Name	Brand Name
Morphine	MS-Contin, Avinza, Kadian
Hydrocodone	Opioid constituent in Vicodin and Lortab
Oxycodone	Opioid constituent in Percocet and OxyContin
Codeine	Opioid constituent in Tylenol 3
Propoxyphene	Opioid constituent in Darvon, Darvocet
Methadone	Dolophine
Fentanyl	Actiq, Duragesic
Hydromorphone	Dilaudid
Tramadol	Ultram, Ultracet

being an opioid combined with a nonopioid analgesic such as acetaminophen). Finally, the route of prescribed administration can also vary and typically is either oral (swallowed), mucosal (absorbed through mouth membranes), parenteral (injected), or transdermal (absorbed through skin).

To understand the range of problematic prescription opioid use, three terms require definition: nonmedical use, abuse, and dependence. *Nonmedical use* refers to licit drugs (in this case, opioids) that are used "even once, that were not prescribed for you, or that you took only for the feeling or experience it caused" (SAMHSA 2003b). Nonmedical use is not a diagnostic category.

Abuse, on the other hand, can be used as a diagnostic category and has been defined by the American Psychiatric Association (APA) in its *Diagnostic and Statistical Manual of Mental Disorders* (DSM-IV-TR) (APA 2000). It is a maladaptive pattern of opioid use that has led to clinically significant impairment or distress (e.g., failure to fulfill major obligations at work, home, or school, or recurrent substance abuse-related legal problems).

Finally, *dependence* has also been defined by the APA in DSM-IV-TR and is a more severe form of opioid misuse. The DSM has seven criteria for the category of dependence, and a person must meet three of the seven criteria to qualify for the diagnosis of dependence (see table 9.2). The criteria include symptoms such as a persistent desire or unsuccessful effort to cut down or control opioid use; spending a great deal of time in activities necessary to obtain the opioid; tolerance; and physical dependence.

There has been a great deal of disagreement about the definitions of abuse and dependence because these terms mean different things to different people and organizations (Rinaldi et al. 1988; Savage et al. 2003;

Zacny et al. 2003). For the sake of consistency, when the terms "abuse" and "dependence" are used in this chapter the modifier "DSM-IV-TR" will be used to indicate when the these definitions are being specifically utilized.

The remainder of this chapter will address the following three issues related to prescription opioid misuse:

1. The epidemiology of nonmedical use and abuse of prescription opioids: How extensive is the problem, and how does it compare with use and abuse of other drugs? Who are the potential subpopulations of people that use prescription opioids nonmedically or abuse them? What personal or societal factors might be related to changing prevalence in abuse of prescription opioids?
2. Potential deterrents to diversion and abuse of prescription opioids: What are some programs that are or might be used to reduce the diversion and abuse of prescription opioids?
3. Treatment of prescription opioid dependence: What treatment modalities or interventions are available to people dependent on prescription opioids?

Epidemiology of Nonmedical Use and Abuse of Prescription Opioids

How Extensive Is the Problem?

Data from several national epidemiologic databases collected in the United States since 2000 indicate that there is a significant problem with nonmedical use and abuse of prescription opioids. These databases include the National Survey on Drug Use and Health (NSDUH), the Drug Abuse Warning Network (DAWN), the Monitoring the Future (MTF) project, and the Treatment Episode Data Set (TEDS). Several key points illuminate the seriousness of the problem.

National Survey on Drug Use and Health

NSDUH (formerly called the National Household Survey on Drug Abuse, or NHSDA) collects data on the incidence and prevalence of abused drugs by administering questionnaires each year to a random sample of the population that live in households (including shelters and rooming houses). Participants are 12 years of age and older. According to the 2002 report, the number of first-time nonmedical users of prescription opioids was estimated to be 2.4 million people, as compared with 0.6 million people in 1985 and 2 million people in 1999 (SAMHSA 2003b). Prevalence of lifetime, past-year, and past-month nonmedical use of prescription opioids in 2002 was estimated to be 12.6 percent, 4.7 percent, and 1.9 percent of the U.S. population, respectively. Two of the more widely abused drugs were hydrocodone combination products (estimated nonmedical users at least once in lifetime, 13.1 million people) and oxycodone single-entity and combination products (estimated nonmedical users at least once in lifetime, 9.7 million people). Estimated lifetime nonmedical use of OxyContin and methadone was less, but certainly not trivial, 1,924,000 and 928,000 people, respectively.

A component of this survey asks the same questions that are used by clinicians when assessing for substance abuse and dependence disorders as defined by the DSM-IV-TR criteria (APA 2000). However, these assessments are not conducted by trained clinicians. In the 2002 report, 573,000 respondents (an estimated 0.2% of the U.S. population 12 years of age and older) who reported nonmedical use of prescription opioids in the past year met DSM-IV-TR criteria for opioid abuse, and 936,000 (an estimated 0.4% of the U.S. population 12 years of age and older) who reported nonmedical use of prescription opioids in the past year met DSM-IV-TR criteria for opioid dependence. These data on rates of DSM-IV-TR abuse and dependence, although important, should be viewed with some caution because the application of these criteria is usually by skilled clinicians rather than through self-report questionnaires.

Monitoring the Future

The MTF project, funded by the National Institute on Drug Abuse (NIDA), surveys a representative sample of eighth, tenth, and twelfth graders in public and private schools in the coterminous United States to ascertain their nonmedical use of drugs (Johnston et al. 2003). Only twelfth graders are asked about their use of psychotherapeutic drugs ". . . on your own—that is, without a doctor telling you to take them." Prevalence of lifetime, past-year, and past-month use of "narcotics other than heroin" among twelfth graders in 2002 was estimated to be 10.1 percent, 7.0 percent, and 3.1 percent, respectively. Compared with 1992, these figures represent an increase of 66 percent for lifetime use, 112 percent for past-year use, and 158 percent for past-month use. Students were also asked about what specific opioids they had used without a doctor's order in the past year: 0.9 percent reported that they had used methadone; comparable exposure rates were 1.6 percent for OxyContin, 1.9 percent for Percocet, 4.1 percent for Vicodin, and 4.4 percent for codeine.

Drug Abuse Warning Network

DAWN collects information on drug-related visits to emergency departments (EDs) at selected hospitals throughout the country (SAMHSA 2003a). The number of mentions of specific psychotropic drugs during drug-related visits to the ED is a key endpoint in this database. From 1995 to 2002, the number of mentions of opioid analgesics (single-entity and combination products) increased from 45,254 to 119,185, an increase of 163 percent. The number of opioid analgesic mentions in 2002 comprised 10 percent of the total number of ED mentions for that year. Broken down into specific drugs, the number of mentions of hydrocodone combination products increased from 1995 to 2002 by 160 percent (from 9,686 to 25,197) and the number of mentions of oxycodone single-entity and combination products increased during this same period by 560 percent (from 3,393 to 22,397). Hydrocodone is prescribed three times as much as oxycodone products (Zacny et al. 2003), but the number of mentions in 2002 is nearly identical. The number of mentions of methadone increased by 176 percent from 1995 (4,247) to 2002 (11,709).

Treatment Episode Data Set

TEDS is a compilation of data on the demographic characteristics and substance abuse problems of those admitted to substance abuse treatment facilities (primarily those receiving some form of public funding) (SAMHSA 2003c, 2004) and includes the primary drug class or drug that brought people into the center for treatment. One of the categories of drugs is "opiates other than heroin" and it is synonymous with prescription opioids (including methadone). The number of treatment admissions because of prescription opioid abuse was relatively stable from 1992 to 1997 (13,555 in 1992 to 16,274 in 1997), but increased markedly to 45,605 admissions by 2002 (SAMHSA 2004). From 1992 to 2002, treatment admissions for "opiates other than heroin" increased by 236 percent. The number of admissions for methadone abuse increased by 109 percent, from 1,198 in 1992 to 2,504 in 2002. Unfortunately, one cannot tell what percentage of admissions came from abuse of liquid methadone (used in methadone maintenance centers) versus methadone tablets (prescribed for pain relief).

How Does the Magnitude of Nonmedical Use of Prescription Opioids Compare to Other Drugs?

Some of the numbers and percentages reported in the previous section are large, but it is useful to put them into the context of non-medical use and abuse of other drugs. Table 23.2 presents data for past year non-medical use (or use in the case of alcohol and tobacco), and past year DSM-IV-TR dependence for drug classes and specific drugs.

From table 23.2 we can see the following:

- Among the psychotherapeutic drug classes examined, opioids were the class with the greatest nonmedical use and dependence.
- Past-year prevalence of alcohol and tobacco use far exceeded non-medical use of prescription opioids, and prevalence of marijuana use was double that of prescription opioids. Similarly, past-year prevalence of alcohol and marijuana dependence exceeded prevalence of dependence on prescription opioids.
- The proportion of nonmedical prescription opioid users who report DSM-IV-TR dependence problems (8.5%) is far lower than the proportion of heroin users who report such problems (49%)

Table 23.2 **Persons Reporting Past-Year Use and Past-Year Dependence for Licit and Illicit Drugs in 2002**

	Past-Year Users		Past-Year Dependence		
	Number (in thousands)	% (pop)	Number (in thousands)	% (pop)	% (users)*
Alcohol	155,476	66.1	8,222	3.5	5.3
Tobacco	84,731	36.0	—†		
Marijuana and hashish	25,755	11.0	2,614	1.1	10.1
Cocaine	5,902	2.5	1,025	0.4	17.4
Heroin	404	0.2	198	0.1	49.0
Hallucinogens	4,749	2.0	136	0.1	2.9
Inhalants	2,084	0.9	47	0.0	2.3
Psychotherapeutic drugs					
Opioids	10,992	4.7	936	0.4	8.5
Tranquilizers	4,849	2.1	251	0.1	5.2
Stimulants	3,181	1.4	259	0.1	8.1
Sedatives	981	0.4	131	0.1	13.4

Source: SAMHSA 2003a, based on data from the National Survey on Drug Use and Health
Note: U.S. population (pop) aged 12 years or older
*Reflects percentage of past-year users who reported past-year dependence
†Data not collected by SAMHSA

and also lower than the proportion of cocaine users with DSM-IV-TR dependence (17.4%).

- The proportion of nonmedical prescription opioid users who report DSM-IV-TR dependence problems (8.5%) is similar to the proportion of users reporting DSM-IV-TR dependence on alcohol (5.3%), marijuana (10.1%), stimulants (8.1%), tranquilizers (5.2%), or sedatives (13.3%) and is somewhat higher than the proportion of those who use hallucinogens (2.9%) and inhalants (2.3%).

Note that heroin use is thought to be underestimated by the NSDUH (GAO 1998). Two other sources place prevalence of heroin dependence at approximately 600,000–800,000 persons (National Consensus Development Panel 1998; ONDCP 1997) rather than the 198,000 indicated in table 23.2. This would suggest that prevalence of heroin and nonprescription opioid use may be more similar than indicated in table 23.2.

Two final pieces of information from the TEDS and DAWN databases lend additional perspective to the data from the NSDUH in table 23.2. In 2002, there were 1,882,584 admissions for substance abuse at treatment centers that collected data for TEDS. Of these admissions, only 2.4 percent were for opiates other than heroin. In contrast, 15 percent and 43 percent of all admissions involved heroin and alcohol abuse, respectively (SAMHSA 2004). This suggests that relatively few people develop problems associated with prescription opioid use that lead them to seek treatment. However, DAWN data provide convincing evidence that nonmedical use and abuse of prescription opioids does have a sizable impact on public health: in the 2002 DAWN report, prescription opioids were mentioned 119,185 times during emergency room visits, similar to the numbers for heroin (93,519) and marijuana (119,472) (SAMHSA 2003a).

What Are the Demographics and Potential Subpopulations That Are Involved in the Nonmedical Use of Prescription Opioids?

Teenagers and adults in their early 20s are more likely than people aged 26 years or older to be nonmedical users and abusers of prescription opioids. From the 2002 NSDUH report, prevalence of past-year nonmedical use of prescription opioids in people aged 12–17 years, 18–25 years, and 26 years or older was 7.6 percent, 11.4 percent, and 3.1 percent, respectively (SAMHSA 2003b). Prevalence of past-year dependence for the three age groups was 0.5 percent, 0.8 percent, and 0.3 percent, respectively. Females were as likely to report lifetime nonmedical use as males. The TEDS database contains demographic data on those people admitted into treatment centers for abuse or dependence on "opiates other than heroin" (i.e., prescription opioids). For 2002, the average age on admission was 35 years and males comprised 54 percent of these admissions (SAMHSA 2004). Of patients admitted for "opiates other than heroin," 88 percent were white (non-Hispanic). Whether the same racial/ethnicity make-up exists in nonmedical users and abusers of prescription opioids not seeking treatment is unknown. Seventy-five percent of patients reported abusing prescription opioids via the oral route.

The population that abuses prescription opioids may be composed of several distinct subpopulations, as discussed in a position paper on the nonmedical use and abuse of prescription opioids written by the College on Problems of Drug Dependence (CPDD) taskforce (Zacny et al. 2003). These subpopulations may include:

1. persons who abuse or are dependent on only prescription opioids;
2. heroin users who use prescription opioids to supplement or substitute for heroin;
3. users or abusers of others drugs who concomitantly use prescription opioids;
4. methadone maintenance patients;
5. patients with pain who develop de novo problems with abuse or dependence on prescription opioids in the course of legitimate treatment; and
6. patients with chronic nonmalignant pain who have a history of substance abuse.

Data support the existence of the first four subpopulations. For example, a study conducted in Ontario, Canada, provides support for the first two subpopulations (Brands et al. 2004). In that study, retrospective chart reviews were conducted on new admissions that entered methadone treatment centers between 1997 and 1999 for either prescription opioid or heroin dependence. Two subgroups of prescription opioid abusers emerged: those who used prescription opioids only (24% of the entire group), and those who had used heroin but then began abusing prescription opioids when heroin was not available or when they tried to withdraw from heroin (35% of the entire group). Similarly, in TEDS data from 2001, 43 percent of treatment admissions for "narcotics other than heroin" involved people who did not abuse other substances (SAMHSA 2003c).

The TEDS database also provides evidence for the existence of the third subpopulation, polysubstance abusers. Fifty-seven percent of admissions for "narcotics other than heroin" in the year 2001 involved people who also reported abuse of another drug, and the drugs most frequently mentioned were alcohol, marijuana, and tranquilizers (SAMHSA 2003c). Additional support for the polydrug pattern of abuse comes from DAWN. In 2002, 31 percent of ED visits that involved nonmedical use of hydrocodone and 33 percent of the ED visits involving oxycodone also involved the use of alcohol. Thus, one in three people coming into the ED with problems related to oxycodone and hydrocodone had also ingested alcohol.

Methadone maintenance patients are a fourth potential subpopulation of nonmedical users and abusers of prescription opioids. Evidence that prescription opioids are being used illicitly by some methadone maintenance patients comes from a program run by the Office on National Drug Control Policy (ONDCP) called Pulse Check (www.whitehousedrugpolicy .gov/publications/drugfact/pulsechk/january04/index.html). In brief, Pulse Check consists of four sources: ethnographers, epidemiologists, treatment providers, and law enforcement officials; they provide a snapshot of drug abuse patterns in 25 cities in the United States. In the fall of 2002, a methadone treatment provider from each of the cities was asked, "What drugs do clients in a methadone program use?" Of the 20 providers who answered this question, 15 mentioned illicit use of prescription opioids. In many cases the percentages given were small (5%) and usually involved OxyContin or hydrocodone products. However, in some cities, including Atlanta, Cincinnati, and Tampa/St. Petersburg, percentages of OxyContin abuse cited were at 30 percent or greater.

A great deal of controversy exists regarding the fifth potential subpopulation of nonmedical users and abusers of prescription opioids: patients with pain without a history of substance abuse problems who may develop new problems with abuse or dependence on prescription opioids in the course of legitimate treatment for their pain problems. The controversy is whether this group should be considered at risk for problems with prescription opioids. Unfortunately, few data are available that estimate the prevalence of prescription opioid abuse in patients with pain who have no addiction history. In the study by Brands et al. (2004), the researchers found that 86 percent of persons who only abused prescription opioids had cited pain as the initial reason for using the drugs. In another study in which current methadone maintenance patients were interviewed ($N = 248$), 61.3 percent of the patients reported chronic pain, and of these patients, 44 percent believed that opioids prescribed for their pain had led to an addiction process (Jamison et al. 2000). Because many of these patients reported life-long problems with substance abuse, however, their substance abuse history may have predisposed them to become addicted to opioids. Because of the public health significance of the issue, there has been a call for studies to explicitly address the question of whether opioids prescribed for pain can engender new cases of addiction in individuals without substance abuse histories (Sellers 2003).

A final related subpopulation at potential risk for nonmedical use and abuse of prescription opioids is patients with chronic nonmalignant pain who have a history of current or past substance abuse and are receiving prescription opioids as part of the pain treatment plan. Here, too, there has been insufficient research to address the issue. One small-sample study examined prevalence of prescription opioid abuse in patients with prior histories of substance abuse. In that study, 20 patients with a dual history of chronic nonmalignant pain and substance abuse were treated at a pain clinic with chronic opioid therapy for at least a year (Dunbar and Katz 1996). The substances abused before clinic treatment included alcohol, injectable opioids, and prescription opioids (chiefly oxycodone). Nine of the 20 patients showed behaviors, usually early in the course of therapy, that suggested opiate abuse (e.g., losing or reporting prescriptions as "stolen"). These patients were more likely to have had a recent history of polysubstance abuse and oxycodone abuse than patients who did not display such potential drug-seeking behaviors. The latter patients, who did not display drug-seeking behaviors, were more likely to have abused only alcohol and to be active members of Alcoholics Anonymous. This study needs to be replicated with a much larger sample, so that more definitive conclusions can be drawn about what types and patterns of prior substance abuse are risk factors for opioid abuse when opioids are prescribed for the treatment of chronic pain. Also, studies are needed to examine the relative risk of prescription opioid abuse in patients with a history of substance abuse compared with those without such a history (Savage 1999).

The general consensus in the chronic pain treatment community is that patients with chronic nonmalignant pain who are current or past substance abusers may be at increased risk for misusing or abusing prescription opioids that are part of their treatment program (Compton and Athanasos 2003; Portenoy 1996; Savage 1999; Weaver and Schnoll 2002), compared with patients without a substance abuse history. There also appears to be a consensus, however, that patients with substance abuse problems should be given opioid therapy if medically indicated (Miyoshi and Leckband 2001; Passik 2001; Savage 1999; Weaver and Schnoll 2002), but that the physician in charge of the opioid therapy needs to monitor these patients more closely than patients without a history of substance abuse (Passik and Kirsh 2004; Weaver and Schnoll 2002). Explicit guidelines exist for how to monitor these patients, including the use of a medication agreement, monitoring urine drug screens, and pill counts (Passik and Kirsh 2004; Weaver and Schnoll 2002).

What Factors Might Be Related to Changing Prevalence in the Abuse of Prescription Opioids?

Because of fears surrounding the potential for opioid addiction, pain tends to be undertreated (Cleeland et al. 1994; Marks and Sachar 1973; Tamayo-Sarver et al. 2003). During the past 10 years, there has been increased emphasis on providing appropriate treatment for pain, both acute and chronic, treatment that in some cases involves opioid therapy (JCAHO 2003; Joranson et al. 2002b). This increased emphasis on appropriate management of pain has no doubt played a role in the increased amount of opioids produced for distribution to medical facilities and retail and mail-order pharmacies (Zacny et al. 2003). As the quantity of drugs available for licit purposes increases, availability for illicit purposes also may increase.

The relationship between availability and prevalence of abuse was examined in one retrospective study that compared the amount of morphine, fentanyl, oxycodone, and hydromorphone distributed at the retail level with the number of DAWN mentions (as a proxy for drug abuse) for each of those drugs between 1990 and 1996 (Joranson et al. 2000). Amount of drug available for licit purposes increased during that period, but the number of ED mentions remained relatively stable. In 2003, the CPDD taskforce on nonmedical use and abuse of prescription opioids did a similar analysis, again comparing DAWN data with the number of prescriptions dispensed for five drugs, the four listed here and hydrocodone (Zacny et al. 2003). The period from 1994 to 2001 was examined. The number of prescriptions dispensed for each of the drugs increased across that period, as did the number of DAWN mentions. The reason for the discrepancy between the two studies is not clear, but it may suggest that the rise in prescription opioid abuse is a relatively recent phenomenon.

A causal relationship between availability and illicit use may be impossible to demonstrate, but it appears that availability may be a factor that is related to the increase in nonmedical use and abuse of prescription opioids. Another plausible factor, but also one that is hard to document, is that media attention surrounding abuse of drugs such as OxyContin and Vicodin may serve to inform people with a propensity to abuse drugs about the local availability of prescription opioids. These issues create a tension between the desire to have medications available for legitimate use in medical practice and the public health problems created when these medications are diverted for illicit use.

STRATEGIES TO REDUCE THE DIVERSION AND NONMEDICAL USE AND ABUSE OF PRESCRIPTION OPIOIDS

Because opioids are available for legitimate use, there are several ways in which they can be obtained for misuse or abuse. Diversion methods include prescription forgeries, pharmacy robberies, and "doctor shopping" (individuals who routinely visit multiple doctors with the same ailment to obtain multiple prescriptions). Pharmacists or pharmacy technicians may falsify records and subsequently sell the drugs, patients may sell their prescription opioids to others, people may steal opioids out of medicine cabinets, and doctors may sell prescriptions to abusers or drug dealers (Zacny et al. 2003). In the United States, several federal, state, and local agencies, as well as committees and subcommittees in federal and state legislations, are addressing the problem of diversion and abuse of prescription opioids. To describe all these efforts is beyond the scope of this chapter. Rather, a selected number of initiatives will be described briefly.

In the Unites States, three federal agencies involved in preventing and reducing the diversion and abuse of prescription opioids are the Drug Enforcement Administration (DEA), the Food and Drug Administration (FDA), and the Office of National Drug Control Policy (ONDCP).

Drug Enforcement Administration

The federal DEA, part of the Department of Justice, administers the Controlled Substances Act (CSA) of 1970. Medications are categorized by the DEA according to their abuse potential through criteria laid out in the CSA. Those drugs with high abuse potential and no currently accepted use in medical treatment in the United States are placed in the highest or most restricted category (Schedule I). Drugs with low abuse potential and currently accepted medical use are in the lowest category (Schedule V). Prescription opioids such as morphine and oxycodone are categorized in Schedule II and have special restrictions placed on them because of their high potential for abuse. These restrictions include a requirement that the prescription is hand written (i.e., no telephone or internet orders are accepted), and no refill option is allowed. The mere existence of a scheduling system is thought to be an important deterrent to diversion. Another mandate of the CSA is to prevent, detect, and investigate the diversion of legally manufactured substances. To that end, the DEA Office of Diversion Control is engaged in multiple activities, including but not limited to coordinating major investigations, establishing national drug production quotas, fulfilling U.S. obligations under drug control treaties, designing and proposing national legislation, controlling imports and exports of drugs and chemicals, monitoring and tracking the distribution of certain controlled drugs, and providing of distribution intelligence to the states. Although one of the charges of the DEA is to prevent and reduce drug diversion, including diversion of prescription opioids, the DEA also is responsible for ensuring the widespread availability of these opioids for the medical community and patients who need these medications for pain relief.

Food and Drug Administration

The Food and Drug Administration (FDA) is responsible for protecting the public health by assuring the safety, efficacy, and security of drugs used by humans. Once a drug is approved by the FDA and is available to physicians, a voluntary postmarketing surveillance system called MedWatch allows doctors, patients, and the sponsor (i.e., drug manufacturer) to report adverse events to the FDA. MedWatch has been criticized for underestimating adverse events, including abuse-related events (Arfken and Cicero 2003). The FDA though utilizes several other means for ongoing assessment of a drug's safety profile (or its abuse), including data from the World Health Organization, federal databases such as DAWN, and FDA contracts and grants. Another process under development by the FDA is risk management. The FDA will most likely require sponsors of prescription opioids that have abuse potential (or that have been abused in other countries) to submit risk management plans (RMPs) with strategies for (1) monitoring the use of these drugs, (2) identifying potential abuse and diversion problems, and (3) developing plans to address those abuse and diversion problems. Monitoring the licit use of drugs could come from governmental sources such as the DEA, or industry, such as IMS Health, a for-profit company that collects quantitative data on prescription drugs that are dispensed from various licit channels of trade (i.e., retail pharmacies, long-term care, and mail order) (www.imshealth.com, accessed June 1, 2004). Monitoring the abuse/diversion of these drugs might be accomplished via the Internet (chat rooms), surveys of entrants into drug treatment programs, surveys of law enforcement agencies and physicians, "key informant" networks, and "street" ethnographers. Strategies to prevent and reduce diversion might include educational efforts designed for pharmacists, physicians, and patients about potential misuse or abuse of these drugs, as well as involvement of the DEA and law enforcement agencies. At present there are no established guidelines for risk management plans or how their efficacy would be evaluated (Balster and Bigelow 2003).

Office of National Drug Control Policy

The Office of National Drug Control Policy (ONDCP), an umbrella organization originating from the White House, is charged with leading the U.S. efforts against drug abuse by developing policy and initiatives to reduce both the supply and demand of illicit drugs and the abuse and nonmedical use of prescription drugs. In March 2004, ONDCP along with the Surgeon General of the United States, the DEA, and the FDA released the President's National Drug Control Strategy (www.whitehousedrugpolicy .gov/news/press04/030104.html). One of the principal aims of this strategy is to outline the extent of prescription drug abuse and initiate federal programs designed to address the problem. The DEA and FDA, for example, will address the proliferation of internet e-pharmacies that inappropriately prescribe drug, including opioids, to people who may abuse and/or sell them.

In addition to these three federal agencies, two other stakeholder programs are involved in monitoring prescription opioid abuse:

State Prescription-Monitoring Programs

The purpose of prescription-monitoring programs (PMPs) is to reduce the diversion of prescription controlled substances. These programs are state initiated and components can vary but usually include a computer-based system that collects prescribing and dispensing data from pharmacies, conducts reviews and analyses of the data, and disseminates them to appropriate regulatory and law enforcement agencies. By using PMPs, certain diversion methods such as "doctor shopping," scams, and illicit prescribing and dispensing can be identified (Joranson et al. 2002a). Unfortunately, as of March 2004, only 20 states have PMPs (www .deadiversion.usdoj.gov/faq/rx_monitor.htm#1) and there is a lack of uniformity and coordination between them (Manchikanti et al. 2002). One of two recent initiatives to address this problem is a call for a nationwide federally run PMP (Manchikanti et al. 2002); the other, a PMP

Model Act, provides a statutory framework to establish new and update existing PMPs based on the best practices of the states that currently run PMPs (www.nascsa.org/rxmonnascsa.htm).

The Pharmaceutical Industry

The risk management plans (RMPs) discussed earlier have sometimes been a joint collaboration between pharmaceutical industries and the FDA—this is one way the industry is involved in preventing abuse and diversion of prescription opioids. Another way is by developing new formulations of existing opioids with the intent to reduce their abuse liability by making them more tamperproof than products already on the market. Some of those new formulations include sequestering drugs in a polymer/cross-linking matrix so that crushing a tablet or pill does not make the entire amount of the drug immediately available. Another approach is to add an opioid antagonist that is poorly absorbed when taken orally but that precipitates withdrawal in physically dependent users upon injection (such as the buprenorphine/naloxone combination, Suboxone). Yet another innovation is to add irritants such as capsaicin to a formulation; this is innocuous if the drug is swallowed whole, but if crushed and then swallowed, snorted, or injected, the capsaicin can produce extreme pain (Woolf and Hashmi 2004).

TREATMENT OF INDIVIDUALS DEPENDENT ON PRESCRIPTION OPIOIDS

The first issue that must be addressed in considering treatment is the level of abuse and dependence shown by the individual using prescription opioids. A careful clinical interview aimed at determining abuse and dependence diagnosis is needed to determine the need for treatment. A second issue that must be taken into account is whether the individual has a history or current diagnosis of abuse or dependence on other drugs (e.g., cocaine). If a positive history and/or current abuse exists, then treatment for co-occurring dependencies is warranted.

A third issue is whether the person dependent on prescription opioids is in chronic pain. If the person dependent on prescription opioids is in chronic pain, in some cases they can be tapered off prescription opioids and other pain management therapies can be used (e.g., nonopioid pharmacotherapy). In other cases this may not be an option, because nonopioid therapies are ineffectual. In these circumstances, and as discussed briefly earlier in this chapter, the physician can prescribe opioids but should monitor the patient more closely. This includes establishing a written contract or agreement designed to prevent drug-seeking behavior and escalation of prescription opioid use. Recommended components in a contract include: the patient should be seen by only one doctor (or a single practice) and use only one pharmacy; if a prescription is lost, misplaced, or stolen, or if it is used up sooner than prescribed, the prescription is not replaced; the patient agrees to deliver urine samples at periodic unannounced times to ascertain adherence to the plan of care as well as a screen for other psychoactive drugs not prescribed by the pain management physician; the patient also agrees to active participation in an addiction recovery program; and the physician has the right to taper the patient off the opioid therapy if the patient does not comply with the rules in the contract (Fishman et al. 1999; Passik and Kirsh 2004; Weaver and Schnoll 2002).

For people who are dependent on prescription opioids but not in chronic pain, the current treatment options for them are the same options used to treat heroin dependence. To date, there have been no specialized treatments developed for people dependent on prescription opioids. One pharmacotherapy option for them is methadone maintenance. For patients entering a methadone program, special care should be taken during the induction phase by increasing the methadone dose cautiously, because levels of tolerance and dependence may be difficult to predict based on reports of prescription opioid use obtained from the patient. The evidence shows that some patients entering treatment for prescription opioid dependence do enroll in methadone maintenance programs; in the 2002 TEDS report, 19.2 percent of prescription opioid abusers interviewed reported entering a program that had methadone planned as part of the treatment. Another recently available pharmacotherapy option is office-based buprenorphine therapy (see chap. 12). Other treatment options include naltrexone maintenance (see chap. 14), opioid detoxification (see chap. 16), and drug-free programs (12-step, therapeutic communities; chap. 15). In general, treatment outcomes have not been tracked for prescription opioid abusers entering community treatment programs. Research is clearly needed to evaluate what treatments are most efficacious for prescription opioid dependence.

Conclusions

Prescription opioids are important for the treatment of acute and chronic pain, but they are subject to misuse and abuse. In this chapter, the epidemiology of the nonmedical use and abuse of prescription opioids, current and proposed methods to reduce diversion and abuse of prescription opioids, and treatment options for prescription opioid abusers were discussed. The problem of nonmedical use and abuse of prescription opioids has increased in the last several years, and there is little indication that the problem is abating. Several different subpopulations may abuse prescription opioids (e.g., heroin abusers, polydrug abusers, patients receiving methadone, and patients with pain and histories of drug abuse). Several organizations have developed or are in the process of developing programs aimed at reducing diversion and abuse of prescription opioids. There are a number of treatment options for those dependent on prescription opioids, but research is needed to determine what options are efficacious.

In closing, the word "balance" has been used frequently when discussing prescription opioids as both licit drugs with a clear clinical indication and as drugs that are used illicitly (Hoffman and Tarzian 2003; Joranson et al. 2002a; Regan and Alderson 2003; Zacny et al. 2003; www.deadiversion.usdoj.gov/pubs/pressrel/painrelief.pdf). Extreme restriction on their availability (to control abuse) runs the risk of limiting their appropriate clinical use in a population with pain that can benefit from their appropriate use. On the other hand, ready availability may increase the chance of diversion and abuse. The emphasis on reducing prescription opioid abuse needs to be balanced with the need to make these drugs readily available to physicians and patients for the treatment of pain (WHO 2000). This balance can be best achieved through shared understanding of the issues through combined and coordinated efforts of medical prescribers, regulatory agencies, and treatment providers.

Acknowledgment
The preparation of this chapter was funded by USPHS Grant R37 DA08573.

References
APA (2000). *Diagnostic and Statistical Manual of Mental Disorders, 4th ed. Text Revision.* Washington, DC: American Psychiatric Association.
Arfken CL, Cicero TJ (2003). Postmarketing surveillance for drug abuse. *Drug Alcohol Depend* 70: S97–S105.
Balster RL, Bigelow GE (2003). Guidelines and methodological reviews concerning drug abuse liability assessment. *Drug Alcohol Depend* 70: S13–S40.
Brands B, Blake J, Sproule B, Gourlay D, Busto U (2004). Prescription opioid abuse in patients presenting for methadone maintenance treatment. *Drug Alcohol Depend* 73: 199–207.
Cleeland CS, Gonin R, Hatfield AK, Edmonson JH, Blum RH, Stewart JA, Pandya KJ (1994). Pain and its treatment in outpatients with metastatic cancer. *N Engl J Med* 330: 592–6.

Compton P, Athanasos P (2003). Chronic pain, substance abuse and addiction. *Nurs Clin North Am* 38: 525–37.

Dunbar SA, Katz NP (1996). Chronic opioid therapy for nonmalignant pain in patients with a history of substance abuse: report of 20 cases. *J Pain Symptom Manage* 11: 163–71.

Fishman SM, Bandman TB, Edwards A, Borsook D (1999). The opioid contract in the management of chronic pain. *J Pain Symptom Manage* 18: 27–37.

GAO (1998). *Drug Abuse Treatment: Data Limitations Affect the Accuracy of National and State Estimates of Need.* Washington, DC: U.S. General Accounting Office.

Hoffman DE, Tarzian AJ (2003). Achieving the right balance in oversight of physician opioid prescribing pain: the role of state medical boards. *J Law Med Ethics* 31: 21–40.

Jamison RN, Kauffman J, Katz NP (2000). Characteristics of methadone maintenance patients with chronic pain. *J Pain Symptom Manage* 19: 53–62.

JCAHO (2003). *Approaches to Pain Management: An Essential Guide for Clinical Leaders.* Lombard, IL: Joint Commission Resources.

Johnston LD, O'Malley PM, Bachman JG (2003). Monitoring the Future National Survey Results on Drug Use, 1975–2002. Vol. I: Secondary School Students. NIH Pub. No. 03-5375. Bethesda, MD: National Institute on Drug Abuse.

Joranson DE, Carrow GM, Ryan KM, Schaefer L, Gilson AM, Good P, Eadie J, Peine S, Dahl JL (2002a). Pain management and prescription monitoring. *J Pain Symptom Manage* 23: 231–8.

Joranson DE, Gilson AM, Dahl JL, Haddox JD (2002b). Pain management, controlled substances, and state medical board policy: a decade of change. *J Pain Symptom Manage* 23: 138–47.

Joranson DE, Ryan KM, Gilson AM, Dahl JL (2000). Trends in medical use and abuse of opioid analgesics. *JAMA* 283: 1710–4.

Manchikanti L, Brown KR, Singh V (2002). National All Schedules Prescription Electronic Reporting Act (NASPER). *Pain Physician* 5: 294–319.

Marks RM, Sachar EJ (1973). Undertreatment of medical inpatients with narcotic analgesics. *Ann Intern Med* 78: 173–81.

Miyoshi HR, Leckband SG (2001). Systemic opioid analgesics. In: Loeser JD, ed. *Bonica's Management of Pain*, 1682–1709. Philadelphia: Lippincott, Williams and Wilkins.

National Consensus Development Panel on Effective Medical Treatment of Opiate Addiction. (1998). Effective medical treatment of opiate addiction. *JAMA* 280: 1936–43.

ONDCP (1997). *What America's Users Spend on Illegal Drugs: 1988–1995.* Rockville, MD: Office of National Drug Control Policy.

Passik SD (2001). Responding rationally to recent report of abuse/diversion of Oxycontin. *J Pain Symptom Manage* 21: 359.

Passik SD, Kirsh KL (2004). Opioid therapy in patients with a history of substance abuse. *CNS Drugs* 18: 13–25.

Portenoy RK (1996). Opioid therapy for chronic nonmalignant pain: a review of the critical issues. *J Pain Symptom Manage* 11: 203–17.

Regan JJ, Alderson A (2003). OxyContin: maintaining availability and efficacy while preventing diversion and abuse. *Tenn Med* 96: 88–90.

Rinaldi RC, Steindler EM, Wilford BB, Goodwin D (1988). Clarification and standardization of substance abuse terminology. *JAMA* 259: 555–7.

SAMHSA (2001). Summary of Findings from the 2000 National Household Survey on Drug Abuse. DHHS Pub. No. (SMA) 01-3549. Rockville, MD: Substance Abuse and Mental Health Services Administration, Office of Applied Studies.

SAMHSA (2003a). Emergency Department Trends from the Drug Abuse Warning Network, Final Estimates 1995–2002. DHHS Pub. No. (SMA) 03-3780. Rockville, MD: Substance Abuse and Mental Health Services Administration, Office of Applied Studies.

SAMHSA (2003b). Overview of Findings from the 2002 National Survey on Drug Use and Health. DHHS Pub. No. (SMA) 03-3774. Rockville, MD: Substance Abuse and Mental Health Services Administration, Office of Applied Studies.

SAMHSA (2003c). Treatment Episode Data Set (TEDS): 1992–2001. National Admissions to Substance Abuse Treatment Services. DHHS Pub. No. (SMA) 03-3778. Rockville, MD: Substance Abuse and Mental Health Services Administration, Office of Applied Studies.

SAMHSA (2004). Treatment Episode Data Set (TEDS). Highlights–2002. DHHS Pub. No. (SMA) 04-3946. Rockville, MD: Substance Abuse and Mental Health Services Administration, Office of Applied Studies.

Savage SR (1999). Opioid therapy of chronic pain: assessment of consequences. *Acta Anaesthesiol Scand* 43: 909–17.

Savage SR, Joranson DE, Covington EC, Schnoll SH, Heit HA, Gilson AM (2003). Definitions related to the medical use of opioids: evolution towards universal agreement. *J Pain Symptom Manage* 26: 655–67.

Sellers EM, Expert Panel (2003). Abuse liability assessment of CNS drugs: conclusions, recommendations, and research priorities. *Drug Alcohol Depend* 70: S107–S114.

Tamayo-Sarver JH, Hinze SW, Cydulka RK, Baker DW (2003). Racial and ethnic disparities in emergency department analgesic prescription. *Am J Public Health* 93: 2067–73.

Weaver M, Schnoll S (2002). Abuse liability in opioid therapy for pain treatment in patients with an addiction history. *Clin J Pain* 18: S61–S69.

WHO (2000). *Achieving Balance in National Opioids Control Policy. Guidelines for Assessment.* Geneva, Switzerland: World Health Organization.

Woolf CJ, Hashmi M (2004). Use and abuse of opioid analgesics: potential methods to prevent and deter non-medical consumption of prescription opioids. *Curr Opin Investig Drugs* 5: 61–66.

Zacny J, Bigelow G, Compton P, Foley K, Iguchi M, Sannerud C (2003). College on Problems of Drug Dependence taskforce on prescription opioid non-medical use and abuse: position statement. *Drug Alcohol Depend* 69: 215–32.

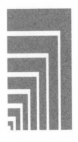

24

Pain Management in Addicted Patients

Mitchell J.M. Cohen, M.D., and Samar A. Jasser

This chapter reviews the current status of treatment for acute and chronic noncancer pain. It discusses the evaluation and treatment principles that should be used for pain in patients with addictions and provides a focused update on the use of opioids as a component of the treatment plan for this population. Using opioids to treat acute pain in nonaddicted patients is generally well accepted, but using opioids to treat acute pain in patients with addiction is less well accepted and when attempted is often ineffective. Similarly, although there is a growing consensus regarding the appropriateness of opioid use to treat chronic pain, less agreement exists on this practice in the context of addiction. This chapter reviews active concerns about opioid treatment, in general, and in patients with addictions, in particular. These issues of pain and addiction are particularly difficult to evaluate and treat when present in the same patient—although chronic pain and addictive disorders are independent and often poorly understood and managed, the risk of unavailable or inadequate treatment is magnified when a patient presents with both problems (Kamerow et al. 1986; Turk et al. 1994).

Clinicians regularly encounter patients with addiction and chronic pain. This chapter addresses the relationship between chronic pain and addiction syndromes, and it reviews guidelines for effective management of pain in patients with addictions. Although guidelines for opioid treatment of chronic pain in nonaddicts have become widely accepted and available (ASA 1997; AAPM and APS 1997; Ballantyne and Mao 2003; FSMB 1998; Jovey et al. 2003; Portenoy 1990), guidelines for the treatment of chronic pain in patients with addictions are less well developed (Breitbart et al. 1996; Jacox and Carr 1994; Schug and Large 1995). In addition to its other objectives, this chapter is intended to help fill that void.

As a result of a tradition of separately studying cancer-related versus noncancer pain, and because of the limitations of space, this chapter will address nonmalignant chronic pain and most citations will be drawn from the noncancer literature. Nevertheless, most of the clinical issues discussed here regarding pain and psychiatric comorbidities, the relationship between pain and addiction syndromes, and the guidelines for the use of opioids with patients with addictions are applicable to patients with cancer pain. Another initial clarification involves the use of terms describing substance use disorders. We choose to avoid the confusion generated by the DSM-IV-TR term *substance dependence,* with its implication of physical dependence (APA 2000). Among patients longitudinally treated with opioids for pain, physical dependence is inevitable and does not serve to distinguish a patient using analgesics effectively from the analgesic abuser (Compton et al. 1998; Sees and Clark 1993). As others have done, we will use *addiction* throughout this chapter to connote substance use that causes harm to the user, is compulsive, and has escaped the user's control (Chabal et al. 1997; Portenoy 1996a). For clarity and accuracy in our use of citations, we will use *substance abuse* as a milder form of the same behavioral syndrome, with less compulsive use and less severe personal, social, and occupational consequences (Miotto et al. 1996).

RELATIONSHIPS BETWEEN CHRONIC PAIN AND ADDICTION

Chronic pain and addiction syndromes have much in common: both tend to be misunderstood conditions that are underdiagnosed and often treated inadequately (Breitbart et al. 1996; Portenoy et al. 1997; Rosenblum et al. 2003; Scimeca et al. 2000). Chronic pain and addiction also commonly coexist in patients; chronic pain is often found among patients with addictions (Rosenblum et al. 2003; Scimeca et al. 2000). The co-occurrence of these two conditions can produce particular problems in clinical management. For example, compared with nonaddicted patients with chronic pain, patients with chronic pain and addiction use more prescribed and nonprescribed drugs and show a higher prevalence of other physical and psychiatric disorders (Jamison et al. 2000). Patients with both chronic pain and addiction represent a particularly symptomatic population in terms of physical and mental life complaints (Rosenblum et al. 2003). Addiction in a patient with chronic pain can perhaps be best thought of as one of many social, behavioral, mental, and physical factors that inten-sify the intrusiveness of chronic pain (Compton et al. 2000; Rosenblum et al. 2003).

Comorbidity of pain and addiction develops for many reasons. In general, one mental life disorder always raises the risk of a second disor-der. Patients with addictions are also at particular risk for development of pain as a result of accidents (e.g., motor-vehicle accidents, falls) and med-ical illnesses (e.g., HIV infection, hepatitis, neuropathies, pancreatitis, head and neck cancers) associated with substance abuse (Jacox and Carr 1992; Miotto et al. 2002; Savage 1993). Patients with opioid addiction also may have decreased pain tolerance (Compton et al. 2000, 2001), or increased pain sensitivity (Doverty et al. 2001), and thus may be more prone to develop chronic pain.

Once established in a patient, each of these two syndromes affects management of the other. As shown in figure 24.1, destabilization of ad-diction can create physiologic and psychosocial stressors that can, in turn, increase pain levels. Similarly, failure of pain control or worsening of the medical condition causing pain can lead to recurrent substance abuse as the patient attempts to reduce or escape increasing physical pain and the associated emotional suffering (Compton et al. 2000; Jacox and Carr 1994; Miotto et al. 1996; Savage 1999a; Weaver and Schnoll 2002). Con-versely, these syndromes can improve together with treatment of each problem, and under certain circumstances this may be accomplished with the same agent. Opioids, for example, may treat both an addiction and pain in the patient with addiction who develops pain (Savage 1999a), al-

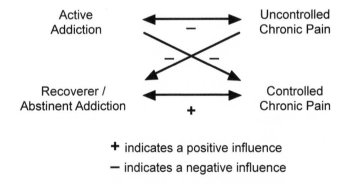

+ indicates a positive influence
− indicates a negative influence

Figure 24.1. Relationship between chronic pain and addiction syndromes. Among patients with chronic pain and addiction, stabilization of one syndrome enhances con-trol of the other. Conversely, when either problem symptomatically escalates, control of the other problem is jeopardized.

though the dose and frequency of use for the prescribed opioid may differ for the two problems (Scimeca et al. 2000).

General agreement also exists regarding the validity of the frequent observation that higher opioid doses are required to control pain for patients with a history of opioid addiction, compared with nonaddicted patients with pain (Compton et al. 2000; Jacox and Carr 1994; Scimeca et al. 2000). The need for higher doses of opioids in addicts raises the risk of underdosing with opioid analgesics. Underdosing can provoke drug-seeking behaviors as the patient obtains partial relief from medication, but experiences end-of-dose analgesic failure and breakthrough pain. In the context of underdosing, drug-seeking behaviors such as requesting higher dosages and approaching additional physicians for analgesics may actually be treatment seeking and give a false appearance of addiction or "pseudoaddiction" (Weissman and Haddox 1989). Similarly, there may be a need for higher doses of methadone to treat opioid addiction when the patient also has chronic pain (Jamison et al. 2000), but this may not occur as predictably as the higher analgesic dose requirement in addicts (Rosenblum et al. 2003).

Treatment of chronic pain routinely involves pharmacotherapy with three or more medications, usually from various drug classes, to adequately control pain and associated problems such as sleep, anxiety, and depressive disorders. These combinations are developed through serial trials of agents and are highly individualized. This practice is often referred to as "rational polypharmacy" and can involve prescription of opioids, nonsteroidal anti-inflammatory drugs, anticonvulsants, antidepressants, anxiolytics, sedative-hypnotics, and psychostimulants. These complex medication regimens, though often effective on target symptoms and functional impairment, also raise the risk of substance abuse and addiction in patients with pain (Kouyanou et al. 1997). Substance use issues most often arise related to the use of opioids as well as sedative-hypnotics, anxiolytics, and psychostimulants, which frequently can be used appropriately in this population (Weaver and Schnoll 2002). Rational polypharmacy can increase the risk of addiction to multiple substances, because addictive disorders can generalize across substances (Miotto et al. 1996), possibly via shared reward pathways (Longo et al. 2000; Nedeljkovic et al. 2002; Sees and Clark 1993).

Other factors can simultaneously destabilize both pain and addiction, including mood and anxiety disorders, sleep disorders, marital stress, occupational and financial problems, and traits such as neuroticism and impulsivity (Compton et al. 2000; Dunbar and Katz 1996; Rosenblum et al. 2003).

Comorbidity of Pain and Addiction

Patients with addiction who develop pain problems appear to be a highly symptomatic, functionally impaired population. They spend longer periods in medical and addiction treatment and typically require larger opioid doses to treat addiction and pain problems. The prevalence of chronic pain in patients with addictions appears to be much higher than the prevalence of chronic pain in the general population. Patients with addictions and pain frequently report that medications used to treat pain lead to addiction and that they need to take their pain medication not just for analgesia, but to feel normal (Nedeljkovic et al. 2002). These features are rarely described by nonaddicted patients with pain.

A study of patients receiving methadone maintenance in three opioid treatment programs found significant chronic pain problems in 61 percent of subjects (Jamison et al. 2000), most of these having pain in more than one pain site. Comparing the subjects with patients receiving methadone maintenance without pain, these investigators found that subjects were more likely to be unemployed, receive disability benefits, receive higher methadone doses, and have a longer duration of methadone maintenance treatment. Pain complaints in patients with addiction closely mirrored the most common pain complaints found in nonaddicts: low-back pain, leg pain, generalized total body pain, and headache. The only difference in this profile of complaints is that nonaddicted patients had a much lower frequency of diffuse body pain as a primary pain complaint.

Some data are available on the prevalence of new-onset addiction in populations of opioid-treated patients with pain. As opioid pain treatment came back into practice during the past quarter century, iatrogenic addiction in noncancer patients with pain was expected to be low based on the extensive experience using opioids in the treatment of cancer pain, in which new-onset addiction is infrequent (Portenoy 1996a; Savage 1999a). In fact, published prevalence rates of prescription and illicit substance abuse and addiction in noncancer patients have varied widely. Reports have differed in terms of patient populations, definitions of substance use and dependence (Savage 1999a; Sees and Clark 1993), and study design, which helps to explain the divergent results. Some authors have reported rates for new-onset opioid addiction among patients treated for pain that are as low as 0–5 percent; however, such findings raise questions about the validity of these results, because they are lower than general population rates for new-onset opioid addiction (McCarberg and Barkin 2001; Taub 1982; Tennant and Uelman 1983; Zenz et al. 1992). Other authors have reported prevalence in proportion to population rates, ranging from 3 to 19 percent (Dunbar and Katz 1996; Fishbain et al. 1992; Kouyanou et al. 1997).

The prevalence of new-onset addiction appears to be clearly consistent with population rates when patients with a history of substance abuse and patients treated in tertiary pain programs, two psychiatrically enriched samples, are excluded from these calculations (Dunbar and Katz 1996). Careful interpretation of these varied findings suggests that the prevalence of opioid abuse and addiction in opioid-treated patients appears to be in the 6–12 percent range, although a precise number remains elusive (Portenoy and Foley 1986; Savage 1999a; Schofferman 1993; Weaver and Schnoll 2002).

Abuse of prescribed opioids in the general population, including patients with pain, is a relatively minor part of the national drug problem, but it is a growing problem as would be expected with more regular prescribing and an increased supply of opioid analgesics in the community. In the United States, the Drug Abuse Warning Network (DAWN) emergency room (ER) admissions database reports that opioid analgesics were involved in 10 percent of total drug abuse-related visits in 2002 (SAMHSA 2003). From 1995 to 2002 opioid analgesic prescribing for chronic pain moved from discouraged to acceptable practice. During this same period opioid abuse-related analgesic ER visits increased 163 percent (SAMHSA 2003). From 1997 to 2002 medical prescription of oxycodone increased 403 percent, fentanyl prescriptions increased 227 percent, hydromorphone prescriptions increased 96 percent, and morphine prescriptions increased 73 percent (Gilson et al. 2004). These data suggest that predictable increased abuse is occurring with increased dispensing of opioid analgesics, but the increased abuse is not in proportion with the increased prescribing. In other words, increases in abuse of prescribed opioids have not been in proportion with significant increases in medical prescribing (Joranson et al. 2000), which could be interpreted as a relative decrease in abuse of available opioids.

Opioid analgesics are rarely the only substance involved in the DAWN-reported visits; 71 percent of these visits involve simultaneous abuse of other substances, including alcohol, cocaine, and marijuana. These data make the case for aggressive substance abuse treatment before initiating opioid therapy in patients with pain who have histories of addiction, and for random urine testing for abusable drugs once opioid analgesics are started. Because most patients with pain who abuse their prescribed opioids are likely to be abusing other drugs, many of these patients will be picked up with random urine testing. Because continued increased opioid prescribing is likely, pain and addiction specialists along with appropriate governmental agencies must work together to better understand diversion routes for prescribed analgesics and stem their increasing abuse.

Although the exact prevalence of new-onset addiction and abuse of opioids by patients treated for pain is unclear, available data suggest that most patients with pain who are maintained on chronic opioids do not manifest psychological or behavioral characteristics of addiction. The minority of patients who develop abuse or addiction deserve and have received considerable attention in the medical literature and an approach to management of these patients is described later in this chapter (Miotto et al. 1996) and in chapter 23.

FUNDAMENTALS OF PAIN MANAGEMENT IN PATIENTS WITH ADDICTION

Pain treatment for patients with any serious psychiatric comorbidity requires access to clinicians specialized in the management of pain and serious psychiatric illness, perhaps the most significant barrier to treatment. Physicians' attitudes toward patients with chronic pain and addictive disorders have often been demonstrated to be dismissive and judgmental. Moreover, many physicians have minimal training and experience in the diagnosis and treatment of these disorders (Cohen et al. 2002; Kamerow et al. 1986; Turk et al. 1994).

Whether chronic pain coexists with major depression, posttraumatic stress disorder, panic disorder, or addiction, the psychiatric comorbidity should be treated aggressively and stabilized before launching a full pain management plan (Cohen 1995; Savage 1993; Scimeca et al. 2000). An untreated psychiatric disorder can distort the perception of pain and reduce the efficacy of otherwise helpful pain treatments. In addition, patients may misuse or overuse prescribed analgesics in an attempt to control symptoms of comorbid disorders such as depression, anxiety, or sleep disturbance when more appropriate, targeted treatments for such psychiatric disorders are not in place.

Once psychiatric comorbidity is diagnosed and stabilized, the next step in pain management is to identify pain generators, when possible, followed by categorization and treatment of the various pain etiologies. Pain management, however, is rarely successful if pain reduction or elimination is the sole focus of treatment (Cohen 1995; Portenoy 1996a). Pain can be nociceptive, meaning the pain conduction system is intact, or neuropathic, meaning pain is transmitted through a damaged pain transmission system in the peripheral nervous system, central nervous system, or both. Nociceptive and neuropathic pains are both seen in patients with addictive disorders.

Nociceptive pains suffered by patients with addiction include mechanical spinal pain from degenerative disease, traumatic compression fractures secondary to poor nutrition and osteoporosis, inflammatory pain secondary to cellulites, and joint destruction resulting from avascular necrosis or osteomyelitis. Nociceptive pain also includes focal or generalized myofascial pain and visceral pain, the latter manifesting in the addicted population in syndromes such as liver pain and tenderness related to hepatitis or abdominal pain associated with pancreatitis and alcoholism.

Neuropathic pain syndromes are characterized by burning, dysesthestic, and spontaneous pains, often occurring with trivial or no stimulation of the affected body region. Neuropathic pain does not follow dermatomal sensory nerve innervation, often raising misguided concerns about malingering or other abnormal illness behavior. Neuropathic pain syndromes encountered in the addicted population include idiopathic peripheral neuropathies and diagnostically clearer peripheral neuropathies, such as those occurring with diabetes or HIV infection. Central pain following stroke in patients dependent on cocaine or resulting from head trauma are particularly difficult nerve-injury pain syndromes, sometimes affecting a full side of the body. Spinal cord injury with constant pain below the level of the injury and paralysis, paresis, and loss of sexual, bowel, and bladder functions is another difficult complication of injury that occurs while intoxicated or in withdrawal. Chronic daily headache, provoked and sustained by short-acting opioid, barbiturate, benzodiazepine, and alcohol abuse, as well as sleep disorders, are also common pain complaints in this population (Harden and Cohen 2003).

Identification of pain generators then leads to targeted treatments. For example, nociceptive pains can be treated with mechanical supports, body mechanics, and postural work, nonsteroidal anti-inflammatory drugs, the more specific cyclo-oxygenase type II inhibitors (COX-2 drugs) such as celecoxib and valdecoxib, steroids, and control of underlying diseases such as hepatitis or cellulitis. Neuropathic pains can also be controlled with treatment of underlying diseases such as HIV infection and sleep disorders. Neuropathic pains also respond to tricyclic antidepressants, various anticonvulsants (e.g., gabapentin, carbamazepine, and oxcarbazepine), $alpha_2$-adrenergic agonists (e.g., clonidine), NMDA-type glutamate receptor antagonists (e.g., ketamine), and topical and systemic anesthetics (e.g., lidocaine) (McCarberg and Barkin 2001; Weaver and Schnoll 2002).

Opioid analgesics also have been demonstrated to help in both nociceptive and neuropathic pains (Ballantyne and Mao 2003; Watson and Babul 1998). This substantial array of pharmacotherapies continues to expand and leads to the rational polypharmacy that often characterizes optimal treatment of many patients with chronic pain. As described earlier, state-of-the-art pharmacotherapy brings with it increased risk of addiction. All patients must be seen frequently and monitored closely for signs of medication abuse or addiction, such as mental status or behavioral changes from overuse or withdrawal, requests for early medication refills, or functional deterioration. Patients with a history of addiction deserve the closest monitoring.

In addition to these targeted therapies, nonspecific multidisciplinary-based treatments are critical to successful pain management. These approaches include relaxation training, appropriate exercise programs, physical therapy, manipulation of taut muscles, and biofeedback. Goals beyond pain reduction should be developed, such as increasing standing and walking endurance, becoming able to sit through a movie or tolerate longer automobile rides to visit family, finding meaningful activity in the face of occupational disability, and maintaining satisfying human relationships. These latter goals can be addressed in individual cognitive-behavioral, supportive, or insight-oriented psychotherapy, as well as group therapy or marital counseling.

All these components require careful introduction and integration into the treatment plan, and the efficacy of such nonspecific approaches can vary greatly between patients. Identifying physical therapists, psychotherapists, and other clinicians who are comfortable and competent in working with patients with chronic pain alone is often difficult, and this becomes even harder when the patient with chronic pain also has an addiction. Nevertheless, the most controversial component of a full pain management program remains the use of opioid analgesics, especially in those patients with comorbid pain and addiction.

STATUS OF OPIOID USE IN THE TREATMENT OF NONMALIGNANT PAIN

During the past 25 years, a consensus has steadily formed regarding the appropriateness of ongoing opioid treatment for chronic nonmalignant pain (Moulin et al. 1996; Portenoy 1996a, 1996b; Zenz et al. 1992). Many prominent professional and regulatory groups, such as the American Pain Society, American Society of Anesthesiologists, and the Federation of State Medical Boards, have endorsed opioid therapy in the treatment of chronic noncancer pain (ASA 1997; AAPM and APS 1997; FSMB 1998). Additionally, opioids have been advocated for an increasing number of painful conditions (Arkinstall et al. 1995; Jamison et al. 1998; Jovey et al. 2003; Moulin et al. 1996; Portenoy 1990; Portenoy and Foley 1986; Schofferman 1999). However, although the consensus view holds that chronic opioid therapy is a responsible approach in many painful conditions, clinical reports have varied widely in the clinical outcomes described and the patients reported most likely to benefit. Furthermore, few validated guidelines for selection of good candidates for opioid treatment have been published, and many patients are selected on a case-by-case basis (Nedeljkovic et al. 2002; Portenoy 1996a).

Acute pain control with opioids is less controversial but is often poorly done. It is common to find confusion over the prescribing that is appropriate for acute pain in a patient who is treated with a chronic opioid analgesic or is in methadone maintenance treatment. The best clinical practice approach in these situations is actually straightforward: the chronic opioid analgesic or methadone should be continued at the current dose, and additional opioids for the acute pain should be added, at doses similar to or slightly higher than those used for patients with the same acute pain syndrome who are not taking chronically prescribed opioids. Patients on mixed agonist-antagonist drugs (e.g., pentazocine, buprenorphine, buprenorphine/naloxone) are best converted to methadone at an equianalgesic dose roughly 60 percent that of the mixed agonist-antagonist before administering additional opioids for acute pain.

Controversies Surrounding Opioid Treatment of Chronic Pain

Despite consensus regarding opioid treatment holding value for many patients with nonmalignant nociceptive and neuropathic pain syndromes, various controversies remain. Although use of this treatment in patients with addictions may be among the most intensely debated controversies, it should be understood in the context of other important remaining questions. First we consider addiction-related issues and then provide perspective by giving an overview of other concerns about chronic opioid therapy.

Concerns about abuse and addiction are the most prominent controversies related to opioid treatment of nonmalignant pain, but others remain. Some authors have suggested that opioids ought to be provided at doses high enough to control symptoms, as long as side effects are tolerable (McCarberg and Barkin 2001; Portenoy 1996a; Scimeca et al. 2000;

Weaver and Schnoll 2002). At the same time, unresolved issues regarding long-term therapy include relatively scant long-term outcome data, and the possible pronociceptive effects of long-term, high-dose opioid therapy (Ballantyne and Mao 2003; Compton et al. 2000, 2001; Doverty et al. 2001; Mao 2002; Mao et al. 1995a, 1995b; Portenoy 1996c). The neurobiology of opioid tolerance and pathophysiology of neuropathic pain also share critical features, including the sensitization of neuronal NMDA receptors and the activation of second messenger phosphokinase C (Levitt and Ovelmen-Levitt 1996; Mao 1999; Mao et al. 1995a; Price et al. 2000), raising the possibility of tolerance and neuropathic pain driving each other during the course of opioid treatment of neurogenic pain.

These concerns about possible long-term complications of high-dose opioid therapy are especially germane in patients with addiction and pain who frequently require higher-than-standard doses for relief. Current best practice is to balance these long-term potential and theoretical risks with the significant known medical complications of undertreated pain. If the decision is made to use opioids as part of the pain-treatment plan, it is best to increase the dose until pain is reduced enough to allow progress to occur in functional goals agreed on by the patient and treating clinician. Partial or undertreatment leads to frustration and confusion on both sides of the treatment relationship and can provoke emergence of pseudo-addiction.

Concerns about immunosuppressive effects of opioids arise from the presence of mu opioid receptors on lymphocytes, but this does not appear to be a clinical concern for most patients (Ballantyne and Mao 2003; Portenoy 1996a, 1996c; Savage 1999b). Patient populations in which the potential for immunosuppression merits further study include those with poor general health, HIV infection, and other treatments or conditions causing baseline immunosuppression. Patients with pain who have histories of addiction are often members of these populations. (See chap. 6 for further review of methadone's effects on immune functioning.)

OPIOID THERAPY AS PART OF THE PAIN MANAGEMENT PLAN

Selecting patients with chronic pain who have histories of addiction for opioid therapy must involve a comprehensive evaluation of the status of the addiction, ongoing substance abuse treatment, involvement in support groups, and a full psychosocial evaluation. Patients with stable treatment of anxiety and mood disorders (Jacox and Carr 1992; Miotto et al. 1996; Nedeljkovic et al. 2002; Scimeca et al. 2000), good psychosocial supports, more remote histories of addiction, alcohol as the abused substance, and active participation in Alcoholics Anonymous or Narcotics Anonymous do better with opioid pain treatment than other patients with addiction and pain (Dunbar and Katz 1996).

For all patients placed on ongoing opioid therapy, the analgesic must be one component of a comprehensive treatment plan as described previously, including other interventions appropriate for the particular patient (such as physical therapy, occupational therapy, individual and family counseling, relaxation training, postural and body mechanics education, and exercise training) (Portenoy 1996a). Use of nonopioid adjuvants (e.g., anticonvulsants and tricyclic antidepressants) can enhance pain control, improve sleep, and reduce the required effective dose of opioid (Cohen et al. 2000; Harden and Cohen 2003; Menefee et al. 2000). Patients must collaborate with the treating physician in designing the treatment plan and adhere to it. Opioid therapy alone may not result in significant functional gains, attitudinal changes, adaptation to chronic illness, or maximally restored quality of life (Moulin et al. 1996; Portenoy and Foley 1986).

Opioid therapy for pain is best managed by a prescribing physician who also serves as the case manager, referring the patient for other treatments required and who maintains communication with clinicians providing those treatments (Green and Coyle 1989; Jacox and Carr 1994; Miotto et al. 1996; Portenoy and Foley 1986; Scimeca et al. 2000). A single physician managing the patient allows for consistent observation of the patient's behavior over time, which is crucial for distinguishing pseudoaddiction from true addiction (Weaver and Schnoll 2002). Pain and addiction each require multifaceted treatment plans that include various interventions, participation of family members, and ongoing monitoring and clinical assessment. The patient with addiction and pain must have access to pain and addiction experts and treatment programs, both of which are often in short supply. Ideally, a single physician with expertise in both pain and addiction medicine would oversee treatment, but such clinicians are rare and will not be available for many patients (Miotto et al. 1996; Portenoy et al. 1997).

Opioid treatment should always be started as a trial, with an exit strategy in place should pain fail to respond, side effects be problematic, function deteriorate, or abuse of medication occur. The exit strategy should be explicit and include a responsible taper of the opioid analgesic, control of withdrawal symptoms when possible (for example, through the use of clonidine), and continuation of other components of the treatment plan that have proven beneficial (Katz 2004; Portenoy 1996a; Savage 1999a). A clear exit strategy presented at the start of opioid therapy will

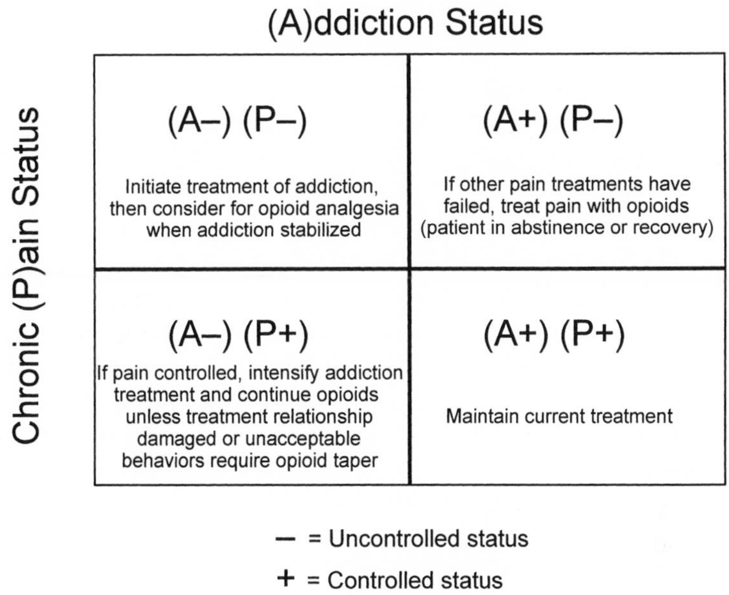
(A)ddiction Status
Chronic (P)ain Status
(A–) (P–)
Initiate treatment of addiction, then consider for opioid analgesia when addiction stabilized
(A+) (P–)
If other pain treatments have failed, treat pain with opioids (patient in abstinence or recovery)
(A–) (P+)
If pain controlled, intensify addiction treatment and continue opioids unless treatment relationship damaged or unacceptable behaviors require opioid taper
(A+) (P+)
Maintain current treatment
– = Uncontrolled status
+ = Controlled status

Figure 24.2. Clinical approach to the patient with chronic pain and addiction. In the patient with active pain and addiction (left upper quadrant), addiction should be stabilized before opioid therapy of pain is considered or initiated. Opioids for treatment of pain should be considered in the patient with addiction if addiction is stable and other approaches to pain control have not provided adequate relief (right upper quadrant). If a patient receiving opioids for pain with good response has a relapse in addiction, intensify addiction interventions and maintain opioid therapy unless the treatment relationship has become tenuous or unacceptable behaviors are occurring (e.g., prescription theft, prescription forgery, medication diversion). In the latter instances, opioid analgesics will require tapering through the exit strategy discussed at the start of opioid treatment for pain (left lower quadrant).

help offset charges of abandonment patients may consider when opioids must be tapered (ASA 1997).

Addiction should be treated before the initiation of opioid pain treatment whenever possible (Savage 1993; Scimeca et al. 2000). If a patient has a relapse in addiction during the course of successful pain reduction with opioids, the addiction is best treated as a relapsing/remitting chronic disorder that the physician manages (fig. 24.2). Precipitants of the relapsed addiction should be identified, and treatment of the substance use disorder should be initiated or intensified. If the treatment relationship breaks down or criminal behaviors emerge in the context of recurrent addiction, opioid taper will be necessary (Miotto et al. 1996; Weaver and Schnoll 2002).

OPIOID ANALGESICS TO USE AND AVOID IN THE CONTEXT OF CHRONIC PAIN AND ADDICTION

Long-acting opioid agents or preparations have advantages over short-acting opioids when treating a patient with chronic pain and addiction. In addition to providing more stable opioid blood levels and more consistent pain control (McCarberg and Barkin 2001), long-acting opioids do not produce the rapid onset of action noted to be associated with development of addiction in vulnerable individuals (Fishman et al. 2002; Longo et al. 2000; Scimeca et al. 2000; Weaver and Schnoll 2002). Use of fixed dosing schedules "by the clock," without rescue or as-needed doses (Savage 1999a) will decrease the patient's focus on medications and lessen opportunities for excessive dosing (Kouyanou et al. 1997; Scimeca et al. 2000). The fentanyl transdermal patch is a novel approach to timed-released opioid therapy that reduces pill focus and interrupts the cueing of medication abuse that may occur with the swallowing of a pill (McCarberg and Barkin 2001; Weaver and Schnoll 2002).

Agonist-antagonist and partial agonist opioid medications (e.g., butorphanol, buprenorphine, and pentazocine), in general, should be avoided because of the risk of precipitating a pain flare as dosages are increased and antagonist action becomes more pronounced. Such pain flares in the context of prescribed or even patient-initiated medication increases tend to confuse the patient and clinician and can destabilize the addiction and pain problems (Jacox and Carr 1992; Scimeca et al. 2000; Weaver and Schnoll 2002). Meperidine and propoxyphene should be avoided because prolonged, high-dose therapy can result in the accumulation of neurotoxic metabolites (McCarberg and Barkin 2001; Scimeca et al. 2000).

Methadone is a long-acting opioid that often has particular benefit as a long-term opioid for chronic neuropathic pain (Fishman et al. 2002; Scimeca et al. 2000). Methadone is commercially produced as a racemic mixture that includes an isomer that binds to mu opioid receptors and an isomer that does not. This latter isomer acts as an antagonist at NMDA-type glutamate receptors (Ballantyne and Mao 2003; Davis and Inturrisi 1999; Fishman et al. 2002; Scimeca et al. 2000), which play a role in sensitization of pain pathways and opioid tolerance (Mao 1999; Mao et al. 1995a, 1995b). Methadone may also function as a central serotonin reuptake inhibitor. For these reasons methadone is often successfully used in the treatment of chronic pain over long periods and when other opi-

Table 24.1 Guidelines for the Opioid Treatment Plan in Patients with a History of Addiction

1. Opioids are one component of a full pain-treatment program developed in collaboration with the patient (Portenoy 1996a).
2. Present initiation of treatment with opioids as a treatment trial, delineating treatment goals and a clear exit strategy (Portenoy 1996a; Savage 1999a; Katz 2004).
3. Identify a pain medicine physician to serve as the opioid analgesic prescriber and treatment coordinator (Portenoy and Foley 1986; Jacox and Carr 1994; Scimeca et al. 2000; Miotto et al. 1996; Green and Coyle 1989).
4. Identify expert substance abuse treatment if the opioid prescriber is not expert in the treatment of addiction.
5. Treat addiction before treating pain when possible (Savage 1993; Scimeca et al. 2000).
6. Require and arrange assessment and treatment of comorbid psychiatric disorders (Jacox and Carr 1992; Nedeljkovic et al. 2002; Scimeca et al. 2000; Miotto et al. 1996).
7. Establish clear prescribing limits, which should be discussed and printed in a pain-treatment agreement, providing a structure for treatment.
8. Pain-treatment agreements specify practice limits, including an acceptable number of missed office visits (e.g., 1–3), use of a single pharmacy, medication being taken only for the chronic pain for which it was prescribed, opioids not being sought in emergency rooms or from other physicians, early refills not being provided, and lost or stolen prescriptions being replaced at the discretion of the prescriber and only one to three times (Jacox et al. 1994; Miotto et al. 1996; Weaver and Schnoll 2002; Kennedy and Crowley 1990; Green and Coyle 1989; Scimeca et al. 2000).
9. Frequent office visits are required during initiation of opioids and during dose-escalation periods (weekly or biweekly) (Dunbar and Katz 1996).
10. Higher opioid doses will usually be required for pain control in patients with addiction (Jacox and Carr 1994; Compton et al. 2000; Scimeca et al. 2000).
11. Patients must agree to periodic opioid dose reductions after a period of dose and pain stabilization at the physician's discretion (Green and Coyle 1989).
12. Patients must remain in addiction treatment, including attendance at NA, AA, or Rational Recovery meetings (Dunbar and Katz 1996; Nedeljkovic et al. 2002; Weaver and Schnoll 2002). Patients must agree to random urine toxicology (Jacox and Carr 1994; Miotto et al. 1996; Scimeca et al. 2000; Weaver and Schnoll 2002).
13. Family members must attend office visits periodically to be educated regarding treatment goals and to serve as outside historians (Katz 2004; Miotto et al. 1996; Weaver and Schnoll 2002).
14. Long-acting opioids should be used (McCarberg and Barkin 2001; Scimeca et al. 2000; Longo et al. 2000; Fishman et al. 2002; Weaver and Schnoll 2002).
15. Use fixed "by-the-clock" dosing schedules without rescue or "as needed" doses (Savage 1999a; Kouyanou et al. 1997; Scimeca et al. 2000).
16. Avoid agonist-antagonist (and partial agonist) drugs (Jacox and Carr 1992; Scimeca et al. 2000; Weaver and Schnoll 2002).
17. Avoid meperidine and propoxyphene due to the accumulation of neurotoxic metabolites (McCarberg and Barkin 2001; Scimeca et al. 2000).

oids fail or tolerance develops (Fishman et al. 2002; Kennedy and Crowley 1990; Taylor et al. 2000). Table 24.1 provides a summary of the treatment principles described in the preceding sections and other desirable components of the opioid treatment plan.

SUMMARY

Pain management for patients with addiction is a relatively common challenge for physicians who specialize in the treatment of addiction. Patients with pain and addiction, however, always require expertise in evaluation and treatment of both problems for optimal treatment outcomes. Unfortunately, physician training in each of these areas historically has been inadequate and must continue to improve if these patients are to be treated effectively. Acute pain management with opioids in patients with addictions has become less controversial in the practice of medicine, although there are gaps in training and the use of opioids in such situations is frequently not carried out according to ideal practice standards. Management of chronic pain is most effective when broad functional and meaningful goals are pursued, rather than a narrow focus on pain reduction.

Provision of opioid therapy for chronic nonmalignant pain continues to gain acceptance as a useful component of a comprehensive treatment plan for intractable pain syndromes. Questions regarding long-term outcome and side effects of this treatment remain, but at this time there is expert consensus that opioid pain management can be safely carried out for patients with a history of addiction and is an ethical responsibility for clinicians (Cohen et al. 2002). In providing opioid analgesia to these patients, clinicians must pay special attention to their increased risk of recurrent addiction, greater prevalence of comorbid psychiatric illness, and higher analgesic dose requirements. Opioid treatment in this population also requires an explicit treatment plan specifying goals and limits, compliance with all aspects of addiction management, and an exit strategy if treatment proves unhelpful or problematic. For patients with chronic pain and addiction, stabilizing each syndrome improves the management of the other, with the greatest barrier to care often being limitations on access to clinical expertise in pain management and addiction medicine.

References

AAPM, APS (1997). *The Use of Opioids for the Treatment of Chronic Pain: A Consensus Statement from the American Academy of Pain Medicine and the American Pain Society.* Glenview, IL: American Academy of Pain Medicine and the American Pain Society, pp. 4.

APA (2000). *Diagnostic and Statistical Manual of Mental Disorders, 4th Ed. Text Revision.* Washington, DC: American Psychiatric Association.

Arkinstall W, Sandler A, Goughnour B, Babul N, Harsanyi Z, Darke AC (1995). Efficacy of controlled-release codeine in chronic non-malignant pain: a randomized, placebo-controlled clinical trial. *Pain* 62: 169–78.

ASA (1997). Practice Guidelines for Chronic Pain Management. A report by the American Society of Anesthesiologists Task Force on Pain Management, Chronic Pain Section. *Anesthesiology* 86: 995–1004.

Ballantyne JC, Mao J (2003). Opioid therapy for chronic pain. *N Engl J Med* 349: 1943–53.

Breitbart W, Patt RB, Passik SD, Reddy KS, Lefkowitz M (1996). Pain in AIDS: a call for action. *Pain Clin Updates* 4: 1–9.

Chabal C, Erjavec MK, Jacobson L, Mariano A, Chaney E (1997). Prescription opiate abuse in chronic pain patients: clinical criteria, incidence, and predictors. *Clin J Pain* 13: 150–55.

Cohen MJ (1995). Psychosocial aspects of evaluation and management of chronic low back pain. In: *Physical Medicine and Rehabilitation: State of the Art Reviews, Vol. 9.* Philadelphia: Hanley and Belfus, 725–46.

Cohen MJ, Jasser S, Herron PD, Margolis CG (2002). Ethical perspectives: opioid treatment of chronic pain in the context of addiction. *Clin J Pain* 18: S99–S107.

Cohen MJM, Menefee LA, Doghramji K, Whitney RA, Frank ED (2000). Sleep in pain: problems and treatments. *Int Rev Psychiatry* 12: 113–26.

Compton P, Charuvastra VC, Kintaudi K, Ling W (2000). Pain responses in methadone-maintained opioid abusers. *J Pain Symptom Manage* 20: 237–45.

Compton P, Charuvastra VC, Ling W (2001). Pain intolerance in opioid-maintained former opiate addicts: effect of long-acting maintenance agent. *Drug Alcohol Depend* 63: 139–46.

Compton P, Darakjian J, Miotto K (1998). Screening for addiction in patients with chronic pain and "problematic" substance use: evaluation of a pilot assessment tool. *J Pain Symptom Manage* 16: 355–63.

Davis AM, Inturrisi CE (1999). d-Methadone blocks morphine tolerance and N-methyl-D-aspartate-induced hyperalgesia. *J Pharmacol Exp Ther* 289: 1048–53.

Doverty M, White JM, Somogyi AA, Bochner F, Ali R, Ling W (2001). Hyperalgesic responses in methadone maintenance patients. *Pain* 90: 91–96.

Dunbar SA, Katz NP (1996). Chronic opioid therapy for nonmalignant pain in patients with a history of substance abuse: report of 20 cases. *J Pain Symptom Manage* 11: 163–71.

Fishbain DA, Rosomoff HL, Rosomoff RS (1992). Drug abuse, dependence, and addiction in chronic pain patients. *Clin J Pain* 8: 77–85.

Fishman SM, Wilsey B, Mahajan G, Molina P (2002). Methadone reincarnated: novel clinical applications with related concerns. *Pain Med* 3: 339–48.

Federation of State Medical Boards (FSMB) (1998). Model Guidelines for the Use of Controlled Substances for the Treatment of Pain. Available at www.fsmb.org.

Gilson AM, Ryan KM, Joranson DE, Dahl JL (2004). A reassessment of trends in the medical use and abuse of opioid analgesics and implications for diversion control: 1997–2002. *J Pain Symptom Manage* 28: 176–88.

Green J, Coyle M (1989). Methadone use in the control of nonmalignant chronic pain. *Pain Manag* 2: 241–46.

Harden N, Cohen M (2003). Unmet needs in the management of neuropathic pain. *J Pain Symptom Manage* 25: S12–S17.

Jacox A, Carr DB (1992). Acute Pain Management: Operative or Medical Procedures and Trauma. DHHS Pub. No. 92-0032. Rockville, MD: U.S. Department of Health and Human Services, Agency for Health Care Policy and Research (AHCPR).

Jacox A, Carr DB (1994). Management of Cancer Pain. DHHS Pub No. 94-0592. Rockville, MD: U.S. Department of Health and Human Services, Agency for Health Care Policy and Research.

Jamison RN, Kauffman J, Katz NP (2000). Characteristics of methadone maintenance patients with chronic pain. *J Pain Symptom Manage* 19: 53–62.

Jamison RN, Raymond SA, Slawsby EA, Nedeljkovic SS, Katz NP (1998). Opioid therapy for chronic noncancer back pain. A randomized prospective study. *Spine* 23: 2591–2600.

Joranson DE, Ryan KM, Gilson AM, Dahl JL (2000). Trends in medical use and abuse of opioid analgesics. *JAMA* 283: 1710–14.

Jovey RD, Ennis J, Gardner-Nix J, Goldman B, Hays H, Lynch M, Moulin D (2003). Use of opioid analgesics for the treatment of chronic noncancer pain—a consensus statement and guidelines from the Canadian Pain Society, 2002. *Pain Res Manag* 8 Suppl A: 3A–28A.

Kamerow DB, Pincus HA, Macdonald DI (1986). Alcohol abuse, other drug abuse, and mental disorders in medical practice. Prevalence, costs, recognition, and treatment. *JAMA* 255: 2054–57.

Katz NP (2004). Opioids for chronic pain: a question of balance. *Pain Manag Today* 4: 10.

Kennedy JA, Crowley TJ (1990). Chronic pain and substance abuse: a pilot study of opioid maintenance. *J Subst Abuse Treat* 7: 233–38.

Kouyanou K, Pither CE, Wessely S (1997). Medication misuse, abuse and dependence in chronic pain patients. *J Psychosom Res* 43: 497–504.

Levitt M, Ovelmen-Levitt J (1996). Neuropathic pain: lessons from opioid tolerance/dependence. *Pain* 67: 227–29.

Longo LP, Parran T, Jr., Johnson B, Kinsey W (2000). Addiction. Part II. Identification and Management of the Drug-Seeking Patient. *Am Fam Physician* 61: 2401–8.

Mao J (1999). NMDA and opioid receptors: their interactions in antinociception, tolerance and neuroplasticity. *Brain Res Brain Res Rev* 30: 289–304.

Mao J (2002). Opioid-induced abnormal pain sensitivity: implications in clinical opioid therapy. *Pain* 100: 213–17.

Mao J, Price DD, Mayer DJ (1995a). Experimental mononeuropathy reduces the antinociceptive effects of morphine: implications for common intracellular mechanisms involved in morphine tolerance and neuropathic pain. *Pain* 61: 353–64.

Mao J, Price DD, Mayer DJ (1995b). Mechanisms of hyperalgesia and morphine tolerance: a current view of their possible interactions. *Pain* 62: 259–74.

McCarberg BH, Barkin RL (2001). Long-acting opioids for chronic pain: pharmacotherapeutic opportunities to enhance compliance, quality of life, and analgesia. *Am J Ther* 8: 181–86.

Menefee LA, Cohen MJ, Anderson WR, Doghramji K, Frank ED, Lee H (2000). Sleep disturbance and nonmalignant chronic pain: a comprehensive review of the literature. *Pain Med* 1: 156–72.

Miotto K, Compton P, Ling W, Conolly M (1996). Diagnosing addictive disease in chronic pain patients. *Psychosomatics* 37: 223–35.

Miotto K, McCann M, Basch J, Rawson R, Ling W (2002). Naltrexone and dysphoria: fact or myth? *Am J Addict* 11: 151–60.

Moulin DE, Iezzi A, Amireh R, Sharpe WK, Boyd D, Merskey H (1996). Randomised trial of oral morphine for chronic non-cancer pain. *Lancet* 347: 143–47.

Nedeljkovic SS, Wasan A, Jamison RN (2002). Assessment of efficacy of long-term opioid therapy in pain patients with substance abuse potential. *Clin J Pain* 18: S39–S51.

Portenoy RK (1990). Chronic opioid therapy in nonmalignant pain. *J Pain Symptom Manage* 5: S46–S62.

Portenoy RK (1996a). Opioid therapy for chronic nonmalignant pain. *Pain Res Manage* 1: 17–28.

Portenoy RK (1996b). Opioid therapy for chronic nonmalignant pain: a review of the critical issues. *J Pain Symptom Manage* 11: 203–17.

Portenoy RK (1996c). Opioid therapy for chronic nonmalignant pain: clinician's perspective. *J Law Med Ethics* 24: 296–309.

Portenoy RK, Dole V, Joseph H, Lowinson J, Rice C, Segal S, Richman BL (1997). Pain management and chemical dependency. Evolving perspectives. *JAMA* 278: 592–93.

Portenoy RK, Foley KM (1986). Chronic use of opioid analgesics in non-malignant pain: report of 38 cases. *Pain* 25: 171–86.

Price DD, Mayer DJ, Mao J, Caruso FS (2000). NMDA-receptor antagonists and opioid receptor interactions as related to analgesia and tolerance. *J Pain Symptom Manage* 19: S7–S11.

Rosenblum A, Joseph H, Fong C, Kipnis S, Cleland C, Portenoy RK (2003). Prevalence and characteristics of chronic pain among chemically dependent patients in methadone maintenance and residential treatment facilities. *JAMA* 289: 2370–78.

SAMHSA (2003). Emergency Department Trends from the Drug Abuse Warning Network, Final Estimates 1995–2002. DHHS Pub. No. (SMA) 03-3780. Rockville, MD; Substance Abuse and Mental Health Services Administration, Office of Applied Studies.

Savage SR (1993). Addiction in the treatment of pain: significance, recognition, and management. *J Pain Symptom Manage* 8: 265–78.

Savage SR (1999a). Opioid therapy of chronic pain: assessment of consequences. *Acta Anaesthesiol Scand* 43: 909–17.

Savage SR (1999b). Opioid use in the management of chronic pain. *Med Clin North Am* 83: 761–86.

Schofferman J (1993). Long-term use of opioid analgesics for the treatment of chronic pain of nonmalignant origin. *J Pain Symptom Manage* 8: 279–88.

Schofferman J (1999). Long-term opioid analgesic therapy for severe refractory lumbar spine pain. *Clin J Pain* 15: 136–40.

Schug SA, Large RG (1995). Opioids for chronic noncancer pain. *Pain Clin Updates* 3: 1–7.

Scimeca MM, Savage SR, Portenoy R, Lowinson J (2000). Treatment of pain in methadone-maintained patients. *Mt Sinai J Med* 67: 412–22.

Sees KL, Clark HW (1993). Opioid use in the treatment of chronic pain: assessment of addiction. *J Pain Symptom Manage* 8: 257–64.

Taub A (1982). Opioid analgesics in the treatment of chronic intractable pain of non-neoplastic origin. In: Kitahata LM, Collins JG, eds. *Narcotic Analgesics in Anesthesiology*, 199–208. Baltimore: Williams and Wilkins.

Taylor WF, Finkel AG, Robertson KR, Anderson AC, Toomey TC, Abashian SA, Mann JD

(2000). Methadone in the treatment of chronic nonmalignant pain: a 2-year follow-up. *Pain Med* 1: 254–59.

Tennant F, Uelman G (1983). Narcotic maintenance for chronic pain: medical and legal guidelines. *Postgrad Med J* 73: 81–94.

Turk DC, Brody MC, Okifuji EA (1994). Physicians' attitudes and practices regarding the long-term prescribing of opioids for non-cancer pain. *Pain* 59: 201–8.

Watson CP, Babul N (1998). Efficacy of oxycodone in neuropathic pain: a randomized trial in postherpetic neuralgia. *Neurology* 50: 1837–41.

Weaver MF, Schnoll SH (2002). Opioid treatment of chronic pain in patients with addiction. *J Pain Palliat Care Pharmacother* 16: 5–26.

Weissman DE, Haddox JD (1989). Opioid pseudoaddiction—an iatrogenic syndrome. *Pain* 36: 363–66.

Zenz M, Strumpf M, Tryba M (1992). Long-term oral opioid therapy in patients with chronic nonmalignant pain. *J Pain Symptom Manage* 7: 69–77.

Index